A Crisis Call
for New
Preventive
Medicine

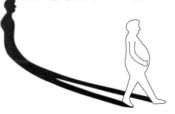

Emerging Effects of Lifestyle on
Morbidity and Mortality

A Crisis Call
for New
Preventive
Medicine

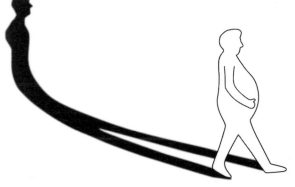

Emerging Effects of Lifestyle on
Morbidity and Mortality

Joseph A Knight, MD

University of Utah School of Medicine, USA

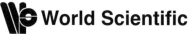 World Scientific

NEW JERSEY · LONDON · SINGAPORE · BEIJING · SHANGHAI · HONG KONG · TAIPEI · CHENNAI

Published by

World Scientific Publishing Co. Pte. Ltd.

5 Toh Tuck Link, Singapore 596224

USA office: Suite 202, 1060 Main Street, River Edge, NJ 07661

UK office: 57 Shelton Street, Covent Garden, London WC2H 9HE

Library of Congress Cataloging-in-Publication Data
Knight, Joseph A., 1930–
    A crisis call for new preventive medicine : emerging effects of lifestyle on morbidity and
mortality / Joseph A Knight.
        p. cm.
    Includes bibliographical references and index.
    ISBN 981-238-700-5 (alk. paper)
        1. Medicine, Preventive. 2. Health behavior. I. Title.

    RA425.K577 2004
    616.07--dc22

                                                                    2004041971

British Library Cataloguing-in-Publication Data
A catalogue record for this book is available from the British Library.

Typeset by Stallion Press.

Printed by Fulsland Offset Printing (S) Pte Ltd, Singapore

Contents

Preface

Over 200 years ago, Benjamin Franklin wrote: "There are few things which are appreciated more in their absence and less in their presence than health. When we have it, we take it for granted, giving little care to its preservation. When we do not have it, there is precious little we would not do to get it back."

The average life expectancy in the industrialized nations has increased greatly since the beginning of the 20th century, primarily due to improvements in sanitation and the accompanying reduction of communicable bacterial and parasitic diseases, as well as immunization against various viral infections. The discovery of penicillin and other antibiotics during the mid-1900s also significantly added to the life expectancy. Thus, the average life expectancy in the United States increased from about 47 years in 1900 to 77 years in 2000 (slightly higher in Japan and some European countries).

With this increasing life expectancy, the impending "elder boom" as the post-World War II "baby boomers" approach retirement, as well as the dramatic negative changes in lifestyle over the past 50 years, we face highly challenging medical and financial crises unless we make significant changes in the way we live. For example, the incidence of obesity has more than doubled over the past four to five decades. As a result, there has been a corresponding increase in obesity-associated diseases and disorders (e.g. accelerated aging, type 2 diabetes, coronary heart disease, cerebrovascular disease, hypertension and various cancers). Not only have our diets become less nutritious, but we have become less physically active due to changes in the workplace and increased use of computers and television watching, as well as the numerous modern household electronic conveniences. There has also been a significant reduction in physical education in the public schools. Furthermore, lifestyle factors including smoking, substance abuse and excess alcohol intake, as well as various potentially harmful workplace and environmental factors (e.g. heavy metals, organic solvents, sun radiation, pesticides, ozone, etc.) are also associated with increased morbidity and mortality, as well as medical costs.

Physicians have always been trained to diagnose and treat disease and physical and psychiatric disorders. Thus, our healthcare system is a treatment-oriented system, as physicians and other healthcare providers too often encounter people only when they are sick or have signs and/or symptoms of a disease. Yet, at least 65% of the major causes of disease and death are lifestyle-related. Unfortunately, managed care programs too infrequently allow adequate professional counseling time for improved nutrition, weight control, increased physical activity, and the serious problems of smoking, alcohol and drug abuse, and other potential problems. Yet, this would not only increase the life expectancy and quality of life, but it would save billions of healthcare dollars each year.

Can there be any doubt that disease and disability prevention are far better than disease or disability treatment? There is truly a "Crisis Call for New Preventive Medicine." Hopefully, physicians and other healthcare providers, managed care executives, public school teachers, and federal and local government officials will become more active in educating the general public on the importance of "wellness," disease prevention, and the promotion of health. Indeed, there are pearls in the words of Thomas Edison: "The doctor of the future will give no medicine, but will interest his patient in the care of the human frame, in diet, and in the prevention of disease."

In this book I have attempted to present information from significant and relevent peer-reviewed studies showing that a healthy lifestyle can significantly decrease the risk of numerous diseases and disorders. Moreover, the life expectancy and the quality of life will be significantly increased while the burdensome healthcare costs will decrease.

Acknowledgments

This book is based entirely on specific evidence obtained from published studies in numerous peer-reviewed medical and other scientific journals. Indeed, none of the material came from the often biased and false claims that commonly appear in newspapers and magazines.

I am especially indebted to Dr. John F. Wilson; friend, colleague and former pediatric pathology partner who suggested the book's title. I also appreciate the thoughtful remarks and suggestions of Dr. Dean Sorenson who reviewed most of the material. Moreover, I want to thank my wife, Pauline, who fully supported me during the months needed to complete the book.

1

Life Expectancy, Disease Prevention and Wellness Assessment

Introduction

It is truly amazing that over 200 years ago Benjamin Franklin wrote, "There are few things which are appreciated more in their absence and less in their presence than health. When we have it, we take it for granted, giving little care to its preservation. When we do not have it, there is precious little we would not do to get it back."[1] Unfortunately, many of us still take our good health for granted until we are diagnosed with a serious disease that might have been prevented. We stop smoking, begin to exercise, lose weight, improve our diet, or give up alcohol/ drugs *after* we have had a heart attack or diagnosed with cirrhosis, diabetes mellitus, hypertension, cancer or some other serious disease/ disorder. Unfortunately these diseases are not reversible; we have them for life. They decrease both our life expectancy and the quality of life. Unless we, as a nation, change our lifestyles and stress the importance of wellness, health promotion and disease prevention, there will be very difficult personal, as well as national, financial problems.

We face a tremendous impending "elder boom" as the post-World War II "baby boomers" grow old (persons born between 1946 to 1963).

1

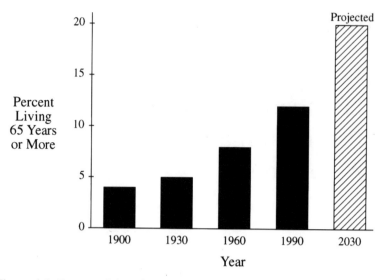

Figure 1.1: Percent of Americans age 65 years and over from 1900 to 2030.

In 1900, about 4% of the United States population was 65 or more years old; today that figure is 12.4%, and by the year 2030 it is expected to reach 19.6% (Fig. 1.1).[2] Thus, a recent US census indicated that in 1960 there were 16.6 million Americans 65 years or older and in 1980 there were 25.6 million. It was estimated that in the years 2000, 2020 and 2040 there will be 34.7 million, 53.2 million and 75.2 million people 65 years or older, respectively.[3] Of all humans who have ever lived to age 65, it is estimated that at least half are alive today.[4] The fastest growing group in the US reportedly comprises those over age 85.[5] In 1990 approximately 1% of the US population was 85 years or over; by 2030 it is estimated to be 3% and will increase to 5% by 2050. However, the fastest growing group might actually be those 100 years and over. In 1960 the estimated number of Americans 100 years and over was 3600; in 1998 it was 54,000 and is estimated to reach 200,000 by the year 2020 and 400,000 by 2040.[6] Importantly, the health prospects for these unusual individuals is not as bleak as generally thought. Thus, at age 85 years men can expect that 80% of their remaining life will be free of serious disability; for women, the estimated disability-free time is 65%.[7] As a result, the medical costs of increased longevity beyond age 65 will probably not be as great as some have predicted.[8] Rather, total costs will be primarily affected by the increase in absolute number of older individuals. These investigators reported that proportionate health care costs reached a maximum at 75 years, after which the older the people were, the lower their proportionate lifetime health care costs became. Thus, the average Medicare payments in the last two years of life for those dying in their 60s was US$22,590 compared to an average of US$8296 for those who died at 101 years or older. Perls and Wood[9] also concluded that in the acute hospital setting, costs peaked in the 70- to 79-year-old age group and subsequently declined with increasing age; patients in their 80s, 90s and 100 and over, all incurred lower costs per hospital stay than patients in their 60s and 70s. For those who died while in the hospital, the average cost per discharge decreased from US$16,886 for the 60- to 69-year-old group to US$6523 for the centenarians.

More recently, Spillman and Lubitz[10] compared the effect of longevity on the costs for acute and long-term care. They found that the effect of longevity on expenditures for acute care differs significantly from its effects for long-term care. Thus, acute care costs, primarily for hospital care and physicians' services, increase at a reduced rate as the age at death increases. On the other hand, long-term care costs increase at an accelerated rate. They concluded that although increases in longevity after age 65 years results in higher long-term care costs, the increased number of elderly has a more important effect on total costs. How about sex differences in the use of health care services and the expenses incurred? Mustard *et al.*[11] studied the age- and sex-specific per capita use of health care resources for a one-year period during 1994 and 1995 in the Canadian province of Manitoba. They found that health care expenditures were similar for males and females after differences in reproductive biology and higher age-specific mortality rates for men were accounted for.

Fries[12] proposed that a healthy lifestyle, improved medical care, and a higher standard of living would compress morbidity into a significantly shorter period of time rather than expand disability. He and co-workers[13] later demonstrated that all people can compress their morbidity. In this study, 1741 college alumni were first surveyed in

1962 at an average age of 43 years. Each person's health status was rated on the basis of weight, smoking and exercise habits. In 1994, at an average age of 75 years, the importance of these health habits were apparent. Those who exercised regularly, controlled their weight, and avoided smoking in midlife and later adulthood lived significantly longer. In addition, disability was postponed and compressed into fewer years at life's end. More recently, these researchers provided further evidence that a healthy lifestyle will delay the onset of age-related diseases and compress the time of illness into a short period at the end of their lives.[14] Moreover, it is never too late to promote a healthy lifestyle, even in older persons. In agreement with these studies, Perls and Silver[6] found that most centenarians are healthy throughout most of their lives and the great majority are healthy into their 90s and in some who are over 100. In short, they reported that morbidity could be compressed into 4% of the total lifespan. This is reasonable since these older individuals have generally escaped the major age-related diseases which are, to a very significant degree, lifestyle related (Table 1.1). Interestingly, these

Table 1.1: Fifteen Most Common Causes of Death in the US (2000)[20]

Disease/Disorder	Number of Deaths	Total Percent
Heart disease	709,894	29.5
Cancer	551,833	22.9
Cerebrovascular disease	166,028	6.9
Chronic obstructive pulmonary disease	123,550	5.1
Accidents/adverse effects	93,592	3.9
Diabetes mellitus	8662	2.9
Pneumonia/influenza	67,024	2.8
Alzheimer's disease	49,044	2.0
Nephritis/nephrosis/nephrotic syndrome	37,672	1.6
Septicemia	31,613	1.3
Suicide	28,332	1.2
Chronic liver disease/cirrhosis	26,219	1.1
Essential hypertension/hypertensive renal disease	17,964	0.7
Pneumonitis due to solids/liquids	16,659	0.7
Homicide	16,137	0.7

latter authors proposed a "Life Expectancy Calculator" which is based on the assumption that the average person has adequate "longevity genes" to live to age 85 or more; those with an appropriate lifestyle may add an additional ten or more years. They suggested that the major factors, in addition to genetics, in living to 100 are the following: not smoking, eat modest amounts of meat and fatty foods, eat plenty of fruits, vegetables and bran, supplement the diet with vitamin E and selenium, take an aspirin daily, control your weight (BMI $\leq$ 24 kg/m^2), exercise regularly, avoid stress and live close to family members.

Pronk *et al.*[15] reported that adverse health risks (i.e. physical inactivity, increased body mass index, current smoking, and/or history of previous tobacco use) were related to significantly higher health care costs. For example, those who never smoked, had a body mass index (BMI) of 25 kg/m^2 or less (overweight 25–29.9 kg/m^2; obese $\geq$ 30 kg/m^2), and exercised three days a week had mean health care charges over an 18-month period of about 49% lower than physically inactive smokers with a BMI of 27.5 kg/m^2. Others[16] reported that beyond the biological effects of aging, much of the illness and disability associated with older individuals is related to risk factors present in midlife. Thus, the most consistent predictors of healthy aging were low blood pressure, low serum glucose, not smoking cigarettes, and not being obese.

What are the economic costs of obesity and physical inactivity? Colditz[17] recently reported that physical inactivity leads to a significant increase in numerous chronic diseases/disorders including coronary heart disease (CHD), hypertension, type 2 diabetes (non-insulin dependent diabetes mellitus; NIDDM), colon cancer, depression, osteoporotic hip fractures and obesity. Increasing adiposity is, itself, related to type 2 diabetes, hypertension, CHD, gall bladder disease, osteoarthritis and cancer of the breast, endometrium and colon. He found that the direct cost of physical inactivity, in terms of 1995 dollars, was US$2.4 billion/year (2.4% of total health care costs) while obesity (BMI $\geq$ 30 kg/m^2) costs US$70 billion a year.

Together, these two lifestyle-related conditions accounted for 9.4% of the total US health care expenditures.

Schneider[18] recently suggested that the issue most likely to affect the quality of life is their future health needs. Their health will not only affect future health care costs but will also have major consequences on their economic, housing and transportation needs. He proposed the following two possible scenarios that define "the most likely range of future health changes."

(1) Appropriate funding for aging research, disease prevention and improved treatment will result in the triumph of the current major causes of disease and disability of older individuals. As a result, the health of an 85-year-old person in the year 2040 would resemble that of a 70-year-old today.

(2) Continue at the current relatively low levels for research support, prevention and treatment such that current health trends continue to show small, if any, improvements in the average health of the elderly. As a result, the future 85+ age group in the year 2040 will not be significantly different from that of a current person in the same age group with its considerable needs for both acute and long-term care.

Life Expectancy

The estimated life expectation at birth represents the average number of years that a group of newborns would be expected to live if, throughout their lifetime, they were to experience the age-specific prevailing death rates during the year of their birth. In this regard, the average life expectancy of a Roman citizen 2000 years ago was about 22 years.[19] In 1900, the average life expectancy (birth to death) was 47 years; in 2000 it had increased to a record high of 76.9 years: white females, 80.0 years; black females, 75.0 years; white males 74.8 years; and black males, 68.3 years[20] (Fig. 1.2). Olshansky *et al.*[21,22] suggested that the average life expectancy would not exceed 85 years "in the absence of scientific breakthroughs that modify the

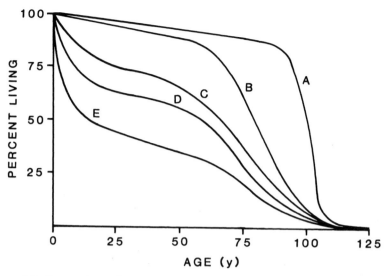

Figure 1.2: Comparison of approximate percent of surviving Americans at various periods of time (B) 1990, (C) 1920, (D) 1900 with the "ideal" life span (A) and those living in Rome 2000 BC (E) (adapted from Fries).[12]

basic rate of aging." However, a recent publication suggests an even more optimistic outlook for increased life expectancy, especially for women.[23] These authors projected, on the basis of recent information from experimental studies, that in established market economies the average life expectancy for women will be about 90 years by 2020 and about 80 years for men.[24,25] Thus, humans appear to be approaching the maximum attainable average life expectancy of 95 years as proposed by Lohman *et al.*[26] which is approximately ten years more than suggested by Olshansky and associates.[21,22]

As noted above, Fries[12] hypothesized that a healthy lifestyle would result in a compression of morbidity. Thus, a person could live a vigorous, productive and healthy life for 85 or more years and then, over a very short period of time, would become ill and die (Curve A, Fig. 1.2). This compression of morbidity would result in the following: (1) the percent of very old people would not increase; (2) the average period of decreased physical activity and vigor would decrease; (3) chronic diseases would involve a smaller percent of the life span; and (4) medical care needs in later life would decrease. He emphasized that postponement of chronic illness would result in rectangularization, not only of the mortality curve, but also the morbidity curve (Fig. 1.2).[12,27,28] As a result, most individuals would be healthy and active until a relatively short time before the final illness; death would rapidly follow. Moreover, medical expenses would be significantly lowered.

Others,[29] however, came to different conclusions and suggested that: (1) the number of very old people is rapidly increasing; (2) the average period of decreased vigor will likely increase; (3) chronic disease will occupy a larger percent of our lifespan; and (4) the needs for medical care in later life are likely to increase. In support of these latter authors, by not anticipating the marked decline in mortality in the elderly that has occurred over ther past two decades, previous US Census Bureau projections underestimated the growth of the oldest age groups, which surpassed even projections based on the lowest mortality assumptions.[30] In addition, Rakowski and Hickey[31] reported a general tendency to attribute various diseases, as well as mortality, to "aging" rather than to treatable but undiagnosed disorders. This tendency may itself carry an adverse risk since some may delay seeking medical care, a problem that exceeds 60% for some medical disorders.[32]

Nevertheless, a recent report strongly supports the importance of lifestyle habits in the compression of morbidity.[14] In this study, 418 deceased people of an aging cohort were observed over a 12-year period during which their functional status, in relationship to lifestyle-related risk factors, was observed. The results showed a distinct reduction and postponement of disability in persons with healthier lifestyles (i.e. not being overweight, being physically active and not smoking).

Major life expectancy risk factors

There is a common conception among the general public, as well as many physicians and other health professionals, that the very elderly frequently die of "old age." This is well illustrated by examining death certificates and newspaper obituaries. Moreover, the fact that there is a maximum lifespan suggests that the incredible human machine eventually wears out, although exactly what stops the "clock of life" is often an enigma. Nevertheless, aging and disease are not the same; aging predisposes one to various diseases. John and Koelmeyer[33] clarified the answer to the question, "do people die of old age?" to a significant degree in their recent report on death in nonagenarians and centenarians. In this forensic autopsy study of 319 cases of people 90 years and older, they found that 272 cases (85%) were natural and of these, only 13 (5%) could be attributed to old age or senile debility. The most common causes of death were as follows: ischemic heart disease, 74 cases (23%); bronchopneumonia, 37 cases (12%); fractures and related complications, 28 cases (9%); acute myocardial infarction, 25 cases (8%); cerebrovascular accident, 19 cases (6%); and ruptured aneurysm, 17 cases (5%). Forty-seven deaths (15%) were considered unnatural (i.e. 43 accidents due mainly to falls, three suicides and one homicide). Thus, it is apparent that most of the very elderly do not die of "old age." As more is learned about the aging process, the relationship between aging and disease will be further clarified. At that time, perhaps all natural deaths can be related to a single disease or a combination of diseases.

The overall improvement in the health of Americans from 1900 to 2000 is exemplified by two highly significant trends: (1) the age-adjusted death rate declined by about 74%, while (2) life expectancy increased 56%.[34] In 1900, the ten most common causes of death were, in order of frequency, pneumonia, tuberculosis, diarrhea, heart disease, stroke, liver disease, accidents, cancer, senility and diphtheria. Thus, over the past 100 years, the major causes of death shifted from infectious diseases to chronic diseases. For example, in 1900 infectious respiratory diseases accounted for about 25% of all deaths. In 2000, heart disease accounted for 29.5% and cancer 22.9% of all deaths (Table 1.1).[20] It is apparent, therefore, that a "crisis call" for new preventive medicine exists; the "call" is for improved lifestyles. Importantly, the fifth leading cause of death may actually be due to adverse drug reactions, even when the drugs are properly prescribed and administered.[35] In this report, there were an estimated 2,216,000 serious drug reactions and 106,000 drug-related deaths in 1994. The major causes of death are, to a significant degree, lifestyle-related. The eighth most common cause of death in 1995 was AIDS. This lifestyle-related disease dropped out of the top 15 causes of death in 1998, primarily due to improved treatment. Furthermore, tobacco use, poor diet and physical inactivity have been identified as the major contributors to overall mortality in the US, accounting for about one-third of all deaths.[36] More specifically, these authors quantified the major external factors that contributed to the most common causes of death in 1990. Almost half of all deaths were attributed to the following: tobacco (400,000); diet and activity patterns (300,000); alcohol (100,000); microorganisms (90,000); toxic agents (60,000); firearms (35,000); sexual activity (30,000); motor vehicles (35,000); and illicit drug use (20,000). Others[37] have also documented that cigarette smoking, obesity, physical inactivity, poor dietary habits and drug abuse are associated with numerous diseases, a significant decrease in the quality of life and a shortened life expectancy.

In 1990, Michigan reportedly had a very high incidence of chronic disease-related mortality.[38] More recently, the prevalence of four healthy lifestyle characteristics [i.e. healthy weight (BMI 18.5–25.0 kg/m^2), adequate intake of fruits and vegetables (five or more servings a day), regular leisure-time physical activity (at least 30 minutes five times or more a week), and not smoking in Michigan residents were analyzed for 1998 and 2000.[39] The findings showed an estimated 37.9% of Michigan adults had a healthy body weight, 22.8% ate the recommended amount of fruits and vegetables, 25.9% engaged in regular leisure-time physical activity, and 72.3% did not smoke. However, 11.2% engaged in none of these practices, 38.6% in one, 33.3% in two, 13.9% in three, and 3.0% in all four. Thus, those who were involved in all four areas was extremely low and was affected by sex, education level and health status. For example, the prevalence of engaging in all four areas was lower in men than women (1.6% versus 4.5%), increased with the level of education (college graduates were three times higher than those with high school education or less), and those with excellent health were higher than those in poor health (7.1% versus 1.0%). Moreover, when compared with other states, the prevalence of obesity and smoking in Michigan were higher than the national average.[40] Conversely, in 2000 the daily consumption of five fruits and vegetables met the national average and the state ranked among the top ten states for participation in regular and sustained physical activity.

It has been reasonably assumed that if these relative risks were eliminated, or at least reduced, the average life expectancy would be significantly increased. Although there has been little previous direct evidence supporting this presumption, a recent study of Seventh-day Adventists, who probably have the highest life expectancy of any formally described population, adds significant support.[41] Here, 34,192 Adventists were followed from 1976 to 1988. The results showed that at age 30 years, California Adventists have higher life expectancies than other white Californians by 7.28 years in men and 4.42 years in women. Moreover, the authors concluded that diet, exercise, tobacco use, body weight and hormone replacement therapy (in women) in combination can change life expectancy up to ten years among Adventists.

These and other reports clearly emphasize the critical need to educate all Americans, including politicians and those in the medical profession, as to the importance of a healthy lifestyle. Longer, happier and more productive lives with greatly fewer medical expenses can become a reality but it will require considerable effort from all. These topics will be discussed in detail in later chapters of this book.

Miscellaneous life expectancy risk factors

Race and socioeconomic status

Differences in health outcomes by socioeconomic status have long been recognized as a persisting and possibly increasing public health problem. For example, Guralnik *et al.*[42] reported that those with lower socioeconomic status, as measured by income, education and occupation, have significantly higher mortality rates than those in higher socioeconomic levels. They also noted that among older blacks and whites, the level of education has a greater effect than race on both total life expectancy and active life expectancy. Interestingly, in the over 85 age group, black women had a total life expectancy of 3.6 years greater than white women. Others have reported significant socioeconomic and racial differences in the incidence of both CHD and ischemic stroke. Here, Barnett *et al.*[43] reported a significant increase in CHD mortality in black men of lower social classes over a ten-year period (1984–1993); however, mortality of upper class black men decreased. CHD mortality for white males in all social classes declined during this time period. Similarly, Rosamond and associates[44] studied ischemic stroke incidence and survival in a large cohort of middle-aged (45–64 years) men and women from 1987 to 1995. The age-adjusted incidence rate/1000 person years was highest in black men (4.44) followed by black women (3.10), white men (1.78) and white women (1.24). After accounting for established baseline risks (hypertension, diabetes, education level and smoking status), blacks still had a 38% greater risk of ischemic stroke compared with whites. Moreover, a recent review of stroke mortality noted that compared with US whites, US blacks have significantly greater mortality rates for every stroke subtype, except perhaps cerebral infarction due to carotid artery occlusion;[45] the number of stroke deaths, between 1992 and 1996, increased in blacks by over 8%.

With respect to education, Timiras[46] proposed that continuing education and learning is an effective means to promote longevity and improve the quality of life in old age. As he pointed out, current evidence supports the idea that education is a strong psychological and biologic tool to attain a longer and more satisfying life. As a Chinese proverb says, "aging begins when we stop learning." In this regard, a recent Dutch longitudinal study[47] examined the role of behavioral (i.e. alcohol, smoking, BMI and physical activity) and material (i.e. financial problems, employment status and income proxy) factors in explaining educational differences in all-cause mortality. The authors concluded that the association between mortality and educational level was largely explained by material factors. Similarly, Wamala and co-workers[48] concluded that the increased risk for

CHD in women with low education is linked to both psychosocial stress (i.e. job stress, social isolation, poor coping and hopelessness) and lifestyle factors (smoking, leisure physical activity and obesity). They further noted that blood lipids, hemostatic factors and hypertension contribute to CHD to a lesser extent.

Others have also shown an inverse relationship between longevity and socioeconomic status. For example, Pappas and associates[49] reported that an inverse relation between mortality and socioeconomic position persisted in 1986 and was even stronger than in 1960. This disparity in mortality rates according to education and income increased for both women and men, whites and blacks, and family members and unrelated persons. On the other hand, in their study of centenarians, Perls and Silver[6] stated, "... we realized that the commonly accepted profile of successful aging, which assumes that the person will be well-educated, employed in a profession, and financially secure, is dangerously flawed." Moreover, Lantz *et al.*[50] noted that a prominent hypothesis regarding social inequalities in mortality is that the increased risk among the lower socioeconomic groups is mainly due to a higher prevalence of lifestyle risk factors (i.e. cigarette smoking, alcohol drinking, sedentary lifestyle and increased body weight). These authors reported, however, that although these factors are important, they explain no more than "12% to 13% of the predictive effect of income on mortality." They concluded that mortality differences are due to a wider array of factors and, therefore, would persist to some extent, even with improved health behaviors among the disadvantaged.

Of further interest regarding the relationship between social status, life expectancy and all-cause mortality, is a recent report of survival among Academy Award-winning actors and actresses.[51] This study analyzed all actors and actresses ever nominated for an Academy Award (n = 762). For each of these, another same sex cast member who was in the same film and born in the same era was identified (n = 887). All 1649 performers were analyzed; the median duration of follow-up time from birth was 66 years. The results showed that life expectancy was 3.9 years longer for Academy Award winners compared with the less recognized performers. Furthermore, those who received additional awards had a 22% relative reduction in death rates; however, additional films and nominations but without awards did not reduce the death rates. The authors concluded that high social status and increased longevity demonstrated in the general public extends to celebrities and is partially explained by success-related factors.

Other possible factors include hostility, depression and social isolation, all of which have been shown to predict increased all-cause mortality.[52] In addition to these important life expectancy risk factors, House *et al.*[53] studied the mortality rate among urban residents compared with suburban and rural/small-town residents. After adjustment for baseline sociodemographic and health variables, city dwellers had a mortality hazard ratio of 1.62 relative to rural/small-town residents; suburbanites had an intermediate but insignificant elevated hazard rate ratio. The mortality risk was particularly significant for non-black men younger than 65 years of age. There was no increased risk for women. The authors concluded that among men, the mortality risk of city residence is as significant as race, low income, smoking and social isolation.

Depression and suicide, heart disease, stroke

Depression is a chronic disorder and often associated with a wide range of other medical problems from alcoholism to CHD. It affects people all over the world and may, in fact, be worse in poorer countries where malnutrition and infectious diseases are particularly widespread.[54] In 1995, depression and other mental disorders accounted for 28% of the total disabilities in the world. It is estimated that depression, which ranked fourth in the world in disability-adjusted life years in 1990, will rank second in 2020, a figure greater than traffic accidents and second only to ischemic heart disease.[54]

Depression in people age 65 years and older is a major public health problem in the US, resulting in decreased quality and length of life.

It is also associated with increased medical costs, decreased worker productivity and increased dysfunctional families. The major risk factors for depression include substance/alcohol abuse, spousal bereavement, financial problems, medical illness/disability, and lack of social support from family and friends. Unfortunately, the early signs of depression (i.e. sleep disturbance, fatigue, guilt feelings, weight loss, decreased interest and enjoyment of normal life pursuits, and recurrent thoughts of death and suicidal ideation) may not always be apparent.

Depression also greatly increases the suicide rate, currently the eighth most common cause of death in the US. According to figures recently released by the Centers for Disease Control (CDC), people over age 65 years committed 19% of all suicides between 1980 and 1992, although they account for only 13% of the population;[55] moreover, men accounted for 81% of these suicides. Although suicide may be declining in women aged 65–74 years, it rises in those aged 75 years and over. Elderly suicides may be even more common than current statistics suggest (e.g. intentional overdoses of prescribed medications, cease taking prescribed medications, stop caring for themselves, delay treatment for medical conditions, stop eating and drinking, etc.).[56]

In addition to increased suicides among depressed people, various studies have shown a direct correlation between depression and several other diseases. For example, depression in women has been associated with decreased bone mineral density, which results in a significant increase in hip fractures.[57] In addition, several lines of evidence suggest that depression is a major risk factor for CHD. Ford *et al.*[58] reported that the cumulative incidence of depression in male medical students at 40-year follow-up was 12%. Multivariate analysis of their data indicated that depression was a significant risk factor for subsequent CHD and myocardial infarction (relative risk 2.12 for both disorders). Others[59] studied depressed men and women and compared them with non-depressed matched controls. Here, the risk for CHD was three times higher among men with depression than in the controls. However, depression was not associated with CHD in women. Conversely, Ferketich and associates[60] found that after controlling for possible confounding factors, depression was associated with an increased risk for CHD in both women and men, although depression directly correlated with increased mortality only in men with CHD.

In persons with known CHD, depression also predicts an increased risk for mortality.[61,62] Similarly, Denollet *et al.*[63] reported that a type-D personality (the tendency to suppress emotional distress), independent of other risk factors, was a significant predictor of long-term mortality in patients with CHD. More recently, depression was reported to be independently associated with a "substantial increase in the risk of heart failure among older persons. ..."[64] After controlling for numerous confounders, including the occurrence of myocardial infarction, depressed persons 60 years and older with isolated systolic hypertension had more than a two-fold higher risk of developing heart failure compared with non-depressed individuals. Still others found that work-related stress is associated with an increased prevalence of atheromatous carotid artery lesions in men but not women.[65] Here, the highest stress quintile showed a 36% presence of carotid lesions compared with 21% among men in the lowest stress quintile.

Two recent studies have also linked cerebrovascular disease with depression.[66,67] This latter six-year prospective study[67] of 2478 older whites and blacks from five North Carolina counties found that increasing scores on the modified Center for Epidemiological Stroke Depression Scale were associated with an increased risk of stroke. Conversely, high levels of positive effect appeared to be protective against stroke.

Various explanations have been proposed to explain the association between depression and the diseases associated with arteriosclerosis. For example, Carney *et al.*[68] suggested that it is directly or indirectly related to poorer health behaviors (e.g. increased smoking, decreased physical activity). Poor nutrition, resulting in an inadequate intake of critical antioxidants and micronutrients, is also likely to play an important role.

Personal longevity traits

Strong, optimistic personalities are typical of long-lived people while depression is uncommon. They are determined to face and over-come obstacles. Thus, rather than taking life easy, these special people take whatever measures are necessary to maintain their physical strength and mental capabilities. They refuse to see age as a limitation on life's enjoyments and strive to avoid lifestyle-related diseases and disorders.[6] In a recent study, Maruta *et al.*[69] examined how people explain events as a risk factor for early death using scores obtained from the Optimism-Pessimism scale of the Minnesota Multiphasic Personality Inventory. After following 839 patients for 30 years, they found that the more pessimistic group had a 19% higher risk for mortality. Earlier reports have also shown that pessimistic individuals are more susceptible to depression,[70] have poorer physical health,[71] and are more frequent users of medical and mental health care facilities.[72] Proneness to anger is also a significant risk factor for CHD morbidity and mortality independent of established biological risk factors.[73] Others[74] found that mental stress (i.e. feelings of tension, frustration and sadness) can more than double the risk of cardiac ischemia in the subsequent hour. Similarly, a study of life satisfaction, defined as interest in life, happiness, loneliness and general ease of living, showed the age-adjusted hazard ratios for all-cause, disease and injury mortality among dissatisfied compared with satisfied men were 2.11, 1.83 and 3.01, respectively.[75] After adjusting for marital status, social class, smoking, alcohol use and physical activity, the risk ratios were reduced to 1.49, 1.35 and 1.93, respectively. Their data did not demonstrate similar associations among women.

Although Alzheimer's disease is the major cause of dementia in older people, few risk factors have been identified. To evaluate the possible association between this disease and cognitively stimulating activities, Wilson *et al.*[76] studied 801 older Catholic nuns, priests and brothers without dementia at baseline. They evaluated the following seven cognitive stimulating activities involving information processing: viewing television; listening to radio; reading newspapers; reading magazines; reading books; playing games (e.g. cards, checkers, crossword and other puzzles); and going to museums. Their findings suggested that frequent participation in these stimulating cognitive activities was associated with a reduced incidence of Alzheimer's disease. Similarly, regular participation in social or leisure activities (e.g. traveling, odd jobs, knitting, etc.) are associated with a lower risk of dementia.[77] Others found that individuals who live alone and those without social ties have an increased risk for developing dementia (relative risk, 1.5)[78] Moreover, compared with married people, the relative risk for those who were single or living alone was 1.9. The risk of dementia with social disengagement is further supported by the work of Bassuk *et al.*[79] After correcting for various confounders, they found that elderly people with no social ties were significantly at risk for cognitive decline compared with those with five or more social ties (odds ratio, 2.24 after three years, 1.91 after six years, and 2.37 after 12 years follow-up).

In addition to these individual characteristics, a growing body of empirical evidence suggests that active religious involvement has a positive effect on health and mortality.[80-86] Oman and Reed[87] analyzed the prospective association between attending religious services and all-cause mortality. After comparing the mortality rate of those who attended religious services with several confounding factors (i.e. demographics, health status, physical functioning, health habits, social functioning and support, and psychological state), they concluded that attendance at religious services was associated with a lower mortality rate but that "we were unable to explain the protection against mortality offered by religious attendance." More specifically, Helm and associates[88] examined the relationship between survival and private religious activity such as prayer, meditation and Bible study. Importantly, they divided the population into religious activity of daily living into impaired and unimpaired groups since physical impairment and stress often lead to increased religious activity. After a 6.3-year average follow-up, and control for multiple confounding variables, their data demonstrated a significant protective effect of private religious activity against mortality in the relatively healthy unimpaired group. However, no protective effect persisted in the physically impaired population suggesting that the impaired group "may have begun private religious activity only in response of declining health. ..."

Other studies are also consistent with the view that religious involvement "is a general protective factor that promotes health through a variety of causal pathways."[89] Moreover, the protective effect of religious attendance may be stronger for women than men.[90] Strawbridge *et al.*[91] also noted that the lower mortality rates among those who are more involved in religious activities are partly explained by improved health practices, increased social activity and more stable marriages. The subject of religious commitment and health status has been reviewed.[92] Interestingly, medical schools have recently become interested in the association between health and spirituality. In 1994, only three medical schools taught courses on religious and spiritual issues. There were 30 in 1997 and in 2000 about half (i.e. 65) of the US medical schools offered "spirituality" courses.[93]

Maximum Lifespan

In contrast to the steady rise in average life expectancy, especially since 1900, it had been widely accepted that the maximum theoretical life span was about 115 years.[12] Thus, in 1980 the oldest authenticated person was a Japanese woman who lived for 114 years.[94] More recently, however, several individuals have significantly exceeded this mark, the current authenticated record being 122 years and 163 days.[95] Here, Jeanne Calment of France was born in 1875 and died in 1997. Interestingly, she remained spirited and mentally sharp, albeit blind during her last few years. As of the fall of 1999, the oldest authenticated living person was Sara (Clark) Knauss of Allentown, PA at 119 years.[96] The oldest documented male is Christian Mortenson (San Francisco, California) who died in 1998 at 115 years.[97] As of the fall of 1999, the oldest known living man (112 years) was Kamato Hongo of Japan.[96]

Is it possible to further extend the human lifespan? Certainly, attempts to increase the human lifespan date as early as 3500 BC; the search for immortality by Ponce de Leon (Fountain of Youth) and Alexander the Great are well known. As such, so-called aging experts have long touted various anti-aging elixirs to the general public. Nevertheless, as recently emphasized by 51 of the world's leading authorities on aging, there is "no truth to the Fountain of Youth."[98] These authors wrote that "the hawking of 'anti-aging' therapies has taken a particularly troubling turn of late. Disturbingly large numbers of entrepreneurs are luring gullible and frequently desperate customers of all ages to 'longevity' clinics, claiming a scientific basis for the anti-aging products they recommend and, often, sell."

In 1981, Harman[99] proposed that the maximum lifespan could be increased by five to ten or more years by weight control and ingesting diets adequate in essential antioxidant nutrients designed to minimize the negative effects of free radical reactions. More recently, Manton and Stallard suggested that lifespan limits are not yet manifested.[100] Using one of their analyses that involved parameters from extinct cohorts, they predicted that the maximum longevity potential could be 130 or more years. There are several things that will increase life expectancy, as well as the quality of life. Indeed, survival to old age is well known to be strongly affected by various environmental and behavioral components.

Major longevity determinants

Although several major factors are involved in longevity, their relative importance and inter-relationships are not well understood.

Genetics

Genetics plays a very important role in the aging process; however, the exact mechanisms are extremely complex and far from being identified. The major support for the role of genetics in human longevity is as follows:

(1) Family Longevity

There is a modest to moderate correlation in life expectancy among family members. Thus, families with centenarians have a greater chance to have equally long-lived members than those without centenarians. In addition, the difference in longevity is, on average, significantly less in identical twins than in fraternal twins. Thus, Perls *et al.*[101] recently analyzed the pedigrees of 449 American centenarian families. Compared with the 1900 cohort, male siblings of centenarians were "at least 17 times as likely to attain age 100 themselves, while female siblings were at least eight times as likely."

(2) Accelerated Aging Syndromes

Progeria (Hutchinson-Gilford syndrome; probable chance mutation in one copy of one gene), Werner's syndrome (autosomal recessive), and Down's syndrome (trisomy 21) are all associated with chromosomal abnormalities and significantly shortened lifespans. However, the subsequent biochemical phenomena are not well understood.

(3) Finite Doubling Potential

In 1965, Hayflick[102] demonstrated that human diploid cells dividing *in vitro* have a limited number of potential cell doublings (50 ± 10), presumably due to a genetic senescence program. Importantly, the cells from individuals with progeria, Werner's and Down's syndromes have significantly fewer divisions than normal cells.

(4) Telomerase

The enzyme telomerase is expressed in some malignant cells but not in normal cells.[103] When each cell divides, the telomeres (chromeric tips of chromosome arms) shorten. Once critically shortened telomere length is reached, the cell stops dividing and becomes senescent. However, in some cancer cells, telomerase stimulates continued cell division by maintaining the telomere length. As a result, new anticancer therapy may be aimed at inhibiting this enzyme.[104] Further studies are also critical to better understand its probable role in aging.

(5) Aging Genes

Although numerous genetically-determined biochemical pathways influence longevity, very few genes that might be involved have been discovered. Those that have been identified have primarily involved the fruit fly *Drosophila melanogaster* and the nematode worm *Caenorhabditis elegans*.[105] Whether these findings are applicable to humans remains to be determined. Nevertheless, a few studies have been done in people. For example, in French centenarians, two variable genes that may be important in postponing aging have been identified.[105] One of these codes for apolipoprotein E (involved in cholesterol transport among other things) while the other codes for angiostensin-converting enzyme (involved in blood pressure regulation). Here, particular alleles, or variants, of the genes are more frequent in centenarians than in the general population. However, exactly how these alleles are related to the aging process is poorly understood.

Free radicals/antioxidants

The free radical theory of aging[106] suggests that naturally occurring, highly reactive chemical species (i.e. free radicals) cause progressive, random damage to enzymes and other proteins, cell membranes (lipid peroxidation), DNA and RNA. Since then, abundant evidence has been presented to indicate that aging correlates with the sum of all free radical reactions produced in all body cells and tissues, or at least is a major contributor of it.[107–110] In addition, numerous naturally occurring protective substances (i.e. antioxidants) have been identified (Table 1.2).

(1) Observational Studies

(a) Metabolic rate: In 1928, Pearl[111] proposed that aging is dependent on the "rate of living." In fact, the metabolic rate theory of aging is part of other theories, particularly the free radical and genetic theories. Thus, a positive correlation was experimentally shown to exist between metabolic rate, aging, lipid peroxidation and the concentration of age-pigments.[112] These variables all support the idea that aging may be modulated by

Table 1.2: Major Antioxidant Defenses

Antioxidant Enzymes
  Catalase
  Glutathione peroxidase
  Glutathione reductase
  Superoxide dismutases (three enzymes)

Metal Binding Proteins
  Ceruloplasmin
  Ferritin
  Hemoglobin
  Lactoferrin
  Metallotheinein
  Myoglobin
  Transferrin

Common Antioxidants (Radical "Scavengers")
  Bilirubin
  Uric acid
  Thiols (R-SH)
  Vitamins A, C, and E
  Carotenoids (beta-carotene, lycopene, etc.)
  Flavonoids (quercetin, rutin, catechin, etc.)

Other Antioxidants
  Antioxidant enzyme co-factors (Zn, Mn, Se and Cu)
  Reduced glutathione (GSH)

the rate of oxygen consumption and hence the formation of oxygen-derived free radicals. In accordance with this, large animals generally have slower metabolic rates than small animals which have lower rates than insects. Thus, large animals generally live longer than small ones; variables such as hibernation and environmental temperature play a role in some cases.

(b) Caloric restriction: McKay *et al.*[113] first demonstrated that by restricting the food intake of young rats, their longevity could be increased. Follow-up studies by others confirmed that restricting laboratory animals to 60% of an *ad libitum* diet, but with adequate vitamins and minerals, results in a 30–50% increased lifespan.[114] Moreover, early data from current on-going studies with non-human primates suggests similar results.[115] Thus, dietary restriction in rhesus monkeys was shown to lower body temperature and thereby slow the metabolic rate,[116] increase physical activity,[117] and slow the postmaturational decline in serum levels of the steroid hormone dehydroepiandrosterone sulfate.[118] Moreover, caloric restriction decreases the load of oxidized proteins, enhances the immune system, has anti-inflammatory effects in the brain, and reduces oxidative stress, among others.[119] These findings also presumably apply to humans. These and other studies should not be surprising since obesity is not only associated with numerous diseases (CHD, stroke, diabetes, cancer, etc.), but it also accelerates the aging process.

(c) Age-pigments: The accumulation of "age-pigments" (lipofuscin and ceroid), mainly in the heart, muscle, liver and brain of the very old has been recognized by pathologists for well over 100 years. This brown fluorescent pigment, located in lysosomes, is formed as a by-product of oxygen free-radical reactions and lipid peroxidation. Its presence suggests inadequate body defenses against the stresses of reactive oxygen species.

(2) Antioxidant Enzymes

A strain of *Drosophila melanogaster* that lives twice as long as the normal strain also has significantly higher levels of superoxide dismutase.[120] Furthermore, a strain of *Caenorhabditis elegans* lives 70% longer than the normal strain and has increased activities of both superoxide dismutase and catalase.[120] In addition, Kellog and Fridovich[121] reported that long-lived mouse strains have significantly higher antioxidant enzyme activities (superoxide dismutase) than short-lived mice. However, de Grey[122] reviewed a series of studies and concluded that there is no correlation between longevity and increased levels of antioxidant enzymes in warm-blooded animals (homeotherms). Further studies are clearly needed to clarify this critical area.

(3) Antioxidants ("Free Radical Scavengers")

The body is well-supplied with naturally occurring protective mechanisms, including antioxidant enzymes and metal-binding proteins, both of which prevent the formation of free radicals.[107–110] In addition, other naturally synthesized substances (i.e. uric acid and bilirubin), as well as antioxidants from fruits and vegetables (vitamins, flavonoids, etc.) neutralize oxyradicals (Table 1.2).

Immunity

A loss of immune function with increasing age is well recognized. Older people are more prone to infectious diseases, autoimmune phenomena, amyloidosis, myelomatosis, chronic lymphocytic leukemia and other malignancies. This decreased immune responsiveness is primarily related to cell-mediated immunity (T-lymphocytes). Thus, with increasing age, the following changes commonly occur:

- decreased interleukin-2 (IL-2) production;
- decreased cellular response to mitogen stimulation;
- decreased antibody production following antigenic stimulation;
- increased production of interleukin-6 (IL-6); and
- increased production of autoantibodies.

Nevertheless, the immune system is negatively influenced by decreased hormone levels (e.g. dehydroepiandrosterone),[123] protein malnutrition, lack of important dietary antioxidants, and physical inactivity, among others.[124] Hence, a close relationship exists between immunity, oxidative stress and the endocrine system.

Hormones

A wide variety of neuroendocrine disorders, including impaired glucose tolerance, hyperthyroidism, hypothyroidism, muscle and organ atrophy due to decreased growth hormone production, gonadal dysfunction and hypertension possibly related to increased sympathetic nervous system sensitivity commonly increase with age. However, which of these are primary factors related to the aging process and which are secondary phenomena is currently not well understood.

Lifestyle

Life expectancy is, to a highly significant degree, lifestyle-related. Thus, as discussed in Chapters 2 to 5, weight control, physical activity, nutrition, various personal characteristics, and occupational and environment factors are all important in longevity, well-being, and health care costs.

Wellness Assessment and Health Promotion

Early recognition of the major risk factors for various diseases, and appropriate steps taken to alter them, can significantly decrease the costs of medical care, improve the quality of life and increase life expectancy. In this regard, the CDC recently reported that at least 60% of all doctor's office visits, hospitalizations and deaths are due to preventable or delayable disorders.[125] Of considerable importance, however, is that physicians are primarily disease-oriented and generally have little interest or training in behavioral counseling, preventive medicine except for infectious diseases, health promotion or nutrition.[126] Rather, they are taught to focus on the "chief complaint," presence of a current illness, physical examination and evaluation of various tests to confirm or rule out possible diseases. Unfortunately, they are often not interested in the patient's lifestyle (i.e. smoking, alcohol, drugs, exercise, diet and weight). Moreover, even when the physician is interested in these matters, managed care has significantly reduced the time available for physicians to counsel patients, a problem that results in far greater personal and financial costs than generally appreciated. For example, if people stopped smoking, exercised regularly, lowered their serum cholesterol levels by 10%, and controlled their blood pressure, it would prevent about 328,000, 178,000, 133,000 and 68,000 annual deaths, respectively.[127] Moreover, it would significantly compress morbidity and markedly reduce medical costs.

McGlynn and associates[128] recently evaluated the quality of health care in the United States. Overall, they reported that only 54.9% of the study participants received current recommended care. The proportions of recommended care for acute and chronic conditions were 53.5% and 56.1%, respectively. Similarly, the participants received only 54.9% of the recommended preventive care. Thus, strategies to reduce these serious deficits, including preventive care, are critical.

Complementary and alternative medical (CAM) therapies

Alternative medical therapies, defined as "interventions neither taught widely in medical schools nor generally available in US hospitals,"[129] have attracted significant national attention from the news media, government agencies, medical community and the general public. Since many people believe that physicians are primarily interested in disease, it is not surprising that an increasing number of adults are using CAM therapies (e.g. herbal medicine, massage, megavitamins, self-help groups, folk remedies, energy healing, acupuncture, chiropractic and homeopathy among others). This more educated and health-conscious group, among other things, believes that physicians are too focused on diagnosing and treating disease and have little interest in improving, or at least maintaining, a person's good health.[130] A 1990 national survey estimated that 34% of American adults (60 million) used at least one alternative therapy in the prior 12 months;[131] in 1997, that proportion increased to 42% (about 80 million persons).[129] Indeed, the estimated number of visits to practitioners of alternative therapies in 1990 was 427,120,000 compared with 387,558,000 visits to all primary care physicians. In 1997, the number who visited primary care physicians remained essentially the same (385,919,000), while visits to alternative practitioners increased significantly (628,825,000).[129] In a more recent study, Kessler and associates[132] reported that 67.6% of the respondents had used some form of CAM at least once. Moreover, lifetime use increased steadily with age. Thus, three of every ten in the pre-baby boom cohort; five of every ten of the baby boom cohort, and seven of every ten in the post-baby boom cohort used some type of CAM therapy by age 33 years.

Although there has been an upward trend in the use of CAM therapies, a recent study indicates that adults who use both CAM and
conventional therapies "tend to be less concerned about their
medical doctor's disapproval than about their doctor's inability to
understand or incorporate CAM therapy use within the context of
their medical management."[133] In this study, 79% of individuals who
visited a physician and used CAM therapy in the previous 12 months
perceived the combination to be superior to either one alone.
Interestingly, confidence in CAM providers was not significantly
different from confidence in physicians.

Physician counseling

How frequent do physicians counsel their patients about important
lifestyle changes to improve their health? CHD is the most common
cause of death in the industrialized countries; well-recognized risk
factors include, among others, lack of exercise, obesity, poor diet
and smoking. Yet, a recent CDC report stated that only 19% of physicians counseled their patients about exercise, 22% about diet and
10% about weight reduction.[125] Moreover, Frolkis *et al.*[134] reported
that physicians are poorly compliant with the National Cholesterol
Education Program (NCEP) guidelines, even with patients at high
risk for coronary heart disease. They found that only 50% of physicians followed NCEP algorithms for lipid screening and many
hyperlipidemic patients remained untreated. Moreover, these authors
noted that only 4% of physicians encouraged their patients to quit
smoking, 14% referred overweight patients to dieticians and 1% recommended exercise. Similarly, Rafferty[135] reported that primary care
physicians spent only 11% of their time on disease prevention (about
seven minutes/patient/year).

A favorable cardiovascular risk-profile not only results in greater
longevity and increased quality of life, but significantly lowers health
care costs.[136] These authors noted that the total annual charges
for men at low risk for cardiovascular disease were less than two-
thirds of the charges for men not at low risk (US$1615 less); charges

for women at low risk were half those for women not at low risk (US$1885 less). Others studied the relationship between patient income and physician counseling.[137] They reported that lower income patients were more likely to be obese and smoke than high-income patients and were less likely to wear seat belts and exercise. However, stress and alcohol consumption increased with income. Interestingly, physicians were more likely to discuss diet and exercise with high-income patients than those with a low-income. However, they were more likely to discuss smoking with low-income than with high-income smokers. The authors concluded that improvement is especially needed in regards to alcohol consumption, safe sex and seat belt use. They also emphasized that physicians need to be more diligent in identifying and counseling low-income patients regarding diet and exercise and high-income smoking patients.

Wee *et al.*[138] also reported that physician counseling about exercise was very low. Unfortunately, they found that physicians tend to counsel only as secondary prevention (i.e. after patients have developed diabetes, had a heart attack, etc.) and are less likely to counsel those at risk for obesity. These authors concluded that "the failure to counsel younger, disease-free adults and those from lower socioeconomic groups may represent important missed opportunities for primary prevention." Indeed, the European EUROASPIRE Study Group conducted a retroactive study of current clinical practice in relation to secondary prevention of CHD in patients 70 years and older.[139] They examined six major modifiable risk factors for CHD that could significantly reduce morbidity and mortality by secondary prevention (cigarette smoking, obesity, hypertension, blood cholesterol, diabetes, and advise relatives of patients with premature CHD to be screened). Although there was a significant reduction in CHD morbidity and mortality over time due to lifestyle improvements, the study group concluded that "there is considerable potential for cardiologists and physicians to further reduce coronary heart disease morbidity and mortality. ..." Thus, even though physicians counsel more often for secondary prevention, there is still significant room for improvement.

Expenditures: disease treatment and health promotion

There has been considerable interest in the amount and types of medical services rendered late in life. The general impression is that a greater proportion of health resources is currently devoted to terminally ill patients than in the past. However, a 12-year evaluation showed no evidence that people in the last year of their lives in 1988 accounted for a greater percent of Medicare expenditures than those in1976.[140] Thus, the yearly percent of the total Medicare budget changed little during this period, fluctuating between 27.2% and 30.6%. Furthermore, Perls and Wood[141] found that acute hospitalization costs peaked in patients aged 70 to 79 years and declined with age after that. Thus, the hospital costs for each admission for the oldest old (i.e. 80 years and older) was less than that for the younger elderly patients. The major reasons for the decreased costs were due to less intense care and admission to non-teaching hospitals.

Unfortunately, despite the overall health improvements achievable by preventive interventions, society continues to be burdened by preventable diseases, injury and disability. For example, in 1988 the annual health care expenditures for CHD alone exceeded US$135 billion, and injury and disability US$170 billion.[142] Yet, only 3% of the national health expenditures was spent on disease prevention. As noted by Furberg,[143] many research projects have shown substantial public health benefits from preventive measures. Yet, due to a marked shortage for funding, as well as the organization of the National Institutes of Health (NIH), prevention research usually receives very low priority. It seems reasonable to assume that managed-care plans, especially capitated Health Maintenance Organizations (HMOs), would provide significantly more comprehensive health education and health promotion benefits and programs to their members than traditional indemnity health insurance and Preferred Provider Organizations (PPOs). One might also assume that large companies would strongly encourage and reward their employees who participate in healthy practices which should lead to decreased company health insurance costs. Unfortunately, there is little evidence that either of these possibilities take place to any significant extent. Indeed, "only

35%–45% of California's HMOs, and no PPO/indemnity plans, assess the impact of health promotion programs on health risks and behaviors, health status or health care costs."[144] Nevertheless, active participation in health promotion strategies to modify risk factors such as smoking, obesity and physical inactivity can result in significant cost reductions. For example, Pronk *et al.*[145] reported that adverse health risks lead to significantly higher health care costs within 18 months. They suggested that health plans and payors interested in minimizing health care charges should consider strategic investments in programs that effectively reduce adverse health risks.

Health assessment and disease susceptibility

Most chronic diseases are usually not recognized until they are relatively well advanced. Thus, an individual develops specific signs and/or symptoms of a disease/disorder and then visits his/her physician. However, the time delay between disease onset and signs/symptoms may be years (e.g. cancer and diabetes) or even decades (e.g. atherosclerosis). Laboratory tests are now far more sensitive, and often more specific, for detecting early disease than simply assessing how one feels, looks or performs. They are also far more sensitive than a history and physical examination in situations in which a positive finding indicates that the disease is already present. It is unfortunate, as stressed by Gambino,[146] that a normal (negative) test result is of highest value to the patient but of "middling" value to the physician who is interested in ruling out a disease; it is of little or no value to the payer, who may mistakenly interpret a "normal" result as a test not warranted and therefore a waste of money. Nevertheless, a "normal" test result usually signifies decreased risk or even absence of a particular disease and, if properly interpreted, may help differentiate among diagnoses that yield normal results with different interpretations.[147]

Physicians and other health care workers, especially those trained in medicine and interested in laboratory medicine, can play a very significant role in reducing the major causes of death by assessing one's current level of "wellness" and susceptibility to various diseases.[148]

In this setting, "wellness assessment," which includes a careful evaluation of a panel of laboratory tests in conjunction with a patient's personal profile consisting of age, sex, family medical history, blood pressure, BMI (weight, kg/height, m²) and lifestyle (diet, physical activity, smoking and alcohol or drug history, etc.) can lead to a reasonable estimate of one's current state of health, as well as their future risk of developing various disorders/diseases. Table 1.3 gives a few examples of a "target" (i.e. minimal premature risk of morbidity/mortality) BMI (Chapter 2 contains a more complete BMI table and discussion of this topic).

Early recognition that a risk factor for various diseases, including coronary and cerebral vascular diseases, cancer, chronic obstructive pulmonary disease, diabetes and liver disease among others, is extremely important to both the individual and society. Moreover, testing is very cost-effective, especially if one adheres to the lifestyle changes or medication necessary to improve one's life expectancy and quality of life, as well as decrease the costs of medical care. The major diseases that may be identified in their early stages, or increased risks for these diseases, by "wellness assessment" are listed in Table 1.4.

In addition to these considerations, every older adult should receive an annual "flu shot." Govaert *et al.*[149] concluded that if healthy

Table 1.3: "Target" BMI* Related to Weight and Height

Height (Feet/Inches)	Weight (Pounds; BMI 20)	Weight (Pounds; BMI 24)
5' 0"	100	125
5' 2"	110	130
5' 4"	115	140
5' 6"	125	150
5' 8"	130	155
5' 10"	140	180
6' 2"	155	190
6' 3"	160	195

*20–24="Target" (minimal premature morbidity/mortality); 25–26=low risk (overweight); 27–29=moderate risk (obese); 30–34=high risk (significant obesity); 35–39=very high risk (morbid obesity); and ≥40=extremely high risk (extreme marked obesity).

Table 1.4: Major Identifiable Diseases/Disorders by Wellness Assessment

Accelerated aging

Atherosclerosis (coronary, cerebral and peripheral vascular diseases)

Cancer (various types)

Chronic obstructive lung diseases (mainly emphysema/chronic bronchitis)

Type 2 diabetes mellitus (non-insulin dependent diabetes mellitus; NIDDM)

Liver disease/cirrhosis

Hemochromatosis

Hypothyroidism and hyperthyroidism

Metabolic syndrome (Syndrome X)

Nutritional deficiencies (proteins, minerals and antioxidants)

Immune deficiencies

Anemia

individuals aged 60 and over received an annual influenza vaccination, their chances of influenza would be reduced by 50%. Importantly, more than 90% of the mortality arising from influenza/pneumonia occurs in this age group[150] (No. 6 cause of death in the US). Nevertheless, the Public Health Service predicted that only about 60% of Americans received influenza vaccinations in the year 2000. Why don't more elderly people get vaccinated? A recent report indicated that these older individuals fear possible vaccination side effects and their own perceived good health.[151] These authors concluded that "better and more specific information about the paucity of systemic side effects" must be emphasized by health care workers. How about influenza vaccination for healthy working adults aged 18–50 years? A recent report found that vaccination is also cost-effective "in most influenza seasons in healthy working adults."[152]

In addition to influenza vaccination, over 50% of elderly people have not received a pneumococcal vaccination (Pneumovax). The estimated annual incidence of pneumococcal bacteremia in those aged 65 years and older is 50–83 cases/100,000. These infections are not only associated with a very high fatality rate (about 40,000/year), but Medicare costs for hospitalizations can reach US$1 billion/year.[153] Importantly, a single life-time vaccination of the elderly against the pneumococcal microorganism is very cost-effective.[154,155] The most recent recommended adult guidelines for Americans are as follows:[156]

Tetanus, diphtheria: A booster dose every ten years for all adults 19 years and older.
Influenza: An annual dose for all adults 50 years and older. Adults aged 19–49 years with medical or occupational indications or household contacts with persons with indications should also receive an annual dose.
Pneumococcal: A single dose for all unvaccinated persons aged 65 years and older and other adults with medical or other indications. Adults with immunosuppressive conditions should be revaccinated.
Hepatitis B: Three doses (zero, one to two months and four to six months) for all adults with medical, behavioral, occupational or other indications.
Hepatitis A: Two doses for adults with medical, behavioral, occupational or other indications.
Meningococcal: One dose for all adults with medical or other indications.

In addition, stools should be regularly tested for blood, women over the age of 40–50 years should have periodic mammograms, and most women should receive a regular "Pap" smear for uterine cervical cancer. Periodic colonoscopies should also be a part of one's health evaluation, especially for those with a family history of colorectal cancer.

It is clearly evident that a much better job educating the general public regarding the health benefits, increased life expectancy, and quality of life associated with the prevention of these common diseases by promoting their health, is extremely important. Only then will we experience longer and more fruitful lives, and health care costs will become far more manageable.

Following objective evaluation of the clinical information and laboratory test results, a "rating" or "risk" profile can be produced which compares prior test results with current ones to indicate possible

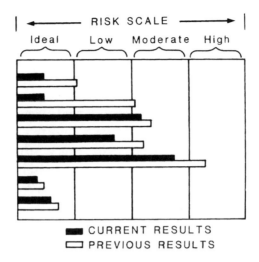

Figure 1.3: Risk/Rating Scale. The bars may represent various tests (i.e. cholesterol, homocysteine, oxidative reserve capacity, etc.) and/or disease risk (CHD, cancer, diabetes mellitus, etc.).

changes (Fig. 1.3). A second similar scale may be used to represent the estimated risk for various diseases (e.g. CHD, cancer, diabetes, etc.). These visual indicators give the patient more specific and useful information as to where they are and where they should be with respect to disease susceptibility. Furthermore, specific written recommendations to accompany each report (i.e. weight reduction, exercise program, specific dietary changes, antioxidant supplements, etc.) would be highly useful. After all, "your patients can't follow instructions if they don't understand."[157] Follow-up appointments should be scheduled to discuss one's progress and for repeat testing and evaluation, the frequency depending on the current risk factors and progress to date.

Wellness Assessment Tests

Oxidative stress

The air we breathe is truly a double-edged sword. We obviously need it to survive, yet each breath results in the formation of highly reactive and potentially destructive chemical species known as free radicals. Although the body has numerous mechanisms to prevent their formation, or neutralize them once formed, there is an imbalance such that free radicals are produced in excess. As such, oxygen-derived free radicals have been associated with over 100 diseases and disorders, as well as having a centrol role in aging.[111] The major medical conditions associated with increased free radical-induced oxidative stress include arteriosclerosis, cancer, cataracts, macular degeneration, type 2 diabetes, immune system deficiencies, various neurodegenerative disorders and ischemia/reperfusion injury, among others.

Tests that measure various aspects of oxidative stress have primarily been limited to research laboratories. However, when the importance of oxidative stress in disease and aging is more widely recognized, quantitative measurements will become common. The substances which undergo oxidative changes and the available tests to measure them, include the following: (1) lipid peroxidation (e.g. malondialdehyde, thiobarbituric acid reactive substances (TBARS), 4-hydroxynonenal, conjugated dienes, lipid hydroperoxides, and breath analysis for pentane and ethane); (2) protein oxidation (e.g. protein carbonyls and nitrotyrosine); (3) DNA damage (e.g. 8-hydroxy-2-deoxyguanosine and other hydroxylated bases);[158] and (4) arachidonyl-containing lipids (e.g. F2-isoprostanes).[159]

Whereas most of the lipid peroxidation tests are excellent biomarkers of lipid peroxidation *in vitro*, they are less reliable as an index of lipid peroxidation *in vivo*. However, F2-isoprostanes are generated in large amounts *in vivo* and are a reliable marker of lipid peroxidation *in vivo*.[159] Importantly, F2-isoprostanes are stable, they can be measured in all body fluids, and the assay is highly precise and accurate. However, a more clinically useful and economically feasible screening test of total body oxidative stress is the measurement of the oxidative reserve capacity;[160] importantly, automation of this technique has been reported.[161] The oxidative reserve capacity is an estimate of one's overall ability to cope with damaging reactive oxygen species and, therefore, might serve as a general risk factor for the major free radical-linked diseases/disorders. Moreover, several more recent tests have been reported which measure total antioxidant capacity.[162] However, these authors emphasized that under certain conditions these tests may be misinterpreted since they do not all measure exactly the same thing. As a result, a "battery" of tests which measure slightly different aspects of the complex oxidative process is more reliable than a single test. Although currently available only in research and a few specialty laboratories, tests that measure oxidative stress will become more accessible as physicians recognize the importance of oxidative stress in aging and disease. A critical review of the various tests that measure antioxidant capacity has been recently published.[163]

Arteriosclerosis (coronary heart and cerebrovascular diseases)

CHD is the leading cause of death and disability in both men and women (Table 1.1); cerebrovascular disease (CVD) is the third leading cause of death. The annual direct and indirect costs of CHD for 1999 were estimated at US$274 billion, including lost productivity.[164] It is an unfortunate misconception that CHD is widely considered a "man's disease" when, in fact, more women died of CHD in 1996 than men.[164] This misconception by the general public, as well as by many physicians, is perhaps due to the fact that men often suffer from CHD during their 40s and early 50s, a time when very few women are affected. However, following menopause, CHD in women parallel the disease in men.[165] To further illustrate the misconception of the relative unimportance of CHD in women, Mosca *et al.*[166] recently reported their findings that women do not perceive heart disease as a major health problem. In this study, which involved 1000 women 25 years and older (65.8% white, 13.0% African American and 12.6% Hispanic), only 8% of the respondents identified heart disease and stroke as their greatest health concern and 33% identified heart disease as the leading cause of death in women. Conversely, about 61% regarded cancer as their greatest health concern. In addition, more than 70% of the partcipants reported that their physicians had not discussed the risks of heart disease with them. Thus, it is apparent that considerably more emphasis regarding the importance of CHD and stroke must be emphasized not only to women, but to physicians as well.

Table 1.5 lists the major arteriosclerotic risk factors, most of which are generally well known [i.e. age, sex, obesity, smoking, physical inactivity, diabetes, hypertension, increased serum total cholesterol (TC), low-density lipoprotein cholesterol (LDL-C; "bad" cholesterol), apolipoprotein B-100, triglycerides, and low serum levels of high-density lipoprotein cholesterol (HDL-C; "good" cholesterol)]. Although less well-known and appreciated, the following are also major risk factors for atherogenesis: increased serum TC/HDL-C ratio, fibrinogen, Factor VII, homocysteine, uric acid, C-reactive protein (C-RP), blood hematocrit, leukocyte count (mainly neutrophil and band counts), albumin, ferritin, and clinical depression.

Perhaps other less appreciated risks for CHD are various socioeconomic factors such as low levels of personal income and education, as well as occupation.[165] Furthermore, a recent report indicated that

Table 1.5: Major Risk Factors For CHD and CVD

Commonly Known/Understood	Less Known/Understood
Age	Albumin
Sex	Cholesterol/HDL-C ratio
Diabetes	C-RP
Hypertension	Depression
Socioeconomic status	Factor VII
Increased TC	Ferritin
Increased LDL-C	Fibrinogen
Decreased HDL-C	Hematocrit
Increased triglycerides	Homocysteine
Overweight/obese	Leukocyte count (neutrophils)
Physically inactive	Neighborhood of residence
Smoking	Uric acid level

neighborhood of residence is also associated with CHD.[167] These investigators found, after controlling for the socioeconomic factors, that living in a disadvantaged neighborhood significantly increased the risk for CHD.

Tests for arteriosclerosis

A 1981 literature review found "at least" 246 risk factors for CHD.[168] Clearly, however, the more important risk factors are far fewer (Table 1.5). Laboratory tests are not only important in the identification of risk factors for CHD, but also in other atherosclerotic diseases such as CVD and peripheral vascular disease (Table 1.6).

(1) Blood Lipid Profile
The Expert Panel of the National Cholesterol Education Program (NCEP) recently updated their recommendations on the detection, evaluation and treatment of elevated blood cholesterol in adults (Adult Treatment Panel III; ATP III).[169] ATP III emphasized that LDL-C was of major importance based on research from experimental animal studies, laboratory investigations, epidemiology and genetic forms of hypercholesterolemia. In addition, recent clinical trials have shown that LDL-C lowering therapy significantly reduces the risk for CHD. As a result, ATP III continues to consider increased plasma LDL levels as the primary target of cholesterol-lowering therapy, although other lipid moities are also recognized as being very important. As such, they recommended that all adults 20 years and older should have a fasting lipoprotein profile every five years (i.e. TC, LDL-C,

Table 1.6: Tests for Arteriosclerosis Risk Factors

Blood lipid profile	
TC	Hematocrit
HDL-C	Ferritin
LDL-C	White blood count
Triglycerides	Homocyst(e)ine
TC/HDL-C ratio	Uric acid
C-RP	Fibrinogen

Table 1.7: 2001 NCEP Lipid Profile Guidelines[169]

LDL Cholesterol (mg/dl)
    <100: Target level
    100–129: Near or above optimal
    130–159: Borderline high
    160–189: High
    ≥190: Very high

Total Cholesterol (mg/dl)
    <200: Desirable
    200–239: Borderline high
    ≥240: High

HDL Cholesterol (mg/dl)
    <40: Low
    ≥60: High

HDL-C and triglycerides). The recommended risk guidelines are presented in Table 1.7.

The panel also recognized that cigarette smoking, hypertension (blood pressure ≥ 140/90), low HDL-C, family history of premature CHD and age (men ≥ 45 years; women ≥ 55 years) are also major risk factors for CHD (see original publication for details regarding recommended LDL-lowering drug therapy[169]).

(2) Total cholesterol/HDL-C Ratio

TC alone misclassifies a person's risk for coronary heart disease about 40% of the time.[146] Castelli and Anderson first emphasized that the TC/HDL-C ratio is a highly reliable risk factor for coronary heart disease.[165] This ratio is, in many ways, the most informative and least expensive routine lipid risk indicator for both coronary and cerebrovascular diseases. Furthermore, it gives more than just a number; it gives a risk level that the patient can readily appreciate, understand and remember. A compromise cutoff ratio of ≥ 4.5 for adults was suggested, although an "ideal" target is 3.5 or less. In this study, the ratio range for most women with CHD was 4.6–6.4, while for men it was 5.5–6.1; a ratio of 7.1 and 9.3 indicated twice the risk for women and men, respectively;[165] the average ratio for vegetarians was 2.8 and 3.4 for Boston marathoners.

Numerous subsequent studies are in agreement that the TC/HDL-C ratio is a highly reliable predictor for CHD. The ratio holds not only in those with increased TC levels, but also in those with "desirable" levels (i.e. < 200 mg/dL),[170–173] as well as in women[174] and the elderly.[175,176] In addition, the ratio was recently shown to be a major baseline atherothrombotic biomarker for the development of peripheral vascular disease.[177]

(3) Fibrinogen

Many studies have shown that an elevated plasma fibrinogen level significantly increases the risk for CHD;[178,179] data from the Framingham Study showed a progressive increase in CHD in men and women with plasma levels above 1.25 g/L.[180] A recent review of 18 prospective studies, including six in patients with either angina pectoris or a history of prior myocardial infarction at baseline, concluded that fibrinogen is a major risk factor for CHD.[181] Coagulation Factor VII has also been shown to be an important risk factor for CHD.[182]

Although the determinants of plasma fibrinogen as a risk factor for CHD are poorly understood, smoking, male gender, low social class and the winter season were all associated with increased plasma fibrinogen levels. These studies suggest that elevated fibrinogen levels directly affect atherogenesis, add to plasma and erythrocyte viscosity, stimulate platelet aggregation, and increase the amount of fibrin deposition. Importantly, strenuous physical activity reportedly lowers both plasma fibrinogen and Factor VII levels.[182]

(4) Homocyst(e)ine

Homocytinuria is a rare inherited recessive disorder of homocysteine metabolism; markedly elevated serum homocyst(e)ine (i.e. the sum of free and bound homocysteine plus homocystine and homocysteine-cysteine mixed disulfide) levels are present. This metabolic disorder was first shown to be associated with severe premature atherosclerosis in children.[183] Subsequent studies revealed that heterozygotes also had elevated homocyst(e)ine levels and an increased incidence of CHD. Numerous recent studies have now shown a significant positive correlation between CHD and stroke with increased plasma homocyst(e)ine levels in persons without a genetic link to homocystinuria.[184–189] Recent studies have also shown that increased homocyst(e)ine levels are associated with common carotid artery wall thickness[190] and stenosis,[191] non-fatal stroke,[192] recurrent venous thrombosis[193] and peripheral arterial occlusive disease.[194] These latter workers also reported a negative correlation between homocysteine levels and vitamin B_{12} and folic acid. Thus, deficiencies of these vitamins, as well as B_6, are all related to increased plasma homocyst(e)ine concentrations;[195,196] vitamin supplementation generally lowers homocysteine plasma levels[197–199] and thereby reduces the risk of these atherosclerotic-related diseases.

(5) Uric Acid

Numerous studies,[200,201] although not all,[202] have suggested that an increased serum uric acid level is a risk factor for CHD. Increased serum uric acid levels have also been associated with obesity, dyslipidemia and hypertension, all of which are associated with increased CHD. Most recently, Fang and Alderman[203] reported that increased serum uric acid is an independent risk factor for cardiovascular mortality. In this report, they found that deaths due to CHD in both men and women increased when serum uric acid concentrations were in the highest quartile compared with the lowest quartile (men > 416 versus < 321 μmol/L; > 7.0 versus < 5.4 mg/dL; risk ratio 1.77; for women > 333 versus < 238 μmol/L;> 5.6versus < 4.0 mg/dL; risk ratio 3.0).

(6) Hematocrit

Blood viscosity depends on a combination of erythrocyte aggregatability and deformability, protein concentration, plasma viscosity and the blood hematocrit. An elevated hematocrit was first recognized as a risk factor of acute myocardial infarction in the early 1960s.[204,205] More recently, there has been further evidence that an increased hematocrit is, indeed, an important risk factor for CHD.[206,207] It has also been correlated with peripheral vascular abnormalities and stroke.[208] These clinical disorders progressively increase as the hematocrit rises above 49%. Hence, individuals with elevated hematocrits should be encouraged to donate blood often enough to maintain levels below 50%. Here, the individual, transfusion service and the anemic hospitalized patient will all benefit.

(7) Leukocyte Count

In 1974, Friedman and associates[209] reported that the total white blood count (WBC) was significantly higher in those who subsequently suffered an acute myocardial infarction (AMI) compared with two control groups: one matched for age, gender and race; the other included these variables as well as other common risk factors (i.e. total serum cholesterol, hypertension, etc.). Zalokar *et al.*[210] prospectively studied 7000 men for an average of 6.5 years. They found that among smokers, the WBC correlated directly with the risk for AMI. Thus, the incidence for AMI was four times greater in smokers whose WBC was 9000/μL compared with smokers whose WBC was 6000/μL or less. Similarly, a study of a Japanese cohort found a significant correlation between the WBC and CHD.[211] In addition, these authors reported that the strongest cellular association was the neutrophil count. A recent publication[181] reviewed 19 prospective studies linking an increased leukocyte count with CHD. The seven largest studies, involving 5337 cases, showed that individuals with leukocyte counts in the top third had a combined risk ratio of 1.4 compared with those in the bottom third.

To further examine the association between the WBC and AMI, Barron *et al.*[212] studied the WBC on admission and 30-day mortality of 153, 213 patients aged 65 years and older who had an AMI. Their findings showed a significantly higher risk for in-hospital events, in-hospital mortality and 30-day mortality. Thus, compared with patients in the lowest quintile, patients in the highest quintile were three times more likely to die at 30 days (10.3% versus 32.3%). After adjustment for various confounders, the WBC was a strong independent predictor for 30-day mortality (odds ratio, 2.37). As the authors noted, their findings "have important clinical implications for risk-stratifying patients with AMI."

(8) C-Reactive Protein (C-RP)

As emphasized by Gambino,[213] serum C-RP is a greatly underutilized and unappreciated screening test for various inflammatory and infectious diseases and tissue injury. Indeed, an increased C-RP level is now recognized as an important risk factor for acute myocardial infarction,[214–216] ischemic stroke,[214,215,217] sudden death from cardiac causes[218] and peripheral arterial disease.[219] In a recent literature review,[181] seven prospective studies were examined, including two whose patients had angina or a history of AMI at baseline. Together, the overall risk ratio for AMI was 1.7 between the highest and lowest third C-RP levels. Ridker and others[214] also reported that the baseline plasma C-RP level predicts the risk of future AMI and stroke. Moreover, they noted that the reduction associated with the use of aspirin and the risk of a first AMI appeared to be directly related to the C-RP value, suggesting that anti-inflammatory agents may have direct clinical benefits in preventing AMI and stroke in addition to their antithrombotic action on blood platelets. These researchers subsequently reported that serum C-RP was an independent risk factor for CHD in women.[216] Their data suggested that the addition of a high sensitivity C-RP test to the routine screening profile may improve the identification of women at risk for cardiovascular events. Indeed, compared with several other major risk factors [HDL-C, LDL-C, TC, apolipoprotein B, homocysteine and lipoprotein (a)], the high sensitivity C-RP measurement was the single strongest predictor of a future vascular event. Others[220] reported that increased C-RP levels are predictors of negative coronary events in those with either stable or unstable angina.

LDL-C is the major focus of current guidelines to determine the risk of cardiovascular disease.[221] Since cardiovascular events often occur in the absence of hyperlipidemia, C-RP and LDL-C were measured at baseline in 27,939 healthy women (Women's Health Study) who were then followed for an average of eight years for the occurrence of myocardial infarction, ischemic stroke, coronary revascularization, or death from cardiovascular causes.[222] After adjusting for the usual confounders (i.e. age, smoking, diabetes mellitus, blood pressure and hormone replacement therapy), the relative risks of first cardiovascular events according to increasing quintile of C-RP, as compared with those in the lowest quintile, were 1.4, 1.6, 2.0 and 2.3. The corresponding relative risks in increasing quintiles of LDL-C compared with the lowest were 0.9, 1.1, 1.3 and 1.5. Thus, the authors concluded that "these data suggest that C-RP level is a stronger predictor of cardiovascular events than LDL-C ..." Importantly, this study's results are consistent with published reports in diverse populations.[223]

An increased serum C-RP value as a predictor of AMI and stroke is presumably related to several recent studies suggesting that arteriosclerosis may be, in part, an infectious process due to microorganisms such as *Chlamydia pneumoniae*.[224,225] If so, it is important to recognize that the "respiratory burst," following phagocytosis, results in the production of highly reactive oxygen-derived free radicals which not only kill microorganisms, but oxidize LDL (i.e. oxidative modification of LDL and the pathogenesis of atherosclerosis).[110]

It should be noted that in addition to several other health benefits, physical activity significantly improves the immune system (Chapter 3). Indeed, Ford[226] recently published data indicating that increased physical activity is associated with lower serum C-RP concentrations. Thus, the odds ratios for elevated C-RP levels were 0.98, 0.85 and 0.53 for individuals who engaged in light, moderate and vigorous physical activity, respectively.

(9) Serum Albumin

Danesh and associates[181] reviewed eight prospective, population-based studies of albumin and CHD involving a total of 3770 cases with a weighted mean age at baseline of 64 years and a mean follow-up of 11 years. These studies were all adjusted for smoking and cholesterol levels; several also adjusted for blood pressure, obesity and socioeconomic status. At baseline, those with serum albumin levels in the lower third (mean 3.8 g/dL), compared with those in the upper third (4.2 g/dL), had a significantly increased risk for CHD (risk ratio 1.5).

The authors noted that although various theories have been proposed to explain the relationship between low serum albumin levels and CHD, none were fully satisfactory. They proposed that the consistency of the association of decreased serum albumin levels and CHD with other diseases is the most probable explanation. However, it should be noted that decreased serum albumin levels are frequent in the elderly and others in whom protein malnutrition is common. As a result, these individuals have a decreased intake of critical antioxidants, which have been repeatedly shown to be inversely associated with increased CHD, stroke, cancer and other diseases[110] (see Chapter 4).

(10) Serum Iron Levels

Based on the theory of oxidative modification of LDL and atherogenesis,[227] it is reasonable to assume that increased serum iron would be associated with an increased risk for CHD. Indeed, Salonen et al.[228] published "the first solid evidence" supporting this theory which was first put forth by Sullivan in 1981.[229,230] Their study indicated that for every 1% rise in serum ferritin, there was a 4% increase in the risk of AMI. More specifically, men with serum ferritin levels of 200 µg/L (200 ng/mL) or more had a 2.2-fold increase in the risk for AMI compared with those whose ferritin levels were less than 200 µg/L. Conversely, two subsequent reports indicated that iron stores were not related to CHD.[231,232] However, two more recent publications have given significant support for this proposal. These studies showed that heterozygosity for hereditary hemochromatosis was associated with an increased risk of cardiovascular disease in both women[233] and men.[234]

Cancer

Since the US has no nationwide cancer registry, the number of new cancer cases are estimated.[235] Thus, there were an estimated 1,284,900 new cancer cases and 555,500 cancer deaths in the United States in 2002.[236] The major forms of cancer and the number of predicted cases in men and women for 2002 are presented in Table 1.8; the estimated number of major cancer deaths in 2002 is presented in Table 1.9. Racial and ethnic minorities account for a disproportionate number of malignant diseases. Indeed, African Americans reportedly have a 10% higher incidence rate and a 30% higher death rate from all cancers combined than whites.[237] The major reasons for this higher cancer incidence and death rate in African Americans include lower socioeconomic status (e.g. lower education level, poor nutrition and decreased health care) and increased risk-promoting lifestyles (e.g. physical inactivity, overweight/obesity and cigarette smoking).

The financial costs of cancer diagnosis and treatment are enormous; several examples will be cited. Will and associates[238] estimated the lifetime costs of breast cancer in a cohort of 17,700 Canadian women diagnosed in 1995. They found that the lifetime treatment cost per case varied by stage, from US$36,340 for Stage IV (metastatic

Table 1.8: Estimated US Cancer Cases in 2002[236]

Site	Men	Women	Total
Oral cavity and pharynx	18,900	10,000	28,900
Digestive system	130,300	120,300	250,600
Lung and bronchus	90,200	79,200	169,400
Breast	1500	203,500	205,000
Prostate	189,000	–	189,000
Uterine cervix	–	13,000	13,000
Uterine corpus	–	39,300	39,300
Ovary	–	23,300	23,300
Urinary system	62,200	28,500	90,700
Brain and nervous system	9600	7400	17,000
Thyroid	4900	15,800	20,700
Non-Hodgkins lymphoma	28,200	25,700	53,900
Leukemia	17,600	13,200	30,800

Table 1.9: Estimated US Cancer Deaths in 2002[236]

Site	Total	Men	Women
Digestive tract	132,300	70,800	61,500
Colon	48,100	23,100	25,000
Pancreas	29,700	14,500	15,200
Liver	14,100	8900	5200
Stomach	12,400	7200	5200
Esophagus	12,600	9600	3000
Respiratory system	161,400	94,100	67,300
Lung and bronchus	154,900	89,200	65,700
Breast	40,000	400	39,600
Genital system	57,100	30,900	26,200
Ovary	13,900	–	13,900
Uterine corpus	6600	–	6600
Uterine cervix	4100	–	4100
Prostate	30,200	30,200	–
Urinary system	24,900	16,200	8700
Brain/nervous system	13,100	7200	5900
Lymphoma	25,800	13,500	12,300
Multiple myeloma	10,800	5500	5300
Leukemia	21,700	12,100	9600

disease) to US$23,275 for Stage 1. The total cost for the 17,700 cases was estimated at over Canadian $454 million. Hospitalization, mainly for initial treatment and terminal care, accounted for 63% of the total costs. Others[239] estimated the annual cost in 1997 for breast and gynecological cancers in American women at US$5 billion. Other reports estimated the average cost/case as follows: colon, US$33,700,[240] rectum US$36,500[240] and prostate US$19,755.[241] In the 1997 cohort of 5.8 million Canadian men, aged 40–80 years, an estimated 701,491would develop prostate cancer; the total direct medical cost was estimated at Canadian $9.76 billion.[242]

Epidemiologic studies indicate that cancer is largely an avoidable disease. Indeed, cigarette smoking and a poor diet account for an estimated 65% of all cancer deaths.[243] The major risk factors for the most common malignancies, in addition to genetics, include smoking (cancer of the lung, oropharynx, kidneys and bladder),[244,245] poor diet [246] with insufficient essential antioxidants (i.e. vitamins C,

E, etc.)[247,248] and other micronutrients (e.g. selenium),[249,250] obesity and high fat intake (cancer of prostate,[251] breast and colon[252,253]), excessive alcohol intake (breast),[254] and overexposure to various transition metals (e.g. nickel),[255] and ultraviolet light (skin),[256] among others (Table 1.10). Moreover, the relationship between oxidative stress and cancer has been repeatedly emphasized by numerous epidemiologic studies reporting a direct relationship between dietary antioxidant intake and the incidence of various malignancies.[257–261]

Floyd and associates[262] first demonstrated that DNA damage by the hydroxyl radical results in the formation of 8-hydroxyguanosine, which can be measured in the urine. This finding has been repeatedly verified and the topic of oxyradicals and cancer has been reviewed.[257,258] Importantly, 8-hydroxyguanosine and other hydroxylated bases may prove to be important markers for cancer susceptibility; however, clinical studies have yet to be reported. Since the oxidative reserve capacity is an overall measure of oxidative stress, this test may also serve as a general guide to cancer susceptibility.[158]

Thyroid dysfunction

Both hypo- and hyperthyroidism increase with age; both disorders are significantly more common in women. Signs and symptoms of these disorders may be atypical or mild and thought to be merely signs of "old age" or represent mild psychiatric problems. Abnormal test results are also commonly present in subclinical cases.

Table 1.10: Major Risk Factors For Cancer

Environmental pollutants
Excess alcohol intake
Genetics
Poor nutrition (inadequate antioxidants, micronutrients, fiber and excess fat)
Obesity
Sedentary lifestyle
Smoking
Transition metals (Ni, Cd, etc.)
Ultraviolet light

Some physican organizations have not recommended routine screening for occult thyroid disease.[263] On the other hand, Danese *et al.*[264] presented important evidence that periodic screening for mild thyroid failure is as cost-effective as estrogen replacement therapy, exercise and breast cancer screening. In addition, their data indicated that it is as favorable a strategy as screening either men or women of comparable ages for hypertension. These investigators recommended periodic measurement of serum thyroid stimulating hormone (TSH) in all patients, especially but not exclusively women, aged 35 years and older who are undergoing periodic health examinations.

More recent reports also support these latter recommendations. Canaris *et al.*[265] in a cross-sectional study involving 25,862 participants, found the prevalence of abnormal thyroid function to be substantial with increased TSH levels in 9.5% of the study group and decreased levels in 2.2%. Moreover, recently reported guidelines from the American Thyroid Association[266] recommend that all adults be screened by measuring serum TSH concentration beginning at age 35 years and every five years thereafter. They emphasized that although screening is particularly important in women, it is also cost-effective in men.

Type 2 diabetes (NIDDM)

There were an estimated 10.4 million Americans with diabetes in 1998, an increase of 2.9 million since 1980;[267] at least six million others have the disease but have not been diagnosed. Of the several types of diabetes, type 2 accounts for about 90% of the total American cases. Unfortunately, these individuals have the disease, on average, at least four to seven years before the diagnosis is made.[268] Boyle and associates[269] recently projected the number of people with diabetes in the US through the year 2050. Their data indicates that the number of Americans with diagnosed diabetes will increase 165% from 11 million in 2000 (prevalence of 4.0%) to 29 million in 2050 (prevalence of 7.2%). They predicted that the largest group will involve those 75 years of age and older. The fastest growing ethnic group will be black males (+363%) followed by black females (+217%), white males (+148%) and white females (+107%). Of the projected increase, 37% will be due to demographic composition, 27% to population growth and 36% to increasing prevalence rates.

Diabetes mellitus is currently listed as the sixth most common cause of death in the US (Table 1.1); it reportedly leads to more than 68,000 deaths/year with an annual total medical cost of at least US$100 billion.[270] However, the true figure is probably significantly higher since type 2 diabetes is a major risk factor for CHD, stroke, renal failure, hypertension and blindness. The major risk factors for type 2 diabetes are a positive family history, obesity and decreased physical activity.[271,272] In 1998, the World Health Organization (WHO) reported that 54% of American adults were overweight; 22.5% were clinically obese compared to 14.5% less than 20 years previously.[271] Indeed, a recent report involving 84,941 female nurses showed that 91% of type 2 diabetes could be attributed to lifestyle.[273] The single most important risk factor was overweight/obesity. Exercise, poor dietary habits and smoking were also significant risk factors even after correcting for BMI. This epidemic of type 2 diabetes and obesity was recently reviewed.[274] Importantly, diabetes is also associated with a significant increase in oxidative stress.[158]

Recent recommendations were made that a fasting plasma glucose level of 110–125 mg/dL (6.1–6.9 mmol/L) indicates impaired glucose tolerance while a fasting plasma level of 126 mg/dL (7.0 mmol/L) is the cut-off level for type 2 diabetes (previous fasting glucose concentration for NIDDM was 140 mg/dL; 7.8 mmol/L).[275] Fasting glucose levels of 110 mg/dL or greater should probably result in automatic testing for glycosylated hemoglobin (HbA$_{1C}$). The WHO criteria for the diagnosis of NIDDM also recommends a fasting glucose level of 126 mg/dL or higher, as well as a two-hour glucose level from an oral glucose tolerance test (OGTT) of 200 mg/dL or higher. In this regard, a recent publication compared the WHO and American Diabetes Association diagnostic criteria for type 2 diabetes.[276] This study involved 18,048 men and 7316 women 30 years of age or older who were followed for a mean of 7.3 years. They used the following criteria for fasting glucose: normal, less than 110 mg/dL; impaired glucose tolerance, 110–125 mg/dL; and diabetes, 126 mg/dL or higher. Using the WHO criteria of fasting glucose level of 126 mg/dL or higher and a two-hour glucose level of 200 mg/dL or more from the OGTT, the hazard ratios for death in those with newly diagnosed diabetes were 2.02 for men and 2.77 for women. The hazard ratios for death in subjects with impaired glucose tolerance (two-hour glucose of 141–200 mg/dL) were 1.51 for men and 1.60 for women. Increased mortality was particularly evident in those with impaired glucose tolerance according to two-hour glucose levels following an OGTT, despite having normal fasting levels. The authors concluded that fasting glucose levels alone do not identify individuals at increased risk of death associated with hyperglycemia. They stated that the OGTT provides additional prognostic information and detects those with impaired glucose tolerance who have the greatest risk of death from hyperglycemia.

Hemochromatosis

Hemochromatosis is a recessively inherited disorder of iron metabolism which is characterized by increased gastrointestinal absorption of iron. Population studies suggest that one in 200–250 Americans have the disease while approximately one in ten are heterozygotes. It has been suggested that the excess iron promotes the production of oxygen-derived free radicals and lipid peroxidation, which damage liposomal membranes with the release of enzymes, which in turn cause cellular injury.[277] The major clinical manifestations of hemochromatosis include hepatic and cardiac dysfunction, diabetes mellitus, arthropathy, endocrine failure and changes in skin pigmentation.

Routine screening for hemochromatosis has been suggested[278] since (1) it is a common disorder and frequently missed until tissue injury has occurred, (2) it has the potential to cause significant morbidity and mortality, (3) there is a long asymptomatic period, (4) there is safe effective therapy (phlebotomy), and (5) simple screening tests are available. Several other studies also reported that adult screening by measuring serum iron and iron binding capacity (transferrin) is cost-effective.[279–281] Edwards and Kushner[278] recommend that the threshold transferrin saturation value after fasting should be set at 60% for men and 50% for women. In these cases, a follow-up serum ferritin concentration greater than twice the upper reference level generally indicates the need for a liver biopsy for morphological study and iron quantitation. Diagnostic and therapeutic algorithms have been suggested.[278,282]

Immune function

Aging is commonly accompanied by a decrease in immune function. However, much of this loss is due to secondary factors and are unrelated to the aging process *per se*. In this regard, protein calorie undernutrition, common in the otherwise healthy elderly, is characterized by serum albumin levels below 3.8 g/dL (also present in hepatic disorders and chronic inflammatory conditions). Serum transferrin levels have also been suggested as an indicator of chronic protein deficiency. Thus, Grant *et al.*[283] found that serum transferrin values of 150–200 mg/dL, 100–150 mg/dL and less than 100 mg/dL are indicative of mild, moderate and severe protein deficiency, respectively. Immune dysfunction is also a phenomenon of protein deficiency and is often characterized by a total lymphocyte count less than 1800 cells/µL (normal 2000–3500 cells/µL). These people often respond poorly to skin tests for mumps and/or Candida antigens and are more prone to become infected with various microorganisms including Mycobacteria, Listeria and Salmonella.[284] Moreover, Chandra[285] found that protein deficiency impairs several complement system components, mucosal secretory IgA antibodies, antibody affinity and phagocyte killing of ingested bacteria and fungi.

Older individuals are also commonly undernourished in various micronutrients (vitamins and minerals) which have been shown to significantly affect the immune system. Thus, supplementation with vitamins A, C and E,[286] only vitamin E,[287] or a multi-vitamin/mineral preparation[288] all improved the immune response in elderly people (i.e. increased IL-2 levels and various T-lymphocyte subsets, improved mitogen responsiveness and antibody response to tetanus vaccine). In addition, zinc is not only important in wound healing, taste acuity, prostaglandin metabolism and as an important antioxidant, but it is important in the immune system.[289] Here, Duchateau *et al.*[290] showed that zinc supplementation resulted in the following: (1) increased number of circulating T-cells; (2) improved delayed hypersensitivity reactions; and (3) increased IgG levels in response to tetanus vaccine.

These studies suggest that the evaluation of serum albumin and transferrin levels, total lymphocyte count and oxidative reserve capacity may all be useful in evaluating one's ability to respond to various antigenic stimuli.

Metabolic syndrome (syndrome X)

The metabolic syndrome is present in individuals meeting three or more of the following criteria:[165,291]

- abdominal obesity: waist circumference >102 cm (40.2 inches) in men and 88 cm (34.6 inches) in women;
- hypertriglyceridemia: ≥150 mg/dL (1.69 mmol/L);
- low HDL-C: <40 mg/dL (1.04 mmol/L) in men and <50 mg/dL (1.29 mmol/L) in women;
- elevated blood pressure: ≥130/85 mm Hg; and
- elevated fasting glucose: ≥110 mg/dL (≥6.1 mmol/L).

Individuals with the metabolic syndrome are at increased risk for developing type 2 diabetes and cardiovascular disease; they are also at increased mortality risk from all causes.

Unfortunately this syndrome is highly prevalent and appears to be steadily increasing. Recently published unadjusted and age-adjusted findings for the syndrome were 21.8% and 23.7%, respectively.[292] The prevalence increased from 6.7% in persons 20–29 years of age to 43.5% and 42.0% for persons aged 60–69 years and 70 or more years, respectively. The age-adjusted prevalence among Mexican Americans was 31.9% (the highest of all groups). The prevalence among men and women were similar (24.0% and 23.4%, respectively), although African American women had a 57% higher prevalence than men and Mexican American women were 26% higher than men. Using the 2000 census data, the authors estimated that 47 million US adults have the metabolic syndrome.

Miscellaneous disorders/laboratory tests

Prostate specific antigen (PSA)

Routine screening for prostate cancer with serum PSA is still controversial despite its obvious popularity.[293–296] There is little question that PSA testing and digital rectal examination can effectively detect prostate cancer in its early stages. Moreover, recent evidence suggests that radical prostatectomy may reduce prostate cancer mortality. However, the balance between the potential benefits (i.e. reduced morbidity and mortality) and harms (i.e. false-positive results, unnecessary biopsies, possible complications and costs) of early surgery remains uncertain. Ongoing clinical trials, the results of which are probably several years away, should help clarify the problem. In the meantime, no US medical organization currently endorses universal or mass screening for any group of men. Indeed, the US Preventive Services Task Force (USPSTF) recently published their recommendation and rationale for prostate cancer screening.[297] They concluded that "Screening is associated with important harms, including frequent false-positive results and unnecessary anxiety, biopsies and potential complications of treatment of some cases of cancer that may never have affected a patient's health. The USPSTF concludes that evidence is insufficient to determine whether the benefits outweigh the harms for a screened population." The issues regarding prostate cancer screening have been recently reviewed.[298,299]

Chemistry profile

A chemistry profile consisting of electrolytes (sodium and potassium), urea nitrogen and creatinine (renal function), aspartate and alanine aminotransferases, lactate dehydrogenase (hepatitis B and C, chronic alcoholism, hemochromatosis and occult malignancy), uric acid (gout and CHD), total protein and albumin (protein malnutrition and chronic inflammatory process), and direct and total biliburin (Gilbert's Syndrome and liver function) is very important in establishing the health status of several organ systems.

Magnesium, zinc and selenium

Serum magnesium is also a very important, albeit greatly under-utilized, analyte; it is a co-factor for over 325 enzymes.[300] Importantly, 10% of the so-called "healthy elderly" were found to be hypomagnesemic when serum was analyzed. When erythrocyte Mg was quantified, however, 20% were hypomagnesemic.[301] The minimum Mg recommended intake is 350 mg/day, although 450–500 mg/day is preferred. The average American reportedly consumes only 175–225 mg/day.[302]

As more is learned and appreciated regarding the pathogenesis of various diseases, as well as the aging process, it may be useful to measure serum zinc and selenium levels since both are commonly decreased in older people. Moreover, the measurement of various antioxidants (i.e. vitamins C and E, carotenoids and flavonoids) to assess deficiencies due to poor nutrition and/or malabsorption may be useful in selected cases. Furthermore, quantitation of the major antioxidant enzymes (i.e. glutathione peroxidase, glutathione reductase, catalase and superoxide dismutase) for identification of genetic deficiencies may also prove beneficial in some individuals.

Chapter Summary

The US faces a tremendous impending "elder boom" as those born in the post-World War II era become older. In addition, people are living much longer than ever before. As a result, medical costs will continue to escalate and quality medical care may become more difficult to obtain. Nevertheless, this scenario need not be the case since the ten most common causes of disease and death in the US are, to a significant extent, lifestyle-related. Hence, we must concentrate our efforts on improving our lifestyles which include the following: increased physical activity, weight control, improved nutrition, better health education and decreased frequency of undesirable personal habits (e.g. smoking, alcohol/drug abuse, unsafe sex, etc.). Moreover, funding for research, treatment, health promotion and patient behavioral counseling must be significantly increased. These actions will not only improve the quality of life and increase the average life expectancy, but significantly decrease medical costs. The US Department of Health and Human Services recently published their health goals for the year 2010 (Healthy People 2010).[303] Hopefully, these recommendations will be widely publicized in such a way that the American people will grasp their importance and put forth the effort to successfully achieve them. After all, as the Greek saying goes, "die young as late in life as possible."

References

1. Franklin B. *The Art of Virtue*, 3rd. Ed. GL Rogers (ed.) Acorn Publishing, Eden Prairie, MN, 1996, p. 181.
2. Goulding MR, Rogers ME, Smith SM. Public health and aging: trends in aging—United States and worldwide. *MMWR* 2003;52:101–106.
3. Lynn G. *USA Today*, 1 October 1999.
4. Rowe JW, Kahn RL. *Successful Aging*. Pantheon Books, New York, 1998.
5. Leaf A. Long-lived populations: extreme old age. *J Am Geriatr Soc* 1982;30:485–487.
6. Perls TT, Silver MH. *Living to 100*. Basic Books, New York, 1999.
7. Campion EW. The oldest old. *N Engl J Med* 1994;330:1819–1820.
8. Lubitz J, Beebe J, Baker C. Longevity and medicare expenditures. *N Engl J Med* 1995;332:999–1003.
9. Perls TT, Wood ER. Acute care costs of the oldest old. *Arch Intern Med* 1996;156:754–760.
10. Spillman BC, Lubitz J. The effect of longevity on spending for acute and long-term care. *N Engl J Med* 2000;342:1409–1415.

11. Mustard CA, Kaufert P, Kozyrskyj A, Mayer T. Sex differences in the use of health care services. *N Engl J Med* 1998;338:1678–1683.

12. Fries JF. Aging, natural death, and the compression of morbidity. *N Engl J Med* 1980;303:130–135.

13. Vita AJ, Terry RB, Hubert HB, Fries JF. Aging, health risks, and cumulative disability. *N Engl J Med* 1998;338:1035–1041.

14. Hubert HB, Bloch DA, Oehlert JW, Fries JF. Lifestyle habits and compression of morbidity. *J Gerontol Med Sci* 2002;57A:M347–M351.

15. Pronk NP, Goodman MJ, O'Connor PJ, Martinson BC. Relationship between modifiable health risks and short-term health care charges. *JAMA* 1999;282:2235–2239.

16. Reed DM, Foley DJ, White LR, *et al.* Predictors of healthy aging in men with high life expectancies. *Am J Public Health* 1998;88:1463–1468.

17. Colditz GA. Economic costs of obesity and inactivity. *Med Sci Sports Exerc* 1999;31 (Suppl 11):S663–S667.

18. Schneider EL. Aging in the third millennium. *Science* 1999;283:796–797.

19. Weiss R. Aging: new answers to old questions. *National Geographic* 1997;192:2–31 (November).

20. Hoyert DL, Freedman MA, Strobino DM, Guyer B. Annual summary of vital statistics: 2000. *Pediatrics* 2001;108:1241–1255.

21. Olshansky SJ, Carnes BA, Cassel CK. The aging of the human species. *Sci Amer*, April 1993, pp. 46–52.

22. Olshansky SJ, Carnes BA, Cassel C. In search of Methuselah: estimating the upper limits to human longevity. *Science* 1990;250:634–640.

23. Murray CJL, Lopez AD. Alternative projections of mortality and disability by cause 1990–2020: global burden of disease study. *Lancet* 1997;349:1498–1504.

24. Carey JR, Liedo P, Orozco D, Vaupel JW. Slowing of mortality rates at older ages in large Medfly cohorts. *Science* 1992;258:457–461.

25. Curtsinger JW, Fukui HH, Townsend DR, Vaupel JW. Demography of genotypes: failure of the limited life-span paradigm in *Drosophila melanogaster*. *Science* 1992;258:461–463.

26. Lohman PHM, Sankaranarayanan K, Ashby J. Choosing the limits of life. *Nature* 1992;357:185–186.

27. National Center for Health Statistics. *US Decennial Life Tables, 1979–1981*. Department of Health and Human Services, Washington, DC, 1985, Publication 85-1150-L.

28. National Center for Health Statistics. *Vital Statistics of the United States, 1987,* US Public Health Service, Washington, DC, 1990.

29. Schneider EL, Brody JA. Aging, natural death, and the compression of morbidity: another view. *N Engl J Med* 1983;309:854–856.

30. Schneider EL, Guralnik JM. The aging of America: impact on health care costs. *JAMA* 1990;263:2335–2340.

31. Rakowski W, Hickey T. Mortality and the attribution of health problems to aging among older adults. *Am J Pub Health* 1992;82: 1139–1141.

32. Gjorup T, Hendriksen C, Lung E, Stromgard E. Is growing old a disease? A study of the attitudes of elderly people to physical symptoms. *J Chron Dis* 1987;40:1095–1098.

33. John SM, Koelmeyer TD. The forensic pathology on nonagenarians and centenarians: do they die of old age? (The Auckland Experience). *Am J Forensic Med Pathol* 2001;22:150–154.

34. Guyer B, Freedman MA, Strobino DM, Sondik EJ. Annual survery of vital statistics: trends in the health of Americans during the 20th century. *Pediatrics* 2000;106:1307–1317.

35. Lazarou J, Pomeranz BH, Corey PN. Incidence of adverse drug reactions in hospitalized patients. *JAMA* 1998;279:1200–1205.

36. McGinnis JM, Foege WH. Actual causes of death in the United States. *JAMA* 1993;270:2207.

37. Fries JF, Green LW, Levine S. Health promotion and the compression of morbidity. *Lancet* 1989;1:481–483.

38. Hahn RA, Teutsch SM, Rothenberg RB, Marks JS. Excess deaths from nine chronic diseases in the United States, 1986. *JAMA* 1990;264: 2654–2659.

39. Reeves MJ, Rafferty A, McGee H, Miller C. Prevalence of healthy lifestyle characteristics—Michigan, 1998 and 2000. *MMWR* 2001; 50:758–761.

40. Centers for Disease Control and Prevention. *Chronic Diseases and Their Risk Factors: The Nation's Leading Causes of Death,* report with expanded state-by-state information. US Department of Health and Human Services, CDC, Atlanta, Georgia, 1999.

41. Fraser GE, Shavlik DJ. Ten years of life: is it a matter of choice? *Arch Intern Med* 2001;161:1645–1652.

42. Guralnik JM, Land KC, Blazer D, Fillenbaum GG, Branch LG. Educational status and active life expectancy among older blacks and whites. *N Engl J Med* 1993;329:110–116.

43. Barnett E, Armstrong DL, Casper ML. Evidence of increasing coronary heart disease mortality among black men of lower social class. *Ann Epidemiol* 1999;9:464–471.
44. Rosamond WD, Folsom AR, Chambless LE, *et al.* Stroke incidence and survival among middle-aged adults: 9-year follow-up of the Atherosclerosis Risk in Communities (ARIC) cohort. *Stroke* 1999;30:736–743.
45. Gillum RF. Stroke mortality in blacks: disturbing trends. *Stroke* 1999;30:1711–1715.
46. Timiras PS. Education, homeostasis, and longevity. *Exp Gerontol* 1995;30:189–198.
47. Schrijvers CTM, Stronks K, van de Mheen HD, Mackenbach JP. Explaining educational differences in mortality: the role of behavioral and material factors. *Am J Public Health* 1999;89:535–540.
48. Wamala SP, Mittleman MA, Schenck-Gustafsson K, Orth-Gomer K. Potential explanations for the educational gradient in coronary heart disease: a population-based case-control study of Swedish women. *Am J Public Health* 1999;89:315–321.
49. Pappas G, Queen S, Hadden W, Fisher G. The increasing disparity in mortality between socioeconomic groups in the United States, 1960 and 1986. *N Engl J Med* 1993;329:103–109.
50. Lantz PM, House JS, Lepkowski JM, *et al.* Socioeconomic factors, health behaviors, and mortality. *JAMA* 1998;279:1703–1708.
51. Redelmeier DA, Singh SM. Survival in Academy Award-winning actors and actresses. *Ann Intern Med* 2001;134:955–962.
52. Williams RB. Lower socioeconomic status and increased mortality. *JAMA* 1998;279:1745–1746.
53. House JS, Lepkowski JM, Williams DR, *et al.* Excess mortality among urban residents: how much, for whom, and why? *Am J Public Health* 2000;90:1898–1904.
54. Holden C. Global survey examines impact of depression. *Science* 2000;288:39–40.
55. Suicide among older persons—United States, 1980–1992. *MMWR* 1996;45:3–6.
56. Devons CAJ. Suicide in the elderly. How to identify and treat patients at risk. *Geriatrics* 1996;51:67–72.
57. Michelson D, Stratakis C, Hill L, *et al.* Bone mineral density in women with depression. *N Engl J Med* 1996;335:1176–1181.
58. Ford DE, Mead LA, Chang PP, *et al.* Depression is a risk factor for coronary artery disease in men. *Arch Intern Med* 1998;158:1422–1426.

59. Hippisley-Cox J, Fielding K, Pringle M. Depression as a risk factor for ischaemic heart disease in men: population based case-control study. *BMJ* 1998;316:1714–1719.
60. Ferketich AK, Schwartzbaum JA, Frid DJ, Moeschberger ML. Depression as an antecedent to heart disease among women and men in the NHANES I study. *Arch Intern Med* 2000;160:1261–1268.
61. Frasure-Smith N, Lesperance F, Talajic M. Depression and 18-month prognosis after myocardial infarction. *Circulation* 1995;91: 999–1005.
62. Barefoot JC, Helms MJ, Mark DB, *et al.* Depression and long-term mortality risk in patients with coronary artery disease. *Am J Cardiol* 1996;78:613–617.
63. Denollet J, Sys SU, Stroobant N, *et al.* Personality as an independent predictor of long-term mortality in patients with coronary heart disease. *Lancet* 1996;347:417–421.
64. Abramson J, Berger A, Krumholz HM, Vaccarino V. Depression and risk of heart failure among older persons with isolated systolic hypertension. *Arch Intern Med* 2001;161:1725–1730.
65. Nordstrom CK, Dwyer KM, Merz CNB, *et al.* Work-related stress and early atherosclerosis. *Epidemiology* 2001;12:180–185.
66. Steffens DC, Helms MJ, Krishman RR, Burke GL. Cerebrovascular disease and depression symptoms in the Cardiovascular Health Study. *Stroke* 1999;30:2159–2166.
67. Ostir GV, Markides KS, Peek MK, Goodwin JS. The association between emotional well-being and the incidence of stroke in older adults. *Psychosom Med* 2001;63:210–215.
68. Carney RM, Rich MW, Freedland KF, *et al.* Major depressive disorder predicts cardiac events in patients with coronary artery disease. *Psychosom Med* 1988;50:627–633.
69. Maruta T, Colligan RC, Malinchoc M, Offord KP. Optimists vs pessimists: survival rate among medical patients over a 30-year period. *Mayo Clin Proc* 2000;75:140–143.
70. Seligman ME, Abramson LY, Semmel A, von Baeyer C. Depressive attributional style. *J Abnorm Psychol* 1979;88:242–247.
71. Peterson C, Seligman ME, Vaillant GE. Pessimistic explanatory style is a risk factor for physical illness: a thirty-five-year longitudinal study. *J Pers Soc Psychol* 1988;55:23–27.
72. Peterson C. Explanatory style as a risk factor for illness. *Cognit Ther Res* 1988;12:119–132.

73. Williams JE, Paton CC, Siegler IC, *et al.* Anger proneness predicts coronary heart disease risk. *Circulation* 2000;101:2034–2039.

74. Gullette ECD, Blumenthal JA, Babyak M, *et al.* Effects of mental stress on myocardial ischemia during daily life. *JAMA* 1997;277:1521–1526.

75. Koivumaa-Honkanen H, Honkanen R, Viinamaki H, *et al.* Self-reported life satisfaction and 20-year mortality in healthy Finnish adults. *Am J Epidemiol* 2000;152:983–991

76. Wilson RS, Mendes de Leon CF, Barnes LL, *et al.* Participation in cognitively stimulating activities and risk of incident Alzheimer Disease. *JAMA* 2002;287:742–748.

77. Fabrigoule C, Letenneur L, Dartigues JF, *et al.* Social and leisure activities and risk of dementia: a prospective longitudinal study. *J Am Geriatr Soc* 1995;43:485–490.

78. Fratiglioni L, Wang H-X, Ericsson K, *et al.* Influence of social network on occurrence of dementia: a community-based longitudinal study. *Lancet* 2000;355:1315–1319.

79. Bassuk SS, Glass TA, Berkman LF. Social disengagement and incident cognitive decline in community-dwelling elderly persons. *Ann Intern Med* 1999;131:165–173.

80. Levin JS. How religion influences morbidity and health reflections on natural history, salutogenesis and host resistance. *Soc Sci Med* 1996;43:849–864.

81. Levin JS. Religion and health: is there an association, is it valid, and is it causal? *Soc Sci Med* 1994;38:1475–1482.

82. Gardner JW, Lyon H. Cancer in Utah Mormon men by lay priesthood level. *Am J Epidemiol* 1982;116:243–257.

83. Enstrom JE. Health practices and cancer mortality among active California Mormons. *J Natl Cancer Inst* 1989;81:1807–1814.

84. Philips RI, Lemon FR, Beeson WL, Kuzma JW. Coronary heart disease mortality among Seventh-Day Adventists with differing dietary habits: a preliminary report. *Am J Clin Nutr* 1978;31:S191–S198.

85. Harris WS, Gowda M, Kolb JW, *et al.* A randomized, controlled trial of the effects of remote, intercessory prayer on outcomes in patients admitted to the coronary care unit. *Arch Intern Med* 1999;159:2273–2278.

86. Mitka M. Getting religion seen as help in being well. *JAMA* 1998;280:1896–1897.

87. Oman D, Reed D. Religion and mortality among the community-dwelling elderly. *Am J Public Health* 1998;88:1469–1475.

88. Helm HM, Hays JC, Flint EP, *et al.* Does private religious activity prolong survival? A six-year follow-up study of 3851 older adults. *J Gerontol Med Sci* 2000;55A:M400–M405.

89. Oman D, Kurata JG, Strawbridge WJ, Cohen RD. Religious attendance and cause of death over 31 years. *Int J Psychiatry Med* 2002;32:69–89.

90. Strawbridge WJ, Cohen RD, Shema SJ. Comparative strength of association between religious attendance and survival. *Int J Psychiatry Med* 2000;30:299–308.

91. Strawbridge WJ, Cohen RD, Shema SJ, Kaplan GA. Frequent attendance at religious services and mortality over 28 years. *Am J Public Health* 1997;87:957–961.

92. Matthews DA, McCullough ME, Larson DB, *et al.* Religious commitment and health status. *Arch Fam Med* 1998;7:118–124.

93. Koenig HG, McCullough ME, Larson DB. *Handbook of Religion and Health.* Oxford University Press, New York, 2001.

94. McWhirter N. *Guiness Book of Records*, 17 Ed. Bantam Books, New York, 1980.

95. Perls TT. The oldest old. *Sci Amer*, January 1995, pp. 70–75.

96. The world's anti-aging experts. *J Anti-Aging Med* 1999;2:315.

97. Wilmoth J, Skytthe A, Friou D, Jeune B. The oldest man ever? A case study of exceptional longevity. *Gerontologist* 1996;36:783–788. (For authentic death date and Wilmoth's personal communication see: *http://demog.berkeley.edu/~jrw/tribute.html*).

98. Olshansky SJ, Hayflick L, Carnes BA. No truth to the Fountain of Youth. *Sci Amer*, June 2002, pp. 92–95.

99. Harman D. The aging process. *Proc Natl Acad Sci* 1981;78: 7124–7128.

100. Manton KG, Stallard E. Longevity in the United States: age and sex-specific evidence on life span limits from mortality patterns 1960–1990. *J Gerontol Biol Sci* 1996;51A:B362–B375.

101. Perls TT, Wilmoth J, Levenson R, *et al.* Life-long sustained mortality advantage of siblings of centenarians. *Proc Natl Acad Sci* 2002;99:8442–8447.

102. Hayflick L. The limited *in vitro* life time of human diploid cell strains. *Exp Cell Res* 1965;37:614–636.

103. Counter CM, Hirte HW, Bacchetti S, *et al.* Telomerase activity in human ovarian carcinoma. *Proc Natl Acad Sci USA* 1994;91: 2900–2904.

104. Haber DA. Clinical implications of basic research: telomerases, cancer, and immortality. *N Engl J Med* 1995;332:955–956.

105. Rose MR. Can human aging be postponed? *Sci Amer* 1999;281: 106–111.
106. Harman D. Aging: a theory based on free radical and radiation chemistry. *J Gerontol* 1956;11:298–300.
107. Harman D. Aging: minimizing free radical damage. *J Anti-Aging Med* 1999;2:15–36.
108. Harman D. Free radical theory of aging: increasing the average life expectancy at birth and the maximum life span. *J Anti-Aging Med* 1999;2:199–208.
109. Beckman KB, Ames BN. The free radical theory of aging matures. *Physiol Rev* 1998;78:547–581.
110. Knight JA. Free radicals: their history and current status in aging and disease. *Ann Clin Lab Sci* 1998;28:331–346.
111. Pearl R. *The Rate of Living.* Knopf, New York, NY, 1928.
112. McArthur MC, Sohal RS. Relationship between metabolic rate, aging, lipid peroxidation, and fluorescent age pigment in milkweed bug, *Orcopeltus fasciatus* (Hemiptera). *J Gerontol* 1982;37: 268–274.
113. McKay CM, Crowell MF, Maynard LA. The effect of retarded growth upon the length of life span and upon the ultimate body size. *J Nutr* 1935;10:63–79.
114. Yu BP, Masoro EJ, Murata I, *et al.* Life span of SPF Fischer 344 male rats fed *ad libitum* or restricted diets: longevity, growth, lean body mass and disease. *J Gerontol* 1982;37:130–141.
115. Weindruch R. Caloric restriction and aging. *Sci Amer*, January 1996, pp. 46–52.
116. Lane MA, Baer DJ, Rumpler WV, Weindruch R, *et al.* Caloric restriction lowers body temperature in rhesus monkeys, consistent with a postulated anti-aging mechanism in rodents. *Proc Natl Acad Sci USA* 1996;93:4159–4164.
117. Weed JL, Lane MA, Roth GS, Speer DL, Ingram DK. Activity measures in rhesus monkeys on long-term caloric restriction. *Physiol Behav* 1997;62:97–103.
118. Lane MA, Ingram DK, Ball SS, Roth GS. Dehydroepiandrosterone sulfate: a bio-marker of primate aging slowed by caloric restriction. *J Clin Endocrinol Metab* 1997;82:2093–2096.
119. Longo VD, Finch CE. Evolutionary medicine: from dwarf model systems to healthy centenarians? *Science* 2003;299:1342–1341.
120. Rusting RL. Why do we age? *Sci Amer* 1992;267:130–141.
121. Kellogg EW, Fridovich I. Superoxide dismutase in the rat and mouse as a function of age and longevity. *J Gerontol* 1976;31:405–408.

122. de Grey ADNJ. Noncorrelation between maximum life span and antioxidant enzyme levels among homeotherms: implications for retarding human aging. *J Anti-Aging Med* 2000;3:25–36.

123. Daynes RA, Araneo BA. Prevention and reversal of some age-associated changes in immunologic responses by supplemental dehydroepiandrosterone sulfate therapy. *Aging Immunol Inf Dis* 1992;3:135–154.

124. Knight JA. Review: free radicals, antioxidants, and the immune system. *Ann Clin Lab Sci* 2000;30:145–158.

125. Centers for Disease Control. Missed opportunities in preventive counseling for cardiovascular disease—United States, 1995. *JAMA* 1998;279:741–742.

126. Scutchfield FD, Hartman KT. Physicians and preventive medicine. *JAMA* 1995;273:1150–1151 (Editorial).

127. Woolf SH. The need for perspective in evidence-based medicine. *JAMA* 1999;282:2358–2365.

128. McGlynn EA, Asch SM, Adams J, *et al.* The quality of health care delivered to adults in the United States. *N Engl J Med* 2003;348: 2635–2645.

129. Eisenberg DM, Davis RB, Ettner SL, *et al.* Trends in alternative medicine use in the United States, 1990–1997. *JAMA* 1998;280: 1569–1575.

130. Fox E. Predominance of the curative model of medical care: a residual problem. *JAMA* 1997;278:761–763.

131. Eisenberg DM, Kessler RC, Foster C, *et al.* Unconventional medicine in the United States. *N Engl J Med* 1993;328:246–252.

132. Kessler RC, Davis RB, Foster DF, *et al.* Long-term trends in the use of complementary and alternative medical therapies in the United States. *Ann Intern Med* 2001;135:262–268.

133. Eisenberg DM, Kessler RC, van Rompay MI, *et al.* Perceptions about complementary therapies relative to conventional therapies among adults who use both: results from a national survey. *Ann Intern Med* 2001;135:344–351.

134. Frolkis, JP, Zyzanski SJ, Schwartz JM, Suhan PS. Physician non-compliance with the 1993 national cholesterol education program (NCEP-ATPH) guidelines. *Circulation* 1998;98:851–855.

135. Rafferty M. Prevention services in primary care: taking time, setting priorities. *West J Med* 1998;169:269–275.

136. Daviglus ML, Liu K, Greenland P, *et al.* Benefits of a favorable cardiovascular risk-factor profile in middle age with respect to Medicare costs. *N Engl J Med* 1998;339:1122–1129.

137. Taira DA, Safran DG, Seto TB, Rogers WH, Tarlov AR. The relation-ship between patient income and physician discussion of health risk behaviors. *JAMA* 1997;278:1412–1417.
138. Wee CC, McCarthy EP, Davis RB, Phillips RS. Physician counseling about exercise. *JAMA* 1999;282:1583–1588.
139. EUROASPIRE Study Group. A European Society of Cardiology sur-vey of secondary prevention of coronary heart disease: principal results. *Eur Heart J* 1997;18:1569–1582.
140. Lubitz JD, Riley GF. Trends in Medicare payments in the last year of life. *N Engl J Med* 1993;328:1092–1096.
141. Perls TT, Wood ER. Acute care costs of the oldest old: they cost less, their care intensity is less, and they go to nonteaching hospitals. *Arch Intern Med* 1996;156:754–760.
142. Centers for Disease Control and Prevention. Estimated national spend-ing on prevention—United States, 1988. *MMWR* 1992;41:529–531.
143. Furberg CD. Challenges to the funding of prevention research. *Prev Med* 1994;23:599–601.
144. Schauffler HH, Chapman SA. Health promotion and managed care: surveys of California's health plans and population. *Am J Prev Med* 1998;14:161–167.
145. Pronk NP, Goodman MJ, O'Connor PJ, Martinson BC. Relationship between modifiable health risks and short-term health care charges. *JAMA* 1999;282:2235–2239.
146. Gambino R. *Wellness Testing: Implementation and Utilization.* Work-shop Manual, ASCP/CAP Fall Meeting, Philadelphia, 1997.
147. Gorry GA, Pauker SG, Schwartz WB. The diagnostic importance of the normal finding. *N Engl J Med* 1978;298:486–489.
148. Knight JA. Wellness assessment: a role for laboratory medicine. *Ann Clin Lab Sci* 2000;30:23–32.
149. Govaert TME, Thijs CTM, Masurel N, *et al.* The efficacy of influ-enza vaccination in elderly individuals. A randomized double-blind placebo-controlled trial. *JAMA* 1994;272:1661–1665.
150. Sprenger MWJ, Mulder PGH, Beyer WEP, van Strik R, Masurel N. Im-pact of influenza on mortality in relation to age and underlying disease, during the period 1967 to 1989. *Int J Epidemiol* 1993;22:334–340.
151. van Essen GA, Kuyvenhoven MM, de Melker RA. Why do healthy elderly people fail to comply with influenza vaccination? *Age Ageing* 1997;26:275–279.
152. Lee PY, Matchar DB, Clements DA, *et al.* Economic analysis of in-fluenza vaccination and antiviral treatment for healthy working adults. *Ann Intern Med* 2002;137:225–231.

153. Centers for Disease Control and Prevention. Pneumococcal and influenza vaccination levels among adult aged ≥65 years—United States, 1995. *JAMA* 1997;278:1306–1308.

154. Sisk JE, Moskowitz AJ, Whang W, *et al.* Cost-effectiveness of vaccination against pneumococcal bacteremia among elderly people. *JAMA* 1997;278:1333–1339.

155. Nichol KL, Baken L, Wuorenma J, Nelson A. The health and economic benefits associated with pneumococcal vaccination of elderly persons with chronic lung disease. *Arch Intern Med* 1999;159:2437–2442.

156. Centers for Disease Control. Recommended adult immunization schedule—United States, 2002–2003. *MMWR* 2002;51:904–905.

157. Opinion. Your patients can't follow instructions they don't understand. *Am Med News*, 16 June 2003, p. 29.

158. Knight JA. *Free Radicals, Antioxidants, Aging, and Disease.* AACC Press, Washington, DC, 1999.

159. Liu TZ, Stern A, Morrow JD. The isoprostanes: unique bioactive products of lipid peroxidation. an overview. *J Biomed Sci* 1998;5:415–420.

160. Ghiselli A, Serafini M, Maiani G, *et al.* A fluorescence-based method for measuring total plasma antioxidant capability. *Free Radic Biol Med* 1994;18:29–36.

161. Cao G, Verdon CP, Wu AHB, *et al.* Automated assay of oxygen radical absorbance capacity with the COBAS FARA II. *Clin Chem* 1995;41:1738–1744.

162. Prior RL, Cao G. *In vivo* total antioxidant capacity: comparison of different analytical methods. *Free Radic Biol Med* 1999;27:1173–1181.

163. Niki E, Naguchi N. Evaluation of antioxidant capacity. What capacity is being measured by which method? *Life* 2000;50:323–329.

164. American Heart Association. *1999 Heart and Stroke Statistical Update.* American Heart Association, Dallas, TX, 1998.

165. Castelli WP, Anderson K. A population at risk: prevalence of high cholesterol levels in hypertensive patients in the Framingham Study. *Am J Med* 1986;80(Suppl 2A):23–32.

166. Mosca L, Jones WK, King KB, *et al.* Awareness, perception, and knowledge of heart disease risk and prevention among women in the United States. *Arch Fam Med* 2000;9:506–515.

167. Roux AVD, Merkin SS, Arnett D, *et al.* Neighborhood of residence and incidence of coronary heart disease. *N Engl J Med* 2001;345:99–106.

168. Hopkins PN, Williams RR. A survey of 246 suggested coronary risk factors. *Atherosclerosis* 1981;40:1–52.

169. Expert Panel on Detection, Evaluation, and Treatment of High Blood Cholesterol in Adults. Executive summary of the third report of the National Cholesterol Education Program (NCEP) expert panel on detection, evaluation, and treatment of high blood cholesterol in adults (Adult Treatment Panel III). *JAMA* 2001;285:2486–2497.

170. Miller M, Mead LA, Kwiterovich PO Jr, Pearson TA. Dyslipidemias with desirable plasma total cholesterol levels and angiographically demonstrated coronary artery disease. *Am J Cardiol* 1990;65:1–5.

171. Ginsburg GS, Safran C, Pasternak RC. Frequency of low serum high-density lipoproten cholesterol levels in hospitalized patients with "desirable" total cholesterol levels. *Am J Cardiol* 1991;68:187–192.

172. Romm PA, Green CE, Reagan K, Rackley CE. Relation of serum lipoprotein cholesterol levels to presence and severity of angiographic coronary artery disease. *Am J Cardiol* 1991;67:479–483.

173. Miller M, Seidler A, Kwiterovich PO, Pearson TA. Long-term predictors of subsequent cardiovascular events with coronary artery disease and "desirable" levels of plasma total cholesterol *Circulation* 1992;86:1165–1170.

174. Hong MK, Romm PA, Reagan K, *et al.* Usefulness of the total cholesterol to high-density lipoprotein cholesterol ratio in predicting angiographic coronary artery disease in women. *Am J Cardiol* 1991;68:1646–1650.

175. Castelli WP, Anderson K, Wilson PWF, Levy D. Lipids and risk of coronary heart disease: the Framingham Study. *Ann Epidemiol* 1992;2:23–28.

176. Corti MC, Guralnik JM, Salive ME, *et al.* HDL cholesterol predicts coronary heart disease mortality in older persons. *JAMA* 1995;274:539–544.

177. Ridker PM, Stampfer MJ, Rifai N. Novel risk factors for systemic atherosclerosis: a comparison of C-reactive protein, fibrinogen, homocysteine, lipoprotein (a), and standard cholesterol screening as predictors of peripheral arterial disease. *JAMA* 2001;285:2481–2485.

178. Handa K, Kono S, Saku K, *et al.* Plasma fibrinogen levels as an independent indicator of severity of coronary atherosclerosis. *Atherosclerosis* 1989;77:209–213.

179. Ernst E. Plasma fibrinogen: an independent cardiovascular risk factor. *J Intern Med* 1990;227:365–372.

180. Kannel WB, Wolf PA, Castelli WP, D'Agostino RB. Fibrinogen and risk of cardiovascular disease: the Framingham Study. *JAMA* 1987;258:1183–1186.

181. Danesh J, Collins R, Appleby P, Peto R. Association of fibrinogen, C-reactive protein, albumin, or leukocyte count with coronary heart disease. *JAMA* 1998;279:1477–1482.

182. Connelly JB, Cooper JA, Meade TW. Strenuous exercise, plasma fibrinogen, and factor VII activity. *Br Heart J* 1992;67:351–354.

183. McCully KS. Vascular pathology of homocysteinemia: implications for the pathogenesis of arteriosclerosis. *Am J Pathol* 1969;56: 111–128.

184. Genest JJ, McNamara JR, Salem DN, *et al.* Plasma homocyst(e)ine levels in men with premature coronary artery disease. *J Am Coll Cardiol* 1990;16:1114–1119.

185. Stampfer MJ, Malinow MR, Willett WC, *et al.* A prospective study of plasma homocyst(e)ine and risk of myocardial infarction in US physicians. *JAMA* 1992;268:877–881.

186. Bots ML, Launer LJ, Lindemans J, *et al.* Homocysteine, atherosclerosis and prevalent cardiovascular disease in the elderly: the Rotterdam Study. *J Intern Med* 1997;242:339–347.

187. Jacobsen DW. Homocysteine and vitamins in cardiovascular disease. *Clin Chem* 1998;44:1833–1843.

188. Wald NJ, Watt HC, Law MR, *et al.* Homocysteine and ischemic heart disease. *Arch Intern Med* 1998;158:862–867.

189. Bots ML, Launer LJ, Lindemans J, *et al.* Homocysteine and short-term risk of myocardial infarction and stroke in the elderly. *Arch Intern Med* 1999;159:38–44.

190. Voutilainen S, Alfthan G, Nyyssonen K, *et al.* Association between elevated plasma total homocysteine and increased common carotid artery wall thickness. *Ann Med* 1998;30:300–306.

191. Selhub J, Jacques P'F, Bostom AG, *et al.* Association between plasma homocysteine concentrations and extracranial carotid-artery stenosis. *N Engl J Med* 1995;332:286–291.

192. Giles WH, Croft JB, Greenlund KJ, *et al.* Total homocyst(e)ine concentration and the likelihood of nonfatal stroke. *Stroke* 1998; 29:2473–2477.

193. den Heijer M, Blom HJ, Gerrits WBJ, *et al.* Is homocysteinaemia a risk factor for recurrent venous thrombosis? *Lancet* 1995;345:882–885.

194. Rassoul F, Richter V, Janke C, *et al.* Plasma homocysteine and lipoprotein pro-file in patients with peripheral arterial occlusive disease. *Angiology* 2000;51:189–196.

195. Malinow MR. Hyperhomocyst(e)inemia: a common and easily reversible risk factor for occlusive atherosclerosis. *Circulation* 1990;81:2004–2006.

196. Ubbink JB, Vermaak HWJ, van der Merwe A, Becker PJ. Vitamin B$_{12}$, vitamin B$_6$, and folate nutritional status in men with hyperhomocysteinemia. *Am J Clin Nutr* 1993;57:47–53.

197. Clarke R & Homocysteine Lowering Trialists' Collaboration. Lowering blood homocysteine with folic acid based supplements: meta-analysis of randomised trials. *BMJ* 1998;316:894–898.

198. Rimm EF, Willett WC, Hu FB, *et al.* Folate and vitamin B$_6$ from diet and supplements in relation to risk of coronary heart disease among women. *JAMA* 1998;279;359–364.

199. Welch GN, Loscalzo J. Homocysteine and atherothrombosis. *N Engl J Med* 1998;338:1042–1050.

200. Fessel WJ. High uric acid as an indicator of cardiovascular disease. *Am J Med* 1980;68:401–404.

201. Freedman DS, Williamson DF, Gunter EW, Byers T. Relation of serum uric acid to mortality and ischemic heart disease. *Am J Epidemiol* 1995;141:637–644.

202. Culleton BF, Larson MG, Kannel WB, Levy D. Serum uric acid and risk for cardiovascular disease and death: the Framingham Heart Study. *Ann Intern Med* 1999;131:7–13.

203. Fang J, Alderman MH. Serum uric acid and cardiovascular mortality. *JAMA* 2000;283:2404–2410.

204. Burch G, DePasquale NP. Erythrocytosis and ischemic myocardial disease. *Am Heart J* 1961;62:139–140.

205. Burch G, DePasquale NP. The hematocrit in patients with myocardial infarction. *JAMA* 1962;180:143–145.

206. Thaulow GE, Sandvik L, Stormorken H, Erikssen J. Hematocrit: a predictor of cardiovascular mortality? *J Intern Med* 1993;234:493–499.

207. Gagnon Dr, Zhang T, Brand FN, *et al.* Hematocrit and the risk of cardiovascular disease: the Framingham Study. *Am Heart J* 1994;127:674–682.

208. Wannamethee G, Perry IJ, Shaper AG. Hematocrit, hypertension and risk of stroke. *J Intern Med* 1994;235:163–168.

209. Friedman GD, Klatsky AL, Siegelaub AB. The leukocyte count as a predictor of myocardial infarction. *N Engl J Med* 1974;290:1275–1278.

210. Zalokar JB, Richards JL, Blaude JR. Leukocyte count, smoking and myocardial infarction. *N Engl J Med* 1981;294:465–468.

211. Prentice RI, Shimizu Y, Lin CH, *et al.* Leukocyte counts and coronary heart disease in a Japanese cohort. *Am J Epidemiol* 1982;116:496–506.

212. Barron HV, Harr SD, Radford MJ, *et al.* The association between white blood count and acute myocardial infarction mortality in patients ≥65 years of age: findings from the cooperative cardiovascular project. *J Am Coll Cardiol* 2001;38:1654–1661.

213. Gambino R. C-reactive protein—undervalued, underutilized. *Clin Chem* 1997;43:2017–2018.

214. Ridker PM, Cushman M, Stampfer MJ, *et al.* Inflammation, aspirin, and the risk of cardiovascular disease in apparently healthy men. *N Engl J Med* 1997;336:973–979.

215. Tracy RP, Lemaitre RN, Psaty BM, *et al.* Relationship of C-reactive protein to risk of cardiovascular disease of the elderly: results from the Cardiovascular Health Study and the Rural Health Promotion Project. *Arterioscler Thromb Vasc Biol* 1997;17:1121–1127.

216. Ridker PM, Hennekins CH, Buring JE, Rifai N. C-reactive protein and other markers of inflammation in the prediction of cardiovascular disease in women. *N Engl J Med* 2000;342:836–843.

217. Rost NS, Wolf PA, Kase CS, *et al.* Plasma concentration of C-reactive protein and risk of ischemic stroke and transient ischemic attack: the Framingham Study. *Stroke* 2001;32:2575–2579.

218. Albert CM, Ma J, Rifai N, *et al.* Prospective study of C-reactive protein, homocysteine, and plasma lipid levels as predictors of sudden cardiac death. *Circulation* 2002;105:2595–2599.

219. Ridker PM, Stampfer MJ, Rifai N. Novel risk factors for systemic atherosclerosis: a comparison of C-reactive protein, fibrinogen, homocysteine, lipoprotein (a), and standard cholesterol screening as predictors of peripheral arterial disease. *JAMA* 2001;285:2481–2485.

220. Haverkate F, Thompson SG, Pyke SDM, *et al.* Production of C-reactive protein and risk of coronary events in stable and unstable angina. *Lancet* 1997;349:462–466.

221. Expert Panel on Detection, Evaluation, and Treatment of High Blood Cholesterol in Adults: Executive Summary of the Third Report of the National Education Program (NCEP) (Adult Treatment Panel III). *JAMA* 2001;285:2486–2497.

222. Ridker PM, Rifai N, Rose L, *et al.* Comparison of C-reactive protein and low density lipoprotein cholesterol levels in the prediction of first cardiovascular events. *N Engl J Med* 2002; 347:1557–1565.

223. Danesh J, Whincup P, Walker M, *et al.* Low grade inflammation and coronary heart disease: prospecitve study and updated meta-analyses. *BMJ* 2000;321:199–204.

224. Muhlestein JB. Chronic infection and coronary artery disease. *Sci Med*, November/December 1998, pp. 16–25.

225. Ross R. Atherosclerosis—an inflammatory disease. *N Engl J Med* 1999;340:115–126.

226. Ford ES. Does exercise reduce inflammation? Physical activity and C-reactive protein among US adults. *Epidemiology* 2002;13:561–568.

227. Knight JA. *Free Radicals, Antioxidants, Aging, and Disease.* AACC Press, Washington DC, 1999, pp. 75–110.

228. Salonen JT, Nyyssonen K, Korpela H, *et al.* High stored iron is associated with excess risk for myocardial infarction in Eastern Finnish men. *Circulation* 1992;86:803–811.

229. Sullivan JL. Iron and the sex difference in heart disease risk. *Lancet* 1981;1:1293–1294.

230. Sullivan JL. The iron paradigm of ischemic heart disease. *Am Heart J* 1989;117:1179–1188.

231. Baer DM, Tekawa IS, Harley LB. Iron stores are not associated with acute myocardial infarction. *Circulation* 1994;89:2915–2918.

232. Sempas CT, Looker AC, Gillum RF, Makuc DM. Body iron stores and the risk of coronary heart disease. *N Engl J Med* 1994;330:1119–1124.

233. Roest M, van der Schouw YT, de Valk B, *et al.* Heterozygosity for a hereditary hemochromatosis gene is associated with cardiovascular death in women. *Circulation* 1999;100:1268–1273.

234. Toumainen T-P, Kontula K, Nyyssonen K, *et al.* Increased risk of acute myocardial infarction in carriers of the hemochromatosis gene Cys282Tyr mutation: a prospective cohort study in men in Eastern Finland. *Circulation* 1999;100:1274–1279.

235. Ghafoor A, Jemal A, Cokkinides V, *et al.* Cancer statistics for African Americans. *CA Cancer J Clin* 2002;52:326–341.

236. Jemal A, Thomas A, Murray T, Thun M. Cancer statistics, 2002. *CA Cancer J Clin* 2002;52:23–47.

237. Ries LAG, Eisner MP, Kosary CL, *et al.* (eds.). *SEER Cancer Statistics Review, 1973–1999.* National Cancer Institute, Bethesda, MD, 2002.

238. Will BP, Berthelot JM, LePetit C, *et al.* Estimates of the lifetime costs of breast cancer treatment in Canada. *Eur J Cancer* 2000;36:724–735.

239. Hoerger TJ, Downs KE, Lakshmanan MC, *et al.* Healthcare use among U.S. women aged 45 and older: total costs and costs for selected post-menopausal health risks. *J Womens Health Gend Based Med* 1999;8:1077–1089.

240. Brown ML, Riley GF, Potosky AL, Etzioni RD. Obtaining long-term disease specific costs of care: application to Medicare enrollees diagnosed with colorectal cancer. *Med Care* 1999;37:1249–1259.

241. Borre M, Nerstrom B, Overgaard J. The dilemma of prostate cancer—a growing human and economic burden irrespective of treatment strategies. *Acta Oncol* 1997;36:681–687.

242. Grover SA, Coupal L, Zowall H, *et al.* The economic burden of prostate cancer.in Canada: forecasts from the Montreal Prostate Cancer Model. *CMAJ* 2000;162:987–992.

243. Bal DG. Cancer statistics 2001: quo vadis or whither goest thou? *CA Cancer J Clin* 2001;51:11–14.

244. Gazdar AF, Minna JD. Molecular detection of early lung cancer. *J Natl Cancer Inst* 1999;91:299–301.

245. Ames BN, Gold LS, Willett WC. The causes and prevention of cancer. *Proc Natl Acad Sci USA* 1995;5258–5265.

246. Doll R, Peto R. The cause of cancer: qantitative estimates of avoidable risks of cancer in the United States today. *J Natl Cancer Inst* 1981;66:1191–1308.

247. Packer L. Vitamin E is nature's master antioxidant. *Sci Med*, March/April 1994, pp. 54–63.

248. Borek C. Antioxidants and cancer. *Sci Med*, November/December 1997, pp. 52–61.

249. Salonen JT, Alfthen G, Huttunen JK, Puska P. Association between serum selenium and the risk of cancer. *Am J Epidemiol* 1984;120:343–349.

250. Willett WC, Polk BJ, Morris JS, *et al.* Prediagnostic serum selenium and risk of cancer. *Lancet* 1983;2:130–134.

251. Kolonel LN, Nomura AMY, Cooney RV. Dietary fat and prostate cancer: current status. *J Natl Cancer Inst* 1999;91:414–428.

252. Statland BE. Nutrition and cancer. *Clin Chem* 1992;38:1587–1594.

253. Simopoulus AP. Obesity and carcinogenesis: Historical perspective. *Am J Clin Nutr* 1987;45:271–276.

254. Wright RM, McManaman JL, Repine JE. Alcohol-induced breast cancer: a proposed mechanism. *Free Rad Biol Med* 1999;26:348–354.

255. Sunderman FW Jr. Nickel carcinogenesis. In: *Nickel.* National Academy of Sciences, Washington, DC, 1975, pp. 144–188.

256. Gilchrest BA, Eller MS, Geller AC, Yaar M. The pathogenesis of melanoma induced by ultraviolet ratiation. *N Engl J Med* 1999; 340:1341–1348.

257. Cerutti PA. Oxy-radicals and cancer. *Lancet* 1994;344:862–863.

258. Knight JA. Oxidative stress and cancer. In: *Free Radicals, Antioxidants, Aging and Disease*. AACC Press, Washington, DC, 1999, pp. 297–328.

259. Borek C. Antioxidants and cancer. *Sci Med*, November/December 1997, pp. 52–61.

260. Blot WJ, Li J-Y, Taylor P-R, *et al.* Nutrition intervention trials in Linxian, China. Supplementation with specific vitamin/mineral combinations, cancer incidence, and disease-specific mortality in the general population. *J Natl Cancer Inst* 1993;85:1483–1492.

261. Giovannucci E. Tomatoes, tomato-based products, lycopene, and cancer: review of the epidemiologic literature. *J Natl Cancer Inst* 1999;91:317–331.

262. Floyd RA, Warson JJ, Wong PK, *et al.* Hydroxyl free radical adduct of deoxyguanosine: sensitive detection and mechanism of formation. *Free Radic Res Comm* 1986;1:163–172.

263. US Preventive Service Task Force. *Guide to Clinical Preventive Services*, 2nd Ed. Williams and Wilkins, Baltimore, 1996.

264. Danese MD, Powe NR, Sawin CT, Ladenson PW. Screening for mild thyroid failure at the periodic health examination. *JAMA* 1996;276:285–292.

265. Canaris GJ, Manowitz NR, Mayor G, Ridgway EC. The Colorado thyroid disease prevalence study. *Arch Intern Med* 2000;160:526–534.

266. Ladenson PW, Singer PA, Ain KB, *et al.* American Thyroid Association guidelines for detection of thyroid dysfunction. *Arch Intern Med* 2000;160:1573–1575.

267. Geiss LS (ed.). *Diabetes Surveillance*. Center for Disease Control and Prevention, US Department of Health and Human Services, Atlanta, GA, 1999.

268. Harris MI, Klein R, Welborn TA, Knuiman MW. Onset of NIDDM occurs at least 4–7 years before clinical diagnosis. *Diabetes Care* 1992;15:815–819.

269. Boyle JP, Honeycutt AA, Narayan KMV, *et al.* Projection of diabetes burden through 2050. *Diabetes Care* 2001;24:1936–1940.

270. Brancati FL, Kao WHL, Folsom AR, *et al.* Incident type 2 diabetes mellitus in African American and white adults. *JAMA* 2000;283: 2253–2259.

271. World Health Organization. Obesity: Preventing and Managing the Global Epidemic. World Health Organization, Geneva, 1998.

272. Helmrich SP, Ragland DR, Leung RW, Paffenberger RS Jr. Physical activity and reduced occurrence of non-insulin-dependent diabetes mellitus. *N Engl J Med* 1991;325:147–152.

273. Hu FB, Manson JE, Stampfer MJ, *et al.* Diet, lifestyle, and the risk of type 2 diabetes in women. *N Engl J Med* 2001;345:790–797.

274. Jovanovic L, Gondos B. Type 2 diabetes: the epidemic of the new millennium. *Ann Clin Lab Sci* 1999;29:33–42.

275. Report of the Expert Committee on the Diagnosis and Classification of Diabetes Mellitus. *Diabetes Care* 1997;20:1183–1197.

276. DECODE Study Group. Glucose tolerance and mortality: comparison of WHO and American Diabetes Association diagnostic criteria. *Lancet* 1999;354:617–621.

277. Bacon BR, Britton RS. The pathology of hepatic iron overload. A free radical mediated process? *Hepatology* 1990;11:127–137.

278. Edwards CQ, Kushner JP. Screening for hemochromatosis. *N Engl J Med* 1993;328:1616–1620.

279. Bulan V, Baldus W, Fairbanks V, *et al.* Screening for hemochromatosis: a cost effectiveness study based on 12,258 patients. *Gastroenterology* 1994;107:453–459.

280. Gambino R. Routine screening for iron status. *Hosp Pract* 1991;26(Suppl 3):41–44.

281. Buffone GJ, Beck JR. Cost-effectiveness analysis for evaluation of screening progrmams: hereditary hemochromatosis. *Clin Chem* 1994;40:1631–1636.

282. Ludwig J, Batts KP, Moyer TP, *et al.* Liver biopsy diagnosis of homozygous hemochromatosis. A diagnostic algorithm. *Mayo Clin Proc* 1993;68:263–268.

283. Grant JP, Custer PB, Thurlow J. Current techniques of nutritional assessment. *Surg Clin North Am* 1981;61:437–463.

284. Terpenning MS, Bradley SF. Why aging leads to increased susceptibility to infection. *Geriatrics* 1991;46:77–80.

285. Chandra RK. The relation between immunology, nutrition, and disease in elderly people. *Age Ageing* 1990;19:525–531.

286. Penn ND, Purkins L, Kelleher J, *et al.* The effect of dietary supplementation with vitamins A, C, and E on cell-mediated immune function in elderly long-stay patients. A randomized controlled study. *Age Ageing* 1991;20:169–174.

287. Meydani SN, Borklund MP, Liu S, *et al.* Vitamin E supplementation enhances cell-mediated immunity in healthy subjects. *Am J Clin Nutr* 1990;52:557–563.

288. Chandra RK. Effect of vitamin and trace-element supplementation on immune responses and infection in elderly patients. *Lancet* 1992;340:1124–1127.

289. Goode HF, Penn ND, Kelleher J, Walker RE. Evidence of cellular zinc depletion in hospitalized but not in healthy elderly subjects. *Age Ageing* 1991;20:345–348.

290. Duchateau J, Delepesse G, Vrijens R, Collet H. Beneficial effects of oral zinc supplementation on the immune response of old perople. *Am J Med* 1981;70:1001–1004.

291. National Institutes of Health. *Third Report of the National Cholesterol Education Program Expert Panel on Detection, Evaluation, and Treatment of High Blood Cholesterol in Adults (Adult Treatment Panel III)*. National Institutes of Health, Bethesda, Md, 2001. NIH Publication 01-3670.

292. Ford ES, Giles WH, Dietz WH. Prevalence of the metabolic syndrome among US adults: findings from the Third National Health and Nutrition Examination Survey. *JAMA* 2002;287:356–359.

293. Krahn MD, Mahoney JE, Eckman MH, *et al.* Screening for prostate cancer. *JAMA* 1994;272:773–780.

294. Babaian RJ, Dinney CPN, Ramirez EI, Evans RB. Diagnostic testing for prostate cancer detection: less is best. *Urology* 1993;41:421–425.

295. Catalona WJ, Smith DS, Ornstein DK. Prostate cancer detection in men with serum PSA concentrations of 2.6 to 4.0 ng/mL and benign prostate examination. *JAMA* 1997;277:1452–1455.

296. Carter HB, Epstein JI, Chan DW, *et al.* Recommended prostate-specific antigen testing intervals for the detection of curable prostate cancer. *JAMA* 1997;277:1456–1460.

297. US Preventive Services Task Force. Screening for prostate cancer: recommendation and rationale. *Ann Intern Med* 2002;137:915–916.

298. Friedrich MJ. Issues in prostate cancer screening. *JAMA* 1999;281:1573–1575.

299. Harris R, Lohr KN. Screening for prostate cancer: an update of the evidence for the US Preventive Services Task Force. *Ann Intern Med* 2002;137:917–929.

300. Altura BM. Introduction: importance of Mg in physiology and medicine and the need for ion selective electrodes. *Scand J Clin Lab Invest* 1994;54(Suppl 217):5–9.

301. Touitou Y, Godard J-P, Ferment O, *et al.* Prevalence of magnesium and potassium deficiencies in the elderly. *Clin Chem* 1987;33: 518–523.
302. Montague TJ, Ikuta RM, Wong RY, *et al.* Comparison of risk and patterns of practice in patients older and younger than 70 years with acute myocardial infarction in a two-year period. *Am J Cardiol* 1991;68:843–847.
303. US Department of Health and Human Services. *Healthy People 2010: Understanding and Improving Health*, 2nd Ed. US Government Printing Office, Washington, DC, 2000.

2 | Overweight and Obesity: Associated Health Risks and Economic Costs

Introduction

Obesity, now acknowledged as an epidemic in industrialized countries, has mainly developed during the last quarter of the 20th century. Moreover, obesity is emerging as a worldwide phenomenon, affecting not only wealthy and middle-income people in developed countries but in countries generally considered to be poor.[1,2] Indeed, about 315 million people worldwide fall under the World Health Organization's (WHO) definition of obesity (body mass index (BMI) $\geq$ 30 kg/m^2),[3] and more than this are undoubtedly overweight (BMI 25–29.9 kg/m^2). Although the prevalence of obesity varies with socioeconomic status, it is not consistently so since in developed countries obesity is associated with a greater prevalence of poverty, especially in women. In developing countries, however, relative affluence carries a greater risk.[4] In addition, overweight during childhood and adolescence is associated with overweight and obesity during adulthood.[5]

Data from the Third National Health and Nutrition Examination Survey (NHANES III; 1988–1994) indicated that approximately

14% of children and 12% of adolescents were overweight.[6] Moreover, compared with previous studies, the prevalence of overweight had increased significantly from 1976–1980 to 1985–1991 (from 7.6% to 10.9% for children; 5.7% to 10.8% for adolescents; and 25.4% to 33.3% for adults). The prevalence of overweight was also higher among blacks than among whites. Recent data indicates that the obesity epidemic continues unabated. For example, Mokdad *et al.*[7] reported a significant increase in obesity from 1991 through 1998. The greatest increase was found in the following groups: 18- to 29-year-olds (7.1–12.1%), those with some post-high school education (10.6–17.8%), and those of Hispanic ethnicity (11.6–20.8%). The increased prevalence also varied by region, ranging from 31.9% for mid-Atlantic to 67.2% for the South Atlantic, as well as by state (11.3% for Delaware to 101.8% for Georgia). Others[8] reported the prevalence and trends of obesity among American adults in 1999–2000. Compared with the NHANES III report, the age-adjusted obesity prevalence increased by 7.6% (22.9% versus 30.5%). Moreover, morbid (Class 3) obesity increased from 2.9% to 4.7%. Morbid obesity was recently reported to be highest among black women (6.0%), persons with less than a high school education (3.4%), and was inversely related to body height in both men and women.[9]

Americans are among the most overweight people in the world. By the most recent findings and stringent definition, about 34% of American adults are overweight and another 27% are obese (total 61%).[10] Of perhaps even greater concern is that the number of obese American adults has increased by more than 50% over the past two decades; the number of overweight children has also doubled.[11] Overweight and obesity in adults not only greatly increase the risk for numerous diseases/disorders (i.e. coronary heart disease (CHD), stroke, diabetes, some cancers, hypertension, gall bladder disease, among others), but place a tremendous economic burden on health care systems (see under "Economic Costs of Obesity and Physical Inactivity"). To alter this obesity trend, strategies and programs for weight control, as well as weight reduction, must become a major national public health priority.

What is the driving force behind the obesity epidemic? Although biology clearly contributes to individual differences in height and weight, the rapid weight gain over the past 20–30 years is primarily the result of environmental changes. Indeed, the current environment in the United States and other industrialized nations encourages the consumption of energy-rich foods and discourages energy expenditure. Thus, the availability of a wide variety of tasty, inexpensive, energy-rich foods served in large portions are a major contributor to the problem. Although portion sizes vary by the food source, the largest portions are consumed at fast food establishments and in the home. Nielsen and Popkin[12] reported that between 1977 and 1998, the energy intake and portion size of salty snacks increased by 93 kcal, soft drinks by 49 kcal, hamburgers by 97 kcal, french fries by 68 kcal, and Mexican food by 133 kcal. Moreover, the reduction in energy expenditure due to extensive television viewing, video games, surfing the Web, reduction in the number of jobs requiring physical labor, and a decrease in leisure-time and school-sponsored physical activity are also very important contributors to the epidemic.

Definitions of Overweight and Obesity

One of the major difficulties in accurately assessing the prevalence and consequences of being overweight or obese is the controversy involving their definitions. As a result, studies are not standardized. Historically, the medical case against obesity began with the Metropolitan Life Insurance Company tables which defined the "normal" weight range.[13] Based on thousands of policy holders, the tables indicated a progressive increase in the risk for premature death with increasing weight above the "desirable weight" [i.e. 126 pounds (57 kg) for a 5'4" (1.65 m) woman and 154 pounds (70 kg) for a 5'10" (1.78 m) man]. These tables, however, have several major limitations including primary reliance on white populations, invalidated estimate of frame size, and the use of data-based mortality figures which may not accurately reflect obesity-related co-morbidities.[14]

Body mass index (BMI)

The relative body weight is related to the body mass index (BMI), which is defined as a person's weight in kg divided by the square of his or her height in meters [BMI = weight (kg)/height (m^2); Table 2.1]. To calculate the BMI using pounds and inches, divide the weight in pounds by the square of the height in inches and multiply the result by 704.5. The 1995 Dietary Guidelines for Americans[15] recommended that a "healthy weight" for adult men and women corresponds to a BMI of 19 to 24.9 kg/m^2. The 1998 National Institutes of Health (NIH) guidelines define overweight when the BMI exceeds 25 kg/m^2 (i.e. 25–29.9 kg/m^2) and obesity of 30 kg/m^2 and above. These latter figures are also consistent with the WHO recommendations.[16] Here, a BMI of 25 to 29.9 kg/m^2 indicates grade 1 obesity (overweight); a BMI of 30 to 39.9 kg/m^2 equals grade 2 obesity (obese); and a BMI of 40 kg/m^2 or more equals grade 3 obesity (morbid obesity). In their recent book *Living to 100*, Perls and Silver[17] suggested the following correlation between the BMI and morbidity/mortality: 25–26 kg/m^2 is mildly overweight and has low risk; 27–29 kg/m^2 is obese with moderate risk; 30–34 kg/m^2 is significant obesity with a high risk; 35–39 kg/m^2 is morbid obesity and very high risk; and 40 kg/m^2 or above is extreme morbid obesity with an extremely high risk. A more general, albeit less accurate, guide is indicated by the data in Table 2.2. These "healthy weight ranges" have been suggested for men and women;[18] the higher weights apply primarily to men, who have more bone and muscle mass, while the lower weights are more applicable to women. From this data, it is apparent that the BMI is a more accurate indicator of adiposity than weight-for-height tables, although neither measures body fat level.[19] In addition, BMI does not incorporate the distribution of body fat, which is also a predictor of health risk. As a result, both body fat distribution and BMI are useful in evaluating health risk. Moreover, since body fat is not measured directly, some muscular individuals may be misclassified as being overweight or even obese using BMI alone.

Defining obesity as a BMI of 30 kg/m^2 and above, Flegal *et al.*[20] reported that about 25% of American women and 20% of American

Table 2.1: Body Mass Index For Various Weights and Heights*

Weight	100	105	110	115	120	125	130	135	140	145	150	155	160	165	170	175	180	185	190	195	200	205	210	215
Height																								
5'0"	20	21	21	22	23	24	25	26	27	28	29	30	31	32	33	34	35	36	37	38	39	40	41	42
5'1"	19	20	21	22	23	24	25	26	26	27	28	29	30	31	32	33	34	35	36	37	38	39	40	41
5'2"	18	19	20	21	22	23	24	25	26	27	27	28	29	30	31	32	33	34	35	36	37	38	38	39
5'3"	18	19	19	20	21	22	23	24	25	26	27	27	28	29	30	31	32	33	34	35	36	37	37	38
5'4"	17	18	19	20	21	21	22	23	24	25	26	27	27	28	29	30	31	32	33	33	34	35	36	37
5'5"	17	17	18	19	20	21	22	22	23	24	25	26	27	27	28	29	30	31	32	32	33	34	35	36
5'6"	16	17	18	19	19	20	21	22	23	23	24	25	26	27	27	28	29	30	31	31	32	33	34	35
5'7"	16	16	17	18	19	20	20	21	22	23	23	24	25	26	27	27	28	29	30	30	31	32	33	34
5'8"	15	16	17	17	18	19	20	21	21	22	23	23	24	25	26	27	27	28	29	30	30	31	32	33
5'9"	15	16	16	17	18	18	19	20	21	21	22	23	24	24	25	26	27	27	28	29	30	30	31	32
5'10"	14	15	16	17	17	18	19	19	20	21	22	22	23	24	24	25	26	27	27	28	29	29	30	31
5'11"	14	15	15	16	17	17	18	19	20	20	21	22	22	23	24	24	25	26	26	27	28	29	29	30
6'0"	14	14	15	16	16	17	18	18	19	20	20	21	22	22	23	24	24	25	26	26	27	28	28	29
6'1"	13	14	15	15	16	17	17	18	19	19	20	20	21	22	22	23	24	24	25	26	26	27	28	28
6'2"	13	13	14	15	15	16	17	17	18	18	19	20	20	21	22	22	23	23	24	25	26	26	27	28
6'3"	12	13	14	14	15	16	16	17	17	18	19	19	20	21	21	22	22	23	24	24	25	26	26	27
6'4"	12	13	13	14	15	15	16	16	17	17	18	18	19	20	20	21	21	22	23	23	24	25	26	26

*Unclothed weight in pounds, barefoot height in feet (') and inches (")

Table 2.2: Healthy Weight Ranges for Adults[*18]

Height	Weight	Height	Weight
5'0"	97–128	5'10"	132–174
5'1"	101–132	5'11"	136–179
5'2"	104–137	6'0"	140–184
5'3"	107–141	6'1"	144–189
5'4"	111–141	6'2"	148–195
5'5"	114–150	6'3"	152–200
5'6"	118–155	6'4"	156–205
5'7"	121–160	6'5"	160–211
5'8"	125–164	6'6"	164–216
5'9"	129–169		

*Unclothed weight in pounds, barefoot in the feet (') and inches (")

men are in the obese category. The prevalence of obesity is even greater in some minority groups; approximately 37% of non-Hispanic black women are obese as are 34% of Mexican American women. These authors also noted that although the percentage of overweight people has remained relatively constant over the past 30 years, the prevalence of obesity has increased more than 50% within the past ten to 15 years. In a subsequent study on the prevalence of obesity and overweight in the US, these researchers[21] reported that the increases in the prevalences of obesity and overweight continued in 1999–2000. Thus, the age-adjusted obesity prevalence was 30.5% in 1999–2000 compared with 22.9% in 1988–1994. The prevalence of overweight (i.e. BMI ≥ 25 kg/m^2) during this time increased from 55.9% to 64.5%. Moreover, extreme obesity (BMI ≥ 40 kg/m^2) increased from 2.9% to 4.7%.

Body fat distribution

Waist circumference

As noted above, body fat distribution is also a major predictor of disease risk. Body fat may distribute primarily around the hips and thighs (gynoid obesity; lower body fat; "pear" shape) or in the abdomen (android obesity; upper body fat; "apple" shape). Numerous reports have emphasized that individuals with the android obesity pattern are particularly susceptable to various metabolic disorders (i.e. hypertension, glucose intolerance and dyslipidemia).[22]

Waist circumference has been suggested as a simple measurement to identify those at health risk both from being overweight and from having a central fat distribution. Lean *et al.*[23] compared waist circumference with BMI and the waist : hip ratio. They found that a waist circumference ≥ 94 cm (≥ 37 inches) for men and ≥ 80 cm (≥ 31.5 inches) for women identified those with high BMI (≥ 25), as well as those with lower BMI but with a high waist : hip ratio (≥ 0.95 for men; ≥ 0.80 for women); the sensitivity was ≥ 96% and the specificity > 97.5%. A waist circumference > 102 cm (> 40.2 inches) for men or ≥ 88 cm (≥ 34.6 inches) for women identified people with BMI of 30 kg/m² or above, as well as those with a lower BMI but with a high waist : hip ratio; again the sensitivity was > 96% while the specificity increased slightly (> 98%). The authors concluded that men with a waist circumference ≥ 94 cm (≥ 37 inches) and women ≥ 80 cm (≥ 31.5 inches) should gain no further weight; men with a waist circumference ≥ 102 cm (≥ 40.2 inches) and women ≥ 88 cm (≥ 34.6 inches) should strongly be encouraged to lose weight.

In a later report, these investigators studied health impairment and quality of life in people with a large waist circumference.[24] They again compared BMI and waist : hip ratio with waist circumference and assessed their relationship to respiratory insufficiency, low back pain, degree of physical function, presence of non-insulin-dependent diabetes, and cardiovascular risk factors. Their results showed that, after adjustment for age and lifestyle, all disease risks and symptoms increased as the waist circumference increased. However, they concluded that "there is no strong evidence to prefer either BMI or waist circumference for categorization of adiposity or prediction of preventable ill health and there are only minor differences in their associations with diseases and symptoms."

Waist-hip ratio

The waist circumference to hip circumference ratio is another commonly used technique for assessing body composition. In 1990, the

Dietary Guidelines for Americans recommended that the waist : hip ratio should not exceed 0.80 for women or 0.95 for men; however, the 1995 guidelines increased this latter ratio to 1.0.[18]

Dual X-ray adsorptiometry

X-ray adsorptiometry, in contrast to BMI, waist circumference, and waist : hip ratio accurately measures total body fat; it also quantifies regional fat in the central and hip and thigh areas.[25] However, this technique is uncommonly used due to its cost, inconvenience and relative unavailability. Moreover, in most cases the more readily available and simple methods described above give clinically reliable results.

The waist : hip ratio and waist circumference reportedly give similar correlations with common risk factors for CHD (i.e. hypertension and serum lipid levels).[26] As a result, the waist circumference may be the most useful because of its greater simplicity. However, in contrast to the BMI, choosing a point on the waist circumference and waist : hip ratio continuum to differentiate overweight from obesity, has not been reported.

An expert panel on overweight and obesity in adults recently suggested that increased risks exist if waist circumference exceeds 102 cm (40 inches) in men and 89 cm (35 inches) in women.[27] Nevertheless, these dimensions are considerable and waist circumferences significantly less than these cutoff points have been associated with increased relative risks of 3 to 5 for non-insulin-dependent diabetes (type 2 diabetes).[28,29] This clearly indicates that these guidelines are very insensitive in predicting risks for this disease. Moreover, others[26] reported that a waist circumference in men of 94 to 102 cm (35 to 40 inches) had a relative risk of 2.2 for having one or more cardiovascular risk factors; in women a waist circumference of 80 to 88 cm (32 to 35 inches) indicated a relative risk of 1.6.

Taylor *et al.*[30] recently published one of the very few studies using receiver operating characteristic curves to compare the BMI with the waist : hip ratio and waist circumference in women. Although their results "strongly support the use of BMI as an index of adiposity in groups of adult women," they concluded that both the BMI and waist circumference provide simple yet sensitive methods to estimate total and central body fat in women. Both methods were clearly more reliable than the waist : hip ratio. Other less commonly used methods for assessing fatness are skinfold thickness and bioimpedance, neither of which is as clinically useful as those discussed above.

Body Weight, Morbidity and Mortality

In 1958, John Kenneth Galbraith wrote "More die in the United States of too much food than of too little" (*The Affluent Society*). Numerous studies have now shown a strong association between relative body weight and increased morbidity and mortality. The increase in mortality rates in relation to relative weight increase is steeper in women and men younger than 50 years than in older persons, and the increase associated with duration of obesity is also steeper.[31] In addition, women and minorities, including Hispanics, African Americans, American Indians and Pacific Islanders are particularly at risk of obesity.[32]

Greater efforts to prevent weight gain should begin in early adulthood and probably during childhood. Approximately 60% of overweight children aged five to ten years already have one associated biochemical or clinical cardiovascular risk factor (i.e. hyperlipidemia, increased blood pressure and insulin resistance) and about 25% have two or more risk factors.[33] In this regard, Williamson and associates[34] reported that persons in their 20s and 30s are at highest risk of becoming overweight and need encouragement to adopt good dietary and exercise habits in order to prevent them from gaining excessive weight later in life. They recommended that special emphasis is needed for young women who are already overweight.

Disease morbidity increases with increasing body weight. For example, Must *et al.*[35] in a study involving 16,884 adults 25 or more years, reported that 63% of the men and 55% of the women were either overweight (BMI 25–29.9 kg/m^2) or obese (BMI $\geq$ 30 kg/m^2). A graded increase in the prevalence ratio with increasing severity of overweight or obesity was found for type 2 diabetes mellitus, gall bladder disease, hypertension and osteoarthritis in both men and women. The prevalence ratios were generally greater in younger than in older adults. In addition, the prevalence of having two or more health conditions increased with increasing weight across all racial and ethnic subgroups. More recently, Sturm and Wells[36] reported that 33% of US adults are overweight and an additonal 23% are obese. In this report, obesity was associated with more chronic conditions and worse physical health-related quality of life than smoking, poverty, or problem alcohol drinking.

In an early study[37] of mortality rates in morbidly obese men (average weight 143.5 kg; about 315 pounds), mortality was 12 times higher in men aged 25 to 34 years and six times higher in men aged 35 to 44 years versus men with healthy weights of the same age. More recently, Manson *et al.*[38] examined the association between BMI and overall mortality and mortality from specific causes in 115,195 US women (Nurses' Health Study), aged 30 to 55 years, who were free of cancer and cardiovascular disease in 1976. They followed the cohort for 16 years and documented the number of deaths from cancer, cardiovascular disease, and various other causes. They concluded that body weight and mortality from all causes were directly related; the lowest mortality rate was noted in those who weighed at least 15% less than the US average for women of similar age. The mortality rate was also lower in those whose weight had been stable since early adulthood.

Of considerable importance is the recent report by Allison and co-workers[39] in which they found that only smoking exceeds obesity in its contribution to total US mortality rates. These researchers evaluated the 1991 data from six major cohort studies involving adults 18 years and older who were classified as overweight (BMI 25–29 kg/m^2), obese (BMI 30–35 kg/m^2) and severely obese (BMI > 35 kg/m^2). The calculated mean number of annual deaths attributable to obesity was approximately 280,000 based on the relative hazard ratio from all subjects and about 325,000 based on a relative hazard ratio from only non-smokers and never-smokers. These numbers are consistent with those reported earlier by McGinnis and Foege (i.e. obesity 300,000/year; smoking, 400,000/year).[40] More recently, however, Sturm[41] reported that obesity now outranks both smoking and alcohol consumption in its deleterious effects on both health and medical costs. Thus, obesity "has roughly the same association with chronic health conditions as does 20 years' aging" and that "this greatly exceeds the associations of smoking or problem drinking." He noted that over the past few decades, both smoking and chronic alcohol intake have received considerably more attention from medical practitioners and public health officials than obesity. Yet, obesity is associated with a 36% increase in both out- and in-patient costs and a 77% increase in medications compared with a 21% increase in out- and in-patient costs and a 28% increase in medications for current smokers and even lower costs for chronic alcoholics.

The effect of age on optimal body weight is poorly understood since few studies have analyzed mortality as a function of weight across various age groups. To extend our knowledge in the area, Stevens and associates[42] recently reported a 12-year study involving 62,112 white men and 262,019 white women. None of the participants had ever smoked, had no history of stroke, heart disease, or cancer and there was no history of recent weight loss. Their results showed that increased BMI was associated with higher mortality from all causes, as well as from cardiovascular disease in both women and men up to age 75 years. The association between BMI and mortality was weaker in individuals over age 75 years. To further evaluate the effect of adult overweight and obesity on life expectancy and increased premature death at age 40 years, Peeters et al.[43] prospectively studied 3457 adults aged 30 to 49 years at baseline. Their results showed a highly significant decrease in life expectancy with both overweight and obesity. Thus, overweight 40-year-old female non-smokers lost 3.3 years of life while 40-year-old male non-smokers lost 3.1 years. However, obese 40-year-old women and men lost 7.1 and 5.8 years, respectively. Compared with normal-weight non-smokers, obese male and female smokers lost 13.7 and 13.3 years of life, respectively.

A recent significantly larger study estimated the number of years of life lost (YLL) due to overweight and obesity across the life span of adults aged 18 to 85 years.[44] These researchers used data from three sources: the 1999 US Life Tables; Third National Health and Nutrition Examination Survey; and the First National Health and Nutrition Epidemiologic Follow-up Study. Their findings showed the following: (1) among whites, a J- or U-shaped association was present between overweight or obesity and YLL; (2) the optimal BMI for greatest longevity was about 23 to 25 kg/m^2 for whites and 23 to 30 kg/m^2 for blacks; (3) younger adults had greater YLL than did older adults; and (4) the maximum YLL for white males aged 20 to 30 years with severe obesity (BMI > 45 kg/m^2) was 13 (a 22% reduction in remaining lifespan) and eight for white females. For severely obese blacks of similar age, the maximum YLL was 20 years for men and five years for women.

Overweight and Obesity in Adults

Aging is well known to be associated with alterations in body weight. Through middle age, there is an increase in body weight associated with a doubling in body fat in both women and men.[45,46] Conversely, body fat commonly decreases in late old age even in healthy individuals. Although the causes of obesity are many (Table 2.3), the exact

Table 2.3: Risk Factors for Overweight and Obesity

Genetics	Psychological factors (e.g. depression)
Excess caloric intake (portion-size inflation and calorically-dense foods)	Decreased resting metabolic rate
	Socioeconomic (lower classes)
Physical inactivity (increased television and computer use)	Stress
	Cultural
Neuroendocrine disorders	Education (lower levels)

mechanisms are not fully understood. The current surge of worldwide obesity reflects a failure of the various mechanisms that regulate body weight to adjust with an environment that promotes overeating and discourages physical activity. However, there is also considerable variation among people regarding their susceptibility to gain weight. Some individuals apparently become obese despite a continuous struggle not to whereas others remain lean without conscious control.

Although heritability studies suggest that up to 70% of the variability in body weight may be accounted for by genetic factors,[47,48] obesity genes are clearly not responsible for the recent obesity epidemic because the gene pool has certainly not changed significantly over the past two to three decades. Nevertheless, heritability for obesity is reportedly as strong as it is for alcoholism, hypertension and schizophrenia.[49] Several genes involved in energy regulation have been identified and cloned. An example is leptin, a signal protein for satiety; it is produced only in adipose tissue.[50] Ready access to good-tasting, high fat foods[51] and decreased physical activity[52] are also highly significant contributors to the problem, as is the increased time devoted to television and computers.

As with any biologic system, the human body obeys the laws of thermodynamics. As such, body weight depends on a balance between energy intake (food and drink) and energy expenditure. An excess of energy (calories) intake over expenditure leads to energy storage (i.e. increased fat). Importantly, only during the past few decades has an imbalance of energy intake and output occurred for such a large proportion of the population. For example, surveys conducted in 1977–1978 and 1994–1996 showed that the average daily caloric intake increased from 2239 to 2455 kcal/day in men and from 1534 to 1646 kcal/day in women.[53,54]

In addition to genetic factors, increased caloric intake and physical inactivity, other important factors which contribute to adult obesity include a decline in resting metabolic rate with age, high fat diets, and various psychosocial and cultural factors (i.e. different attitudes toward body weight in various cultures and among ethnic groups).[55]

Stress-related excess eating and alcohol drinking are also important risk factors.[56] In this latter longitudinal Finnish population-based study of 2359 men and 2791 women born in 1966, stress-driven eaters ate more sausages, hamburgers, pizza and chocolate than other people. They also had a higher alcohol intake. The major predictors of these stress-driven individuals were being divorced or not married, long history of unemployment, and a low level of occupational education.

Advances in transportation have also reduced the need for physical activity in daily life. Additionally, educational level has recently been shown to be a highly important associated factor in determining body weight.[57] In this study, differences in age-adjusted mean BMI between the highest and lowest tertiles of years of schooling were determined for 26 populations in the initial and final WHO surveys, which included 42,000 men and women aged 35 to 64 years in the initial survey (1979–1989) and about 35,000 in the final survey (1989–1996). Their findings showed that lower levels of education was associated with significantly increased BMI in about one-half of the male and almost all of the female populations. Moreover, the differences in relative body weight between educational levels increased significantly over the ten-year study period.

An additional important, but uncommonly appreciated risk for obesity, is that the source from which food is obtained contributes significantly to the increased incidence of obesity, at least in the US.[58] This study suggested that frequent eating away from home, particularly in fast food establishments, is an important contributor to the increase in obesity. McCrory and associates[59] added further support for this association when they studied the dietary intake and frequency of consuming food from seven different restaurant types (fried chicken, burger, pizza, Chinese, Mexican, fried fish, and "others"). In this group of healthy men and women, restaurant food consumption averaged 7.5 times/month. After controlling for age and sex, the frequency of consuming restaurant food was positively associated with body fatness. The strength of the association did not change after controlling for smoking status, alcohol intake or education level. A recent review of this topic[60] stressed that restaurant food tends to be energy-dense (i.e. high in fat, low in fiber). Significantly larger portions of a wide variety of energy-dense palatible foods are also served than in decades past.[12]

The biobehavioral influences affecting increased energy and body weight have been recently reviewed.[61] The major reported factors that negatively affect adult eating behaviors and increase body weight are summarized as follows.

(1) *Dietary variety*: The variety of available foods has increased markedly over the past several decades, mainly "in nutrient poor, high energy dense categories." This increase in food variety results in increased consumption, body weight and fatness.

(2) *Liquid versus solid energy*: The consumption of energy-dense beverages has increased significantly. For example, the US per capita consumption, in gallons of soft drink, reportedly increased by more than 60% between 1977 and 1998.[62]

(3) *Portion size*: The portion sizes served in US restaurants have markedly increased over the past couple of decades. There has also been a trend since the late 1970s to the present toward larger prepackaged foods.[63]

(4) *Taste (palatability)*: Numerous studies have shown that energy intake, independent of other dietary factors, increases with food palatability. Indeed, taste is reportedly the most important single reason people choose the foods they eat.[61]

(5) *Snacking*: Snacking is a very common habit across all age groups. Thus, the number of daily snacks increased from 1.1 in 1977–1978 to 1.6 in 1995 for all people two years and older.[62] Moreover, the snacks are currently higher in energy than in earlier times.

(6) *Restraint and disinhibition*: Dietary restraint (i.e. tendency to restrict the amount and types of foods consumed to maintain or lose weight) and disinhibition (i.e. tendency to overeat certain "appealing" foods) are both important determinants of adult weight gain.[64] Thus, when these two factors "get out of hand," weight gain is imminent.

Overweight and Obesity in Children and Adolescents

Obesity prevalence

Although the BMI is well accepted as a reasonably reliable method to measure adiposity in adults, a consensus measure of childhood and adolescent adiposity has been limited by the lack of data. However, several recent reports[65-67] suggest that BMI also represents a reasonable index of adiposity in both children and adolescents. Thus, using the BMI as an indicator of overweight/obesity, there was a 100% increase in obesity among American children between 1980 and 1994. Here, Troiano *et al.*[65] studied overweight prevalence and trends in children and adolescents aged six to 17 years in each of five separate time periods (1963–1965; 1966–1970; 1971–1974; 1976–1980; and 1988–1991). Their findings showed the greatest increase was from 1976 to 1980, which was similar to that in adults. From 1988 to 1991, the prevalence of overweight was 10.9% based on the 95th percentile and 22% based on the 85th percentile. Importantly, there was an increase in overweight prevalence among all sex and age groups. The Center for Disease Control's (CDC) National Health and Nutrition Examination Survey (NHANES III) of 1988–1991 found that the prevalence of overweight adolescents, aged 12 to 19 years, was 21%, an increase of 6% since their previous survey (NHANES II).[68] Others[69] reported that 11% of children and adolescents were overweight in the years 1988–1994. However, an additional 14% had a BMI between the 85th and 95th percentiles. The prevalence of overweight did not vary systematically with race-ethnicity, family income or education.

The National Longitudinal Survey of Youth later reported results of a prospective cohort study of children aged four to 12 years conducted between 1986 and 1998.[70] They found that obesity increased significantly and steadily among children of all ages. After age 12 years, overweight prevalence was 12.3% in non-Hispanic whites, 21.5% among African Americans, and 21.8% among Hispanics. Overweight also increased more rapidly among minorities and Southerners. More recently, Ogden and associates[71] surveyed a large group of children from birth through age 19 years; the data was collected in 1999–2000. The overweight prevalence was 15.5% among the 12- through 19-year-olds, 15.3% among the six- through 11-year-olds, and 10.4% among the two- through five-year-olds compared with the 1988–1994 NHANES III report (10.5%, 11.3% and 7.2%, respectively). The prevalence of overweight among non-Hispanic black and Mexican American adolescents increased more than 10% between 1988–1994 and 1999–2000.

The rising prevalence of overweight and obese children is not limited to the US. Reilly and associates[72] reported a significant prevalence of overweight and obesity among British children. Using cutoffs for BMI above the 85th percentile to indicate overweight and above the 95th percentile as obese, they reported the following data for both sexes at ages 24, 49 and 61 months, respectively: 15.8% overweight, 6.0% obese; 20.3% overweight, 7.6% obese; and 18.7% overweight, 7.2% obese. In addition, secular trends indicate that Canadian children, aged seven to 13 years, are also becoming progressively overweight and obese.[73] Thus, the prevalence of overweight among girls increased from 15% in 1981 to 23.6% in 1996 and among boys from 15% to 28.8%. The prevalence of obesity in these children more than doubled during the same period of time, from 5% in both sexes to 13.5% for boys and 11.8% for girls. Overweight and obesity are also serious public health problems in the Navajo.[74] These authors reported that overweight and obesity also begin in childhood, and has become more serious over the past decade.

As noted by Freedman *et al.*,[75] there is a significantly higher prevalence of overweight and obesity among black women compared with white women. However, since a similar pattern had not been described in children, they studied 4542 black girls and 4542 white girls, aged five to 17 years, between 1973 and 1994. They found that although black girls were 1 to 3 kg heavier than comparable white girls, they were also 2 to 3 cm taller. After adjusting for differences in height, the mean relative weight of black girls was consistently greater than white girls only after age 13. In addition, sexual maturation was a stronger correlate of relative body weight among black girls. Taking these variables into consideration, they concluded that black girls do not have a higher mean relative weight than white girls until adolescence.

Weight concerns have also increased among the youth. In an attempt to control their weight, there has been a significant increase in cigarette smoking.[76] As these investigators reported, it is very important for parents, physicians and school health programs "to address healthy methods of weight maintenance and to dispel the notion of tobacco use as a method of weight control."

National recommendations for food intake have been established and are outlined in the Food Guide Pyramid (Chapter 4).[77] Briefly, the pyramid recommends the following mean daily servings for children and adolescents two to 19 years of age: grains six to 11; vegetables three to five; fruit two to four; dairy two to three; and five to seven ounces of meat. Unfortunately, most American children and teens do not meet the national recommendations.[78] This report noted that mean daily servings were below minimum recommendations for all food groups except the dairy group for children aged two to 11 years. The percentages of children and teens meeting recommendations ranged from approximately 30% for fruit, grain, meat and dairy to 36% for vegetables; 16% did not meet any recommendations and only 1% met all recommendations. Moreover, the intake of total fat and added sugar accounted for 35% and 15% of energy, respectively.

With regards to added sugar, Ludwig *et al.*[79] recently concluded that the consumption of sugar-sweetened drinks is associated with childhood obesity. In this prospective study, involving 584 ethnically diverse group of children (mean age 11.7 years), they found, after adjustment for anthropometric, demographic, dietary and lifestyle variables, that for each additional serving of a sugar-sweetened drink both BMI and frequency of obesity increased. Furthermore, baseline consumption of these drinks was independently associated with BMI changes. Furthermore, recent reports indicate increasing consumption of soft drinks by children, especially teenagers.[79] Importantly, a 12-ounce can of regular soda contains 40 g of added sugar (about 160 calories). Since girls 12–19 years of age drink, on average, 12 ounces of regular soda each day and boys about 21 ounces per day (280 calories), these "empty calories" are significantly related to the rising obesity rates.[80] Unfortunately, these soft drinks are too readily available in snack bars, school stores and vending machines outside school cafeterias.

Childhood, adulthood and parental obesity

An early study suggested that dietary intake patterns in childhood and adolescence may be predictive of obesity in adulthood.[81] These findings were recently confirmed and expanded.[82] Here, a group of overweight children, mean age 13.3 ± 0.3 years, were re-evaluated at age 21.8 ± 0.3 years. Blood pressure, weight and height were measured at both periods of time. A euglycemic insulin clamp (measure of insulin resistance) was performed in the young adult group, as were fasting lipid levels (total and low-density lipoprotein cholesterol). The results showed that childhood BMI was highly correlated with young adulthood BMI, inversely correlated with young adult glucose utilization (i.e. insulin resistance), and positively correlated with total cholesterol (TC) and low-density lipoprotein cholesterol (LDL-C) levels. Thus, childhood adiposity is a strong predictor of young adult adiposity, altered cardiovascular risk, and early signs of potential diabetes. Whitaker *et al.*[83] also studied the predictability of young adulthood obesity from childhood and parental obesity. They found that obese children less than three years of age without obese parents were at low risk of adulthood obesity. Among older children, however, obesity was an increasingly significant predictor of adult obesity regardless of parental obesity. In addition, parental obesity increased the risk of adult obesity by more than two-fold among both obese and non-obese children less than ten years of age. More recently, Hardy and co-workers[84] investigated the effects of childhood weight and socioeconomic status in Britain on the pattern of BMI change between the ages of 20 and 43 years. Their results indicated that childhood manual social class, defined by the father's occupation and high relative weight at age 14 years, were associated with a higher mean BMI across adult life; these effects increased with age. Moreover, these two risk factors for high adult BMI were independent of subsequent educational attainment and adult social class.

These latter studies indicate that weight gain prevention is very important in childhood. Moreover, parental attitudes and examples are critical. For example, Davison and Birch[85] studied the relationship between weight status and self-concept in 197 five-year-old girls and their parents. They found that those with a higher weight status had lower body esteem and lower perceived cognitive ability than girls who weighed less. Moreover, paternal concern about child overweight was associated with decreased perceived physical ability; maternal concern was associated with both lower perceived cognitive and physical abilities. Furthermore, parental food restriction was also associated with negative self-evaluations. The authors recommended that public health programs regarding overweight children must also provide "constructive and blame-free alternatives for addressing child weight problems" which otherwise may be detrimental to a child's mental health.

Television viewing and body weight

Behavioral modifications, including dietary changes, increased physical activity, and less time spent with video games and television viewing are very important factors in weight control of children and adolescents. For example, Dietz[86] documented that increased television viewing was a significant factor leading to obesity, and Morgan[87] reported that excessive television watching may also lead to decreased school achievement.

The association between television viewing and child and adolescent adiposity was recently confirmed.[88] The author concluded that reducing television, videotape and video game use may be a "promising population-based approach in preventing childhood obesity."

A more recent study further substantiated the relationship between television viewing and risk of being overweight in preschool-aged children.[89] These researchers reported that "a TV in a child's bedroom is an even stronger marker of increased risk of being overweight." They emphasized that since most children watch television by age two, parents should limit television/video viewing and must keep televisions out of a child's bedroom. Moreover, parental marital status, as well as the mass media, significantly influence the onset of eating disorders, at least in girls aged 12 years and older.[90] These latter researchers also concluded that "the habit of eating alone should be considered as a warning sign of eating disorders." A recent study also found that headache, back pain, eye symptoms and sleep problems are more common among children who watch television four or more hours per day compared with those who watch television less than two hours per day.[91]

Increased television watching is also a common risk factor for obesity in adults. Thus, a prospective cohort study of 50,277 women (Nurses' Health Study) showed that for each two hours/day increment in television watching, there was a 23% increase in obesity and a 14% increase in risk of type 2 diabetes.[92] These findings were independent of age, smoking, exercise levels, dietary factors and other covariates.

Breastfeeding and childhood body weight

Of considerable additional importance is the possible association between infant breastfeeding and overweight children and adolescents. Breast milk is clearly the preferred feeding for infants since it has growth, immunologic and developmental benefits.[93,94] Moreover, infants who are breastfed for at least six months were shown to have increased cognitive developmental scores in comparison with infants who were never breastfed.[95] In addition, early reports suggest that breastfeeding may be protective against being overweight during childhood and adolescence,[96,97] although more recent studies have been somewhat inconsistent. For example, Hediger *et al.*[98] found that breastfeeding reduced the risk of being at risk of overweight for ever breastfed children. However, there was no reduced risk of being overweight. They concluded that although breastfeeding is strongly recommended, it may not be as effective as moderating familial factors (i.e. dietary habits and physical activity), since a significant predictor of child overweight status was the mother's concurrent weight. The rate of children being overweight was almost three times if the mother was overweight (i.e. BMI 25.0–29.9 kg/m^2). Conversely, Gillman and associates[99] reported that infants who were breastfed for at least seven months, compared with those who were breastfed for three months or less, had a lower risk for being overweight during older childhood and adolescence.

Childhood/adolescent obesity and psychosocial problems

Although there is a growing awareness of the long-term health risks of childhood and adolescent obesity, the most widespread consequences may be psychosocial.[100] Indeed, obese children and adolescents are at increased risk for lower perceived competencies on social, athletic and appearance domains, as well as overall self-worth.[101] Studies have also consistently shown an association between both adult and adolescent obesity and depression. However, it has not been clear as to whether depression leads to obesity or whether obesity leads to depression. To further understand this association, Goodman and Whitaker[102] prospectively studied 9374 adolescents in school grades 7 through 12. At baseline, 12.9% were overweight, 9.7% were obese and 8.8% had depressed mood. After follow-up one year later, the authors concluded that "depressed adolescents are at increased risk for the development and persistence of obesity during adolescence." Moreover, baseline obesity did not predict follow-up depression. In addition, Schwimmer and associates[103] recently reported that severely obese children and adolescents have more than a five-fold increase of a lower health-related quality of life compared with healthy children. Importantly, the risk is similar to that previously reported for children and adolescents diagnosed with cancer.

Prevention, Management and Treatment of Obesity

Thomas Edison wrote, "The doctor of the future will give no medicine, but will interest his patient in the care of the human frame, in diet and in the prevention of disease." As with many medical disorders, obesity prevention is significantly better than treatment. The prevention and management of overweight/obesity is complex and affected by numerous factors. As such, no single method is applicable to all individuals. Although parents have a key role in preventing overweight/obesity in their children, involvement in obesity prevention by national, state and local public health agencies, as well as schools and health care professionals, is also critical. These groups and organizations must become more actively involved in campaigns regarding the health consequences of being overweight and stressing the importance of a proper diet and regular exercise. Cities and counties should establish safe walking and bicycle lanes and perhaps most important, schools should reinstate daily physical education and health classes. Moreover, physicians and other health care professionals must become proactive in educating the public and counseling their patients about the importance of this serious epidemic.

Caloric intake

As noted previously, body weight depends on a balance between energy intake (i.e. calories) and energy expenditure. Thus, when an imbalance exists, body weight increases. As a result, reduced energy intake is critical in overweight and obese individuals. Moreover, it should be individually tailored to allow normal activities. A daily caloric deficit of 500 to 600 kilocalories (kcal) per day is usually well tolerated and will result in significant weight loss over time (one or more pounds per week). Emphasis on fat intake is essential since the number of kcal per gram of fat (9.0) is slightly over twice that of carbohydrate (4.0) and protein (4.0). Moreover, total fat intake should not exceed 30% of total calories. For example, the participants in a six-month trial entered a research "supermarket" and obtained either fat-reduced or full-fat foods.[104] Those who selected full-fat foods had higher energy intake and gained weight; those who selected fat-reduced foods did not increase their energy intake and had no change in body weight. Thus, dietary restraint protected against the weight-promoting effect of a high fat diet.

A combination of diet and exercise is far more effective than either alone. A recent study reported that more than two-thirds of American adults are trying to lose or maintain weight.[105] Yet, only 20% reported using a combination of engaging in at least 30 minutes per day, five days per week of leisure-time physical activity and eating fewer calories. Interestingly, among those attempting to lose weight, a common strategy is to consume less fat. However, many of these individuals give little attention to the total number of calories obtained from low-fat foods. This suggests that some individuals fail to appreciate that total caloric intake is the major concern regardless of the source. Hence, an over-emphasis on consumption of low-fat foods may inadvertently contribute to an increase in total energy intake.[106]

Metz *et al.*[107] recently assessed the long-term effects of a nutritionally complete pre-packaged prepared meal plan compared with a usual-care diet on weight loss and various cardiovascular risk factors (blood pressure, plasma lipids, glucose and glycosylated hemoglobin). In this clinical trial, 302 overweight and obese adults were randomized to receive either a nutrient-fortified prepared meal plan or a macronutrient equivalent usual-care diet. Their results showed that these long-term dietary interventions induced significant weight loss and improved cardiovascular risk factors in those at high-risk.

The health benefit differences between a low-carbohydrate and a calorie- and fat-restricted diet are of considerable public interest. The conventional dietary approach to weight control is a high-carbohydrate, low-fat diet. However, low-carbohydrate, high-protein, high-fat diets have become increasingly popular among the general public (e.g. Atkin's diet). Nevertheless, randomized trials evaluating the efficacy of these diets had not been evaluated until recently. In 2003, two studies compared a low-carbohydrate with a low-fat diet in obese people. In a six-month study of 79 severely obese subjects,

Samaha *et al.*[108] found that obese individuals lost more weight on a carbohydrate-restricted diet than on a calorie- and fat-restricted diet. There was also a relative improvement in insulin sensitivity and serum triglyceride levels. They noted, however, that due to the small magnitude of overall and between-group differences in weight loss, and the short study period (i.e. six months), the findings "should be interpreted with caution." Foster and associates[109] also reported that a low-carbohydrate diet produced greater weight loss than the conventional diet in 63 obese men and women after three months. However, after one year the differences were not significant. The authors of both reports indicated that longer and larger studies will be required to determine any long-term benefits of a low-carbohydrate diet, as well as the efficacy and safety of these diets. Indeed, in a recent systematic review of the efficacy and safety of low-carbohydrate diets, Bravata *et al.*[110] concluded that "there is insufficient evidence to make recommendations for or against the use of low-carbohydrate diets, particularly among participants older than age 50 years. ..." Moreover, the findings illustrated that low-carbohydrate diets result in weight loss by reducing calorie intake, thus reaffirming the first law of thermodynamics, as well as emphasizing that without carbohydrate-consuming foods in the diet, less fat is ingested because few people eat much fat by itself. As a result, low-carbohydrate diets cause weight loss because they reduce total calorie intake.[111]

High-protein diets are also frequently promoted as a means to successfully lose weight. However, a recent statement from the Nutrition Committee of the Council on Nutrition, Physical Activity, and Metabolism of the American Heart Association raised serious concerns about these diets.[112] The report noted that these diets are generally associated with higher intakes of total fat, saturated fat and cholesterol because the protein is derived mainly from animal sources. For these and other reasons, the committee concluded that "high protein diets are not recommended because they restrict healthful foods that provide essential nutrients and do not provide the variety of foods needed to adequately meet nutritional needs." Thus, in addition to other potential problems (i.e. cardiac, kidney, bone and liver abnormalities), individuals on these diets are at risk for inadequate essential vitamin and mineral intake.

Physical activity

Regular leisure-time physical activity is critical, not only for successful weight loss but for long-term weight maintenance.[113,114] The minimal recommended national guideline for physical activity is 150 minutes per week (30 minutes per day, five days each week).[115] Yet, Serdula *et al.*[105] reported that although two-thirds of those who said they used physical activity as a way for losing weight, only 40% met the minimum exercise level. It should be noted, however, that the amount of exercise necessary for enhancing long-term weight loss and associated health benefits is probably greater than the minimum recommendation.[116,117] Moreover, long-term low intensity exercise, such as walking, may be as effective as high-intensity activities.[118] In agreement with this, Fogelholm and associates[119] reported that a walking training program of moderate intensity, after an initial weight reduction, had a positive but minor effect on weight maintenance; a more intense walking program had no independent effect of weight maintenance. Moreover, Perri *et al.*[120] have repeatedly shown that a maintenance program is effective only as long as the active intervention is ongoing. Thus, it appears likely that long-term health professional contact and support from family, friends and co-workers are the most important factors in maintaining stable weight levels.

Unfortunately, physical activity as a method of weight loss is least common among obese individuals who are less educated, as well as those who are older.[121] The prevalence of physical inactivity among both children and adults is also extremely high.[122] Thus, interventions to help all individuals to become more physically active is a significant challenge and successful strategies for improving participation in physical activity are sorely needed for underactive and inactive individuals. Indeed, several alternative strategies have been investigated.[123] Since many people in developed countries are exposed to a "toxic environment" that reduces opportunities for physical activity, environmental changes are needed to increase the convenience of exercise participation. For example, Sallis *et al.*[124] reported that when exercise facilities are near an individual's home there was a higher participation in physical activity than when individuals were more distant from exercise facilities. Thus, cities can stimulate increased physical activity by providing convenient walking and bicycle lanes, parks and other exercise promoting opportunities.

Lifestyle changes may also be advantageous in changing physical activity behaviors.[123] Thus, the incorporation of behavioral skills training, such as problem solving, may be successful in promoting the adoption and maintenance of physical activity. Others[125] have suggested that lifestyle forms of physical activity such as gardening, house cleaning, etc. may also help maintain body weight. Studies of other alternative approaches to physical activity are needed to evaluate techniques that may be successful in promoting increased physical activity, especially among those who are less inclined to control their weight.

Miscellaneous preventive measures

Other factors are also important for successful weight control and becoming metabolically fit. In addition to motivation, behavior modification, which includes a daily record of physical activity (i.e. time and distance), recording of food intake, professional nutrition advice and separation from various sedentary activities (i.e. excess television watching, computer time, etc.) are important. Psychological help may also be beneficial in selected cases. Although drugs may be useful to curb the appetite, they must be medically supervised. Unfortunately, adults 30 years and younger who are trying to lose weight are more likely to smoke than those not concerned about their weight.[126]

It is an unfortunate fact that obese people tend to regain lost weight. This raises the question as to whether metabolic factors are important contributors to the regulation of body weight. This suspicion led to the set-point theory that suggests the body has a homeostatic feed-back system that controls body fat stores. This system includes an adaptation in the energy efficiency of metabolic processes that main-tain constant fat stores and body weight.[127] However, the suggestion that weight-gain may be secondary to an adaptive down-regulation in resting metabolic rate after weight loss is controversial.[128] A recent study evaluated this hypothesis and found no evidence to support adaptive metabolic changes to explain the tendency of weight-reduced persons to regain the lost weight.[129]

It should be noted that some concern has been raised that weight loss with concomitant caloric restriction may precipitate eating disorders or exacerbate them among those already affected.[130] To investigate this, the National Task Force on Prevention and Treatment of Obesity recently reviewed the literature evaluating relations among dieting, weight loss treatment, weight cycling, eating disorders and psycho-logical functioning in overweight and obese adults.[131] They concluded that "concerns that dieting induces eating disorders or other psycho-logical dysfunction in overweight and obese adults are generally not supported by empirical studies."

Professional counseling

Counseling by physicians and other health professionals can be very effective in improving a patient's lifestyle since most people will follow professional advice, especially if its importance is clearly explained. Counseling about weight reduction should include advice about weight maintenance for all adults and caloric restric-tion and increased physical activity for all overweight persons. Yet, relevent physician advice is clearly not as frequent as it should be. Moreover, obese patients have significantly more confidence in health counseling and treatment of their disorder from non-obese than from obese physicians.[132]

People often cite professional advice as a major motivating factor in their decision to become physically active;[133] however, the degree of motivation depends significantly on the professional's attitude about physical activity. Thus, a 1991 study reported that 59% of primary care physicians believed that regular physical activity was very important for their patients; however, only 24% believed they would be able to modify patient behavior.[134] Unfortunately, 41% of the physicians apparently did not believe that regular physical activity was important.

In a national population-based survey, Wee and associates[135] reported that of the 17,317 respondents, only slightly over half (9299) responded to the question about exercise and physician counseling. Of these, 34% reported being counseled about exercise. Older patients (≥ 30 years) were counseled more often than younger patients; those 40 to 49 years were counseled most often. In addition, patients with annual incomes above US$50,000, those with college degrees, those with higher levels of physical activity, and those who were overweight to obese (BMI > 25 kg/m^2) were more likely to be counseled.

The low proportion of office visits that include dietary counseling is related to physician attitudes about dietary advice.[133] Although about one-half of US adults are overweight, Kuczmarski *et al.*[11] reported that only 10.4% were counseled for weight reduction. Others[136] reported on 12,835 obese adults (BMI > 30 kg/m^2) 18 years and older who had visited their physician during the previous 12 months. Here, 2% of obese patients reported they were advised to lose weight. Those most likely to receive advice were female, middle-aged, more educated, lived in the northeast, reported poorer perceived health, were more obese and had diabetes mellitus.

Importantly, those who received advice to lose weight were significantly more likely to report trying to lose weight than those who did not. Taira and co-workers[137] examined the relationship between patient income, health risk behaviors, the prevalence of physician discussion of these behaviors, and the receptiveness of patients to their physicians' advice. They concluded that physicians need to be more diligent in identifying and counseling low-income patients with regards to diet and exercise. They should also be more diligent in counseling high income patients to stop smoking. In some cases, psychiatric help may be advisable since about one in four persons seeing a primary care physician for weight problems has a psychiatric disorder (mainly depression).[138]

To aid physicians and other health care providers, the American College of Sports Medicine recently published appropriate intervention strategies for weight loss and prevention of regaining weight in adults.[139] The following guidelines were recommended for weight loss treatment and prevention of weight regain.

(1) Overweight individuals (BMI 25–29.9 kg/m^2) should consider reducing their body weight, especially if the increased BMI is accompanied by abdominal adiposity. All obese individuals (BMI $\geq$ 30 kg/m^2) are encouraged to seek weight loss treatment.

(2) Overweight and obese individuals should target reducing their body weight by at least 5 to 10% and maintain at least this amount of weight loss long-term.

(3) Individuals should strive for long-term weight maintenance and prevention of weight regain.

(4) Weight loss programs should target changing both eating and exercise behaviors. Moreover, programs targeting these modifications should incorportate strong behavioral modification strategies to facilitate the adoption and maintenance of the desired behavioral changes.

(5) Overweight and obese individuals should reduce their current level of energy intake by 500 to 1000 kcal/day. Dietary fat should constitute no more than 30% of the total energy intake.

(6) Overweight and obese persons should progressively increase their moderate intensity physical activity to a minimum of 150 minutes/week. However, for long-term weight loss, this leisure-time physical activity should be increased to 200 to 300 minutes/week.

(7) Resistance exercise should supplement the endurance exercise program to improve muscle strength and endurance.

(8) Pharmacotherapy for weight loss should be used only in individuals with a BMI $\geq$ 30 kg/m^2. Moreover, they should only

be used in combination with a strong behavioral intervention program that focuses on eating and exercise modifications.

Adaptation of the treatment model used for smoking cessation into the National Institutes of Health evidence-based obesity guidelines has been developed.[140,141] This weight-loss counseling tool consists of the 5 A's: (1) Assess obesity risk; (2) Ask about readiness to lose weight; (3) Advise in designing a weight-control program; (4) Assist in establishing appropriate intervention; and (5) Arrange for follow-up. These guidelines were recently discussed in detail.[142]

Commercial weight loss programs have also been recommended. However, since their efficacy has only rarely been rigorously evaluated, Heshka *et al.*[143] compared weight loss and health benefits achieved and maintained through a self-help weight-loss program versus a structured commercial program. The self-help program consisted of two 20-minute counseling sessions with a nutritionist and provision of self-help resources (i.e. printed dietary and exercise guidelines, public library materials, websites, etc.). The commercial weight-loss program consisted of a food plan, an activity plan and a cognitive restructuring behavior modification plan at weekly meetings. The authors concluded that the structured commercial plan "provided modest weight loss but more than self-help over a two-year period."

The management of childhood and adolescent obesity is also critical, not only because of the marked increase in the prevalence of obesity in these young people, but to the potentially serious consequences they will face in adulthood. To control the obesity crisis facing American children and adolescents, immediate action is needed. This must include education, research and appropriate intervention directed not only to health care professionals, but toward policy makers, teachers, community leaders and parents, as well as children. In 1996, the Maternal and Child Health Bureau, Health Resources and Services Administration, Department of Health and Human Services, and the National Center for Education in Maternal and Child Health convened an expert committee to recommend the medical, emotional and behavioral evaluations that should precede efforts to control weight and introduce previously proven interventions in behavior programs.[144] The major recommendations included the following:

(1) children with a BMI greater than or equal to the 85th percentile with obesity complications should undergo evaluation;
(2) a BMI greater than or equal to the 95th percentile, with or without complications, should undergo evaluation and possible treatment;
(3) health professionals should be aware of the signs of rare exogenous causes of obesity (e.g. genetic syndromes, endocrine abnormalities, psychologic disorders);
(4) overweight/obese children should be screened for hypertension, dyslipidemias, orthopedic disorders, sleep disorders, gall bladder disease and insulin resistance;
(5) recommendations for a weight-management program should be focused on healthy eating and adequate physical activity;
(6) early treatment should involve the parents; permanent changes should be instituted in a stepwise manner; and
(7) ongoing family support from health care professionals is essential.

A series of articles on the management of overweight children and adolescents was recently published in the journal *Pediatrics*.[145] These studies were undertaken to examine the attitudes and practices of pediatricians, pediatric nurse practitioners and registered dieticians in the assessment and treatment of overweight and obese children and adolescents. This series, as summarized by Barlow and Dietz,[146] recommended the following current and future strategies that may be helpful in alleviating this major healthcare problem.

(1) To improve the thoroughness of medical asssessment, pediatricians and pediatric nurse practitioners may require further education regarding the risks and different obesity-related disorders and the best screening techniques. The screening tests should be implemented during office visits.
(2) Checklists or forms for medical records similar to those prepared for well-child visits could be prepared and tested for their effectiveness.

(3) Providers must assess the readiness of overweight/obese children to change their behavior. A lack of patient motivation must be addressed. Established "wellness" techniques, such as those used by health authorities for regular exercise, smoking cessation and seatbelt use, could be applied for weight control.

(4) Reducing sedentary behavior is critical. The control of television time in clinical and school-based programs has proven successful. Thus, health care providers, schools and communities should aggressively promote this strategy and encourage parents and other family members to engage in collective physical activities to reduce television time.

(5) Media promotion of healthy eating and regular physical activity could be very beneficial, just as it has been for promoting smoking cessation.

(6) Since markedly obese children are at risk for serious health problems, more intensive medical and psychological care is needed.

Surgical intervention

Bariatrics is the field of medicine that specializes in treating obesity. In selected morbidly obese individuals (i.e. BMI $\geq$ 40 kg/m^2), surgical treatment (i.e. bariatric surgery) to restrict gastric volume may be successful in those in whom other attempts have failed.[147] For this purpose, there are currently three types of gastric restrictive operations: gastric banding, stapled gastroplasty and Roux-en-Y gastric bypass. Persons who undergo these procedures must eat very small food portions since the smaller stomach cannot hold a lot of solid food.

These surgical procedures have generally proven to be quite effective. For example, two recent publications[148,149] reported that gastric banding, a minimally invasive surgical procedure, "is a safe and effective new method in the management of severe obesity."[148] This technique reportedly can "noticeably improve the quality of life in obese patients. Half of the excess body weight can be effortlessly lost within two years."[149] The subject of bariatric surgery was recently reviewed and the basic surgical techniques were illustrated.[150] Since the demand for surgical intervention has significantly increased, scientific and ethical questions were recently addressed.[151]

Economic Costs of Obesity and Physical Inactivity

A recent medical literature review of English-language articles on the medical costs of obesity between 1990 and 2001 suggested that obesity accounts for 5.5 to 7.0% of national health expenditures in the US and 2.0 to 3.5% in other countries.[152] Thus, the economic effect of obesity in the US from both societal and payer perspectives is enormous. In 1998, Wolf[153] reported that the relatively recent rapid increase in obesity has resulted in a 50% increase in lost productivity, 36% increase in restricted activity and 28% increase in the number of hospitalized days. Although the cost of obesity is comparable to that of several chronic diseases (e.g. type 2 diabetes, CHD and hypertension), it receives relatively little attention. In addition, overweight and obesity are major risk factors for several chronic diseases. Indeed, adults at even modest levels of adiposity are at increased risk for CHD,[154,155] type 2 diabetes mellitus,[156,157] postmenopausal breast cancer[158] and mortality.[159] Morbidity related to physical inactivity include cardiovascular disease,[160] colon cancer,[161] osteoporosis[162] and type 2 diabetes.[163] Overweight and obesity also exacerbate hypertension, osteoarthritis and elevated serum cholesterol levels.

The estimated US costs attributable to obesity for various medical disorders in 1996 were as follows:[164] US$11.3 billion for type 2 diabetes; US$22.2 billion for cardiovascular disease; US$2.4 billion for gall bladder disease; US$1.5 billion for hypertension; and US$1.9 billion for breast and colon cancer. These figures, although considered to be conservative, totaled US$39.3 billion or 5.5% of the total costs of illness. In 1990, the direct cost of obesity-associated diseases was estimated at US$45.8 billion.[165] The indirect obesity cost was estimated at US$23 billion, bringing the total 1990 economic cost to US$68.8 billion. In a later study, Colditz[166] assessed the economic costs of obesity and physical inactivity for 1995. He reported a conservative estimate of the direct annual costs of lack of physical activity to be US$24 billion; direct costs of obesity totaled US$70 billion per year. These latter costs were independent of those resulting from physical inactivity. He concluded that physical inactivity and obesity accounted for at least 9.4% of the 1995 national health care costs. In a follow-up report, Wolf and Colditz[167] updated and revised the estimates of the economic impact attributable to obesity (BMI $\geq$ 30 kg/m^2) in 1995 dollars. These diseases included type 2 diabetes mellitus, hypertension, CHD, gallbladder disease, osteoarthritis and several cancers (breast, endometrial and colon). Thus, the total 1995 cost attributable to obesity was US$99.2 billion [includes direct medical costs (US$51.64 billion, lost productivity, lost work, bed-days, restricted activity and physician visits)]. The authors concluded that "the economic and personal health cost of overweight and obesity are enormous and compromise the health of the United States." Since the costs of being overweight (BMI 25–29.9 kg/m^2) were not addressed, the total costs were significantly higher. Moreover, since obesity has continued to rise since 1995, the current costs are undoubtedly much greater. However, the economic burden of obesity is not limited to adults. Thus, from 1979–1981 to 1997–1999 the percentage of hospital discharges of youths aged six to 17 years with obesity-associated diseases almost doubled (1.4–2.36%).[168] Based on 2001 constant US dollar value, the obesity-associated annual hospital costs increased more than three-fold (US$35 million in 1979–1981; US$127 million during 1997–1999).

Quesenberry *et al.*[169] reported an association between BMI and annual rates of inpatient days, number and costs of outpatient visits, outpatient pharmacy, laboratory and total costs. They found that relative to a BMI of 20 to 24.9 kg/m^2, mean annual total costs were 25% greater among those with a BMI of 30 to 34.9 kg/m^2 and 44% higher among those with a BMI of 35 kg/m^2 or more. Interestingly, surgical treatments that resulted in a maintained average weight reduction of 16% reportedly will not reduce total hospital costs compared with conventionally treated obese patients, at least over the first six years.[170] However, the authors noted that these costs could possibly be reduced in a ten- to 20-year perspective.

Diseases and Disorders Associated with Excess Body Weight

There are numerous diseases and disorders associated with excess body weight (i.e. BMI > 25.0 kg/m²; Table 2.4). For example, a recent ten-year follow-up (1986–1996) of middle-aged women (Nurses' Health Study) and men (Health Professionals Follow-up Study) found that the risk of developing diabetes, gall stones, hypertension, heart disease, stroke and colon cancer increased significantly with increasing BMI greater than 24.9 kg/m².[171] Moreover, these researchers found that "the dose-response relationship between BMI and the risk of developing chronic diseases was evident even among adults in the upper half of the healthy weight average (i.e. BMI 22.0–24.9 kg/m²)." Thus, to completely minimize the risk of these chronic diseases, the BMI would have to be 18.5 to 21.9 kg/m². In addition, sleep apnea, chronic hypoxia and hypercapnia and degenerative joint disease,[172] as well as ischemic stroke, pulmonary dysfunction, steatohepatitis, osteoarthritis and increased mortality[14] are associated with increased body weight. In the most recent study, Mokdad and associates[173] confirmed the association between overweight and obesity with diabetes, hypertension and inceased plasma cholesterol. Arthritis, asthma and overall poor health status were also significantly associated with excess body weight. Furthermore, the risk of having two or more of these diseases/disorders increase with body weight across all racial and ethnic subgroups.[174]

Table 2.4: Overweight/Obesity-Related Diseases and Disorders

Arthritis	Gout
Asthma	Hypertension
Abnormal blood lipids	Insulin resistance
Adult onset asthma	Ischemic stroke
Cancer (several forms)	Mortality
Coronary heart disease	Psychopathology
Daytime sleepiness	Quality of life
Degenerative joint disease	Respiratory diseases
Type 2 diabetes mellitus	Sleep apnea
Gallbladder disease	Steatohepatitis

The prevalence of obesity-related co-morbidities strongly emphasizes the importance of concerted efforts to prevent and treat overweight/ obese persons rather than just the associated co-morbidities. This would not only decrease the prevalence of these weight-associated disorders and related medical costs, but improve the quality of life (i.e. physical function and vitality and decreased bodily pain),[175] as well as overall life expectancy. To examine this latter point, Gregg and associates[176] studied 6391 overweight and obese persons who were 35 years and older over a nine-year period in which they evaluated both the intention to lose weight and actual weight change. After adjusting for age, sex, ethnicity, education level, smoking, health status, health care utilization and initial BMI, those who reported intentional weight loss had a 24% lower all-cause mortality rate than those not trying to lose weight and had no weight loss.

Hypertension

The lifetime risk statistic is the probability that a person will develop hypertension over the course of his or her remaining lifetime. To estimate the residual lifetime risk for hypertension in older Americans, Vasan *et al.*[177] studied 1298 individuals aged 55 to 65 years who were free of hypertension at baseline. From their data, they estimated that the residual lifetime risk for developing hypertension (i.e. $\geq$140/90 mm Hg) for individuals 55 years and older is 90%.

The relationship between obesity and hypertension has been recognized since 1923;[178] numerous subsequent epidemiologic studies have confirmed this close association.[179] However, a complete understanding of this relationship is not currently known. An early Framingham study provided strong evidence that hypertensive persons gain weight more readily than normotensive individuals.[180] Their data suggested that about 78% of essential hypertension in men and 65% of essential hypertension in women was directly attributed to obesity. Moreover, they reported that weight gain during early adult life was an important risk factor for the subsequent development of hypertension. In a cross-sectional study (1976–1980) involving a representative sample of Americans, van Italle[181] reported that the prevalence of hypertension among overweight adults was 2.9 times that of non-overweight adults; the risk was 5.6 times greater in people aged 20 to 44 years than in those 45 to 74 years. In this study, the BMI cut-off was 27.8 kg/m^2 for men and 27.3 kg/m^2 for women (levels $\geq$ 25–29.9 kg/m^2 overweight; $\geq$30 kg/m^2 obese). A similar cross-sectional study found that for individuals who are 20% or more overweight, the prevalence of hypertension is double that of persons of normal weight.[182]

It is also now apparent that the association between obesity and hypertension is not limited to adults. Indeed, once considered rare, primary hypertension in obese children has become "a problem of epidemic proportions." Thus, in a recent literature review, Sorof and Daniels[183] reported that obese children are "at approximately a three-fold higher risk for hypertension than non-obese children." Moreover, childhood hypertension increases across the entire range of BMI values.

Although obesity is associated with various factors, including neuroendocrine disorders, increased cardiac output, blood volume, sodium stores and possible neural abnormalities, none of them fully differentiate between hypertensive and normotensive people.[184] Masuo and associates[185] recently evaluated the contribution of sympathetic nervous system activity to weight gain-induced blood pressure elevation and concluded that sympathetic nervous activation with weight gain is a major mechanism of increased blood pressure. There is also a significant heritable component to blood pressure levels and hypertension. Heritability estimates of resting systolic and diastolic blood pressures, based on family studies, reportedly vary from 15 to 35%; twin study estimates are approximately 30 to 40% for women and 60% for men.[186] Moreover, a heritable component to salt sensitivity has been reported in blacks where numerous studies have reported a significantly higher prevalence of hypertension than in whites in the US.[187] A recent report by Larson *et al.*,[188] however, revealed no association between hypertension status of any of three physiologically important candidate gene mutations. This lack of association persisted after stratification of this sample of African Americans by gender and body size.

Various studies have demonstrated that nutritional changes with weight loss have resulted in a significant reduction in blood pressure. Stamler *et al.*[189] reported that nutritional therapy may substitute for drugs in a significant proportion of hypertensives. This four-year trial assessed whether nutritional therapy in less severe hypertensives can result in discontinuance of antihypertensive drugs. The participants were divided into three groups: (1) discontinue drug therapy, reduce body weight, excess salt and alcohol; (2) discontinue drug therapy with no nutritional changes; and (3) continue drug therapy without nutritional changes. Their data showed that 30% of group 1 lost and maintained at least a ten-pound (4.5 kg) weight reduction; sodium intake fell 36%, and there was a modest reduction of alcohol intake. At four years, 39% of group 1 remained normotensive without drug therapy compared with 5% of group 2. Others recently confirmed that weight loss and sodium reduction is a feasible, effective and safe non-pharmacologic therapy for hypertension in older individuals.[190]

Masuo *et al.*[191] reported that weight loss in obese hypertensives was associated with favorable metabolic improvements. Moreover, these improvements were amplified when combined with pharmacologic treatment. In addition, Ben-Dov and associates[192] recently reported that marked weight reduction in morbidly obese people (BMI > 40 kg/m^2) lowers both resting and exercise blood pressures. They further recommended that gastroplasty should be considered in markedly obese hypertensive people who are not well controlled with conventional therapies and who fail to lose or maintain a reduced weight by diet alone.

Current recommendations for the primary prevention of hypertension consist of a population-based approach and an intensive target strategy focused on those who are at high risk for hypertension.[193] These complementary strategies emphasize the following six proven approaches in preventing blood pressure elevation: (1) maintain normal body weight (BMI ≤ 24.9 kg/m^2); (2) engage in moderate physical activity; (3) limit alcohol consumption; (4) reduce sodium intake; (5) maintain adequate potassium intake; and (6) consume a diet rich in fruits and vegetables, low-fat dairy products, and reduced saturated and total fat.

Coronary heart disease

Although the recent decline in the mortality rate attributed to CHD is encouraging, this disease remains the leading cause of death in Western societies among both men and women. The pathogenesis of CHD is complex and multifactorial. The commonly recognized risk factors include, in addition to advancing age and male sex until women reach menopause, the following: serum lipid levels (i.e. increased total cholesterol, low density lipoprotein and triglycerides, decreased high density lipoprotein, and others), increased blood pressure, diabetes mellitus, cigarette smoking, physical inactivity, and being overweight/obese. Less well appreciated risk factors are blood levels of homocysteine, C-reactive protein, uric acid, fibrinogen and hematocrit, among others (Chapter 1).

The role of obesity in CHD morbidity and mortality has been somewhat controversial. Questions regarding its specific role in this disorder have been raised since obesity enhances various major risk factors for CHD including elevated blood cholesterol and triglyceride levels, decreased high density lipoprotein levels, diabetes mellitus and hypertension. Nevertheless, obesity has been shown to be an independent risk factor for CHD.[194] Long-term observational studies have also provided evidence that overweight is an independent predictor of overall mortality, as well as coronary atherosclerosis, in both men and women.[195,196] In addition, this increase in relative risk begins at overweight levels often considered clinically insignificant.

Body mass index and CHD

Rimm *et al.*[197] reported a 72% increased risk for non-fatal or fatal CHD in middle-aged men with a BMI of 25 to 29 kg/m^2 (i.e. overweight) compared with men having a BMI of less than 23 kg/m². More specifically, they found that among men younger than 65 years, the relative risk was 1.72 for a BMI of 25.0 to 28.9 kg/m², 2.61 for BMI 29.0 to 32.9 kg/m² and 3.44 for those with a BMI of 33 kg/m² or more compared to men with a BMI of 23 kg/m² or less. Among men 65 years and older, the association between BMI and CHD risk was weaker. However, the waist-to-hip ratio was a much stronger risk predictor than BMI (relative risk 2.76 between the extreme quintiles).

Overweight is also a major risk factor for CHD in women. In a recent longitudinal study,[198] 115,886 women (Nurses' Health Study) 30–55 years old and free of CHD, stroke or cancer were followed for eight years. They found that a higher BMI was associated with the occurrence in each category of CHD. After adjustment for age and smoking, the relative risk for non-fatal myocardial infarction and fatal CHD were as follows: 1.0 for BMI less than 21 kg/m², 1.3 for BMI 21 to less than 25 kg/m², 1.8 for BMI 25 to less than 29 kg/m² and 3.3 for BMI greater than 29 kg/m². Although controlling for a history of hypertension, diabetes mellitus and increased serum cholesterol levels attenuated the strength of the association, even mild-to-moderate overweight increased the risk for CHD. Other important data linking BMI and CHD involved non-smoking male Seventh-day Adventists[199] who were followed for 26 years. Here, three important findings were emphasized: (1) there was no increased mortality rate in the leanest group; (2) a significant trend toward increasing mortality rate with increasing BMI for all end points studied was noted; and (3) survival analysis showed the protective effect associated with low BMI decreased with advancing age and disappeared by 90 years of age. Others reported the protective effect associated with the lowest BMI quintile for CHD death significantly decreased with advancing age; however, the effect remained greater than 1.0 for men at all ages.[200]

Obesity has also been shown to be an important risk factor in non-Caucasian populations. Although CHD used to be rare among American Indians, there has been a highly significant increase in recent years. Howard and associates[201] recently reported their findings involving 13 American Indian communities in Arizona,

Oklahoma and North/South Dakota. They found that the prevalence rate of CHD among American Indian men and women was about two-fold higher than those reported in the Atherosclerosis Risk Communities Study.[202] The significant CHD risk factors, in addition to age, were obesity, increased blood lipid levels, diabetes and hypertension. In addition, Lee et al.[203] recently reported the relationship between obesity and cardiovascular disease in a cross-sectional clinical study of Hong Kong Chinese subjects. Using a BMI of 19.0 to 20.9 kg/m^2 as the reference interval, the lowest CHD risk was associated with a BMI of less than 23.0 kg/m^2; the risk increased to 3.1 with a BMI of 23.0 to 24.9 kg/m^2 and 5.0 with a BMI greater than 25.0 kg/m^2. To further evaluate the association between obesity and atherosclerosis, McGill et al.[204] studied the arteries (e.g. coronary and renal), blood lipid levels, other tissues and the BMI from about 3000 forensic autopsies performed on persons aged 15 to 34 years dying of external causes. Although BMI was not statistically associated with coronary atherosclerosis in young women, albeit there was a trend, obesity was significantly associated with accelerated coronary atherosclerosis in adolescent and young adult males.

Abdominal adiposity has also been associated with increased cardiovascular morbidity and mortality through mechanisms suggesting a link between the metabolic disorder and platelet and vascular abnormalities. To further investigate this possible association, Davi et al.[205] studied the clinical and biochemical determinants of lipid peroxidation (i.e. urinary 8-isoprostaglandin $F_{2\alpha}$ and 11-dehydrothromboxane B_2), plasma levels of the inflammation marker C-reactive protein, plasma insulin and leptin. Their results showed that abdominal obesity was associated with increased lipid peroxidation (i.e. oxidative stress associated with increased free radicals) and persistant platelet activation, which may lead to thrombosis. The authors concluded that "these abnormalities are driven by inflammatory triggers related to the degree of abdominal adiposity and are, at least in part, reversible with a successful weight-loss program." Similarly, Esposito et al.[206] conducted a multidisciplinary program aimed at reducing body weight in obese women through lifestyle changes. In those who consumed more foods rich in complex carbohydrates, monounsaturated fat and fiber, and had a lower ratio of omega-6 to omega-3 fatty acids, lower saturated fat and cholesterol intake, there was a significant decrease in BMI, interleukin-6, interleukin-18 and C-reactive protein while adiponectin levels increased. In addition to the improvement in these vascular inflammation markers, there was a reduction in insulin resistance.

Obesity and heart failure

According to the American Heart Association, heart failure is a major health problem of increasing concern.[207] As such, the prevention of heart failure by identification of the major risk factors and preclinical phases of the disorder is very important. Numerous studies have shown that obesity is consistently associated with left ventricular hypertrophy and dilatation, which are well-known precursors of heart failure.[208,209]

To further evaluate the relationship between obesity and the risk of heart failure, Kenchaiah and associates[210] investigated the relation between the BMI and the incidence of heart failure among 5881 individuals from the Framingham Heart Study (mean age, 55 years; 54% women). After adjustment for established risk factors, the risk of heart failure was 5% for men and 7% for women for each increment of one in BMI. Thus, compared to those with a normal BMI, obese subjects (BMI $\geq$ 30 kg/m^2) had twice the risk of heart failure. For women, the hazard ratio was 2.12; for men it was 1.90. Moreover, there was a graded increase in heart failure risk across categories of BMI.

Abdominal adiposity and CHD

As demonstrated above, obesity is generally defined by the BMI. However, whether regional fat distribution, as measured by the waist-to-hip ratio (WHR) or waist circumference (WC), is an independent risk factor has been debated. However, several reports have demonstrated that the WHR is an independent risk factor for CHD in men[197,211,212] and probably in women.[212,213] To better clarify the role of abdominal obesity as an independent risk factor in women, Rexrode and associates[214] studied 44,702 women (Nurses' Health Study) aged 40 to 65 years over an eight-year period. After adjusting for BMI and other common CHD risk factors, they found that women with a WHR of 0.88 or higher had a relative risk of 3.25 for CHD compared with women with a WHR of less than 0.72. In those with a WC of 38 inches (96.5 cm) or more, the risk ratio was 3.06. Those with a WHR of 0.76 or more or a WC of 30 inches (76.2 cm) or greater had more than a two-fold higher risk for CHD. Moreover, the WHR and WC were independently associated with an increased risk for CHD in women with a BMI of 25 kg/m^2 or less. Other adiposity measures and their relationship to CHD have also been reported. For example, Folsom and associates[215] found a significant increase in the prevalence of CHD in 45- to 65-year-old black men and women where obesity was defined by using the sum of subscapular and triceps skin fold measurements. Additional analyses also showed that abdominal adiposity increased the risk for CHD. As a result of these and other studies, the American Heart Association reclassified obesity as a major modifiable risk factor for CHD in 1998.[216]

Prevention of CHD

Although considerable effort has focused on the pharmacologic treatment of increased blood lipid levels, diabetes mellitus and hypertension, these treatments may be associated with side effects, require considerable medical intervention, and are expensive. Importantly, changes in diet and lifestyle are also highly effective in the treatment and prevention of CHD. For example, Katzel *et al.*[217] carried out a randomized controlled trial involving 170 obese (BMI 30 $\pm$ 1 kg/m^2) middle-aged and older men which involved three nine-month interventions: diet-induced weight loss, aerobic exercise training and a weight maintenance control group. They found that weight loss significantly improved lipoprotein concentrations, glucose tolerance, blood pressure and postprandial insulin levels. Aerobic exercise, in the absence of weight loss, had significantly fewer beneficial effects on these risk factors. Others[218] assessed the validity of the 1990 US weight guidelines for women that support a significant weight gain at about 35 years of age. The guidelines recommend a BMI range of 21 to 27 kg/m^2 in terms of CHD risk. However, this report, which included 115,818 women (Nurse's Health Study) and used a BMI reference of 21 kg/m^2 or less, found a risk of 1.19 for a BMI of 21 kg/m^2 to 22.9 kg/m^2; 1.46 for a BMI of 23 to 24.9 kg/m^2; 2.06 for a BMI of 25 to 28.9 kg/m^2; and 3.56 for a BMI of 29 kg/m^2 or higher. In women who gained weight after 18 years of age, compared with those with no weight gain, the relative risks were 1.25 for a 11 to 17 pound (5–7.9 kg) gain; 1.64 for a 17 to 24 pound (8 to 10.9 kg) gain; 1.92 for a 24 to 42 pound (11–19 kg) gain; and 2.65 for a gain of 44 pounds (20 kg) or more. The authors concluded that the current guidelines "may be falsely reassuring to the large proportion of women older than 35 years who are within the current guidelines. ..."

This, and other reports, strongly encourage the prevention of fat accumulation by improved diet and lifestyle. In this regard, a recent report[219] from the Nurses' Health Study defined subjects at low risk as those who were not currently smoking, had a BMI less than 25 kg/m^2, consumed an average of at least half a drink of alcoholic beverage each day, were actively involved in moderate-to-vigorous physical activity (30 minutes/day minimum), and scored in the highest 40% of the cohort for a healthy diet (i.e. high in cereal fiber, marine n-3 fatty acids and folate, high ratio of polyunsaturated fatty acids to saturated fatty acids, low trans fatty acids and glycemic load). Their results indicated that although many of these factors were correlated, each was independent in predicting the risk of CHD after adjustment for age, family history, blood pressure, increased blood total cholesterol level and menopausal status. Women in the low-risk category had a relative risk of CHD of 0.17 compared with all other women. In addition, 82% of the coronary events during the study could be attributed to lack of adherence to this low-risk pattern.

With regards to prevention, a 1995–1996 survey of patients with CHD in nine European countries found substantial potential for risk reduction (EUROASPIRE I).[220] A follow-up survey (EUROASPIRE II) was carried out in 1999–2000 to determine whether the risks for

CHD had decreased.[221] There were 3569 patients with CHD in the first survey and 3379 in the second. The findings were as follows: (1) obesity (BMI $\geq$ 30 kg/m^2) increased from 25.3% to 32.8%; (2) smoking remained essentially unchanged (19.4% versus 20.8%); (3) hypertension remained essentially unchanged (55.4% versus 53.9%); (4) increased total serum cholesterol ($\geq$5.0 mmol/L; about 200 mg/dL) decreased significantly (86.2% to 58.8%); and (5) aspirin or other antiplatelet therapy was unchanged (83.9%). The study panel concluded that adverse lifestyle trends in Europeans with CHD remained serious and that there was "a collective failure of medical practice in Europe to achieve the substantial potential among patients with CHD to reduce the risk of recurrent disease and death." These same problems are probably even greater for Americans since they are significantly more overweight and obese than the Europeans.

Blood lipid levels

The association between atherosclerosis and increased serum cholesterol levels was first reported in 1938 when an increased prevalence of premature CHD and acute myocardial infarction was recognized in patients with hereditary xanthomatosis.[222,223] Since then numerous studies in both men and women have shown that, in addition to total cholesterol (TC), other lipid fractions are also correlated with CHD;[224] these include increased blood levels of low-density lipoprotein cholesterol (LDL-C), triglycerides, lipoprotein (a) and apolipoprotein B, decreased high-density lipoprotein cholesterol (HDL-C) and increased TC to HDL-C ratio.

Although several early reports suggested a correlation between body weight and TC, they involved very few subjects whose relative weights were usually calculated from their observed weight and an expected weight based on age, sex and height. Perhaps one of the most complete early studies of the relationship between serum cholesterol and body fatness was reported in 1966 when Montoye and associates[225] studied these parameters in an entire community of 6500 male and female subjects aged four to over 80 years. They concluded that "a low but statistically significant relationship was found between serum cholesterol levels and body fatness, even at an early age and particularly among male subjects."

Serum HDL levels are strongly and inversely correlated with CHD.[226] In addition, the concentration of plasma HDL-C correlates inversely with body mass.[227] This latter study, involving 6865 white children and adults (males, females about equal), found that overall weight, weight/height, weight/height^2 and weight/height^3 were significantly associated with triglyceride levels and inversely associated with HDL-C. After multiple regression analysis which included cigarette smoking, alcohol intake and exogeneous estrogen use, the weight/height^2 index was significantly and inversely correlated with HDL-C levels in both children and adults of both sexes.

Several studies have shown a direct relationship between abdominal obesity and CHD which is partially mediated through altered dyslipidemia metabolism. In a recent report,[228] dyslipidemia (defined as TC/HDL-C ratio > 5.0) was compared with waist-to-hip ratio (WHR) and waist circumference (WC) [abdominal obesity: WHR ≥ 0.90 in men, 0.80 in women; WC ≥ 94 cm in men (42.7 inches), >80 cm in women (36.4 inches)]; the data showed a consistent direct association between abdominal obesity and dyslipidemia. Moreover, these findings held for caucasians from two different regions and for persons of black descent. The authors emphasized that since the data was consistent across ethnicities and environments, the hypothesis of a common etiopathological mechanism is strengthened.

Others[229] also reported an inverse relationship between serum HDL-C levels and visceral obesity, while hyperinsulinemia, increased plasma triglycerides and small dense LDL particles were directly associated. Pouliot *et al.*[230] also reported an inverse relationship between abdominal obesity and plasma HDL-C and a positive correlation with plasma triglyceride and insulin levels. The glucose and insulin areas under the curves measured during an oral glucose tolerance test also correlated with abdominal fat.

Importantly weight loss has been shown to improve lipid profiles in postmenopausal obese women.[231] This study, which extended over a nine-month period, showed that women who reduced their body weight by 14% significantly lowered their plasma concentrations of LDL-C and triglycerides and raised their plasma HDL-C levels. The TC/HDL-C ratio was also significantly decreased. Childhood and adolescent obesity has also been associated with increased plasma levels of TC, triglycerides and LDL-C.[232] These authors reported that in a multidisciplinary weight reduction program, a combination of diet, behavior modification and exercise was effective in lowering these lipid levels in both boys and girls. They also noted that obese girls were more susceptible than boys to decreases in their plasma LDL-C concentrations.

Type 2 diabetes mellitus

Type 2 diabetes mellitus (non-insulin-dependent diabetes; late-onset diabetes), which comprises at least 90% of all diabetics, has increased dramatically over the past few decades and is now the sixth leading cause of death in the US,[233] but may actually be higher since it is an important risk factor for numerous medical conditions. Thus, diabetics are at risk for the development of diabetic ketoacidosis, hyperglycemic hyperosmolar non-ketotic coma and hypoglycemia, as well as neurologic deficits and skin disorders. Diabetes is also a major risk factor for premature CHD and stroke and is a leading cause of blindness, kidney failure and limb amputation. In the year 2000, there were an estimated 110 million people worldwide with diabetes; in 2010, an estimated 220 million people will be diabetic.[234]

Harris *et al.*[235] estimated that the prevalence of diagnosed diabetes in 1988–1994 was about 5.1% of American adults 20 or more years of age. When extrapolated to the 1997 American population, the total was 10.2 million people; an additional 5.4 million Americans were estimated to be diabetic but undiagnosed. Moreover, the number of individuals with impaired fasting glucose was estimated to be 13.4 million. A more recent study[236] reported that the prevalence of diabetes rose from 4.9% in 1990 to 6.5% in 1998 — an increase of 33% in eight years. This translates into about 13 million known diabetics in 1998, and presumably more than the 5.3 million undiagnosed cases noted above. These authors reported increases in both sexes and all ages, ethnic groups, education levels and in most states. Hispanics had a 38% increase compared with 27% of whites and 26% of blacks. They, among others, emphasized that the prevalence of diabetes is highly correlated with the prevalence of obesity. These latter authors sought to determine whether this increase was continuing.[237] Using 1999 data from the Behavioral Risk Factor Surveilance System, they found the prevalence increased to 6.9% in 1999, a 6% increase in just one year. The average weight also increased from 76.2 kg in 1998 (167.4 pounds) to 76.7 kg (168.7 pounds) in 1999. By the year 2050, an estimated 29 million Americans will suffer from type 2 diabetes.[238] The largest percent increase in diagnosed diabetes is expected in individuals aged 75 years and older.

African American men are reportedly 20 to 50% more likely and African American women greater than 100% more likely to develop type 2 diabetes than white men and women, respectively.[239,240] There has also been a marked increase in the prevalence of diabetes in American Indians. For example, the prevalence of diabetes in Navajos over the past several decades has markedly increased. In 1981 an estimated 10% of Navajos over age 45 years had diabetes; in 1996 the prevalence was 21.2%.[241] Furthermore, a survey conducted between 1931 and 1936 reported only one case of diabetes in 6331 Navajo hospital admissions.[242] Major risk factors in both African Americans and Navajos include being overweight and physically inactive. Others[243] reported that the number of Native Americans and Alaskan Natives of all ages diagnosed with diabetes increased from 43,262 to 64,474 between 1990 and 1997. In 1997, the age-adjusted prevalence among these two groups was 8.0%. Although the prevalences of diabetes during 1990–1997 was higher among women, the rate of increase was greater among men (37% versus 25%). Interestingly, the 1997 age-adjusted prevalence varied by region, ranging from 3% in Alaska to 17% in the Atlantic region.

In 1986, it was conservatively estimated that the annual medical costs of diabetes were US$11.6 billion.[244] In 1992 total costs rose to about US$45.2 billion,[245] which was almost 15% of the national health care expenditures,[246] and in 1997 the estimated total diabetic costs had risen to US$77.7 billion.[247] The current annual costs are at least US$100 billion[248] and will continue to rapidly escalate unless widespread lifestyle changes occur.

Valdmanis and co-investigators[249] assessed the cost and burden of diabetes in broad terms of economic status as reflected in income, employment, general health, disability days, general health status and medical care access. Their findings for diabetics, compared with controls matched for age, sex and race/ethnicity for the most recent 30 days, were respectively as follows: (1) poor physical health, 8.3 versus 3.0 days; (2) poor mental health, 2.8 versus 1.8 days; (3) total disability, 5.2 versus 1.3 days; and (4) lower general health status, 50% versus 20%. In addition, among persons with diabetes, 16% had no health insurance compared with 10% of the matched group; 22% of persons with diabetes needed a physician but were unable to pay for the services compared with 11% for the matched group; and 16% of diabetics were unemployed compared with 3% of the comparison group. Thus, in this Oklahoma study, persons with diabetes were disadvantaged on all measures of well-being compared with the matched control group.

Body weight and diabetes mellitus

The hallmark of type 2 diabetes is insulin resistance, a defect in the body's ability to remove glucose from the bloodstream despite the presence of normal or even elevated insulin levels. Thus, recent studies suggest that the disease is triggered when the delicate balance between insulin responsiveness and insulin production goes awry.[250] The exact mechanism whereby this occurs is still poorly understood. However, the current epidemic of type 2 diabetes has generally been attributed to an increasingly sedentary lifestyle and Westernized diet in genetically susceptible populations.

An association between the average weight of population groups and the prevalence of type 2 diabetes has been repeatedly observed. In an early report, the risk of diabetes was two-fold in mildly obese, five-fold in moderately obese and ten-fold in severely obese people compared with those of normal weight.[251] Moreover, both men and women are affected equally. Colditz *et al.*[252] reported on the relationship between BMI and risk of diabetes in a cohort of 113,861 American women aged 30 to 55 years in 1976; the follow-up period was eight years. Here, women with a BMI of 23.0 to 23.9 kg/m^2 were 3.6 times more likely to develop diabetes than women with a BMI of 22 kg/m^2. Moreover, the risk continued to increase as the BMI increased beyond 24 kg/m^2. In addition, after age 18 years, an increase of 20 to 35 kg (44–77 pounds) resulted in a relative risk of 11.3 and for an increase of more than 35 kg, the relative risk was 17.3. Importantly, adjustment for a family history of diabetes did not appreciably affect the relationship between BMI and diabetes. A subsequent study by the same scientific group, involving 114,281 female nurses,[253] showed similar results. In addition, the authors emphasized the importance of maintaining constant body weight throughout adult life. They also noted that the 1990 US Department of Agriculture guidelines that allow a substantial weight gain in women after age 35 years are misleading.

Chan and associates[254] investigated the relation between obesity, fat distribution and weight gain through adulthood and the risk of diabetes from a cohort of 51,529 American men. Not surprisingly, their results also showed a strong positive association between BMI and risk of diabetes in men of all ages. However, the strongest association between diabetes and weight involved the 50- to 59-year-old group. Here, the multivariate relative risk (RR) compared with a BMI of less than or equal to 23.0 kg/m^2 were as follows: BMI 24.0–24.9 kg/m^2, RR 2.9; BMI 27.0–28.9 kg/m^2, RR 13.3; BMI 31.0–32.9 kg/m^2, RR 23.0; and BMI $\geq$ 35 kg/m^2, RR 42.6. Although the RR was less for men under age 50 and over age 60, it was still highly significant in both groups. The BMI at age 21 years and absolute weight gain throughout adulthood were also significant risk factors for diabetes. On the other hand, the WHR was a good predictor of diabetes only among the top 5% while the WC was positively associated only among the top 20%. Similarly, others[255] recently reported a direct correlation between increased weight and diabetes from a national cohort of American adult men and women. However, there was no evidence that the results differed by age, sex or race. They predicted that the increase in BMI of American adults that occurred during the 1980s may portend a significant increase in type 2 diabetes with important subsequent public health consequences. Interestingly, Shaper *et al.*[256] concluded, from their study of the effects of body weight on diabetes, CHD and stroke in middle-aged men, that the healthiest BMI was about 22 kg/m^2.

Anthropometric measures of overall and central obesity as predictors of type 2 diabetes have not been studied as thoroughly as BMI, especially in women. As a result, Carey and co-workers[257] recently reported that in American women the measurement of waist circumference, with or without hip circumference, is a potentially useful and simple tool for counseling patients regarding their risk for type 2 diabetes. They found that a BMI of ≥29.9 kg/m^2, compared with a BMI of 20.1 kg/m^2, increased the risk ratio to 11.2; the risk for a waist to hip ratio of 0.86 versus 0.70 was 3.1; and the risk of a waist circumference of 36.2 inches versus 26.2 inches was 5.1. In addition, Boyko *et al.*[258] compared visceral (intra-abdominal) and regional (thoracic and thigh areas) adiposity by computed tomography in both second- and third-generation Japanese American men. They concluded that increased visceral adiposity precedes the onset of type 2 diabetes and that it is independent of fasting insulin and blood glucose levels, total and regional adiposity and family history of diabetes.

Type 2 diabetes and hypertension have both been associated with a decline in cognitive function.[259] The Atherosclerosis Risk in Communities biracial cohort, which consisted of 8729 white persons and 2234 black persons, underwent cognitive assessments on two occasions separated by six years. Subjects ranged from 47 to 70 years at the first assessment. In multivariate analysis, controlled for demographic factors, the presence of diabetes at baseline was associated with greater decline in both the digit symbol subtest (DSS) and word fluency test; those with hypertension at baseline were associated with a greater decline in the DSS alone. The association of diabetes with cognitive decline persisted when analysis was restricted to the 47- to 57-year-old subgroup. The authors suggested that control of these two disorders before age 60 may decrease the burden of cognitive impairment in later years.

Unfortunately, the prevalence of obesity and diabetes continues to increase significantly among American adults. A recent report[260] estimated the prevalence of obesity (BMI $\geq$ 30 kg/m^2), diabetes and use of weight control strategies among American adults in 2000. Here, the Behavioral Risk Factor Surveillance System was used to conduct a random survey in all states involving 184,450 persons 18 years and older. Their results showed the following: (1) obesity prevalence was 19.8%; (2) diabetes prevalence was 7.3%; (3) Mississippi had the highest rate of obesity (24.3%) and diabetes (8.8%); (4) Colorado had the lowest rate of obesity (13.8%); (5) Alaska had the lowest rate of diabetes (4.4%); (6) 27% did not engage in any physical activity; (7) 28.2% were not regularly active; and (8) only 24.4% consumed five or more servings of fruits and vegetables daily. These authors, along with others, emphasized the critical national need for interventions to improve diet and increase physical activity and thereby control the current obesity epidemic.

Type 1 diabetes (insulin-dependent diabetes; juvenile diabetes) usually begins in late childhood or early adolescence, the peak age of onset being about 12 years. The disease most often begins somewhat abruptly and is characterized by insulinopenia, dependence on exogenous insulin, and a tendency to develop ketoacidosis. Although the etiology is unknown, the lack of insulin production may be due to injury to the pancreatic islet beta cells, possibly secondary to a genetic predisposition to a viral infection or to autoimmunity. However, recent studies suggest that other factors may be involved. For example, Hypponen et al.[261] recently reported an association between infant weight gain and the development of type 1 diabetes. Moreover, others[262,263] previously noted that children with juvenile diabetes were taller than non-diabetic children up to several years before the development of diabetes. In addition, a more recent study found that both obesity and rapid linear growth appear to be important risk factors for type 1 diabetes.[264] These studies suggest that the progressive increase in the number of overweight and obese children over the past few decades may be an important factor in explaining the corresponding increase in type 1 diabetes.

Type 2 diabetes in children and adolescents

Until relatively recently, type 1 diabetes was the only relatively common form of diabetes in children (1–2% of diabetic children had type 2 diabetes or another rare form). Recent studies, however, indicate that the current childhood and adolescent obesity epidemic is associated with a dramatic increase in type 2 diabetes (previously referred to as "late onset diabetes"). Indeed, estimates suggest that type 2 diabetes may now represent about 50% of all new cases of diabetes in certain pediatric populations.[265] This very costly diabetic epidemic is primarily attributable to the increased rates of childhood obesity. Indeed, the annual obesity-related hospital costs in 6- to 17-year-olds has been estimated at US$127 billion.[266]

A recent multiethnic study of obese children and adolescents showed that impaired glucose tolerance (IGT) is highly prevalent, irrespective of ethnic group.[267] Thus, IGT was present in 25% of obese children aged four to ten years and 21% of obese adolescents aged 11–18 years. However, impaired glucose tolerance is not limited to obese American children and adolescents. For example, a recent study of 710 grossly obese Italian children and adolescents, aged six to 18 years, found that glucose intolerance was present in 4.5%.[268] In addition, insulin resistance, impaired insulin secretion and diastolic blood pressure "were significantly and independently related to 2-h postload glucose values." The prevalence of type 2 diabetes is also rapidly increasing in Canadian[269] and Asian-Indian[270] children and adolescents.

The American Diabetes Association recently reviewed the literature regarding the significant increase in type 2 diabetes in children and adolescents and noted the following:[271]

(1) 8–45% of children/adolescents recently diagnosed with diabetes had type 2 (the variation in percentages depended on race/ethnicity and sampling differences);
(2) the peak age of type 2 diabetes in children was mid-puberty;
(3) in white children, total adiposity accounted for about 55% of variance in insulin sensitivity;
(4) obese children were hyperinsulinemic and had about 40% lower insulin-stimulated glucose metabolism;
(5) the inverse relationship between abdominal fat and insulin sensitivity was stronger for visceral than for subcutaneous fat; and
(6) African-American children aged seven to 11 years had significantly higher insulin levels than age-matched white children. Published data suggested that minority children may have a genetic predisposition to insulin resistance.

Testing (fasting blood glucose) for type 2 diabetes was recommended for the following children and adolescents:[271]

(1) Overweight (BMI > 85th percentile for age, sex).
(2) Plus any two of the following:

   (a) family history of type 2 diabetes in first- and second-degree relatives;
   (b) belong to a specific race or ethnic group (African-American, American Indian, Hispanic American and Asian/South Pacific Islander); and
   (c) signs of insulin resistance or conditions associated with insulin resistance (acanthosis nigricans, hypertension and dyslipidemia).

Prevention of type 2 diabetes

Type 2 diabetes mellitus is, to a highly significant degree, a preventable disease. Several recent reports will serve as examples. It has long been assumed that type 2 diabetes is due primarily to obesity, a sedentary lifestyle and a positive family history. To evaluate these factors, Tuomilehto and associates[272] randomly assigned a large group of middle-aged, overweight and obese men and women (mean BMI 31 kg/m^2) with IGT, a well-known significant risk for type 2 diabetes, to either an intervention or control group. Each person in the intervention group was counseled to reduce their weight and intake of total and saturated fat, and to increase their fiber intake and physical activity (i.e. moderate exercise at least 30 minutes/day). After four years, the cumulative incidence of diabetes was 11% of the counseled group compared with 23% of the control group (a 58% reduction). Similarly, a large Chinese study was reported in which 110,660 men and women were initially screened for IGT and diabetes in 1986.[273] Of these, 577 were classified as having IGT (WHO criteria) and were randomized either to a control group or to one of three active treatment groups: diet only, exercise only or diet plus exercise. Regular follow-up evaluations were carried out over a six-year period. The cumulative incidence of diabetes at six years was 67.7% in the control group. After adjusting for differences in baseline BMI and fasting glucose, the diet, exercise and diet-plus-exercise interventions were associated with 31%, 46% and 42% reductions, respectively in the risk of developing diabetes.

More recently, the results of a large scale study involving a diverse group of overweight men and women with IGT was reported.[274] This three-year study involved 3234 participants aged 25 to 85 years; 45% were minorities. Compared with the control group, those who lost just ten to 15 pounds (5–7% of body weight) and walked briskly for 30 minutes five days/week, decreased their risk by 58%; those 60 years and older reduced their risk by 71%. A second group of non-dieting, non-exercising participants who took 850 mg of metformin, an antihyperglycemic agent, twice daily reduced their risk by 31% compared with the control group. The percent of persons who developed type 2 diabetes during the study period is shown in Fig. 2.1. Similarly, Hu and associates[275] recently reported their findings on the association of diet and lifestyle with type 2 diabetes in 84,941 female nurses who were followed for 16 years. Their results

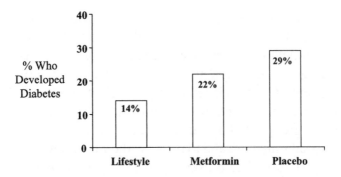

Figure 2.1: Lifestyle, metformin and type 2 diabetes mellitus.[274]

showed that overweight or obesity was the single most important predictor of type 2 diabetes. In addition, lack of exercise, a poor diet and
current smoking and excess alcohol intake were all associated with a
significantly increased risk of type 2 diabetes independent of BMI.
Of prime importance is that 91% of the 3300 new cases of type 2
diabetes were attributed to an unhealthy lifestyle and were, therefore, preventable.

These recent publications make it clear that weight control (maintain
BMI < 25 kg/m^2), proper nutrition and moderate daily exercise would
markedly decrease the risk for this common, highly destructive and
extremely costly disease. It would also improve the quality of life,
increase life expectancy and substantially decrease medical costs.

Cancer

Cancer is the second leading cause of death in the US and other
industrialized countries. In 2002, the estimated number of new
cancer cases and deaths in the US was 1,284,900 and 555,500,
respectively.[276] The relationship between overweight or obesity and
cancer has been studied for many decades and several forms of cancer have been associated with excess body weight (Table 2.5). In
1959, the American Cancer Society began a 12-year prospective study
involving about 750,000 male and female volunteers.[277] They compared the death rates for persons of average weight with those who

Table 2.5: Excess Body Weight and Associated Cancers

Breast	Liver	Prostate
Colon	Multiple myeloma	Rectum
Endometrial	Non-Hodgkin's lymphoma	Stomach
Gallbladder	Ovary	Uterine cervix
Kidney	Pancreas	

were considered both overweight and underweight. Men who were considered 40% or more overweight had a cancer mortality ratio of 1.33; the ratio for women was 1.55. Overweight men had significantly higher mortality ratios for colorectal and prostate cancers while overweight women had increased rates for endometrial, ovarian, cervical, gall bladder and breast cancers. In a recent prospective study, more than 900,000 American adults (404,576 men; 495,477 women) who were free of cancer in 1982 were followed for 16 years.[278] After controlling for other risk factors, the authors estimated "that current patterns of overweight and obesity in the US could account for 14% of all deaths from cancer in men and 20% of those in women."

A report of physicians' failure to screen obese women for cancer is also of considerable importance.[279] In this study, overweight and obese women were less likely to be screened for both cervical and breast cancer with Papanicolaou (pap) smears and mammography than normal weight women. This is particularly unfortunate since overweight women have higher mortality rates for these two cancers and should, therefore, be targeted for increased screening.

Breast cancer

Breast cancer is the second most common worldwide malignancy among women; it is the most common female cancer in developed countries. In 2002, an estimated 205,000 new breast cancer cases were diagnosed in the US (1500 were men).[276] However, early diagnosis and treatment greatly improves the prognosis (about 40,000 deaths/year; 19.5% of total cases). In addition to the American Cancer Society's study,[277] several other studies have also shown a correlation between the degree of obesity and increased mortality for breast cancer in postmenopausal women.[280-284] Almost 50% of breast cancer cases among postmenopausal women reportedly occur in those with a BMI of 29 kg/m^2 or greater.[285] In addition, women in the Nurse's Health Study gaining more than 9 kg (20 pounds) from age 18 to midlife doubled their risk for breast cancer compared with those whose weight was stable during this time period.[286] Similarly, Li and associates[287] reported the following: (1) women who gained 70 pounds or more since age 18 had a significantly increased risk for breast cancer relative to those whose weight remained within ten pounds of their weight at age 18; (2) women with a BMI below what is usually considered healthy (i.e. ≤18 kg/m^2) had a significantly reduced breast cancer rate; and (3) women with BMI in the obese range (i.e. ≥30 kg/m^2) had an increased risk of breast cancer.

Other studies have reported on the association between waist circumference and waist-to-hip ratio and breast cancer risk. For example, a recent report from the Nurses' Health Study[288] (47,382 women) found that in postmenopausal, but not premenopausal, women who had never received hormone replacement therapy, the risk for the highest quintile of waist circumference (36–55 inches) versus the lowest quintile (< 27.9 inches) was 1.88. A similar direct association was noted between waist-to-hip ratio and breast cancer risk.

For both colon and breast cancer, and presumably others, there is some controversy regarding the competing etiologic roles of high-fat diets versus obesity.[289] That is, does obesity, which reflects an individual's lifestyle (high calorie intake and physical inactivity) result in the increased cancer rate or is it the nature of the diet (e.g. high fat and low antioxidants)? The hypothesis that a high intake of dietary fat may increase the risk for breast cancer came mainly from animal studies. Here, experiments with rats and mice showed that high fat intake increases the incidence of breast cancer.[290] In agreement with the animal studies, Wakai *et al.*[291] conducted a case-controlled study with Indonesian women from 1992 to 1995. They found that in the pre-marriage period, the greater the fat intake the greater the breast cancer risk while increased carbohydrate intake during this period decreased the risk. A similar, albeit not quite as strong, association in the post-marriage period was also noted.

Colorectal cancer

Colon cancer is the third most common cancer among both men and women in the US; it is the second most common cause of cancer deaths. In 2002, there were an estimated 107,300 newly diagnosed cases of colon cancer in the US (50,000 men; 57,300 women) and 48,100 deaths (23,100 men; 25,000 women).[276] In addition, there were an estimated 41,000 cases of rectal cancer (22,600 men; 18,400 women) with 8500 deaths (4700 men; 3800 women).[276]

There is consistent and strong evidence that obesity is associated with an increased risk of colorectal cancer, as well as a diet high in red meat and animal fat, and a low intake of vegetables, whole grain cereals and fish. Although up to 50% of colon cancers have a strong inherited factor, the remaining cases are primarily related to diet and lifestyle. Thus, the largest prospective study showed that mortality from colorectal cancer was significantly elevated in men who were 40% or more overweight; however, no such increase was noted in women.[292] Ford,[293] however, reported that excess body weight is a strong colon cancer risk factor for both men and women. Compared with individuals whose BMI was ≤ 22 kg/m^2, the hazard ratios for increased BMI was 1.79, 1.86, 2.47, 3.72 and 2.79 respectively for those with BMI (kg/m^2) 22–23.9, 24–25.9, 26–27.9, 28–29.9 and >30.

Because study results have been somewhat conflicting, Shike[292] suggested that being overweight is likely a surrogate and that other risk factors, including high fat diet, energy-dense food, inadequate fruits and vegetables, and lack of physical activity are the major risk factors. Conversely, several important studies have shown that body weight is directly associated with colon cancer. For example, Giovannucci *et al.*[294] studied the association between obesity, physical inactivity and colon cancer and adenomas in 47,723 male professionals (Health Professionals Follow-up Study). Their results showed that physical activity was inversely associated with colon cancer. However, BMI was also directly associated with increased risk of colon cancer and was independent of the level of physical activity. Waist circumference and waist-to-hip ratio were also strong colon cancer risk factors. These latter associations also persisted after adjustment for physical activity and BMI. Similar associations were noted for colon adenomas 1.0 cm or more in diameter, but not in smaller ones.

Recent Italian studies have also shown that excessive weight at various ages predict an increased risk for colorectal cancer in men while in women, abdominal obesity indicated by increased waist-to-hip ratio, was a more reliable risk indicator.[295] Others studied the association between obesity, weight gain and large weight changes and colorectal adenomatous polyps.[296] Compared with subjects in the lowest BMI quartile, these authors reported increasingly higher odds ratios for those in increasingly higher BMI quartiles as follows: 2.1, 1.8 and 1.7 compared with subjects with a net weight loss during the ten years before sigmoidoscopy. Those with net weight gains of 1.5 to 4.5 kg (3.3–9.9 pounds) or greater than 4.5 kg (> 9.9 pounds) had odds ratios of 2.5 and 1.8, respectively. Thus, BMI, weight gain, unstable weight, waist circumference and waist-to-hip ratio may all be independent risk factors for colorectal cancer.

Although the association between body weight and colorectal cancer is strong for men, studies have been inconsistent in women. However, this inconsistency may have been explained in a recent study of 89,835 women aged 40 to 59 years during an average of 10.6 years follow-up (Canadian National Breast Screening Study).[297] The results showed that obesity (BMI $\geq$ 30 kg/m^2) was associated with about a two-fold increased risk of colorectal cancer among women who were premenopausal at baseline. However, there was no association among women who were postmenopausal at baseline.

It is also of considerable importance to note the similarity of lifestyle and environmental risk factors for colon cancer and type 2 diabetes (increased BMI and central obesity, physical inactivity and increased intake of refined carbohydrates). Although this relationship is not fully understood, diabetics reportedly have slightly elevated rates of colorectal cancer.[298–300] In a recent prospective study with 13 years follow-up, Will and co-workers[301] found a significant positive correlation between type 2 diabetes and colorectal cancer in men; a weaker but non-significant positive association was noted in women. However, Hu *et al.*[302] recently reported data from their prospective study supporting the hypothesis that diabetes may be an independent risk factor for colorectal cancer in women (Nurses' Health Study). After a follow-up period of 18 years and adjustment for age, BMI and physical activity, the relative risk for diabetics was significant at 1.43 for colorectal cancer, 1.49 for colon cancer, 1.11 for rectal cancer, 1.56 for advanced colorectal cancer and 2.39 for fatal colorectal cancer.

Prostate cancer

Prostate cancer is the most common malignancy in American men. In 2002, there were an estimated 189,000 new cases and 30,200 deaths.[276] The incidence was highest among Black Americans and lowest in the population from Eastern Asia.[303] However, little is currently known regarding its causes. Many studies have linked obesity, physical inactivity and diet with prostate cancer. Obesity has also been associated with endocrine changes (i.e. decreased testosterone and increased estrogen blood levels) which have been implicated in prostate carcinogenesis. Hence, an association between body weight and risk for prostate cancer may be expected.

Following the National Cancer Society's report linking obesity with prostate cancer,[283] Snowdon and associates[304] reported similar findings in white male Seventh-day Adventists. They reported that overweight men had a significantly higher risk of fatal prostate cancer than those near their "desirable" weight; the relative risk was 2.5 for those who were overweight. Their data also suggested a positive correlation between fatal prostate cancer and increased consumption of milk, cheese, eggs and meat in that the relative risk for prostate cancer was 3.6 for those who consumed large quantities of all four animal products.

A more recent population based case-controlled Swedish study[305] found that high BMI and total food consumption are independent risk factors for prostate cancer. More specifically, an odds ratio of 2.22 was found for those who consumed somewhat more and 3.89 for those who consumed much more food than men in general. The increased trend for BMI showed an odds ratio of 1.44 for BMI of 26 to 29 kg/m² and 1.80 for those whose BMI was over 29 kg/m² compared to men with a BMI of 23 kg/m². Multivariate analysis showed that both total food consumption and BMI remained as independent risk factors. In addition, neither tobacco nor alcohol use changed the risk for prostrate cancer.

Others have also reported a direct association between body weight and prostate cancer. In the Iowa 65+ Rural Health Study, Cerhan et al.[306] reported a risk ratio of 1.7 for men with a BMI greater than 27.8 kg/m² compared with a BMI less than 23.6 kg/m². In addition, the percent change in BMI after age 50 was positively associated with an increased risk. In this study, cigarette smoking and physical inactivity were also independent risk factors for prostate cancer.

Anderson and others[307] studied the relationship between body size (BMI, weight, height and lean body mass) and prostate cancer among 135,006 Swedish men. They found that all anthropometric measurements were positively associated with the risk of prostate cancer. Moreover, these factors were more strongly associated to cancer mortality than to incidence. The excess risk of death from prostate cancer was also significant in all BMI categories above the reference category (relative risk 1.4). Both height and lean body mass were also directly associated with the incidence of prostate cancer, although BMI was not.

Endometrial cancer

In 2002, there were an estimated 39,300 new cases of endometrial cancer with 6600 deaths in the US.[276] Several early clinical investigations found that excess body weight was common in women with endometrial carcinoma. For example, in 1959 Kottmeier[308] reported that 29% of a series of Swedish women weighed 180 pounds or more;

an additional 7% weighed over 220 pounds. The incidence of obesity and endometrial cancer from seven additional early reports varied from 21% to 64%.[309]

In an Italian case-controlled study to evaluate endometrial cancer risk factors, the use of non-contraceptive estrogens was found to be of moderate risk.[310] Obesity, however, was noted to be the most important single risk factor related to endometrial carcinoma. More recently, an estimated 34% to 56% of cases of endometrial cancer has been attributed to increased body weight (BMI > 29 kg/m^2).[288] Others[311] recently reported that increased body weight, BMI and waist-to-hip ratio were significantly higher in postmenopausal women with endometrial adenomatous and atypical hyperplasia than in controls. However, after multivariate analysis, only BMI remained statistically associated with precancerous adenomatous hyperplasia. It should also be noted that, as with other epithelial tumors, an increased incidence of endometrial cancer has been associated with type 2 diabetes.[312] However, as these authors noted, the increased risk may be confounded by obesity.

Renal cancer

Renal cell cancer accounts for about 2% of all cancers worldwide. There was an estimated 31,800 new cases of kidney and renal pelvis cancers in the US in 2002 (19,100 men; 12,700 women) with 11,600 deaths (7200 men; 4400 women).[276] McLaughlin and Lipworth[313] recently reviewed the epidemiology of renal cell cancer and reported the following: (1) renal cell carcinoma accounts for about 2% of worldwide cancers; (2) the incidence of renal cell cancer has been increasing in North America and northern Europe but not in other countries; (3) in recent years the rate has increased in the US by about 3% per year; (4) cigarette smoking is an important risk factor; (5) obesity and increased relative body weight are major determinants of renal cancer, especially in women.

Mellemgaard and co-workers[314] reported their results from an international multicenter population-based case-control study of renal cell cancer. They considered BMI, height, physical activity and use of amphetamines as possible risk factors for renal cancer. BMI was found to be a significant risk factor among women but to a lesser extent in men. A three-fold increased risk was observed for women with a relative weight in the top 5% compared with those in the lowest quartile. The rate of weight change per year was an independent risk factor for women but not men. Physical activity and height were unrelated to renal cancer regardless of the BMI. Interestingly, the use of amphetamines was associated with an increased risk among men. In their review of the epidemiology of renal cell cancer, Tavani and LaVecchia[315] also concluded that an elevated BMI, mainly in women, is an established risk factor for renal cell carcinoma. More recently, a study of 363,992 Swedish men, who were physically examined at least once from 1971 to 1992, were followed until their death or the end of 1995.[316] Compared with men in the lowest three-eighths for BMI, men in the middle three-eighths had a 30% to 60% greater risk for renal-cell carcinoma, and men in the highest two-eighths had almost twice the risk. A direct association between higher blood pressure and increased risk for renal-call cancer was also noted to be an independent risk factor.

Ovarian cancer

There were an estimated 23,300 newly diagnosed cases of ovarian cancer with 13,900 deaths in the US in 2002.[276] Mink and associates[317] investigated the association of epithelial ovarian cancer with waist-to-hip ratio, physical activity, reproductive factors and family cancer history in a prospective cohort involving 31,396 postmenopausal women. Multivariate-adjusted relative risks for the upper three quartiles of waist-to-hip ratios, compared with the lowest quartile, were 2.0, 1.6 and 2.3, respectively. A family history of ovarian cancer in a first-degree relative had a relative risk of 2.5. Similarly, after controlling for the effects of potential confounders, the odds ratio of ovarian cancer in Japanese women across increasing quartiles of the heaviest body weight were 1.0, 1.15, 1.71 and 2.29.[318] In addition, significantly increased risks were noted in diabetics and for those with a family history of ovarian cancer.

Interestingly, Fairfield and co-workers[319] recently assessed the association between ovarian cancer and current weight, weight at age 18 years, and adult weight changes among 109,445 women covering the period 1976 to 1996 (Nurses' Health Study). Although their findings showed no association between recent BMI and ovarian cancer, there was a two-fold increase in premenopausal ovarian cancer risk associated with a BMI at age 18 of 25 kg/m² or higher compared with a BMI of 20 kg/m².

Pancreatic cancer

Pancreatic cancer represents the fifth leading cause of cancer-related deaths in the US.[320] In 2002, there were an estimated 30,300 cases of pancreatic cancer in the US (14,700 men; 15,600 women), 98% of which resulted in death (14,500 men; 15,200 women).[276] Although several epidemiologic studies on the relationship between pancreatic cancer and obesity have been reported, the results have been conflicting. However, Silverman *et al.*[321] recently published the results of their population-based case-controlled study based on direct interviews with individuals 30 to 79 years of age. They found that obesity was associated with a statistically significant 50% to 60% increased risk of pancreatic cancer. Moreover, there was a significant positive risk with increasing caloric intake with those in the highest quartile caloric intake experiencing a 70% higher risk than those in the lowest quartile. In addition, those in the highest quartile of both BMI and caloric intake had a 180% higher risk compared with those in the lowest quartile. The authors concluded that obesity is a significant risk factor for pancreatic cancer in both white and black individuals although it contributes to a higher risk among blacks than among whites, particularly among women.

Michaud and co-workers[322] reported their data regarding obesity and pancreatic cancer from two recent cohort studies, the Health Professionals Follow-up Study and the Nurse's Health Study. The cohorts consisted of a total of 46,648 men, aged 40 to 75 years, and 117,041 women, aged 30 to 55 years, who were free of prior cancer at baseline and had complete height and weight data. The authors found that both men and women with BMI $\geq$ 30 kg/m² (i.e. obese) had a significantly elevated risk of pancreatic cancer compared to those with BMI < 23 kg/m² (relative risk 1.72). More specifically, obese individuals were 72% more likely to develop pancreatic cancer than those who were neither overweight or obese. Moreover, overweight and obese persons who were involved in sustained regular exercise of moderate intensity (i.e. walking and hiking) were less likely to develop pancreatic cancer compared with inactive persons.

Cancer incidence and diabetes mellitus

Diabetes mellitus also appears to be an important risk factor for various cancers. As noted above, Japanese diabetic women have an increased risk for ovarian cancer.[318] Diabetes has also been associated with an increased incidence of colorectal[301] and pancreatic cancers.[323] In this latter meta-analysis, the authors examined 30 case-controlled and cohort studies of diabetes mellitus and pancreatic cancer published between 1975 and 1994.[323] The pooled relative risk ratio and 95% confidence interval of pancreatic cancer for diabetics, relative to non-diabetics, was 2.1; in those with a diabetic history of at least five years the risk ratio was 2.0.

A recent report of diabetics in Denmark showed increased rates for renal, endometrial, biliary tract, liver and pancreatic cancers.[324] Here, the incidence ratios for liver cancer, after exclusion of hepatitis and cirhosis, were 4.0 and 2.1 in men and women, respectively. For renal cancer, the incidence ratios were 1.4 in males and 1.7 in females. The authors indicated that the elevated risks for endometrial and kidney cancers may be confounded by obesity.

Miscellaneous obesity-associated diseases/disorder

An increased incidence of several other diseases/disorders has also been associated with obesity. These include ischemic stroke, adult-onset asthma, gallbladder disease, sleep apnea, daytime sleepiness, gout and psychological problems.

Ischemic and hemorrhagic stroke

As discussed earlier in this chapter, excess body weight is a well-documented risk factor for CHD, hypertension and type 2 diabetes. However, the question of whether obesity is an important risk factor for stroke has been somewhat inconclusive, especially in women. In men, several earlier studies indicated that obesity significantly increases the risk of ischemic stroke.[325-327] The association between excess body weight and stroke in men has recently been further solidified. In a recent prospective cohort study among 21,414 American male physicians (Physician's Health Study), there were 747 documented strokes (631 ischemic, 104 hemorrhagic and 12 undefined) during 12.5 years of follow-up.[328] Compared to men with BMI < 23 kg/m^2, those with BMIs $\geq$ 30 kg/m^2 had an adjusted relative risk of 2.00 for total stroke, 1.95 for ischemic stroke and 2.15 for hemorrhagic stroke. When the BMI was evaluated as a continuous variable, an increase in each BMI unit resulted in a significant 6% increase in the relative risks for total, ischemic and hemorrhagic stroke. After adjustment for hypertension, diabetes and hypercholesterolemia, there was only a slight risk attenuation for total and ischemic stroke, but not for hemorrhagic stroke.

Few studies, primarily epidemiologic, have been carried out on the association between obesity and stroke in women; the results have been somewhat inconsistent. However, Rexrode *et al.*[329] recently reported the results of their 16-year prospective study of 116,759 women (Nurses' Health Study). Multivariate analysis adjusted for age, smoking, postmenopausal hormone use and menopausal status showed that women with BMI $\geq$ 27 kg/m^2 had a significantly increased risk for ischemic stroke. The relative risks, compared to women with BMI $\geq$ 27 kg/m^2 had a significantly increased risk for ischemic stroke. The relative risks, compared to women with BMI < 21 kg/m^2, were as follows: BMI 27–28.9 kg/m^2, 1.75; BMI 29–31.9 kg/m^2, 1.90; and BMI $\geq$ 32 kg/m^2, 2.37. In addition, weight gain after age 18 years was associated with a relative risk of 1.69 for a gain of 11 to 19.9 kg (24–44 pounds) and 2.52 for a gain of 20 kg or more ($\geq$44 pounds).

Asthma

Asthma reportedly affects about 5% of the US population; the associated medical costs exceed US$6 billion a year.[330] The increasing
prevalence of asthma is a major health concern. Moreover, since the
increased prevalence of asthma and obesity have occurred concomi-
tantly, they appear to be causally related. To investigate whether BMI
and weight change are associated with adult-onset asthma, Camarego
et al.[330] carried out a prospective cohort study involving 85,911 women
aged 26 to 46 years (Nurses' Health Study II). The relative risks of
asthma for six increasing categories of BMI were 0.9, 1.0 (reference),
1.1, 1.6, 1.7 and 2.7. In addition, women who gained weight after age
18 were at a significantly greater risk for developing asthma during
the four-year follow-up period. Others recently studied the relationship between asthma-like symptoms and obesity in a general population of children.[331] The prevalence and incidence of asthma, skin tests
and BMI were determined in 688 children, mean age 6.3 years and
600 children mean age 10.9 years. Lung function, bronchodilator
responsiveness and daily peak flow variability were measured at age
11 years. Their findings showed that females, but not males, who
became overweight or obese between six and 11 years of age significantly increased their risk of developing asthma-like symptoms at
age 11 and 13 years. The increased association of obesity and asthma
in females was also previously noted.[332] Possible explanations for the
increased prevalence in females are as follows:[331] (1) obesity may
influence female sex hormones which in turn increase the risk of
asthma; and (2) the presence of a subgroup of girls with genetic
alterations in receptor responsiveness to female sex hormones. The
authors suggested that both genetic and environmental factors are
probably important in this association.

Gall bladder disease

Obesity has long been recognized as a risk factor for gall bladder
disease. In the Framingham longitudinal study,[333] the prevalence of
gall bladder disease increased significantly with increasing weight.
In addition, the presence of gallstones was three to four times more

common in obese than non-obese persons.[333,334] More recently, these latter authors studied 59,306 women (Nurses' Health Study) and concluded that there is a strong association between symptomatic gallstones and obesity. They suggested that women who are only moderately overweight may also have an increased risk. Numerous other studies have reportedly shown that obesity is a strong risk factor for gallstones.[335] More recently, a longitudinal prospective Nurses' Health Study[336] showed that severely obese women are particularly at risk for gallstones. Here, women with BMI > 45 kg/m^2 had a seven-fold excess risk compared with those whose BMI was < 24 kg/m^2. Those with a BMI of $\geq$ 30 kg/m^2 had a yearly symptomatic gallstone incidence rate over 1%; in those whose BMI was $\geq$ 45 kg/m^2 the rate was about 2%.

Respiratory disorders

Both increased chest wall and abdominal fat negatively affect respiration which results in decreased compliance of the respiratory system.[337,338] In those who are severely obese, a ventilation-perfusion abnormality occurs and hypoxia may develop.[339] Sleep-disordered breathing (SDB), a condition characterized by repeated episodes of apnea and hypopnea events during sleep, is common in Western countries. Peppard *et al.*[340] evaluated 690 randomly selected adults, mean age 46 at baseline (56% males), twice at four-year intervals for SDB. They found that relative to stable weight, a 10% weight gain resulted in an approximate 32% increase in the apnea-hypopnea index (AHI: apnea events + hypopnea events/hour of sleep). This weight gain also predicted a six-fold increase in the odds of developing moderate-to-severe SDB. Conversely, a 10% weight loss resulted in a 26% decrease in AHI.

Kopelman *et al.*[341] reported that a modest but significant fall in hemoglobin oxygen saturation without apnea occurs during sleep in premenopausal obese women whereas no such abnormality occurs in normal weight women of similar age and menstrual status. However, both obese and normal weight postmenopausal women and obese men reportedly develop oxygen desaturation and occasional apneic episodes during sleep.[342] These latter investigators studied respirations during sleep in 20 asymptomatic obese men (age range 18–59 years; mean weight 125 kg; 275 pounds) and compared them with 20 normal weight (67 kg; 147 pounds) men aged 19 to 67 years old. Their findings showed that disordered sleep breathing with severe hypoxia and apnea were common in the obese men of all ages. They suggested that these abnormalities result from mechanical impedence of breathing due to increased abdominal fat combined with abnormal central respiratory control.

Daytime sleepiness and fatigue are also frequent problems in obese people, including those who do not have sleep apnea.[343] In this study, daytime sleepiness was found to be "a morbid characteristic of obese patients." The authors stressed that daytime sleepiness has a potentially significant impact on their lives and on public safety. They attributed this phenomenon to a metabolic and/or circadian abnormality.

Gout

Increased serum uric acid levels and gout have long been associated with excess body weight. In an early cross-sectional survey of Canadian men,[344] serum uric acid levels greater than 0.416 mmol/L (7.05 mg/dL) increased from 7% to 31% as the BMI increased from 21 to 31 kg/m^2. In one study,[345] uric acid levels reportedly did not increase in women until the BMI reached 31 kg/m^2, although an earlier report by Rimm *et al.*[346] showed a direct correlation between uric acid levels and body weight in women. More recent studies have also shown a direct correlation between hyperuricemia and body weight. Cigolini and associates[347] studied a random group of 38-year-old healthy non-diabetic adults without a history of gout. Their results showed that serum uric acid levels were significantly higher in men than women. After adjustment for sex, serum uric acid levels were directly associated with BMI, waist : hip girth, waist : thigh girth, and subscapula : triceps skinfold ratios.

Others[348] studied various clinical features of black South African patients with gout, 79% of whom were from the lower income groups of workers ("blue collar," pensioners and unemployed); 44.4% had polyarticular gout. Case control analysis showed that obesity (odds ratio 7.8), "white collar" occupation (odds ratio 6.4), hypertension (odds ratio 4.9) and alcohol intake (odds ratio 3.5) were significant risk factors for gout in men. However, only alcohol intake correlated with the presence of gout in women (odds ratio 5.0). The authors suggested that in a population where gout was previously rare, changing dietary habits, lifestyle and improved socioeconomic conditions have contributed significantly to its increasing prevalence.

Dessein *et al.*[349] recently reported on the beneficial effects of weight loss and various dietary changes on serum uric acid levels in patients with gout. At the study onset, the average BMI was 30.5 kg/m^2. The dietary recommendations consisted of calorie restriction to 1600 kcal/day with 40% derived from carbohydrates, 30% from protein and 30% from fat. In addition, refined carbohydrates were replaced by complex ones and saturated fats with mono- and polyunsaturated ones. Weight loss averaged 7.7 kg (16.9 pounds) and the incidence of gouty attacks decreased from 2.1 to 0.6 per month. The mean serum uric acid levels decreased from 0.57 to 0.47 mmol/L (9.7 to 8.0 mg/dL) and were normalized in 58% of the subjects.

Osteoarthritis

Several early studies reported an increased prevalence of osteoarthritis in overweight persons.[350,351] Since then, numerous studies have verified this relationship. Overweight people are particularly at risk for developing osteoarthritis of the knees, although other joints are often involved (i.e. hand and hip).[352] In addition, being overweight accelerates disease progression. These latter authors noted that increased joint stress due to obesity generally explains the strong relationship between obesity and knee osteoarthritis. However, it does not fully explain why obese women are at higher risk than men for knee disease or why obese individuals have a higher risk for osteoarthritis in the hand. Although studies are few, weight loss in obese people suggests it has favorable effects.

Cooper *et al.*[353] studied the risk factors for the incidence and progression of radiographic knee osteoarthritis. After adjusting for age and sex, the risk of incident radiographic knee osteoarthritis was significantly increased in those with BMI in the highest versus lowest third (odds rato 18.3), previous knee injury (odds ratio 4.8), and a history of active sports participation (odds ratio 3.2). Another recent report assessed the association between obesity and osteoarthritis of the knee, hip and hand, and whether the arthritis was bilateral or generalized.[354] In this group, 85% had bilateral disease, 26% generalized disease and 31% were obese (BMI $\geq$ 30 kg/m^2). The odds ratios for obesity and overweight (BMI 25–29 kg/m^2) were both strongly associated with bilateral knee osteoarthritis (odds ratios 8.1 and 5.9, respectively). No association between obesity and bilateral hip or generalized osteoarthritis was found. They concluded that obesity "seems to be a mechanical rather than a systemic risk factor for osteoarthritis." Conversely, others[355] reported that both obesity and hip injury are important risk factors for hip osteoarthritis in both men and women. In agreement with this latter study, Oliveria *et al.*[356] studied cases of symptomatic osteoarthritis involving the hip, knee and hand in women aged 20 to 89 years. After controlling for estrogen use, smoking, height and health care use, they found that body weight was a predictor of incident osteoarthritis of all three joints. Odds ratios ranged from 3.0 to 10.5 for women in the upper weight tertile compared with those in the lowest tertile. Similar associations were reported for BMI.

Cataract

Recognizing that obesity is associated with increased oxidative stress, glycosylation and osmotic stress, Weintraub and associates[357] examined the association between increased body weight and the incidence of cataract extraction. This prospective study involved 87,682 women (Nurses' Health Study) and 45,549 men (Health Professionals Follow-up Study) aged 45 years and older who did not have cataract diagnosis at baseline. After adjusting for smoking, age and lutein/ zeaxanthin intake, those who were obese (i.e. BMI $\geq$ 30 kg/m^2) had a 36% greater risk of any type of cataract compared with individuals whose BMI was ≥ 23 kg/m^2. In addition, obesity was primarily associated with posterior subcapsular cataract; obesity was not significantly associated with nuclear cataract.

Maternal obesity and birth defects

Maternal obesity is associated with various fetal complications, including an increased risk of birth defects.[358,359] Recent studies have also shown that obese pregnant women are at increased risk for neural tube defects.[360-362] A recent study added further evidence that the risk of birth defects is increased in obese pregnant women.[363] Not only was the association between maternal obesity and neural tube defects confirmed, but these researchers also "found an association for omphalocele, heart defects and multiple anomalies among infants of obese women."

Psychological effects

In their review of the psychological aspects of obesity, Wadden and Stunkard[364] concluded that the "epidemiological and clinical studies refute the popular notion that overweight persons as a group are emotionally disturbed." In a more recent study of the psychological aspects of severe obesity in patients seeking treatment, these authors concluded "that this population does not report greater levels of general psychopathology than do average-weight control subjects."[365] They also emphasized that there is great psychological heterogeneity in obese individuals. However, a wide variety of studies are in support of an increased incidence of depression among obese individuals compared with the non-obese. The 1985 Consensus Conference on Obesity concluded that obesity creates an enormous psychological burden on these individuals.[366] Moreover, several recent studies also support an increased incidence of depression among the obese compared with the non-obese. Several examples will be cited.

In a community-based study (Alameda County Study, 1994–1995),[367] depression was measured using the outcome measures covered in the

Diagnostic and Statistical Manual of Mental Disorders. The covariates were age, sex, education level, marital status, social isolation and social support, chronic medical disorders, functional impairment, life events and financial strain. Although the results were mixed, cross-sectional analysis showed that an increased risk (odds ratio 1.73) for depression was present in the obese (defined as BMI scores ≥ 85th percentile). Analysis of the data, with obesity defined as a BMI ≥ 30 kg/m², showed similar results. The authors concluded that although their study did not resolve the role of obesity as a major risk factor for depression, it suggests an association between the two. They also noted that there is no support for the "jolly fat" hypothesis that suggests obesity reduces the risk of depression. Moreover, Riva *et al.*[368] concluded that psychopathological aspects, mainly depression, are strongly linked to the eating attitudes of the clinically obese and highlights the need for psychological support in diet therapy.

Carpenter and associates[369] studied the relationships between relative body weight and clinical depression, suicide ideation and suicide attempts in 40,086 African Americans and Caucasians in the US. The outcome measures were diagnosed according to the *Diagnostic and Statistical Manual of Mental Disorders*, Fourth Edition. Their results showed that relative body weight was associated with major depression, suicide attempts and suicide ideation. These relationships, however, differed between men and women. Among men, lower BMI was associated wth major depression, suicide attempts and suicide ideation while in women, increased BMI was directly associated with depression and suicide ideation. There were no racial differences.

Others[370] examined how education and gender moderate the association between obesity and cynical hostility and depression. Here, education was found to moderate the positive association between cynical distrust and obesity among women. That is, cynical distrust was not related to BMI or waist-to-hip ratio among highly educated women. However, depression did have a positive association with waist-to-hip ratio among both genders; BMI was associated with depression only among women. BMI, eating attitudes and depression may also be clinically important in the postpartum period. For example, a recent study[371] found that although symptoms of anxiety and depression were not correlated with eating attitudes or BMI during pregnancy, overweight women were at moderate risk for increased anxiety at four months and depression at both four and 14 months postpartum.

Overweight and Alzheimer disease

Dementia is a major personal and public health problem that is increasing rapidly as people live longer. By age 85 years, the incidence of dementia approaches 10%,[372] and its prevalence is about 30%.[373] The most common form of dementia is Alzheimer's disease (AD), a neurodegenerative disorder; the second most common dementia is vascular dementia which is a consequence of cerebrovascular disease. Importantly, several recent studies have shown an association between AD and various vascular disorders.[374,375] Recognizing that overweight is a major risk factor for coronary heart and cerebrovascular disorders, Gustafson *et al.*[376] studied the association between AD and dementia risk in a cohort of 392 nondemented Swedish adults aged 70 to 88 years. After an 18-year follow-up, women who developed dementia between ages 79 and 88 years were overweight with a higher BMI at age 70 years (27.7 versus 25.7 kg/m²), 75 years (27.9 versus 25.0 kg/m²) and 79 years (26.9 versus 25.1 kg/m²) compared with nondemented women. Additionally, a higher degree of overweight was observed in women who developed AD at age 70 years (29.3 kg/m²), 75 years (29.6 kg/m²), and 79 years (28.2 kg/m²) compared with nondemented women. Thus, the risk for AD increased by 36% for every 1.0 increase in BMI at age 70 years. Interestingly, these associations were not present in men.

Obstructive sleep apnea

Obstructive sleep apnea is a common condition with multiple symptoms, as well as repeated episodes of upper airway obstruction during sleep that results in episodes of hypoxia. Moreover, population-based epidemiologic studies have consistently shown that even mild obstructive sleep apnea may be associated with significant morbidity. Thus, a recent literature review found that undiagnosed obstructive sleep apnea has been independently associated with an increased risk of hypertension, stroke, CHD, daytime sleepiness, motor vehicle accidents and decreased quality of life.[377] Although obstructive sleep apnea has been associated with various modifiable risk factors including obesity, alcohol intake, smoking and nasal congestion, "the only intervention strategy supported with adequate evidence is weight loss."

Socioeconomic status

The early seminal literature review by Sobal and Stunkard[378] showed that people in the lower socioeconomic status in all industrialized nations were at higher risk of becoming obese, especially among women. To explain this phenomenon, Stunkard and Sorensen[379] proposed the following possibilities: (1) socioeconomic status influences obesity; (2) obesity influences socioeconomic status; or (3) a common factor(s) influences both obesity and the socioeconomic level.

A recent English study compared the odds ratios for obesity in men and women by education, occupation and two economic markers after controlling for age, ethnicity and marital status.[380] Their results showed that obesity risk was greater among both men and women with fewer years of education and poorer economic circumstances. In addition, the risk of obesity was greater in women, but not men, of lower occupational status. Moreover, an earlier study found a significantly lower prevalence of obesity among college students; this was particularly striking in womens' colleges.[381] Examination of academic qualifications for admission among the obese and non-obese groups showed no objective differences that would account for the lower acceptance rate of obese students. Similarly, no relation was found between social class and obesity. These authors concluded that discrimination, albeit unconscious, was exercised by high school teachers and college interviewers against the obese applicants.

Gortmaker *et al.*[382] studied the social and economic consequences of obesity in adolescents and young adults. This study, begun in 1981 and concluded in 1988, found that women who were overweight at baseline completed fewer years of school, were less likely to marry, had lower household incomes, and had higher rates of household poverty than women who were not overweight at baseline. This data was independent of socioeconomic status and aptitude-test scores. Overweight men at baseline were less likely to be married. Importantly, those with other chronic disorders did not differ from the non-overweight subjects. The study confirmed earlier reports correlating the socioeconomic status with obesity. For example, an early prospective study[383] controlled for various baseline characteristics and followed up for 12.5 years showed a higher occupational level in non-obese versus obese men (e.g. ranking of 0 for unskilled, manual labor to 7 for judge, professor, etc.). Here, only 30% of the obese attained a position above social class 2 compared with 51% of the non-obese control group. These findings were independent of parental social class, intelligence and education. In an earlier study, Goldblatt and associates[384] reported that 22% of downwardly mobile persons were obese whereas only 12% of upwardly mobile people were obese.

Oxidative stress

Oxidative stress due to excess free radical formation has been implicated in the pathogenesis of numerous diseases including atherosclerosis, cancer, inflammation, cataract and neurodegenerative disorders, among others. It is also a major theory of aging.[385] Moreover, obesity has been associated with increased oxidative stress. Keaney *et al.*[386] examined 2828 individuals from the Framingham Heart Study and measured urinary 8-epi-PGF$_{2\alpha}$ as a systemic oxidative stress marker. Their results showed that smoking, diabetes and body mass index were all "highly associated with systemic oxidative stress" and that the effect of body mass index "may suggest an important role of oxidative stress in the deleterious impact of obesity on cardiovascular disease."

Chapter Summary

Overweight (BMI 25–29.9 kg/m²) and obesity (BMI ≥ 30 kg/m²) are now major public health problems in both developed and developing countries. Obesity, now acknowledged as an epidemic in industrialized nations, has mainly developed during the past 25 years. It affects not only wealthy and middle-income people, but also the poor. An extensive study of the relationship between overweight/obesity and various chronic diseases/disorders was very recently published that further documented the significant relationship between body weight and various diseases. Here, Field and co-workers[387] evaluated the risks of overweight/obesity on the development of several diseases/disorders involving 73,690 women (Nurses' Health Study) and 46,060 men (Professionals Follow-up Study) during a ten-year period. They found that the incidence of diabetes, gallstones, hypertension, heart disease, colon cancer and stroke (men only) increased with the degree of overweight in both men and women. Perhaps most surprising was that the dose-response relationship between the risk of developing these medical conditions and BMI was present even among those in the upper half of the generally accepted healthy weight range (i.e. BMI 22.0–24.9 kg/m²). Their data suggested that a BMI of 18.5 to 21.9 kg/m² would be needed to fully minimize the risk of these and possibly other chronic weight-related diseases/disorders.

The economic costs of obesity, independent of those associated with physical inactivity and the numerous medical diseases/disorders associated with obesity, are striking; they now equal or exceed those due to smoking.[36] Thus, in terms of 1995 dollars, Wolf and Colditz[167] estimated that the economic impact attributable to obesity was US$99.2 billion dollars per year. Moreover, the personal costs of obesity such as lower socioeconomic status, decreased self-esteem, discrimination, depression and suicide are all very common and lead to an untold number of additional problems.

It is apparent that, although genetics is an important determinant of obesity, the major factors are excess caloric intake and physical inactivity. As noted by Jebb,[388] "despite decades of intensive research, there is relatively little evidence of genetic or metabolic defects to explain the majority of cases of human obesity. Instead, we must look to behavioral and/or environmental factors which may be underpinning the current epidemic of obesity." More intense education of the general public, public officials, the education system and professional health community regarding the medical and economic consequences of excess body weight is critical.

References

1. van Italle TB. Worldwide epidemiology of obesity. *PharmaEcon* 1994;5(Suppl 1):1–7.
2. Popkin BM, Doak CM. The obesity epidemic is a worldwide phenomenon. *Nutr Rev* 1998;56:106–114.
3. Caterson ID, Gill TP. Obesity: epidemiology and possible prevention. *Best Pract Res Clin Endocrinol Metab* 2002;16:595–610.
4. Sobal J, Stunkard A. Socioeconomic status of obesity: a review of the literature. *Psychol Bull* 1989;105:260–275.
5. Guo SS, Roche AF, Chumlea WC, *et al.* The predictive value of childhood body mass index values for overweight at age 35 years. *Am J Clin Nutr* 1994;59:810–819.
6. Update: prevalence of overweight among children, adolescents, and adults — United States, 1988–1994. *MMWR* 1997;46:199–202.
7. Mokdad AH, Serdula MK, Dietz WH, *et al.* The spread of the obesity epidemic in the United States, 1991–1998. *JAMA* 1999;282:1519–1522.
8. Flegal KM, Carroll MD, Ogden CL, Johnson CL. Prevalence and trends in obesity among US adults, 1999–2000. *JAMA* 2002;288:1723–1727.
9. Freedman DS, Khan LK, Serdul MK, *et al.* Trends and correlates of Class 3 obesity in the United States from 1990 through 2000. *JAMA* 2002;288:1758–1761.
10. Yanovski SZ, Yanovski JA. Obesity. *N Engl J Med* 2002;346:591–601.
11. Kuczmarski RJ, Flegal KM, Campbell SM, Johnson CL. Increasing prevalence of overweight among US adults. *JAMA* 1994;272:205–211.
12. Nielsen SJ, Popkin BM. Patterns and trends in food portion sizes, 1977–1998. *JAMA* 2003;289:450–453.
13. Metropolitan Life Insurance Company. Metropolitan height and weight tables. *Stat Bull Met Life Ins Co* 1983;64:2–9.
14. National Task Force on the Prevention and Treatment of Obesity. Overweight, obesity, and health risk. *Arch Intern Med* 2000;160:898–904.

15. US Department of Agriculture/Department of Health and Human Services. *Dietary Guidelines for Americans*, 4th Ed. Home and Garden Bulletin 232, US Department of Agriculture/Department of Health and Human Services, Washington, DC, 1995.

16. van Italle TB. Prevalence of obesity. *Endocrinol Metab Clin North Am* 1996;25:887–905.

17. Perls TT, Silver MHJ. *Living to 100*. Basic Books, New York, 1999.

18. Fumento M. Weight after 50. *Modern Maturity* 1998;May–June:34–41.

19. Kraemer H, Berkowitz RI, Hammer LD. Methodological difficulties in studies of obesity, I: measurement issues. *Ann Behav Med* 1990;12:112–118.

20. Flegal KM, Carroll MD, Kuczmarski RJ, Johnson CL. Overweight and obesity in the United States: prevalence and trends, 1960–1994. *Int J Obes Relat Metab Disord* 1998;22:39–47.

21. Flegal KM, Carroll MD, Ogden CL, Johnson CL. Prevalence and trends in obesity among US adults, 1999–2000. *JAMA* 2002;288:1772–1773.

22. Kissebah AH, Krakower GR. Regional adiposity and morbidity. *Physiol Rev* 1994;74:761–811.

23. Lean MEJ, Han TS, Morrison CE. Waist circumference as a measure for indicating need for weight management. *BMJ* 1995;311:158–161.

24. Lean MEJ, Han TS, Seidell JC. Impairment of health and quality of life in people with large waist circumference. *Lancet* 1998;351:853–856.

25. Mazess RB, Barden HS, Bisek JP, Hanson J. Dual-energy x-ray absorptiometry for total-body and regional bone-mineral and soft-tissue composition. *Am J Clin Nutr* 1990;51:1106–1112.

26. Han TS, van Leer EM, Seidell JC, Lean MEJ. Waist circumference action levels in the identification of cardiovascular risk factors: prevalence study in a random sample. *BMJ* 1995;311:1401–1405.

27. NHLBI Obesity Education Initiative Expert Panel on the Identification, Evaluation, and Treatment of Overweight and Obesity in Adults. *Clinical Guidelines on the Identification, Evaluation, and Treatment of Overweight and Obesity in Adults*. National Heart, Lung, and Blood Institute, Bethesda, MD, 1998.

28. Chan JM, Rimm EB, Colditz GA, Stampfer MJ, Willett WC. Obesity, fat distribution and weight gain as risk factors for clinical diabetes in men. *Diabetes Care* 1994;17:961–969.

29. Carey VJ, Walters EE, Colditz GA, *et al.* Body fat distribution and risk of non-insulin-dependent diabetes mellitus in women: the Nurses' Health Study. *Am J Epidemiol* 1997;145:614–619.

30. Taylor RW, Keil D, Gold EJ, Williams SM, Goulding A. Body mass index, waist girth, and waist-to-hip ratio as indexes of total and regional adiposity in women: evaluation using receiver operating characteristic curves. *Am J Clin Nutr* 1998;67:44–49.
31. Bjorntorp P. Classification of obese patients and complications related to the distribution of surplus fat. *Nutrition* 1990;6:131–137.
32. Kumanyika SK. Special issues regarding obesity in minority populations. *Ann Intern Med* 1993;119:650–654.
33. Freedman DS, Dietz WH, Srinivasin SR, Berenson GS. The relation of overweight to cardiovascular risk factors among children and adolescents: the Bogalusa Heart Study. *Pediatrics* 1999;103:1175–1182.
34. Williamson DF, Kahn HS, Remington PL, Anda RF. The 10-year incidence of overweight and major weight gain in US adults. *Arch Intern Med* 1990;150:665–692.
35. Must A, Spadano J, Coakley EH, *et al.* The disease burden associated with overweight and obesity. *JAMA* 1999;282:1523–1529.
36. Sturm R, Wells KB. Does obesity contribute as much to morbidity as poverty or smoking? *Public Health* 2001;115:229–235.
37. Drenick EJ, Bale GS, Seltzer F, Johnson DG. Excessive mortality and cause of death in morbidly obese men. *JAMA* 1980;243:443–445.
38. Manson J, Willett WC, Stampfer MJ, *et al.* Body weight and mortality among women. *N Engl J Med* 1995;333:677–685.
39. Allison DB, Fontaine KR, Manson JE, Stevens J, van Italle TB. Annual deaths attributable to obesity in the United States. *JAMA* 1999;282:1530–1538.
40. McGinnis JM, Foege WH. Actual causes of death in the United States. *JAMA* 1993;270:2207–2212.
41. Sturm R. The effects of obesity, smoking, and drinking on medical problems and costs. Health Aff (Millwood) 2002;21:245–253.
42. Stevens J, Cai J, Pamuk ER, *et al.* The effect of age on the association between body-mass index and mortality. *N Engl J Med* 1998;338:1–7.
43. Peeters A, Barendregt JJ, Willekens F, *et al.* Obesity in adulthood and its consequences for life expectancy: a life-table analysis. *Ann Intern Med* 2003;138:24–32.
44. Fontaine KR, Redden DT, Wang C, *et al.* Years of life lost due to obesity. *JAMA* 2003;289:187–193.
45. Shimokata H, Tobin JD, Muller DC, *et al.* Studies in the distribution of body fat: I. Effects of age, sex, and obesity. *J Gerontol* 1989;44:M66–M73.
46. Steen B. Body composition and aging. *Nutr Rev* 1988;46:45–51.

47. Stunkard AJ, Harris JR, Pedersen NL, McClearn GE. The body-mass index of twins who have been reared apart. *N Engl J Med* 1990;322:1483–1487.

48. Allison DB, Kaprio J, Korkeila M, *et al.* The heritability of body mass index among an international sample of monozygotic twins reared apart. *Int J Obes Relat Metab Disord* 1996;20:501–506.

49. Bouchard C, P'russe L, Leblanc C, Tremblay A, Theriault G. Imheritance of the amount and distribution of human body fat. *Int J Obesity* 1988;12:205–215.

50. Zhang Y, Proenca R, Maffei M, *et al.* Positional cloning of the mouse obese gene and its human homologue. *Nature* 1994;372:425–432.

51. Rolls BJ, Hammer VA. Fat, carbohydrate, and the regulation of energy intake. *Am J Clin Nutr* 1995;62 (Suppl):1086S–1095S.

52. Hill JO. Physical activity, body weight and body fat distribution. In: *Physical Activity and Cardiovascular Health: A National Consensus.* A Leon (ed) Human Kinetics, Champaign, Ill, 1997, p. 272.

53. Centers for Disease Control and Prevention. Prevalence of sedentary leisuretime behavior among adults in the United States. Available at *http://www.cdc.gov/inchswww/products/pubs/pubd/hestats/3and4/ sedentary.htm.* Accessed 4 October 1999.

54. Koplan JP, Dietz WH. Caloric imbalance and public health policy. *JAMA* 1999;282:1579–1581.

55. Grundy SM. Multifactorial causation of obesity: implications for prevention. *Am J Clin Nutr* 1998;67(Suppl):563S–572S.

56. Laitinen J, Ek E, Sovio U. Stress-related eating and drinking behavior and body mass index and predictors of this behavior. *Prev Med* 2002;34:29–39.

57. Molarius A, Seidell JC, Sans S, *et al.* Educational level, relative body weight and changes in their association over 10 years: an international perspective from the WHO MONICA project. *Am J Public Health* 2000;90:1260–1268.

58. Binkley JK, Eales J, Jekanowski M. The relation between dietary change and rising US obesity. *Int J Obes* 2000;24:1032–1039.

59. McCrory MA, Fuss PJ, Hays NP, *et al.* Overeating in America: association between restaurant food consumption and body fatness in healthy adult men and women ages 19 to 80. *Obes Res* 1999;7:564–571.

60. McCrory MA, Fuss PJ, Saltzman E, Roberts SB. Dietary determinants of energy intake and weight regulation in healthy adults. *J Nutr* 2000;130:(Suppl):276S–279S.

61. McCrory MA, Suen VMM, Roberts SB. Biobehavioral influences on energy intake and adult weight gain. *J Nutr* 2002;132:3830S–3834S.

62. Economic Research Service, US Department of Agriculture. *America's Eating Habits: Changes and Consequences*. USDA/Economic Research Service, Washington, DC, 1999.

63. Young LR, Nestle MN. The contribution of expanding portion sizes to the US obesity epidemic. *Am J Pub Health* 2002;92:246–249.

64. McCrory MA, Fuss PJ, Saltzman E, Roberts SB. Dietary determinants of energy intake and weight regulation in healthy adults. *J Nutr* 2000;130:276S–279S.

65. Troiano RP, Flegal KM, Kuczmarski RJ, Campbell SM, Johnson CL. Overweight prevalence and trends for children and adolescents: the National Health and Nutrition Surveys, 1963 to 1991. *Arch Pediatr Adolesc Med* 1995;149:1085–1091.

66. Poskitt EME. Defining childhood obesity: the relative body mass index (BMI). *Acta Paediatr* 1995;84:961–963.

67. Pietrobelli A, Faith MS, Allison DB, *et al.* Body mass index as a measure of adiposity among children and adolescents: a validation study. *J Pediatr* 1998;132:204–210.

68. Centers for Disease Control and Prevention Report. Prevalence of overweight among adolescents — United States, 1988–1991. *MMWR* 1994;43/44:818–821.

69. Troiano RP, Flegal KM. Overweight children and adolescents: description, epidemiology, and demographics. *Pediatrics* 1998;101:497–504.

70. Strauss RS, Pollack HA. Epidemic increase in childhood overweight, 1986–1998. *JAMA* 2001;286:2845–2848.

71. Ogden CL, Flegal KM, Carroll MD, Johnson CL. Prevalence and trends in overweight among US children and adolescents. *JAMA* 2002;288:1728–1732.

72. Reilly JJ, Dorosty AR, Emmett PM. Prevalence of overweight and obesity in British children. *BMJ* 1999;319:1039.

73. Tremblay MS, Willms JD. Secular trends in the body mass index of Canadian children. *CMAJ* 2000;163:1429–1433.

74. Eisenmann JC, Katzmarzyk PT, Arnall DA, *et al.* Growth and overweight of Navajo youth: secular changes from 1955 to 1997. *Int J Obesity* 2000;24:211–218.

75. Freedman DS, Kettel-Khan L, Srinivasan SR, Berenson GS. Black/white differences in relative weight and obesity among girls: the Bogalusa heart study. *Prev Med* 2000;30:234–243.

76. Tomeo CA, Field AE, Berkey CS, *et al.* Weight concerns, weight control behaviors, and smoking initiation. *Pediatrics* 1999;104:918–924.

77. US Department of Agriculture. *The Food Guide Pyramid*. US GPO, Washington, DC, 1992.

78. Munoz KA, Krebs-Smith SM, Ballard-Barbash R, Cleveland LE. Food intake of US children and adolescents compared with recommendations. *Pediatrics* 1997;100:323–329.

79. Ludwig DS, Peterson KE, Gortmaker SL. Relation between consumption of sugar-sweetened drinks and childhood obesity: a prospective, observational analysis. *Lancet* 2001;357:505–508.

80. Nestle M. Soft drink "pouring rights": marketing empty calories. *Public Health Rep* 2000;115:308–319.

81. Kemm JR. Eating patterns in childhood and adult health. *Nutr Health* 1987;4:205–215.

82. Steinberger J, Moran A, Hong C-P, *et al.* Adiposity in childhood predicts obesity and insulin resistance in young adulthood. *J Pediatr* 2001;138:469–473.

83. Whitaker RC, Wright JA, Pepe MS, Seidel KD, Dietz WH. Predicting obesity in young adulthood from childhood and parental obesity. *N Engl J Med* 1997;337:869–873.

84. Hardy R, Wadsworth M, Kuh D. The influence of childhood weight and socioeconomic status on change in adult body mass index in a British national birth cohort. *Int J Obes* 2000;24:725–734.

85. Davison KK, Birch LL. Weight status, parent reaction, and self-concept in five-year-old girls. *Pediatrics* 2001;107:46–53.

86. Dietz WH. Television, obesity, and eating disorders. *Adolesc Med State Art Rev* 1993;4:543–549.

87. Morgan M. Television and school performance. *Adoles Med State Art Rev* 1993;4:607–622.

88. Robinson TN. Reducing children's television viewing to prevent obesity: a randomized controlled trial. *JAMA* 1999;282:1561–1567.

89. Dennison BA, Erb TA, Jenkins PL. Television viewing and television in bedroom associated with overweight risk among low-income preschool children. *Pediatrics* 2002;109:1028–1035.

90. Martinez-Gonzalez MA, Gual P, Lahortiga F, *et al.* Parental factors, mass media influences, and the onset of eating disorders in a prospective population-based cohort. *Pediatrics* 2003;111:315–320.

91. Toyran M, Ozmert E, Yurdakok K. Television viewing and its effect on physical health in schoolage children. *Turk J Pediatr* 2002;44:194–203.

92. Hu FB, Li TY, Colditz GA, *et al.* Television watching and other sedentary behaviors in relation to risk of obesity and type 2 diabetes mellitus in women. *JAMA* 2003;289:1785–1791.

93. American Academy of Pediatrics, Work Group on Breast-feeding. Breast-feeding and the use of human milk. *Pediatrics* 1997;100:1035–1039.

94. Raisler J, Alexander C, O'Campo P. Breastfeeding and infant illness: a dose-response relationship? *Am J Public Health* 1999;89:25–30.

95. Anderson JW, Johnstone BM, Remley DT. Breastfeeding and cognitive development: a meta-analysis. *Am J Clin Nutr* 1999;70:525–535.

96. von Kries R, Koletzko B, Saurwald T, *et al.* Breast feeding and obesity: cross-sectional study. *BMJ* 1999;319:147–150.

97. Tulldahl J, Pettersson K, Andersson SW, Hulthen L. Mode of infant feeding and achieved growth in adolescence: early feeding patterns in relation to growth and body composition in adolescence. *Obes Res* 1999;7:431–437.

98. Hediger ML, Overpeck MD, Kuczmarski RJ, Ruan WJ. Association between infant breastfeeding and overweight in young children. *JAMA* 2001;285:2453–2460.

99. Gillman MW, Rifas-Shiman SL, Camargo CA, *et al.* Risk of overweight among adolescents who were breastfed as infants. *JAMA* 2001;285:2461–2467.

100. Dietz WH. Health consequences of obesity in youth: childhood predictors of adult disease. *Pediatrics* 1998;101:518–525.

101. Banis HT, Varni JW, Wallander JL, *et al.* Psychological and social adjustment of obese children and their families. *Child Care Health Dev* 1988;14:157–173.

102. Goodman E, Whitaker RC. Prospective study of the role of depression in the development and persistence of adolescent obesity. *Pediatrics* 2002;109:497–504.

103. Schwimmer JB, Burwinkle TM, Varni JW. Health-related quality of life of severely obese children and adolescents. *JAMA* 2003;289:1813–1819.

104. Westerterp-Plantenga MS, Wijckmans-Duijsens NEG, Verboeket-van de Venne WPG, *et al.* Energy intake and body weight effects of six months reduced or full fat diets, as a function of dietary restraint. *Int J Obes* 1998;22:14–22.

105. Serdula MK, Mokdad AH, Williamson DF, *et al.* Prevalence of attempting weight loss and strategies for controlling weight. *JAMA* 1999;282:1353–1358.

106. Allred JB. Too much of a good thing? *J Am Diet Assoc* 1995; 95:417–418.

107. Metz JA, Stern JS, Kris-Etherton P, *et al.* A randomized trial of improved weight loss with a prepared meal plan in overweight and obese patients. *Arch Intern Med* 2000;160:2150–2158.

108. Samaha FF, Iqbal N, Seshadri P, *et al.* A low-carbohydrate as compared with a low-fat diet in severe obesity. *N Engl J Med* 2003; 348:2074–2081.

109. Foster GD, Wyatt HR, Hill JO, *et al.* A randomized trial of a low-carbohydrate diet for obesity. *N Engl J Med* 2003;348:2082–2090.

110. Bravata DM, Sanders L, Huang J, *et al.* Efficacy and safety of low-carbohydrate diets: a systematic review. *JAMA* 2003;289:1837–1850.

111. Bray GA. Low-carbohydrate diets and realities of weight loss. *JAMA* 2003;289:1853–1855.

112. St. Jeor ST, Howard BV, Prewitt TE, *et al.* Dietary protein and weight reduction: a statement for healthcare professionals from the Nutrition Committee of the Council on Nutrition, Physical Activity, and Metabolism of the American Heart Association. *Circulation* 2001;104:1869–1874.

113. King AC, Tribble DL. The role of exercise in weight regulation of nonathletes. *Sports Med* 1991;11:331–349.

114. Bouchard C, Depres JP, Tremblay A. Exercise and obesity. *Obes Res* 1993;1:133–147.

115. National Institutes of Health, National Heart, Lung, and Blood Institute. Obesity Education Initiative. *Clinical Guidelines on the Identification, Evaluation, and Treatment of Overweight and Obesity in Adults.* National Institutes of Health, Bethesda, MD, June 1998.

116. Klem ML, Wing RR, McGuire MT, Seagle HM, Hill JO. A descriptive study of individuals successful at long-term maintenance of substantial weight loss. *Am J Clin Nutr* 1997;66:239–246.

117. Schoeller DA, Shay K, Kushner RF. How much physical activity is needed to minimize weight gain in previously obese women? *Am J Clin Nutr* 1997;66:551–556.

118. Despres JP, Lamarche B. Effects of diet and physical activity on adiposity and body fat distribution: implications for the prevention of cardiovascular disease. *Nutr Res Rev* 1993;6:1–23.

119. Fogelholm M, Kukkonen-Harjula K, Nenonen A, Pasanen M. Effects of walking training on weight maintenance after a very-low-energy diet in premenopausal obese women. *Arch Intern Med* 2000;160:2177–2184.

120. Perri MG, McAllister D, Gange JJ, *et al.* Effects of four maintenance programs on the long-term management of obesity. *J Consult Clin Psychol* 1988;56:529–534.

121. Centers for Disease Control and Prevention Editorial Report. Prevalence of leisure-time physical activity among overweight adults — United States, 1998. *JAMA* 2000;283:2650–2651.

122. US Department of Health and Human Services. *Physical Activity and Health: A Report of the Surgeon General.* Centers for Disease Control and Prevention, National Center for Chronic Disease Prevention and Health Promotion, Atlanta, GA, 1996.

123. Jakicic JM. The role of physical activity in prevention and treatment of body weight gain in adults. *J Nutr* 2002;132:3826S–3829S.

124. Sallis JF, Hovell MF, Hofstetter CR, *et al.* Distance between homes and exercise facilities related to frequency of exercise among San Diego residents. *Public Health Rep* 1990;105:179–185.

125. Anderson R, Wadden T, Bartlett S, *et al.* Effects of lifestyle activity versus structured aerobic exercise in obese women: a randomized trial. *JAMA* 1999;281:335–340.

126. Wee CC, Rigotti NA, Davis RB, Phillips RS. Relationship between smoking and weight control efforts among adults in the United States. *Arch Intern Med* 2001;161:546–550.

127. Bennett WA. Beyond overeating. *N Engl J Med* 1995;332:673–674.

128. Flatt JP. Body composition, respiratory quotient, and weight maintenance. *Am J Clin Nutr* 1995;62(Suppl):1107S–1117S.

129. Weinsier RL, Nagy TR, Hunter GR, *et al.* Do adaptive changes in metabolic rate favor weight regain in weight-reduced individuals? An examination of the set-point theory. *Am J Clin Nutr* 2000;72:1088–1094.

130. Polivy J, Herman CP. Dieting and binging: a causal analysis. *Am Psychol* 1985;40:193–201.

131. National Task Force on the Prevention and Treatment of Obesity. Dieting and the development of eating disorders in overweight and obese adults. *Arch Intern Med* 2000;160:2581–2589.

132. Hash RB, Munna RK, Vogel RL, Bason JJ. Does physician weight affect perception of health choices? *Prev Med* 2003;36:41–44.

133. Macera CA, Croft JB, Brown DR, Ferguson JE, Lane MJ. Predictors of adopting leisure-time physical activity among a biracial community cohort. *Am J Epidemiol* 1995;142:629–635.

134. Yeager KK, Donehoo RS, Macera CA, Croft JB, Heath GW, Lane MJ. Health promotion practices among physicians. *Am J Prev Med* 1996;12:238–241.

135. Wee CC, McCarthy EP, Davis RB, Phillips RS. Physician counseling about exercise. *JAMA* 1999;282:1583–1588.

136. Galuska DA, Will JC, Serdula MK, Ford ES. Are health care professionals advising patients to lose weight? *JAMA* 1999;282:1576–1578.

137. Taira DA, Safran DG, Seto TB, Rogers WH, Tarlov AR. The relationship between patient income and physician discussion of health risk behaviors. *JAMA* 1997;278:1412–1417.
138. Lamberg L. Psychiatric help may shrink some waistlines. *JAMA* 2000;284:291–293.
139. American College of Sports Medicine, Position Stand. Appropriate intervention strategies for weight loss and prevention of weight regain for adults. *Med Sci Sports Exerc* 2001;33:2145–2156.
140. National Institutes of Health. Clinical guidelines on the identification, evaluation, and treatment of overweight and obesity in adults: the evidence report. *Obes Res* 1998;6(Suppl. 2):S51–S209.
141. Simkin-Silverman LR, Wing RR. Management of obesity in primary care. *Obes Res* 1997;5:603–612.
142. Serdula MK, Khan LK, Dietz WH. Weight loss counseling revisited. *JAMA* 2003;289:1747–1750.
143. Heshka S, Anderson JW, Atkinson RL, *et al.* Weight loss with self-help compared with a structured commercial plan: a randomized trial. *JAMA* 2003;289:1792–1798.
144. Barlow SE, Dietz WH. Obesity evaluation and treatment: expert committee recommendations. *Pediatrics* 1998;102:626 (Abstract).
145. Treatment of overweight children and adolescents: a needs assessment of health practitioners. *Pediatrics* 2002;110(Suppl):205–238.
146. Barlow SE, Dietz WH. Management of child and adolescent obesity: summary and recommendations based on reports from pediatricians, pediatric nurse practitioners, and registered dieticians. *Pediatrics* 2002;110(Suppl):236–238.
147. Kral JG. Surgical treatment of obesity. In: *Obesity* P Bjorntorp, BN Brodoff (eds.) Lippincott, Philadelphia, 1992, pp. 731–742.
148. Ceelen W, Walder J, Cardon A, *et al.* Surgical treatment of severe obesity with a low-pressure adjustable gastric band: experimental data and clinical results in 625 patients. *Ann Surg* 2003;237:10–16.
149. Zinzindohoue F, Chevallier JM, Douard R, *et al.* Laparoscopic gastric banding: a minimally invasive surgical treatment for morbid obesity (prospective study of 500 consecutive patients). *Ann Surg* 2003;237:1–9.
150. Brolin RE. Bariatric surgery and long-term control of morbid obesity. *JAMA* 2002;288:2793–2796.
151. Mitka M. Surgery for obesity: demand soars amid scientific, ethical questions. *JAMA* 2003;289:1761–1762.
152. Thompson D, Wolf AM. The medical-care cost burden of obesity. *Obes Rev* 2001;2:189–197.

153. Wolf AM. What is the ecomomic case for treating obesity? *Obes Res* 1998;6(Suppl 1):2S–7S.
154. Rimm EB, Stampfer MJ, Giovannucci E, *et al.* Body size and fat distribution as predictors of CHD among middle-aged and older US men. *Am J Epidemiol* 1995;141:1117–1127.
155. Willett WC, Manson JE, Stampfer MJ, *et al.* Weight, weight change, and CHD in women: risk within the "normal" weight range. *JAMA* 1995;273:461–465.
156. Chan JM, Rimm EB, Colditz MJ, Stampfer, Willett WC. Obesity, fat distribution, and weight gain as risk factors for clinical diabetes in men. *Diabetes Care* 1994;17:961–969.
157. Colditz Ga, Willett WC, Rotnitzky A, Manson JE. Weight gain as a risk factor for clinical diabetes in women. *Ann Intern Med* 1995; 122:481–486.
158. Huang Z, Hankinson SE, Colditz GA, *et al.* Dual effects of weight and weight gain on breast cancer risk. *JAMA* 1997;278:1407–1411.
159. Manson JE, Willett WC, Stampfer MJ, *et al.* Body weight and mortality among women. *N Engl J Med* 1995;333:677–685.
160. Berlin J, Colditz G. A meta-analysis of physical activity in the prevention of CHD. *Am J Epidemiol* 1990;132:612–628.
161. Colditz G, Cannuscio C, Frazier A. Physical activity and reduced risk of colon cancer: implications for prevention. *Cancer Causes Control* 1997;8:649–667.
162. Henderson N, White C, Eisman J. The role of exercise and fall risk reduction in the prevention of osteoporosis. *Endocrinol Metab Clin North Am* 1998;27:369–387.
163. US Department of Health and Human Services, Centers for Disease Control and Prevention, National Center for Chronic Disease Prevention and Health Promotion and The President's Council on Physical Fitness and Sports. *Physical Activity and Health: A Report of the Surgeon General*, Office of the Surgeon General, Washington, DC, 1996, pp. 43–45.
164. Colditz GA. Economic costs of obesity. *Am J Clin Nutr* 1992;55: 503S–507S.
165. Wolf AM, Colditz GA. The cost of obesity: the US perspective. *Pharma Econ* 1994;5(Suppl 1):34–37.
166. Colditz GA. Economic costs of obesity and inactivity. *Med Sci Sports Exerc* 1999;31(Suppl 11):S663–S667.
167. Wolf AM, Colditz GA. Current estimates of the economic cost of obesity in the United States. *Obes Res* 1998;6:97–106.
168. Wang G, Dietz WN. Economic burden of obesity in youths aged 6 to 17 years: 1979–1999. *Pediatrics* 2002;109(e81):949–950.

169. Quesenberry CP, Caan B, Jacobson A. Obesity, health service use, and health care costs among members of a health maintenance organization. *Arch Intern Med* 1998;158:466–472.

170. Agren G, Narbro K, Jonsson E, *et al.* Cost of in-patient care over seven years among surgically and conventionally treated obese patients. *Obes Res* 2002;10:1276–1283.

171. Field AE, Coakley EH, Must A, *et al.* Inpact of overweight on the risk of developing common chronic diseases during a 10-year period. *Arch Intern Med* 2001;161:1581–1886.

172. Pi-Sunyer FX. Medical hazards of obesity. *Ann Intern Med* 1993; 119:655–660.

173. Mokdad AH, Ford ES, Bowman BA, *et al.* Prevalence of obesity, diabetes, and obesity-related health risk factors, 2001. *JAMA* 2003; 289:76–79.

174. Must A, Spadano J, Coakley EH, *et al.* The disease burden associated with overweight and obesity. *JAMA* 1999;282:1523–1529.

175. Fine JT, Colditz GA, Coakley EH, *et al.* A prospective study of weight change and health-related quality of life in women. *JAMA* 1999;282:2136–2142.

176. Gregg EW, Gerzoff RB, Thompson TJ, Williamson DF. Intentional weight loss and death in overweight and obese US adults 35 years of age and older. *Ann Intern Med* 2003;138:383–389.

177. Vasan RS, Beiser A, Seshadri S, *et al.* Residual lifetime risk for developing hypertension in middle-aged women and men: the Framingham Heart Study. *JAMA* 2002;287:1003–1010.

178. Symonds B. The blood pressure of healthy men and women. *JAMA* 1923;80:232.

179. US Department of Health, Education and Welfare. *Report of the Hypertension Task Force*, Vol. 9. NIH Publication 79-1631 Washington, DC, 1979, pp. 59–77.

180. Kannel WB, Brand N, Skinner JJ, Jr., Dawber TR, McNamara PM. Relationship of adiposity to blood pressure and development of hypertension: the Framingham study. *Ann Intern Med* 1967;67: 49–59.

181. van Italle TB. Health implications of overweight and obesity in the United States. *Ann Intern Med* 1985;103:983–988.

182. Havlik RJ, Hubert HB, Fabsitz RR, Feinleib M. Weight and hypertension. *Ann Intern Med* 1983;98:855–859.

183. Sorof J, Daniels S. Obesity hypertension in children: a problem of epidemic proportions. *Hypertension* 2002;40:441–447.

184. Dustan HP. Mechanisms of hypertension associated with obesity. *Ann Intern Med* 1983;98:860–864.

185. Masuo K, Mikami H, Ogihara T, Tuck ML. Weight gain-induced blood pressure elevation. *Hypertension* 2000;35:1135–1140.

186. Williams RR, Hunt SC, Hucstedt SJ, *et al.* Are there interactions and relations between genetic and environmental factors in predisposing to high blood pressure? *Hypertension* 1991;18(Suppl 1):1–29.

187. Svetky LP, McKeown SP, Wilson AF. Heritability of salt sensitivity in black Americans. *Hypertension* 1996;28:854–858.

188. Larson N, Hutchinson R, Boerwinkle E. Lack of association of three functional gene variants with hypertension in African Americans. *Hypertension* 2000;35:1297–1300.

189. Stamler R, Stamler J, Grimm R, *et al.* Nutritional therapy for high blood pressure in final report of a four-year randomized controlled trial—the Hypertension Control Program. *JAMA* 1987;257: 1454–1491.

190. Whelton PK, Appel LJ, Espeland MA, *et al.* Sodium reduction and weight loss in the treatment of hypertension in older persons. A randomized controlled trial of nonpharmacologic interventions in the elderly (TONE). *JAMA* 1998;279:839–846.

191. Masuo K, Mikami H, Ogihara T, Tuck ML. Weight reduction and pharmacologic treatment in obese hypertensives. *Am J Hypertens* 2001;14:530–538.

192. Ben-Dov I, Grossman E, Stein A, Shachor D, Gaides M. Marked weight reduction lowers resting and exercise blood pressure in morbidly obese subjects. *Am J Hypertens* 2000;13:251–255.

193. Whelton PK, He J, Appel LJ, *et al.* Primary prevention of hypertension: clinical and public health advisory from the National High Blood Pressure Education Program. *JAMA* 2002;288:1882–1888.

194. Feinleib M. Epidemiology of obesity in relation to health hazards. *Ann Intern Med* 1985;103:1019–1024.

195. Manson JE, Wikllett WC, Stampfer MJ, *et al.* Body weight and mortality among women. *N Engl J Med* 1995;333:677–685.

196. Garrison RJ, Castelli WP. Weight and 30-year mortality of men in the Framingham Study. *Ann Intern Med* 1985;103:1006–1009.

197. Rimm EB, Stampfer MJ, Giovannucci E, *et al.* Body size and fat distribution as predictors of coronary heart disease among middle-aged and older US men. *Am J Epidemiol* 1995;141:1117–1127.

198. Manson JE, Colditz GA, Stampfer MJ, *et al.* A prospective study of obesity and risk of coronary heart disease in women. *N Engl J Med* 1990;322:882–889.

199. Lindsted K, Tonstad S, Kuzma JW. Body mass index and patterns of mortality among Seventh-day Adventist men. *Int J Obes* 1991;15:397–406.

200. Higgens M, Kannel W, Garrison R, Pinsky J, Stokes J, 3rd. Hazards of obesity: the Framingham experience. *Acta Med Scand Suppl* 1988;723:23–36.

201. Howard BV, Cowan LD, Devereux RB, *et al.* Rising tide of cardiovascular disease in American Indians. The Strong Heart Study. *Circulation* 1999;99:2389–2395.

202. Chambless LE, Heiss G, Folsom AR, *et al.* Association of coronary heart disease incidence with carotid arterial wall thickness and major risk factors. The Atherosclerosis Risk in Communities (ARIC) Study, 1987 to 1993. *Am J Epidemiol* 1997;146:483–494.

203. Lee ZSK, Critchley JAJH, Chan JCN, *et al.* Obesity is the key determinant of cardiovascular risk factors in the Hong Kong Chinese population: cross-sectional clinic-based study. *Hong Kong Med J* 2000; 6:13–23.

204. McGill HC Jr., McMahan A, Herderick EE, *et al.* Obesity accelerates the progression of coronary atherosclerosis in young men. *Circulation* 2002;105:2712–2718.

205. Davi G, Guagnano MT, Ciabattoni G, *et al.* Platelet activation in obese women: role of inflammation and oxidant stress. *JAMA* 2002; 288:2008–2014.

206. Esposito K, Pontillo A, DiPalo C, *et al.* Effect of weight loss and lifestyle changes on vascular inflammatory markers in obese women. *JAMA* 2003;289:1795–1804.

207. American Heart Association. *2002 Heart and Stroke Statistical Update.* American Heart Association, Dallas, 2001.

208. Vasan RS, Larson MG, Benjamin EJ, *et al.* Left ventricular dilatation and the risk of congestive heart failure in people without myocardial infarction. *N Engl J Med* 1997;336:1350–1355.

209. Gardin JM, McClelland R, Kitzman D, *et al.* M-mode echocardiographic predictors of six- to seven-year incidence of coronary heart disease, stroke, congestive heart failure, and mortality in an elderly cohort (the Cardiovascular Health Study). *Am J Cardiol* 2001;87:1051–1057.

210. Kenchaiah S, Evans JC, Levy D, *et al.* Obesity and the risk of heart failure. *N Engl J Med* 2002;347:305–313.

211. Larsson B, Svardsudd K, Welin L, *et al.* Abdominal adipose tissue distribution, obesity, and risk of cardiovascular disease and death. *BMJ* 1984;288:1401–1404.

212. Freedman DS, Williamson DF, Croft JB, Ballew C, Byers T. Relation of body fat distribution to ischemic heart disease. *Am J Epidemiol* 1995;142:53–63.

213. Prineas R, Folsom A, Kaye SA. Central adiposity and increased risk of coronary artery disease mortality in older women. *Ann Epidemiol* 1993;3:35–41.

214. Rexrode KM, Carey VJ, Hennekens CH, *et al.* Abdominal adiposity and coronary heart disease in women. *JAMA* 1998;280:1843–1848.

215. Folsom AR, Burke GL, Byers CL, *et al.* Implications of obesity for cardiovascular disease in blacks: the CARDIA and ARIC studies. *Am J Clin Nutr* 1991;53:1604S–1611S.

216. Eckel RH, Krauss RM. American Heart Association call to action: obesity as a major risk factor for coronary heart disease. *Circulation* 1998;97:2099–2100.

217. Katzel LI, Bleecker ER, Colman EG, *et al.* Effects of weight loss versus aerobic exercise training on risk factors for coronary disease in healthy, obese, middle-aged and older men. *JAMA* 1995;274: 1915–1921.

218. Willett WC, Manson JE, Stampfer MJ, *et al.* Weight, weight change, and coronary heart disease in women: risk within the "normal" weight range. *JAMA* 1996;273:461–465.

219. Stampfer MJ, Hu FB, Manson JE, Rimm EB, Willett WC. Primary prevention of coronary heart disease in women through diet and lifestyle. *N Engl J Med* 2000;343:16–22.

220. EUROASPIRE Study Group. EUROASPIRE: a European Society of Cardiology survey of secondary prevention of coronary heart disease, principal results. *Eur Heart J* 1997;18:1569–1582.

221. EUROASPIRE I and II Group. Clinical reality of coronary prevention guidelines: a comparison of EUROASPIRE I and II in nine countries. *Lancet* 2001;357:995–1001.

222. Muller C. Xanthoma, hypercholesterolemia, angina pectoris. *Acta Med Scand Suppl* 1938;89:75–84.

223. Thannhauser SJ, Magendantz H. The different clinical groups of xanthomatous disease: a clinical physiological study of 22 cases. *Ann Intern Med* 1938;11:1662–1746.

224. Knight JA. *Laboratory Medicine and the Aging Process*. ASCP Press, Chicago, 1996, pp. 111–143.

225. Montoye HJ, Epstein FH, Kjeldsberg MO. Relationship between serum cholesterol and body fatness: an epidemiologic study. *Am J Clin Nutr* 1966;8:397–406.

226. Gordon T, Castelli WP, Hjortland MC, Kannel WB, Dawber TR. High-density lipoprotein as a protective factor against coronary heart disease: the Framingham Study. *Am J Med* 1977;62: 707–714.

227. Gluek CJ, Taylor HL, Jacob SD, *et al.* Plasma high-density lipoprotein cholesterol: association with measurement of body mass: the Lipid Research Clinics Program Prevalence Study. *Circulation* 1980;62 (Suppl IV):62–69.

228. Paccaud F, Schluter-Fasmeyer V, Wietlisbach V, Bovet P. Dyslipidemia and abdominal obesity: an assessment in three general populations. *J Clin Epidemiol* 2000;53:393–400.

229. Tchernof A, Lamarche B, Prud'Homme D, *et al.* The dense LDL phenotype: association with plasma lipoprotein levels, visceral obesity, and hyperinsulinemia in men. *Diabetes Care* 1996;19: 629–637.

230. Pouliot M-C, Despres J-P, Nadeau A, *et al.* Visceral obesity in men: associations with glucose tolerance, plasma insulin, and lipoprotein levels. *Diabetes* 1992;41:826–834.

231. Cordero-MacIntyre ZR, Lohman TG, Rosen J, *et al.* Weight loss is correlated with an improved lipoprotein profile in obese postmenopausal women. *J Am Coll Nutr* 2000;19:275–284.

232. Sothern MS, Despinasse B, Brown R, *et al.* Lipid profiles of obese children and adolescents before and after significant weight loss: differences according to sex. *South Med J* 2000;93:278–282.

233. Hoyert DL, Freedman MA, Strobino DM, Guyer B. Annual summary of vital statistics — 2000. *Pediatrics* 2001;108: 1241–1255.

234. Zimmet P. Globalization, coca-colonization and the chronic disease epidemic: can the Doomsday scenario be arrested? *J Intern Med* 2001;247:301–310.

235. Harris MI, Flegal KM, Cowie CC, *et al.* Prevalence of diabetes, impaired fasting glucose, and impaired glucose tolerance in US adults: the Third National Health and Nutrition Examination Survey, 1988–1994. *Diabetes Care* 1998;21:518–524.

236. Mokdad AH, Ford ES, Bowman BA, *et al.* Diabetes trends in the US: 1990–1998. *Diabetes Care* 2000;23:1278–1283.

237. Mokdad AH, Ford ES, Bowman BA, *et al.* The continuing increase of diabetes in the US. *Diabetes Care* 2001;24:412.

238. Boyle JP, Honeycutt AA, Narayan KMV, *et al.* Projection of diabetes burden through 2050. *Diabetes Care* 2001;24:1936–1940.

239. Lipton RB, Liao Y, Cao G, *et al*. Determinants of incident non-insulin-dependent diabetes mellitus among blacks and whites in a national sample: the NHANES I Epidemiologic Follow-up Study. *Am J Epidemiol* 1993;138:826–839.

240. Resnick NE, Valsania P, Halter JB, Lin X. Differential effects of BMI on diabetes risk among black and white Americans. *Diabetes Care* 1998;21:1828–1835.

241. Glass M. Diabetes in Navajo Indians. *Fed Practitioner* 1996;13:41–48.

242. Salsbury CG. Disease incidence among the Navajos. *Southwest Med* 1937;21:230–233.

243. Burrows NR, Geiss LS, Engelgau MM, Acton KJ. Prevalence of diabetes among Native Americans and Alaska Natives, 1990–1997. *Diabetes Care* 2000;23:1786–1790.

244. Huse DM, Oster G, Killen AR, *et al*. The economic costs of non-insulin dependent diabetes mellitus. *JAMA* 1989;262:2708–2713.

245. Ray N, Willis S, Thamer M. *Direct and Indirect Costs of Diabetes in the United States in 1992*. American Diabetes Association, Alexandria, VA, 1993.

246. Rubin RJ, Altman WM, Mendelson DN. Health care expenditures for people with diabetes mellitus, 1992. *J Clin Endocrinol Metab* 1994;78:809A–809F.

247. American Diabetes Association. Economic consequences of diabetes mellitus in the US in 1997. *Diabetes Care* 1998;21:296–309.

248. Brancati FL, Kao WHL, Folsom AR, *et al*. Incident type 2 diabetes mellitus in African American and white adults. *JAMA* 2000;283:2253–2259.

249. Valdmanis V, Smith DW, Page MR. Productivity and economic burden associated with diabetes. *Am J Public Health* 2001;91:129–130.

250. Alper J. New insights into type 2 diabetes. *Science* 2000;289:37–39.

251. United States National Commission on Diabetes. *Report of the National Commission on Diabetes to the Congress of the United States*, Vol. 1. US Department of Health, Education and Welfare, Bethesda, Maryland, 1975, Publication No. 76-1021.

252. Colditz GA, Willett WC, Stampfer MJ, *et al*. Weight as a risk factor for clinical diabetes in women. *Am J Epidemiol* 1990;132:501–512.

253. Colditz GA, Willett WC, Rotnitzky A, Manson JE. Weight gain as a risk factor for clinical diabetes mellitus in women. *Ann Intern Med* 1995;122:481–486.

254. Chan JM, Rimm EB, Colditz GA, *et al*. Obesity, fat distribution, and weight gain as risk factors for clinical diabetes in men. *Diabetes Care* 1994;17:961–969.

255. Ford ES, Williamson DF, Liu S. Weight change and diabetes incidence: findings from a national cohort of US adults. *Am J Epidemiol* 1997;146:214–222.

256. Shaper AG, Wannamethee SG, Walker M. Body weight: implications for the prevention of coronary heart disease, stroke, and diabetes mellitus in a cohort study of middle aged men. *BMJ* 1997;314: 1311–1317.

257. Carey VJ, Walters EE, Colditz GA, *et al.* Body fat distribution and risk of non-insulin-dependent diabetes mellitus in women. The Nurses' Health Study. *Am J Epidemiol* 1997;145:614–619.

258. Boyko EJ, Fujimoto WY, Leonetti DL, Newell-Morris L. Visceral adiposity and risk of type 2 diabetes. *Diabetes Care* 2000;23:465–471.

259. Knopman D, Boland LL, Mosley T, *et al.* Cardiovascular risk factors and cognitive decline in middle-aged adults. *Neurology* 2001;56:42–48.

260. Mokdad AH, Bowman BA, Ford ES, *et al.* The continuing epidemics of obesity and diabetes in the United States. *JAMA* 2001;286: 1195–1200.

261. Hypponen E, Kenward MG, Virtanen SM, *et al.* The Childhood Diabetes in Finland (DiMe) Study Group: infant feeding, early weight gain, and risk of type 1 diabetes. *Diabetes Care* 1999;22:1961–1965.

262. Blom LG, Persson LA, Dahlquist GG. A high linear growth is associated with an increased risk of childhood diabetes. *Diabetologia* 1992;35:528–533.

263. Price DE, Burden AC. Growth of children before onset of diabetes. *Diabetes Care* 1992;15:1393–1395.

264. Hypponen E, Virtanen SM, Kenward MG, *et al.* Obesity, increased linear growth, and risk of type 1 diabetes in children. *Diabetes Care* 2000;23:1755–1760.

265. Ludwig DS, Ebbeling CB. Type 2 diabetes mellitus in children: primary care and public health considerations. *JAMA* 2001;286: 1427–1430.

266. Goran MI, Ball GD, Cruz ML. Obesity and risk of type 2 diabetes and cardiovascular disease in children and adolescents. *J Clin Endocrinol Metab* 2003;88:1417–1427.

267. Sinha R, Fisch G, Teague B, *et al.* Prevalence of impaired glucose tolerance among children and adolescents with marked obesity. *N Engl J Med* 2002;346:802–810.

268. Invitti C, Guzzaloni G, Gilardini L, *et al.* Prevalence and concomitants of glucose intolerance in European obese children and adolescents. *Diabetes Care* 2003;26:118–124.

269. Ball GD, McCarger LJ. Childhood obesity in Canada: a review of prevalence estimates and risk factors for cardiovascular disease and type 2 diabetes. *Can J Appl Physiol* 2003;28:117–140.

270. Ramachandran A, Snehalatha C, Satyavani K, *et al.* Type 2 diabetes in Asian-Indian urban children. *Diabetes Care* 2003;26:1022–1025.

271. American Diabetes Association. Type 2 diabetes in children and adolescents. *Diabetes Care* 2000;23:381–389.

272. Tuomilehto J, Lindstrom J, Eriksson JG, *et al.* Prevention of type 2 diabetes mellitus by changes in lifestyle among subjects with impaired glucose tolerance. *N Engl J Med* 2001;344:1343–1350.

273. Pan X-R, Li G-W, Hu Y-H, *et al.* Effects of diet and exercise in preventing NIDDM in people with impaired glucose tolerance. *Diabetes Care* 1997;20:537–544.

274. Diabetes Prevention Program Research Group. Reduction in the incidence of type 2 diabetes with lifestyle intervention or metformin. *N Engl J Med* 2002;346:393–403.

275. Hu FB, Manson JE, Stampfer MJ, *et al.* Diet, lifestyle, and the risk of type 2 diabetes mellitus in women. *N Engl J Med* 2001;345:790–797.

276. Jemal A, Thomas A, Murray T, Thun M. Cancer statistics, 2002. *CA Cancer J Clin* 2002;52:23–47.

277. Garfinkel L. Overweight and cancer. *Ann Intern Med* 1985;103:1034–1036.

278. Calle EE, Rodriguez C, Walker-Thurmond K, Thun MJ. Overweight, obesity, and mortality from cancer in a prospectively studied cohort of US adults. *N Engl J Med* 2003;348:1625–1638.

279. Wee CC, McCarthy EP, Davis RB, Phillips RS. Screening for cervical and breast cancer: is obesity an unrecognized barrier to preventive care? *Ann Intern Med* 2000;132;697–704.

280. de Waard F. Breast cancer incidence and nutritional status with particular reference to body weight and height. *Cancer Res* 1975;35:3351–3356.

281. Paffenbarger RS Jr, Kampert JB, Chang HG. Characteristics that predict risk of breast cancer before and after menopause. *Am J Epidemiol* 1980;112:258–268.

282. Lubin F, Ruder AM, Wax Y, Modan B. Overweight and changes in weight throughout adult life in breast cancer etiology. A case-control study. *Am J Epidemiol* 1985;122:579–588.

283. Ballard-Barbash R, Schatzkin A, Taylor PR, *et al.* Association of change in body mass with breast cancer. *Cancer Res* 1990;50:2152–2155.

284. Schapira DV, Kumar NB, Lyman GH, *et al.* Abdominal obesity and breast cancer risk. *Ann Intern Med* 1990;112:182–186.

285. Ballard-Barbash R, Swanson CA. Body weight: estimation of risk for breast and endometrial cancers. *Am J Clin Nutr* 1996; 63(Suppl):437S–441S.

286. Huang Z, Hankinson SE, Colditz GA, *et al.* Dual effects of weight and weight gain on breast cancer risk. *JAMA* 1997;278:1407–1411.

287. Li CI, Stanford JL, Daling JR. Anthropometric variables in relation to risk of breast cancer in middle-aged women. *Int J Epidemiol* 2000;29:208–213.

288. Huang Z, Willett WC, Colditz GA, *et al.* Waist circumference, waist : hip ratio, and risk of breast cancer in the Nurses' Health Study. *Am J Epidemiol* 1999;150:1316–1324.

289. Pi-Sunyer FX. Medical hazards of obesity. *Ann Intern Med* 1993; 119:655–660.

290. Freedman LS, Clifford C, Messina M. Analysis of dietary fat, calories, body weight, and the development of mammary tumors in rats and mice: a review. *Cancer Res* 1990;50:5710–5719.

291. Wakai K, Dillon DS, Ohno Y, *et al.* Fat intake and breast cancer risk in an area where fat intake is low: a case-control study in Indonesia. *Int J Epidemiol* 2000;29:20–28.

292. Shike M. Body weight and colon cancer. *Am J Clin Nutr* 1996; 63(Suppl):442S–444S.

293. Ford ES. Body mass index and colon cancer in a national sample of adult US men and women. *Am J Epidemiol* 1999;150:390–398.

294. Giovannucci E, Ascherio A, Rimm EB, *et al.* Physical activity, obesity, and risk for colon cancer and adenoma in men. *Ann Intern Med* 1995;122:327–334.

295. Giacosa A, Franceschi S, La-Vecchia C, *et al.* Energy intake, overweight, physical exercise and colorectal cancer risk. *Eur J Cancer Prev* 1999;9(Suppl):S53–S60.

296. Bird CL, Frankl HD, Lee ER, Haile RW. Obesity, weight gain, large weight changes, and adenomatous polyps of the left colon and rectum. *Am J Epidemiol* 1998;147:670–680.

297. Terry PD, Miller AB, Rohan TE. Obesity and colorectal cancer risk in women. *Gut* 2002;51:191–194.

298. Kessler H. Cancer mortality among diabetics. *J Natl Cancer Inst* 1970;44:673–686.

299. Ragozzino M, Melton LJ 3rd, Chu CP, Palumbo PJ. Subsequent cancer risk in the incidence cohort of Rochester, Minnesota, residents with diabetes mellitus. *J Chronic Dis* 1982;35:13–19.

300. Adami HO, McLaughlin J, Ekbom A, *et al.* Cancer risk in patients with diabetes mellitus. *Cancer Causes Control* 1991;2:307–314.

301. Will JC, Galuska DA, Vinicor F, Calle EE. Colorectal cancer: another complication of diabetes mellitus? *Am J Epidemiol* 1998; 147:816–825.

302. Hu FB, Manson JE, Liu S, *et al.* Prospective study of adult onset diabetes mellitus (type 2) and risk of colorectal cancer in women. *J Natl Cancer Inst* 1999;91:542–547.

303. Ekman P. Genetic and environmental factors in prostate cancer genesis: identifying high-risk cohorts. *Eur Urol* 1999;35:362–369.

304. Snowdon DA, Phillips RL, Choi W. Diet, obesity, and risk of fatal prostate cancer. *Am J Epidemiol* 1984;120:244–250.

305. Gronberg H, Damber L, Damber J-E. Total food consumption and body mass index in relation to prostate cancer risk: a case-control study in Sweden with prospectively collected exposure data. *J Urol* 1996;155:969–974.

306. Cerhan JR, Torner JC, Lynch EC, *et al.* Association of smoking, body mass, and physical activity with risk of prostate cancer in the Iowa 65+ Rural Health Study. *Cancer Causes Control* 1997;8:229–238.

307. Anderson SO, Wolk A, Bergstrom R, *et al.* Body size and prostate cancer: a 20-year follow-up study among 135006 Swedish construction workers. *J Natl Cancer Inst* 1997;89:385–389.

308. Kottmeier HL. Carcinoma of the corpus uteri — diagnosis and therapy. *Am J Obstet Gynecol* 1959;78:1127–1140.

309. Wynder EL, Escher GC, Mantcl N. An epidemiological investigation of cancer of the endometrium. *Cancer* 1966;19:489–520.

310. LaVecchia C, Franceschi S, Gallus G, *et al.* Prognostic features of endometrial cancer in estrogen users and obese women. *Am J Obstet Gynecol* 1982;144:387–390.

311. Gredmark T, Kvints, Havel G, Mattsson L. Adipose tissue distribution in postmenopausal women with adenomatous hyperplasia of the endometrium. *Gynecol Oncol* 1999;72:138–142.

312. Wideroff L, Gridley G, Mellemkjaer L, *et al.* Cancer incidence in a population-based cohort of patients hospitalized with diabetes mellitus in Denmark. *J Natl Cancer Inst* 1997;89:1360–1365.

313. McLaughlin JK, Lipworth L. Epidemiologic aspects of renal cell cancer. *Semin Oncol* 2000;27:115–123.

314. Mellemgaard A, Lindblad P, Schkhofer B, *et al.* International renal-cell cancer study. III. Role of weight, height, physical activity, and use of amphetamines. *Int J Cancer* 1995;60:350–354.

315. Tavani A, LaVecchia C. Epidemiology of renal-cell carcinoma. *J Nephrol* 1997;10:93–106.
316. Chow W-H, Gridley MS, Fraumeni JF, Jarvholm B. Obesity, hypertension, and the risk of kidney cancer in men. *N Engl J Med* 2000;343:1305–1311.
317. Mink PJ, Folsom AR, Sellers TA, Kushi LH. Physical activity, waist-to-hip ratio, and other risk factors for ovarian cancer: a follow-up study of older women. *Epidemiology* 1996;7:38–45.
318. Mori M, Nishida T, Sugiyama T, *et al.* Anthropometric and other risk factors for ovarian cancer in a case-control study. *Jpn J Cancer Res* 1998;89:246–253.
319. Fairfield KM, Willett WC, Rosner BA, *et al.* Obesity, weight gain, and ovarian cancer. *Obstet Gynecol* 2002;100:288–296.
320. Cancer Facts and Figures, 2000. American Cancer Society Inc., Atlanta, GA, 2000.
321. Silverman DT, Swanson CA, Gridley G, *et al.* Dietary and nutritional factors and pancreatic cancer: a case-controlled study based on direct interviews. *J Natl Cancer Inst* 1998;90:1710–1719.
322. Michaud DS, Giovannucci E, Willett WC, *et al.* Physical activity, obesity, height, and the risk of pancreatic cancer. *JAMA* 2001;286:921–929.
323. Everhart J, Wright D. Diabetes mellitus as a risk factor for pancreatic cancer: a meta-analysis. *JAMA* 1995;273:1605–1609.
324. Wideroff L, Gridley G, Mellemkjaer L, *et al.* Cancer incidence in a population-based cohort of patients hospitalized with diabetes in Denmark. *J Natl Cancer Inst* 1997;89:1360–1365.
325. Abott RD, Behrens GR, Sharp DS, *et al.* Body mass index and thromboembolic stroke in nonsmoking men in older middle age: The Honolulu Heart Program. *Stroke* 1994;25:2370–2376.
326. Shinton R, Shipley M, Rose G. Overweight and stroke in the Whitehall Study. *J Epidemiol Community Health* 1991;45:138–142.
327. Paffenbarger RS, Wing AL. Chronic disease in former college students, XI: early precursors of nonfatal stroke. *Am J Epidemiol* 1971;94:524–530.
328. Kurth T, Gaziano JM, Berger K, *et al.* Body mass index and the risk of stroke in men. *Arch Intern Med* 2002;162:2557–2562.
329. Rexrode KM, Hennekens CH, Willett WC, *et al.* A prospective study of body mass index, weight change, and risk of stroke in women. *JAMA* 1997;277:1539–1545.

330. Camargo CA, Weiss ST, Zhang S, *et al.* Prospective study of body mass index, weight change, and risk of adult-onset asthma in women. *Arch Intern Med* 1999;159:2582–2588.

331. Castro-Rodriquez JA, Holberg CJ, Morgan WJ, *et al.* Increased incidence of asthmalike symptoms in girls who become overweight or obese during the school years. *Am J Respir Crit Care Med* 2001; 163:1344–1349.

332. Chen Y, Dales R, Krewski D, Breithaupt K. Increased effects of smoking and obesity on asthma among female Canadians: the National Population Health Survey, 1994–1995. *Am J Epidemiol* 1999; 150:255–262.

333. Friedman GD, Kannel WB, Dawber TR. The epidemiology of gall bladder disease: observations in the Framingham Study. *J Chronic Dis* 1966;19:273–292.

334. Bray GA. Complications of obesity. *Ann Intern Med* 1985;103:1052–1062.

335. Maclure KM, Hayes KC, Colditz GA, *et al.* Weight, diet, and the risk of symptomatic gallstones in middle-aged women. *N Engl J Med* 1989;321:563–569.

336. Stampfer MJ, Maclure KM, Colditz GA, *et al.* Risk of symptomatic gallstones in women with severe obesity. *Am J Clin Nutr* 1992;55: 652–658.

337. Naimark A, Chernlack RM. Compliance of the respiratory system and its components in health and obesity. *J Appl Physiol* 1960;15: 377–382.

338. Waltemath CL, Bergman NA. Respiratory compliance in obese patients. *Anesthesiology* 1974;41:84–85.

339. Douglas FG, Chong PY. Influence of obesity on peripheral airways patency. *J Appl Physiol* 1972;33:559–563.

340. Peppard PE, Young T, Palta M, *et al.* Longitudinal study of moderate weight change and sleep-disordered breathing. *JAMA* 2000;284: 3015–3021.

341. Kopelman PG, Apps MCP, Cope T, Empey DW. Nocturnal hypoxia and prolactin secretion in obese women. *BMJ* 1983;287:859–861.

342. Kopelman PG, Apps MCP, Cope T, *et al.* Nocturnal hypoxia and sleep apnoea in asymptomatic obese men. *Int J Obes* 1986;10:211–217.

343. Vgontzas AN, Bixler EO, Tan T-L, *et al.* Obesity without sleep apnea is associated with daytime sleepiness. *Arch Intern Med* 1998; 158:1333–1337.

344. Canada. *Health Promotion Directorate, Canadian Guidelines for Healthy Weights*. Minister of National Health and Welfare, Ottawa, 1988.

345. Health and Welfare Canada. *Canada Health Survey, Ottawa*. Health and Welfare Canada, 1978.

346. Rimm AH, Werner LN, Yserlov BV, Bernstein RA. Relationship of obesity and disease in 73,532 weight-conscious women. *Public Health Rep* 1975;90:44–54.

347. Cigolini M, Targher G, Tonoli M, *et al.* Hyperuricaemia: relationships to body fat distribution and other components of the insulin resistance syndrome in 38-year-old healthy men and women. *Int J Obes Relat Metab Disord* 1995;19:91–96.

348. Tikly M, Bellingan A, Lincoln D, Russell A. Risk factors for gout: a hospital-based study of urban black South Africans. *Rev Rhum Engl Ed* 1998;65:225–231.

349. Dessein PH, Shipton EA, Stanwix AE, *et al.* Beneficial effects of weight loss associated with moderate calorie/carbohydrate restriction, and increased proportional intake of protein and unsaturated fat on serum urate and lipoprotein levels in gout: a pilot study. *Ann Rheum Dis* 2000;59:539–543.

350. Leach RE, Baumgard S, Broom J. Obesity: its relationship to osteoarthritis of the knee. *Clin Orthop* 1973;93:271–273.

351. Goldin RH, McAdam L, Louie JS, *et al.* Clinical and radiological survey of the incidence of osteoarthrosis among obese patients. *Ann Rheum Dis* 1976;35:349–353.

352. Felson DT, Chaisson CE. Understanding the relationship between body weight and osteoarthritis. *Baillieres Clin Rheumatol* 1997; 11:671–681.

353. Cooper C, Snow S, McAlindon TE, *et al.* Risk factors for the incidence and progression of radiologic knee osteoarthritis. *Arthritis Rheum* 2000;43:995–1000.

354. Sturmer T, Gunther KP, Brenner H. Obesity, overweight and patterns of osteoarthritis: the Ulm Osteoarthritis Study. *J Clin Epidemiol* 2000;53:307–313.

355. Cooper C, Inskip H, Croft P, *et al.* Individual risk factors for hip osteoarthritis: obesity, hip injury, and physical activity. *Am J Epidemiol* 1998;147:516–522.

356. Oliveria SA, Felson DT, Cirillo PA, *et al.* Body weight, body mass index, and incident symptomatic osteoarthritis of the hand, hip, and knee. *Epidemiology* 1999;10:161–166.

357. Weintraub JM, Willett WC, Rosner B, *et al.* A prospective study of the relationship between body mass index and cataract extraction among US women and men. *Int J Obes Relat Metab Disord* 2002;26:588–595.

358. Galtier-Dereure F, Boegner C, Bringer J. Obesity and pregnancy: complications and cost. *Am J Clin Nutr* 2000;71:1242S–1248S.

359. Prentice A, Goldberg G. Maternal obesity increases congenital malformations. *Nutr Rev* 1996;54:146–150.

360. Waller DK, Mills JL, Simpson JL, *et al.* Are obese women at higher risk for producing malformed offspring? *Am J Obstet Gynecol* 1994;170:541–548.

361. Shaw GM, Velie EM, Schaffer D. Risk of neural tube defect-affected pregnancies among obese women. *JAMA* 1996;275:1093–1096.

362. Kallen K. Maternal smoking, body mass index, and neural tube defects. *Am J Epidemiol* 1998;147:1103–1111.

363. Watkins ML, Rasmussen SA, Honein M, *et al.* Maternal obesity and risk for birth defects. *Pediatrics* 2003;111:1152–1158.

364. Wadden TA, Stunkard AJ. Psychopathology and obesity. *Ann NY Acad Sci* 1987;499:55–65.

365. Stunkard AJ, Wadden TA. Psychological aspects of severe obesity. *Am J Clin Nutr* 1992;55:524S–532S.

366. National Institute of Health Consensus Development Panel on the Health Implications of Obesity. Health complications of obesity. *Ann Intern Med* 1985;103:1073–1077.

367. Roberts RE, Kaplan GA, Shema SJ, Strawbridge WJ. Are the obese at greater risk for depression? *Am J Epidemiol* 2000;152:163–170.

368. Riva R, Ragazzoni P, Molinari E. Obesity, psychopathology and eating attitudes: are they related? *Eat Weight Disord* 1998;3:78–83.

369. Carpenter KM, Hasin DS, Allison DB, Faith MS. Relationships between obesity and DSM-IV major depressive disorder, suicide ideation, and suicide attempts: results from a general population study. *Am J Public Health* 2000;90:251–257.

370. Haukkala A, Uutela A. Cynical hostility, depression, and obesity: the moderating role of education and gender. *Int J Eat Disord* 2000;27:106–109.

371. Carter AS, Baker CW, Brownell KD. Body mass index, eating attitudes, and symptoms of depression and anxiety in pregnancy and the postpartum period. *Psychosom Med* 2000;62:264–270.

372. Aevarsson O, Skoog I. A population-based study on the incidence of dementia disorders between 85 and 88 years of age. *J Am Geriatr Soc* 1996;44:1455–1460.

373. Skoog I, Nilsson L, Palmertz B, *et al.* A population-based study of dementia in 85-year-olds. *N Engl J Med* 1993;328:153–158.
374. Hofman A, Ott A, Breteler MMB, *et al.* Atherosclerosis, apolipoprotein E, and prevalence of dementia and Alzheimer's disease in the Rotterdam Study. *Lançet* 1997;349:151–154.
375. Skoog I, Kalaria RN, Breteler MM. Vascular factors and Alzheimer disease. *Alzheimer Dis Assoc Disord* 1999;13(Suppl 3):S106–S114.
376. Gustafson D, Rothenberg E, Blennow K, *et al.* An 18-year follow-up of overweight and risk of Alzheimer disease. *Arch Intern Med* 2003;163:1524–1528.
377. Young T, Peppard PE, Gottlieb DJ. Epidemiology of obstructive sleep apnea: a population health perspective. *Am J Respir Crit Care Med* 2002;165:1217–1239.
378. Sobal J, Stunkard AJ. Socioeconomic status and obesity: a review of the literature. *Psychol Bull* 1989;105:260–275.
379. Stunkard AJ, Sorensen TIA. Obesity and socioeconomic status — a complex relation. *N Engl J Med* 1993;329:1036–1037.
380. Wardle J, Waller J, Jarvis MJ. Sex differences in the association of socioeconomic status with obesity. *Am J Public Health* 2002;92: 1299–1304.
381. Canning H, Mayer J. Obesity — its possible effect on college acceptance. *N Engl J Med* 1966;275:1172–1174.
382. Gortmaker SL, Must A, Perrin JM, *et al.* Social and economic consequences of overweight in adolescence and young adulthood. *N Engl J Med* 1993;329:1008–1012.
383. Sonne-Holm S, Sorensen TIA. Prospective study of attainment of social class of severely obese subjects in relation to parental social class, intelligence, and education. *BMJ* 1986;292:586–598.
384. Goldblatt PB, Moore ME, Stunkard AJ. Social factors of obesity. *JAMA* 1965;192:1039–1044.
385. Knight JA. The biochemistry of aging. *Adv Clin Chem* 2001;35: 1–62.
386. Keaney JF, Larson MG, Ramachandran S, *et al.* Obesity and systemic oxidative stress: clinical correlates of oxidative stress in the Framingham Study. *Arterioscler Thromb Vasc Biol* 2003;23:434–439.
387. Field AE, Coakley EH, Must A, *et al.* Impact of overweight on the risk of developing common chronic diseases during a 10-year period. *Arch Intern Med* 2001;161:1581–1586.
388. Jebb SA. The Nutrition Society Medical Lecture. Obesity: from molecules to man. *Proc Nutr Soc* 1999;58:1–14.

3

Physical Activity: Its Role in Disease/Disorder Prevention

Introduction

In their struggle for survival, it was critical for early humans to maintain a high level of physical fitness. However, modern day humans are dying from various diseases because of physical inactivity. According to the 1990 Global Burden of Disease Study,[1] physical inactivity was among the top ten risk factors for global health. Indeed, the modern sedentary lifestyle most likely represents an important violation of biological principles to which humans have genetically adapted. As such, it is not surprising that physical fitness and the will to remain fit is associated with health and survival. Thus, in addition to its critical role in weight control strategy, regular exercise has numerous health benefits (Table 3.1). An extensive scientific literature over the past two decades has shown that increased physical activity is a major factor in the prevention/control of numerous diseases/disorders including coronary heart disease (CHD), stroke, type 2 diabetes mellitus, hypertension, osteoporosis, some types of cancer, falls/fractures and blood lipid abnormalities. Exercise also improves the immune system, quality of life and confers a protective benefit against all-cause mortality. Moreover, a sedentary and physically unfit lifestyle leads to various functional limitations as one ages. Furthermore, regular physical activity is associated with

183

Table 3.1: Exercise-influenced Diseases/Disorders

Aging	Hypertension
All-cause mortality	Decreased immunity
Blood lipids	Mental health
Cancer (some forms)	Type 2 diabetes mellitus
Cardiovascular disease	Obesity/weight control
Falls/fractures	Osteoporosis
Functional decline	Quality of life
Gallbladder disease	Sarcopenia (muscle loss)
Gastrointestinal bleeding	Stroke

improved mental health and is used as adjunctive therapy in drug- and alcohol-dependency programs. These studies consistently demonstrate that health benefits begin to accrue at a significant and measurable level when one moves from a sedentary lifestyle to one involving even moderate physical activity. Importantly, these health benefits increase even more with regular vigorous physical activity.

Since many of these facts are widely appreciated, why is it so difficult to get people to exercise? Although the most common New Year's resolutions are to lose weight and exercise more, they are soon discarded for various reasons (i.e. muscle/joint pain, too tired, too busy, don't have time, don't like to exercise, among others). It is suggested that the major problem for most of us is a lack of commitment and persistence. As the sayings go, "one of these days is none of these days" and "hoping and wishing are excuses for not doing."

In 1996, the Centers for Disease Control and Prevention (CDC) reported physical activity data from 105,390 adults in 49 states and the District of Columbia (D.C.).[2] Overall, reported participation in regular physical activity by state varied from 16.0% (D.C.) to 35.7% (Oregon) (median: 26.9%); the ranges among states were similar for men and women (15.8–39.0% and 15.6–38.3%, respectively). However, participation in no leisure-time physical activity ranged from 18.3% (Washington) to 49.3% (D.C.); for men, from 16.0% to 49.1% and for women, from 19.5% to 50.1%. Importantly, insufficient physical activity (i.e. no leisure-time activity and irregular activity combined) estimates ranged from 64.3% to 84.0%. Thus, although there was considerable variation between states, in every state 60% or more of adults did not achieve the minimum, recommended level of physical activity and in about half the states, about 73% of adults were insufficiently active. Since these figures are self-reported, it is probable that the true numbers are significantly higher.

Casperson and Merritt[3] studied the physical activity trends among 26 states involving 34,800 adults aged 18 and older during the years 1986–1990. They scored leisure time physical activity into four patterns: (1) physically inactive, (2) irregularly active, (3) regularly active, not intensive, and (4) regularly active, intensive. Their results indicated that six in ten persons were physically inactive or irregularly active; although almost four in ten were regularly active, less than one in ten was regularly active, intensive. In addition, they found that women and older adults were the most likely to have increased their physical activity during this time period, while non-white populations and the least educated groups were significantly less likely to do so. Similarly, Ransdell and Wells[4] recently reported their findings of physical activity in urban white, African-American and Mexican-American women. Here, only 8% of African-American women, 11% of Mexican-American women and 13% of white women participated in the physical activity level recommended by the surgeon general (i.e. moderate physical activity most days of the week for 30 minutes or longer). Women of color, over age 40, and those without a college education had the lowest levels of participation.

A 1995 CDC report on the changes in physical inactivity among persons aged 65 years and above showed a modest decline during 1987–1992.[5] Those engaging in no physical activity during leisure time declined from 43.2% in 1987 to 38.5% in 1992. However, one of the national health objectives for the year 2000 was to reduce the proportion of physically inactive adults aged 65 years and above to 22%. Unfortunately, based on their data, they projected the 1997 physical inactivity in this age group to be 36–37% and would be well below the 2000 year goal. In fact, as of 1999, only one of the 13 physical activity and fitness objectives for 2000 had been met or exceeded.[6] In 1997, the CDC reported that 65% of adolescents in grades 9 to 12 engaged in at least 20 minutes of vigorous physical activity three or more times per week; only 15% of adults aged 18 years and older engaged in 30 minutes of moderate physical activity five or more days per week (minimal CDC recommendations).[7] The goals of Healthy People 2010 is to increase adolescent activity to 85% and adult activity to 30%.

Gordon-Larsen *et al.*[8] studied the determinants of physical activity and inactivity in adolescents. They found that moderate to vigorous physical activity was lower and inactivity higher for non-Hispanic blacks and Hispanic adolescents compared with white and Asian adolescents. In addition, participation in physical education programs was significantly lower in the former adolescents and decreased with age. This study also found that the level of maternal education was inversely associated with high physical inactivity patterns. However, participation in daily school physical education (PE) classes and use of community recreation centers increased the likelihood of engaging in moderate to vigorous physical activity. Unfortunately, only 21.3% of all adolescent participated in one or more days per week of school PE. Increased crime rates were also associated with a decrease in regular moderate to vigorous physical activity. More recently, Kimm and co-workers[9] further substantiated the decline in physical activity among adolescent girls. Here, leisure time physical activity in black and white girls, followed from ages nine to ten to 16 to 17 years, decreased 100% and 64% respectively. Thus, by age 16 to 17 years, 56% of black girls and 31% of white girls were not involved in any leisure time activity. Although a lower level of parental education was associated with a greater decline in activity for white girls at both ages, it applied only to the older black girls. Pregnancy was associated with a decline in activity only among black girls, whereas smoking was associated with decreased physical activity among white but not black girls. Among both black and white girls, the body mass index (BMI) was inversely associated to physical activity.

The intensity and frequency of physical activity is also very low in preadolescent children. The current health recommendation for children is to have daily school PE classes that engage them in moderate to vigorous physical activity at least 50% of class time. To evaluate these recommendations, 814 third-grade children (414 boys, 400 girls) at ten different sites were observed.[10] The study found that the children averaged 33 minutes in each of 2.1 PE lessons per week. Only 5.9% had daily PE in which they accrued 4.8 very active and 11.9 moderate to vigorous minutes of physical activity per PE lesson (15.0% and 37.0% of lesson time, respectively). Thus, the children were involved in only 25 minutes per week of moderate to vigorous physical activity, a level markedly short of the minimum national recommendation.

Others studied the relationship of physical activity and television watching with body weight and degree of fatness in children.[11] Here, 80% of American children reportedly performed three or more bouts of vigorous physical activity each week. The physical activity rate was lower in non-Hispanic black (69%) and Mexican-American girls (73%). Twenty percent of the children participated in two or less bouts of physical activity each week; the rate was higher in girls (26%) than in boys (17%). Overall, 26% of the children watched four or more hours of television per day while 67% watched at least 2 hours each day. Non-Hispanic black children had the highest rate of television watching per day (42%). Furthermore, girls and boys who watched four or more hours of television each day had significantly greater body fat and higher BMI than those who watched television for two hours or less each day.

To further understand the relationship between health beliefs, self-efficacy, social support and sedentary activities and physical activity levels in children, as well as the relationship between physical activity and self-esteem, Strauss and associates[12] studied 92 children aged ten to 16 years. Their findings were as follows: (1) physical activity significantly decreased between ages ten and 16 years, mainly in girls; (2) pre-teen girls spent about 35% more time in low- and high-level activity than did teenage girls; (3) overall, children were inactive 75.5% of the day (watching television, using a computer and homework); and (4) only 1.4% of the day (mean 12.6 minutes) was spent in vigorous activity. Importantly, time spent in high-level activity correlated with both self-efficacy and social influence scores. High level physical activity was also significantly associated with increased self-esteem.

Physical Activity versus Exercise

The terms "exercise" and "physical activity" are commonly used interchangeably, although their meanings are clearly different when applied to health matters. Physical activity refers to any bodily movement produced by skeletal muscles that burn calories (i.e. gardening, lawn mowing, housework, etc.). Exercise, on the other hand, is considered to be a subcategory of physical activity; it is planned, structured, repetitive and results in the maintenance or improvement of one or more facets of physical fitness. It includes regular activities such as cycling, jogging, brisk walking, swimming, etc. "Aerobics" or "aerobic exercises" refer to endurance activities which increase the heart and breathing rates for an extended period of time. Exercises that build muscles are referred to as "strength training," "resistance training," "weight training," or "weight lifting." Physical fitness is not considered a behavior but rather an individuals' achievement which includes muscular strength or endurance, body composition, aerobic endurance and flexibility. As such, physical activity and exercise are health-related behaviors that can improve or maintain various aspects of physical fitness.

Physician Counseling

A clear understanding of the medical and financial benefits of regular exercise is poorly appreciated, even by many physicians. Indeed, physicians counsel their patients less often about the need for increased physical activity than about most other important lifestyle behaviors. For example, a recent CDC report indicated that only 19% of physicians said they counseled their patients about exercise.[13] Frolkis *et al.*[14] also reported that physicians are poorly compliant with the National Cholesterol Education Program (NCEP) guidelines even

with patients at high risk for CHD. Here, only 1% of physicians recommended exercise, 50% followed the NCEP algorithms for lipid
screening, 4% encouraged patients to quit smoking, and 14%
referred overweight patients to dieticians. Reasons for the failure to
adequately counsel patients include lack of knowledge and preparation, inadequate time, perceived effectiveness and lack of training in
behavioral counseling.[15-17] With respect to exercise, a recent study
not only found that physician counseling was nationally very low,[18]
but that physicians were more likely to counsel as secondary prevention. That is, patients were counseled to become more physically
active after they had developed cardiac disease or diabetes. Furthermore, physicians were less likely to counsel patients at risk for
obesity, younger disease-free adults, those with lower socioeconomic
status and the less educated. The authors concluded that failure to
counsel these latter groups "represent important missed opportunities for primary prevention."

Albright and associates[19] recently reported the effectiveness of physician advice alone compared with physician advice plus behavioral
counseling to increase levels of physical activity in healthy but sedentary patients. Physicians were trained to integrate three to four
minutes of initial physical activity advice into the routine office visit.
This advice included assessment of current physical activities, advising patients about appropriate goals and referrals to a health care
educator. Ninety-nine percent of patients received the initial physician advice about physical activity. Their results showed that 83% of
physicians spent less than five to six minutes providing advice while
46% spent the recommended three to four minutes. Furthermore, there
was little disruption in physician routine and attitudes regarding the
advice protocol were positive and beneficial. Hence, with appropriate education and stimulation, many physicians can and will modify
their practices to address this highly important lifestyle factor. Several recent publications have recommended ways whereby physicians
can more effectively motivate patients to increase their physical
activity.[20-23] Indeed, data from the 1998 National Health Interview
Survey (NHIS)[24] showed that the prevalence of older adults who met
the recommended level of physical activity was significantly higher

among those who were simply asked by their physicians about their activity than among those who were not asked (36% versus 23%).

Deitrick[25] also emphasized that an appropriate exercise program with personal counseling can lead to very effective results. Thus, prior to recommendations for exercise counseling, the physician should do the following:

(1) evaluate the patient's cardiac risk;
(2) establish mutually agreed upon goals;
(3) recognize that health benefits accrue at different levels of physical activity;
(4) emphasize the need for regular exercise (see below);
(5) increase exercise duration prior to exercise intensity; and
(6) recommend low intensity exercise for diabetics and improved mental health.

After evaluation of these items, he recommended the following:

(1) assess patient readiness to participate;
(2) review patient's exercise history and select the most likely successful program;
(3) agree on a specific plan of action;
(4) suggest ways to overcome perceived barriers;
(5) convey a strong conviction as to the value of exercise and educate the patient as to the specific diseases/disorders that can be prevented or delayed; and importantly,
(6) serve as a role model.

Others stressed that community-based programs for older people are also needed to facilitate increased physical activity.[26] The Community Healthy Activities Model Program for Seniors (CHAMPS) is designed to promote lifetime physical activity in older persons and allows them "to choose activities that take into account their health, preferences, and abilities." This study "led to meaningful physical activity increases." Although overweight persons especially benefitted from the program, it was also effective in women, older adults (i.e. 75 years and older) and those who were completely inactive at baseline. Elley *et al.*[27] also recently reported that counseling sedentary patients in general practice on exercise is effective not only in increasing physical activity, but improving the quality of life.

How much exercise does one need? In 1995, the CDC and the American College of Sports Medicine concluded that every adult should accumulate at least 30 minutes of moderate-intensity physical activity "on most, preferably all, days of the week."[28] Here, "physical activity" was defined as "any bodily movement produced by skeletal muscles that results in energy expenditure." Moderate physical activity is the equivalent of walking at three to four miles per hour. Thus, aerobic activity such as brisk walking, cycling, swimming and dancing that gradually increases the heart rate and requires deep breathing without undue strain, is of major benefit. However, it should be emphasized that this activity level is the minimum recommended. Those who already meet it "are likely to derive some additional health and fitness benefits from becoming more physically active."[28] More recently, however, the Institute of Medicine committee recommended that people who want to stay healthy should essentially double these recommendations.[29] More specifically, they recommended at least one hour of moderate physical activity daily, such as walking, swimming, bicycle riding or golfing without a cart.

In an interesting related topic, Allen *et al.*[30] evaluated bed rest as a treatment for various medical conditions. They reviewed 39 clinical trials of bed rest for 15 different conditions (total patients, 5777). In 24 trials following a medical procedure, bed rest did not significantly improve the outcomes and in eight trials, some procedures (lumbar puncture, spinal anesthesia, radiculography and cardiac catheterization) worsened the outcomes. In 15 trials, where bed rest was a primary treatment, no outcomes were significantly improved and in nine trials some conditions worsened (labor, proteinuric hypertension during pregnancy, acute low back pain, myocardial infarction and acute infectious hepatitis). The authors concluded that "we should not assume any efficacy for bed rest."

Are there contraindications to increasing physical activity in older adults? The answer is yes, but these are few and generally related to

Table 3.2: Contraindications for Exercise Training in Elderly People[31,32]

Absolute	Relative
Abdominal aortic aneurysm	Cardiomyopathy
Acute heart failure	Complex ventricular ectopy
Myocardial infarction (recent)	Uncontrolled hypertension
Recent electrocardiogram changes	Uncontrolled metabolic disorder
Third degree heart block	Valvular heart disease
Unstable angina	

cardiac disorders (Table 3.2).[31,32] They include recent electrocardiogram changes or an acute myocardial infarction, unstable angina, uncontrolled arrhythmias and acute congestive heart failure. Other potential contraindications, depending on their control and severity, include uncontrolled hypertension, cardiomyopathy, valvular heart disease and uncontrolled metabolic disorders. Gill *et al.*[33] recently published a detailed set of recommendations to minimize possible adverse cardiac events among previously sedentary elderly people without symptomatic cardiovascular disease. Although an older person generally does not need a treadmill test or stress test prior to beginning a modest exercise program, the physician should inquire about the following:[34] (1) presence of chest pain during physical activity; (2) recent chest pain when not engaged in physical activity; (3) loss of balance because of dizziness; (4) loss of consciousness; and (5) medications for hypertension or a cardiac disorder.

Exercise and Weight Reduction

Due to the significant personal and public health burden of overweight and obesity, it is extremely important to identify interventions that prevent weight gain, as well as weight regain for those who have lost significant weight. Since weight-loss occurs when a person maintains a negative energy balance for a period of time, exercise is an important companion of decreased caloric intake for losing and controlling weight. As such, physically active people are significantly less likely to become overweight than their sedentary peers. Although dietary restriction results in greater weight loss than does exercise, more of the loss is from lean body mass than from fat.[29] Thus, the combination of leisure-time physical activity and caloric reduction produces more weight loss than diet alone. In addition, exercise has a more favorable effect on body fat distribution (i.e. reduction of waist-to-hip ratio).[35] Indeed, numerous studies conducted over the past two decades have clearly shown that without physical activity, weight control is usually not achieved. Conversely, regular physical activity can improve weight control, as well as longevity, even for those with BMIs in the overweight category.[36] Moreover, unlike diet-induced weight loss, exercise-induced weight loss increases cardiorespiratory fitness.[37]

In a study of the association between recreational physical activity and weight change, Williamson *et al.*[38] reported a strong inverse association in both cross-sectional and retrospective analyses over a ten-year period in both men and women. The estimated relative risk of major weight gain for those in the low physical activity levels compared with the highest activity levels at the follow-up survey were 3.1 and 3.8 in men and women, respectively. For those whose activity level was low at both baseline and follow-up, the relative risks were 2.3 for men and 7.1 for women. More recent studies have also shown a positive effect of physical activity for weight control in women. Anderson and associates[39] examined short- and long-term changes in weight and body composition by a low fat diet (about 1200 kcal/d) combined with either structured aerobic exercise or moderate-intensity lifestyle activity in obese women. Their results showed mean weight losses during the 16-week treatment period of 8.3 kg for the aerobic group and 7.9 kg for the lifestyle group. During the one-year follow-up, the aerobic group regained 1.6 kg while the lifestyle group regained 0.08 kg. Thus, the program of low fat diet plus a moderate-intensity lifestyle was equivalent in weight loss to the diet plus aerobic activity in obese women. In addition to an increased risk for various chronic medical disorders, the degree of adiposity in women correlates directly with lower daily physical functioning (e.g. climbing stairs and other moderate activities), as well as lower feelings of well-being and greater burden of pain.[40]

Although walking is a very popular form of exercise, the exact number of calories expended is difficult to determine since the energy cost is not linearly correlated to the walking speed, as it is with running and jogging. However, one can get a rough caloric estimate by comparing the distance walked with the caloric cost obtained from running. Harger et al.[41] noted that a 150-pound (68 kg) person uses 147 calories by jogging 1.5 miles (2.4 km). The authors emphasized that even if the daily caloric expendure is only 100 calories, this translates to a weight loss of about ten pounds per year (3500 calories burn one pound of fat). Alternatively, an extra 100-calorie expenditure per day avoids gaining about ten pounds per year. Others[42] reported that the inclusion of a moderate walking regimen into a weight maintenance program in premenopausal obese women improved maintenance of losses in both total body weight and waist circumference.

Although these and other recent studies[43,44] indicate that physical activity is very important in weight control, others have stressed the need for more randomized controlled trials to more accurately evaluate the effect of increased physical activity and fitness as a tool for the prevention of excess body weight and composition.[45,46] Indeed, Lawlor et al.[47] noted that two-thirds of English women participating in their study were active according to the recent recommended levels. However, if domestic activities were excluded, only 21% were regularly active. After adjusting for the usual confounders, women who walked briskly for at least 2.5 hours per week reduced their odds of being overweight (odds ratio, 0.5), whereas women who participated in at least 2.5 hours of heavy housework per week did not reduce their risk of being overweight (odds ratio, 1.1). The authors emphasized the need for prospective studies in order "to demonstrate an independent health benefit of participating in domestic activities."

Recognizing the importance of randomized controlled trials, Jakicic et al.[48] recently reported their findings from an 18-month randomized trial involving 148 sedentary, overweight or obese women (mean BMI 32.8 kg/m^2) aged 36.7 ± 5.6 years. The women were divided into three groups in which each subject was prescribed a similar volume of exercise five days per week. The long-bout exercise duration progressed from 20 minutes per day (min/d) during weeks 1 to 4 to

30 min/d for weeks 5 to 8 and to 40 min/d for the duration of the study. The short-bout exercise group progressed from 20 min/d to 40 min/d by the ninth week. Rather than exercising continuously for the duration, the exercise period was divided into multiple ten-minute bouts performed at convenient times throughout the day. The prescription for the short-bout group with treadmill was otherwise the same as the short-bout exercise group. The results showed that weight loss was significantly greater in the short-bout with treadmill group (mean 7.4 kg; 16.28 pounds) compared with the short-bout (mean 3.7 kg; 8.14 pounds) and long-bout (mean 5.8 kg; 12.76 pounds) exercise groups. Moreover, subjects in the short-bout exercise plus treadmill group maintained a higher level of exercise than the other groups. The mean weight loss after 18 months was also significantly greater in those exercising more than 200 minutes (3.3 hours) per week (mean 13.1 kg; 28.82 pounds) compared with those exercising 150 to 200 minutes per week (mean 8.5 kg; 18.70 pounds) or less than 150 minutes per week (mean 3.5 kg; 7.70 pounds).

More recently, Irwin and associates[49] carried out a randomized controlled trial from 1997 to 2001 involving 173 sedentary overweight postmenopausal women aged 50 to 75 years. The women were randomly assigned to either an intervention consisting of exercise facility and home-based moderate intensity exercise or to a stretching control group. The exercisers, in which walking was the most frequently reported activity, showed statistically significant differences from the controls in both total weight loss and intra-abdominal fat. There was also a significant dose-response for greater body fat loss with increasing duration of exercise.

Exercise and All-Cause Mortality

Exercise versus physical inactivity

A number of prospective studies have shown lower mortality rates in both physically active men and women compared to those who are sedentary. For example, an early study[50] of 10,269 men aged 45 to

84 years, who were free of any life-threatening diseases at baseline, were followed for 15 years. The authors analyzed changes in their level of physical activity, along with cigarette smoking, blood pressure and body weight. Beginning a moderately vigorous sports activity was associated with a 23% lower risk of death compared with those not starting an exercise program. Similar findings were reported for the other lifestyle characteristics. The authors concluded that beginning a moderately vigorous sports activity, maintaining normal blood pressure, averting obesity and quitting smoking were separately associated with lower death rates for all causes, as well as from CHD. In a later report, Blair and co-workers[51] evaluated the relationship between physical fitness changes and mortality risk in 9777 men with two clinical examinations separated by an average of 4.9 years. The highest age-adjusted all-cause mortality was in men who were unfit at both examinations; the lowest death rate was in those who were deemed physically fit at both examinations. Mortality was reduced by 44% for those who improved from physically unfit to fit relative to those who remained physically unfit at both examinations.

The intensity of exercise also appears to be directly related to all-cause mortality and longevity in men.[52] This prospective study involved 17,321 Harvard University alumni who were initially evaluated in 1962 and 1966 and followed through 1988. The results showed a graded inverse relationship between total physical activity and all-cause mortality. In addition, vigorous physical activities, but not non-vigorous activities, were associated with increased longevity. In a follow-up report from the Harvard Alumni Health Study, covering the years 1977–1992, 13,455 men (mean age 57.5 years) reported their walking, stair climbing and sports/recreation activities.[53] Distance walked and floors climbed were independent predictors of longevity. Although light activities were not associated with a reduced mortality rate, moderate activities were "somewhat beneficial" while vigorous activities "clearly predicted lower mortality rates." In agreement with this, Sarna et al.[54] studied 2613 world-class Finnish male athletes who competed in a wide variety of sports (Olympic games, World or European championships and inter-country competitions) during 1920–1965 and who survived until 1985. The mean life expectancy adjusted for marital status, occupational group and age at entry was as follows: (1) endurance sports (long distance running and cross-country skiing), 75.6 years; (2) team games (soccer, ice hockey, basketball and short-distance runners), 73.9 years; and (3) power sports (boxing, weight-lifting, etc.), 71.5 years. The reference group, which consisted of 1712 men matched for age and area of residence, had a mean life expectancy of 69.9 years.

A graded, inverse correlation between all-cause mortality and physical activity in postmenopausal women has also been reported.[55] In this study involving 40,417 postmenopausal women aged 55 to 69 years, those who reported regular physical activity were at a significantly reduced mortality risk during follow-up compared with those who were not physically active. In addition, increasing the frequency of moderate physical activity during the follow-up period was also associated with a reduced risk of death (i.e. those rarely or never engaging in physical activity to activity at least four times each week). Nevertheless, engagement in moderate activity as infrequently as once each week demonstrated a reduced mortality risk. In general agreement with this report, others[56] conducted a ten-year randomized clinical trial of regular walking and health status in women. Compared with the control group, those involved in regular periods of walking had fewer cardiac problems, hospitalizations, surgeries and falls. More recently, Gregg and associates[57] conducted a prospective cohort study of community-dwelling white women 65 years or older at four United States research centers. The participants were initially evaluated in 1986–1988 and again in 1992–1994 (median time difference, 5.7 years). After controlling for age, smoking, BMI, comorbid conditions and baseline activity level, those who increased their physical activity levels between baseline and follow-up had lower mortality from all causes (hazard rate ratio, 0.52), cardiovascular disease (hazard rate ratio, 0.64) and cancer (hazard rate ratio, 0.49) compared with the continually sedentary women. All-cause and cardiovascular mortality were also significantly lower in women who were physically active at both visits.

Kujala *et al.*[58] studied the relationship of leisure-time physical activity and mortality and sought to determine whether genetic factors might modify this relationship. The study included 7925 healthy men and 7977 healthy women of the Finnish Twin Cohort aged 25 to 64 years. "Conditioning exercisers" included those who exercised at least six times each month with an intensity of at least vigorous walking for a mean duration of 30 minutes. Those who did not participate in any leisure-time physical activity were classified as "sedentary," the others who exercised somewhere between these two groups were classified as "occasional exercisers." The study showed an inverse correlation between the level of exercise and all-cause mortality in both men and women. Moreover, the beneficial effects of physical activity remained even after genetic and other familial factors were considered.

Other reports have shown that physical activity in the elderly also has a positive effect on mortality. For example, Bijnen *et al.*[59] studied the associations between physical activity patterns of elderly men aged 64 to 84 years and mortality from CHD, stroke and all causes. After adjusting for major chronic diseases, cigarette smoking and alcohol consumption, mortality risks from CHD and all causes decreased significantly with increasing physical activity. In addition, except for CHD, time spent in more intense activities was more strongly associated with favorable mortality outcomes than less intense activities. Walking or cycling at least three times per week for 20 minutes also decreased all-cause mortality and CHD. These findings are similar to those more recently reported[60] involving 707 non-smoking retired men aged 61 to 81 years. After adjustment for age, the mortality rate among men who walked two miles or more each day was only half that of men who walked less than one mile per day. After 12 years, the cumulative incidence of death for the most active walkers was reached in less than seven years among those who were least active. In addition, the distance walked each day was inversely related to mortality after adjustment for overall activity measures and other risk factors.

Several recent studies have also shown an inverse relationship between increased physical activity and all-cause mortality.[61–64] For example, Stessman and others[64] studied a community-based cohort of 456 70-year-old subjects born in 1920–1921. Unadjusted mortality at six-year follow-up was significantly greater for those reporting no regular exercise than those walking as little as four hours per week (23.4% versus 9.9%). The significance of these benefits applied to both males (30.28% versus 12.14%) and females (16.9% versus 6.86%). Moreover, increased regularity of activity correlated with declining mortality. Several earlier publications documenting the importance of physical activity and physical fitness in averting premature deaths have been reviewed.[65]

The above studies, among others, clearly show that higher levels of physical activity and increased aerobic fitness are protective against premature mortality. However, the relationship between musculoskeletal fitness and all-cause mortality is less well understood. To increase this understanding, Katzmarzyk and Craig[66] quantified this relationship by studying 8116 men and women aged 20 to 69 years who participated in the Canada Fitness Survey. Musculoskeletal fitness levels were measured by sit-ups, push-ups, grip strength and sit-and-reach trunk flexibility. Their findings showed that sit-ups, a measure of abdominal muscular endurance, was particularly predictive of mortality in both men and women. Here, the relative mortality risks of the lowest quartile compared with the highest quartile were 2.72 and 2.26 for men and women, respectively. Although there was a 49% increased risk of death for men in the lower versus the higher quartile of grip strength, there was no association among women. Neither trunk flexibility nor push-ups were associated with mortality.

Measured indicators of mortality

Exercise testing is well recognized as being important in the following patients with CHD. Thus, exercise blood pressure, heart rate acceleration during exercise and deceleration after stopping exercise are predictors of death from CHD.[67–69] Erikssen *et al.*[70] have shown that changes in fitness are also strongly associated with changes in mortality. More specifically, Cole and associates[69] reported a delayed decrease in the heart rate during the first minute after graded exercise "is a powerful predictor of overall mortality independent of workload, the presence or absence of myocardial perfusion defects and changes in heart rate during exercise." In this study, an abnormal value for heart rate recovery was defined as a reduction of 12 beats or less per minute from the heart rate at peak exercise.

Exercise capacity, also a known prognostic factor in patients with cardiovascular disease, was recently evaluated as a predictor of mortality among 6213 men referred for treadmill exercise testing.[71] The group was followed for 6.2 ± 3.7 years, during which there were 1256 deaths. Those who died were older, had a lower maximal heart rate, lower maximal systolic and diastolic blood pressures and lower exercise capacity. The authors concluded that exercise capacity, measured in metabolic equivalents, was the strongest predictor of the risk of death among both normal subjects and those with cardiovascular disease. Moreover, exercise capacity was "a more powerful predictor of mortality among men than other established risk factors for cardiovascular disease."

From the various studies referred to in this section, one would likely predict that the use of hospital facilities, and therefore medical costs, would be significantly less for the physically active elderly compared with those who are essentially inactive. In this regard, Kujala and coworkers[72] investigated the use of hospital care from all causes among 2049 former elite male athletes and compared them with 1403 male controls. They found that, compared with the controls, all-cause hospital days per person were significantly lower in the former athletes. This difference was primarily related to involvement in those sports that required vigorous aerobic activity.

Exercise and Aging

"Use favors function. Disuse invites decay."[73] Sedentary lifestyles are due to several cultural and environmental factors, including extensive television watching, dependence on the automobile and various "labor-saving" devices, lack of public, as well as the healthcare profession awareness of the importance of exercise, and the false belief that people should "slow down" in their later years. As a result, most older individuals are not physically fit. Indeed, a recent study of 33,466 Swedish men found that total physical activity decreased by 4.1% between ages 45 and 79 years.[74] Moreover, the observed decrease with age was greatest among those who were obese (-8.7%), current smokers (-7.9%) and with a low level of education (-5.6%). Others reported that 70% of women aged 65 years and older were involved in low-intensity activity (50%) or none at all (20%), while 67% indicated six to eight hours of just "sitting" each day.[75] In addition, less than 10% of people 65 years and older engaged in vigorous routine physical activity in 1981;[76] the percentage may well be even lower today.

Unfortunately, many older individuals are reluctant to increase their physical activity, even though they may be aware of the potential health benefits. The reasons for a reluctance to begin exercising vary. Some older adults fear that exercise will harm them; others think they have to join a gym or have special equipment, neither of which they can afford. Still others may feel embarassed to exercise because they believe it is for younger people or for those who "look good" in workout attire. Still others may think that exercise is only for those who are able to play tennis, jog, swim, etc. A recent report[77] on this topic examined 17 possible reasons for avoidance or limitation of physical activties in older people. In women, the lack of an exercise companion was the most common reason given, while lack of interest was the most common for older men. Certainly, most older people can increase the level of their physical activity at little or no cost. Simple things such as regular walking, swimming, dancing, housework, gardening, lawn mowing, etc. are effective ways to increase one's physical activity. A major problem is lack of adequate education as to the benefits of exercise in older people. Organization of exercise programs by public officials, churches and other groups interested in the health of older people would be extremely beneficial. After all, its never too late to promote healthy lifestyles and prevent illness in older people.

Disuse syndrome

Lack of adequate physical activity and its consequences results in the so-called "disuse syndrome" (i.e. premature aging, obesity, cardiovascular vulnerability, musculoskeletal fragility and depression).[78] The author emphasized that this syndrome is experimentally reproducible; however, both preventive and restrictive efforts are inexpensive, safe, accessible and effective. Moreover, these principles apply not just to the young and middle-aged, but also to the older person. We must recognize that age *per se* is not responsible for many disorders attributed to it. Bortz suggested that, "illness as we see it has another component that is due neither to disease *per se* nor to time effects but to disuse, the third dimension."[78]

Several early studies indicated that exercise can retard many of the changes commonly attributable to aging.[73,79] Hodgson[80] studied the effect of age on VO_2max (i.e. the body's ability to extract oxygen from air and transmit it to the circulatory system), a measurement that involves the circulatory, respiratory and blood systems. He showed that VO_2 max progressively decreases as one ages. However, when "moderately active" and "athletic" men were studied, the rate of decline with age was markedly reduced. In fact, there is a decrease of 5% to 15% per decade after 25 years of age.[75] If a 70-year-old person begins a "moderately active" exercise program, there will be a gain of 15 years in VO_2 max; if this individual attains the "athlete" level, the potential improvement would be 40 years.[73] Results from other early reports are in general agreement.[81–83] For example, Dehn and Bruce[82] found that sedentary men had a two-fold greater decline in VO_2max than did physically active men.

Sarcopenia

Physical frailty in elderly people is a state of reduced physiologic reserve associated with increased susceptibility to disability.[84] It is widely recognized that there is an age-related, slow inexorable loss of muscle mass (sarcopenia), even in those who engage in regular aerobic exercise. This phenomenon usually goes unnoticed for decades since the muscle loss is replaced with fatty tissue. For example, there is reportedly a decrease of about 50% of both total muscle mass and urinary excretion of creatinine, a metabolic product of muscle creatine, between the ages of 20 and 90 years.[85] In addition, Imamura *et al.*[86] showed that after age 30, there is a cross-sectional decrease in individual thigh muscles, decreased muscle density and increased intramuscular fat. More recently, Poehlman and associates[87] followed a group of healthy but sedentary premenopausal women aged 44 to 48 years, for six years. After six years follow-up, about half had spontaneously stopped menstruating for at least 12 months. The study results showed that those who experienced menopause, compared with women who remained premenopausal, lost more lean mass, had greater decreases in resting metabolic rate and leisure-time physical activity, and greater increases in fat mass, fasting blood insulin levels and waist-to-hip ratios.

Lack of exercise is particularly detrimental to women who are, on average, smaller and weaker than men. Women also have more body fat and less muscle and bone mass than men. Importantly, strength training can improve the quality of life by increasing muscle power to perform daily activities and remain independent longer. Thus, strength training not only increases muscle mass but preserves bone and improves strength, power and balance which can modify such risk factors for fractures as skeletal fragility, muscle weakness and deteriorating balance. Current standards, guidelines and position statements regarding strength training for healthy sedentary adults, the elderly and cardiac patients were recently published.[88]

The Framingham Disability Study[89] showed that 40% of women aged 55 to 64 years, 45% aged 65 to 74 years and 65% of women aged 75 to 84 years were unable to lift 4.5 kg (9.9 pounds). Moreover, similar percentages were unable to perform some aspects of normal housework. Indeed, both cross-sectional and longitudinal studies indicate a 15% loss of muscle strength per decade in the sixth and seventh decades of life and approximately 30% thereafter.[31] However, increased physical activity in frail elderly persons can preserve lean body mass.[90] These authors carried out a 17-week randomized, controlled intervention trial following a 2×2 factorial design: (1) enriched foods, (2) exercise, (3) both, or (4) neither in 143 frail persons aged 78.6 $\pm$ 5.6 years. Exercise focused on skill training (i.e. strength endurance, coordination and flexibility); food was enriched with multiple micronutrients. Their results showed that exercise significantly preserved lean body mass compared with the non-exercisers, while those receiving micronutrients slightly increased their bone density and mass.

Improvement of physical function is also effective in reversing community-dwelling frailty in very old people.[91] In this nine-month randomized controlled trial, 115 sedentary men and women (mean age, 83 $\pm$ 4 years) were assigned to either a control group that performed a low-intensity home exercise program (flexibility exercises) or an exercise training group consisting of the following: an initial three months flexibility, light resistance and balance training; second three months, resistance training was added; and third three months, endurance training was added. After nine months, the exercise training group showed significantly greater improvements in three of the four primary outcome measures (modified Physical Performance Test, peak oxygen uptake and Functional Status Questionnaire).

Others[92] studied the maximum values for isometric strength dynamic strength and speed of movement in the quadriceps muscle of male subjects between 11 and 70 years. They found that isometric and dynamic strength increased up to the third decade of life and remained essentially constant to the fifth decade, after which they decreased with increasing age. There was no measurable external muscle atrophy to explain the decline in strength. However, microscopic studies of muscle biopsies showed a decrease in the proportion of type II fibers, as well as a selective atrophy of these fibers with increasing age.

The mechanisms leading to sarcopenia are unclear but a combination of several factors are probably responsible for the age-related changes in muscle mass and function.[93] Thus, the various factors responsible for this disorder should, at some point, affect muscle protein turnover and an ultimate imbalance between protein synthesis and breakdown. However, a recent study showed no difference in basal muscle protein turnover between younger men (mean age 22 years) and older men (mean age 70 years).[94] Nevertheless, an inadequate daily intake of dietary protein is very common in those over 65 years, including the so-called "healthy elderly." This protein deficiency, along with lack of physical exercise, is a very important cause of sarcopenia. The current minimum US Recommended Dietary Allowance (RDA) of protein is 0.8 g/kg body weight/day and recent data suggest that the safe protein intake for elderly adults is 1.25 g/kg body weight/day. Thus, the diet of a 70 kg (154 pounds) person should include 70–87.5 g of protein each day.[95]

Disability and functional capacity

A recent literature review reported that 20% of older Americans have chronic disabilities, 7–8% have severe chronic impairments, about 33% have mobility problems, 20% have visual limitations and 33% have a hearing impairment.[96] In the 1994 National Health Interview Survey, 38% of persons aged 65 years and older had at least one functional disorder.[97] In this report, the risk of death associated with decreased functional limitations was 2.5 times greater in persons aged 70 to 79 who were functionally limited compared to those with no limitations. Over time, the decline in chronic disabilities can have major implications for fiscal stability of Medicare and Social Security programs, since the medical cost for a disabled elderly person is, on average, three times that for a non-disabled person.[98] Moreover, in 2000 the long-term expenditures for older disabled Americans, including those receiving community-based and nursing home care, was US$123 billion, about 65% of which was paid by the government.[99]

Numerous studies have shown that increased physical activity can significantly reduce the frequency of these deficiencies. In a cross-sectional study involving 705 community-dwelling Japanese women aged 55 to 93 years, the aim was to determine whether remaining strong, lean and physically active contributes to successful aging (maintaining function and independent living).[100] Multivariate models based on physical methods (i.e. walking speed, chair stands, functional reach, hand and foot reaction times and a "Get Up and Go" test), along with eight questions regarding daily living activities yielded the following results: (1) increases in strength were associated with 2–4% increases in performance compared with the cohort mean; (2) physical activity was independently and positively associated with the most complex test (i.e. "Get Up and Go"); (3) a one standard deviation increase in BMI was negatively associated with a 3–8% reduction in performance; and (4) strength was positively associated with daily living activities. The authors concluded that remaining strong, physically active and lean provides a wide variety of benefits.

Similarly, a group of ambulatory nursing home residents were studied to determine the effects of a 12-week walking program on walk endurance capacity, physical activity level, mobility and quality of life.[101] These individuals had been previously identified as having low physical activity levels and low walk endurance capacities. After 12 weeks, the walking group improved their maximal walk endurance by 77% and distance by 92%; there were no changes in walking speed. There were no significant changes in these variables in the control group. In another study, Fries and associates[102] sought to determine whether regular vigorous running activity is associated with accelerated, unchanged, or postponed disability with increasing age. This longitudinal study involved 451 active members of a runner's club and 330 non-runner community controls; the participants, at the beginning, were 50 to 72 years of age. At baseline, the runners were leaner, had fewer joint complaints, disablity problems, medical disorders and took fewer medications. After eight years of follow-up, those who engaged in vigorous running and other aerobic activities had significantly lower mortality and slower development of disability than the control group. These findings were attributed to the runners' increased aerobic activity, strength, physical fitness and increased organ reserve. Similarly, Wang et al.[103] carried out a 13-year prospective cohort study of 370 members of a runners' club for persons aged 50 years and older and 249 control subjects initially aged 50 to 72 years (mean 59 years). Compared with the control group, the runners' club members had significantly lower disability levels. Reaching a Health Assessment Questionnaire (i.e. deaths and their causes) disability level of 0.75 was postponed by 8.7 years in the runners' club members versus the controls. Participants in other aerobic exercises and the runners' club members were also protected against mortality (rate ratio 0.88 and 0.36, respectively), while male sex and smoking were detrimental (rate ratio 2.4 and 2.2, respectively). The control group also had a 3.3 times higher death rate than the runners' club members in every disease category. Moreover, accelerated disability rates were not seen in the runners' club members. Thus, running and other aerobic exercises were protective against disability and early mortality in elderly runners.

The age-associated decline in muscle strength results in a significant loss in functional capacity, including impaired mobility, with an increased risk of falls, fractures and functional dependency. However, a growing literature indicates that the declines in functional capacity among older people may be significantly improved by exercise training and that interventions that increase muscle strength are successful, even in the very old.[104,105] Indeed, other functional deficiences can also be overcome by exercise to a significant degree. For example, Bassey *et al.*[106] reported a significant direct association between preferred walking speed and muscle strength in elderly men and women. In another report, a group of frail individuals aged 90 ± 1 years undertook an eight-week program consisting of high-intensity resistance training.[107] Their quadriceps strength was negatively correlated with walking time. Upon training completion, strength gain averaged 174%, mid-thigh muscle area increased 9.0% and mean tandem gait speed improved 48%. Others[108] reported similar findings in frail, very elderly people. The results were as follows: (1) muscle strength increased by 113% in the exercisers but decreased 1% in the non-exercisers; (2) gait velocity increased 11.8% in the exercisers but declined 1% in the non-exercisers; and (3) stair-climbing power improved in the exercisers by 25.4% but declined 3.6% in those who did not exercise.

McMurdo and Rennie[109] reported their findings in a controlled trial of seated exercise in elderly persons aged 64 to 91 years who lived in local authority rest homes. After seven months, the changes in the exercise group, compared with the non-exercising control group, showed significant improvements in grip strength, spinal flexion, chair-to-stand up time, activities of daily living and self-rated depression. Another study[110] examined five-year trends in measures of physical performance, and the impact of chronic diseases in community-dwelling persons aged 64 to 94 years. They focused on performance in three areas: musculoskeletal strength, flexibility and cardiovascular fitness Their results showed a gradual improvement in physical performance for the first two to three years after which a gradual decline in performances occurred, irrespective of baseline disease status.

These studies have clearly shown that increased physical activity significantly improves functional capacity and endurance in older persons. Conversely, elderly people who are not otherwise at risk for disabilities in activities of daily living, "restricted activity is an important predictor of functional decline and not just a benign feature of old age."[111] These researchers studied 680 community-living persons 70 years and older who were categorized into three groups (low, intermediate or high) according to their disability risk in activities of daily living. After adjusting for several covariates, including baseline disability risk, the disability score at 18 months worsened by 11.2% for each additional month with restricted activity. For the low- and intermediate-risk groups, the adjusted disability scores increased by 18.7% and 7.5%, respectively, for each additional month of restricted activity. There was no association between functional decline and restricted activity in those at high risk.

Postural stability (balance)

There is considerable evidence that postural stability declines with age.[31] However, studies have shown that increased physical activity improves both postural stability and flexibility and thereby decreases the frequency of imbalance and falls. For example, data from a group of brisk walking postmenopausal women aged 61 to 71 years, showed that postural stability was significantly better than in the age-matched non-walking control group.[112] Furthermore, a dose-response relationship was present between the intensity of walking and postural stability. In addition, Lord *et al.*[113] sought to determine whether a 12-month regular exercise program could improve balance, reaction time, neuromuscular control and muscle strength and thereby decrease the rate of falling in older women aged 60 to 85 years. Compared with the inactive controls, their results demonstrated improved performance in strength measures, reaction time and balance. The findings also suggested that compliance to an exercise program may reduce the frequency of falls, although further studies were recommended.

Other reports suggest that Tai Chi, a Chinese martial art, may be helpful in improving balance and strength. For example, Wolfson and coworkers[114] evaluated the results from 110 healthy people, mean age 80 years, who underwent three months of intensive balance and/or weight training followed by six months of low intensity Tai Chi training for maintenances of the gains. Their findings indicated that balance training restored performance to a level similar to an individual three to ten years younger. In addition, significant gains persisted after six months of Tai Chi, although there was minor decrement. Others[115] evaluated the effects of two exercise programs, Tai Chi and computerized balance training, on primary [i.e. biomedical (strength, flexibility, body composition and cardiovascular endurance), functional and psychosocial frailty indicators] and secondary (frequency of falls) outcomes in 200 persons 70 years and older (mean age 76.2). Three arms in this study consisted of Tai Chi, balance training and education. Their results showed that grip strength declined in all groups and lower extremity range of motion showed limited changes. However, lowered blood pressure before and after a 12-minute walk was present following Tai Chi participation. In addition, Tai Chi resulted in a decrease in responses of both fear of falling and intrusiveness and reduced the risk of multiple falls by 47.5%.

Another potential balance problem is the presence of orthostatic hypotension in frail elderly nursing home residents.[116] This disorder reportedly occurs in over 50% of these individuals and is most prevalent in the morning when they first arise and when the supine blood pressure is highest. Other major risk factors include dizziness or lightheadedness on standing, male sex, medication for Parkinson's disease, time of day and low BMI.[116]

Falls

Falls are among the most common problems affecting the elderly. They are a major public health problem and are associated with significant morbidity, mortality, reduced functioning and early admission to nursing homes. Moreover, fall-related injuries in 1999 reportedly resulted in more than US$8 billion in injury treatment and accounted for 6% of Medicare fee-for-service claims.[117] As the elderly increase in number, fall-related injuries and resulting deaths will likely increase. About 25% of persons aged 65 to 74 years, and at least 33% of those 75 years and older, reportedly have fallen.[118] In addition, approximately 66% of older people who fall will do so again within the following six months.[119] An early study indicated that injury was the sixth leading cause of death in people aged 65 years and older, and most of these fatal injuries were related to falls.[120] More recently, injury was reported as the fifth leading cause of death in older adults and most of the fatal injuries were again reportedly fall-related.[121] Moreover, in 1994 falls were the second leading cause of deaths from unintentional injuries.[122]

In a well-defined white Finnish population, the authors studied all persons aged 50 years and older who were admitted to hospitals from 1970 to 1995 for treatment of a first fall-induced injury.[121] Their findings were as follows: (1) both total and population-adjusted number (i.e. per 100,000) significantly increased; (2) total fall-induced injuries increased by 284%, the rate increased 183%; (3) age-adjusted incidence increased in both women (127%) and men (124%); (4) the number of deaths increased by 80% and the rate increased 34%.

Importantly, the age-adjusted incidence of fall-induced deaths did not show an increasing trend over time.

Fall risk factors

The age-related risk factors for falls are multifactorial and include, among others, gait and balance disorders, strength, various cardiovascular abnormalities, use of sedatives and other medications, cognitive status, vision and lower extremity dysfunction (Table 3.3).[123–128] More specifically, in a multivariate analysis, the authors reported increased odds of two or more future falls for persons who had the following: (1) difficulty standing up from a chair; (2) difficulty performing a tandemwalk; (3) arthritis; (4) Parkinson's disease; (5) multiple falls during the previous year; (6) a fall-related injury during the previous year; and (7) were white.[125] Others[129] reported the major risk factors for falls resulting in a fracture were: (1) fear of falling; (2) abnormal heel-shin test; (3) reduced knee extension strength; (4) reduced grip strength; (5) poor distance visual acuity;

Table 3.3: Fall Risk Factors in Elderly People

Age	Low BMI
Cardiovascular Disorders	Lower Extremity Dysfunction
Arrhythmias	Arthritis
Orthostatic hypotension	Muscle weakness (sarcopenia)
Syncopy	Foot deformities, bunnions, calluses
Cognitive Dysfunction	Medications/Drugs
Dementia	Alcohol
Depression	Antidepressants
Gait and Balance Impairments	Antihypertensives
Cerebellar	Benzodiazopines
Hypothyroidism	Diuretics
Parkinson's disease	Narcotics/other addicting drugs
Postural instability	Sedatives
Sedentary lifestyle	Sex (females > males)
General Frailty	Visual Problems
Hearing Disorders	Cataracts
History of Previous Falls	Macular degeneration

(6) low supine pulse rate; (7) inability to carry a 5 kg (11-pound) load 100 meters; (8) not doing heavy outdoor work; and (9) no regular exercise.

Although depression is a risk factor for falls in elderly people, it can also occur after a fall-related injury.[130] In this prospective cohort study, 159 patients who sustained various kinds of fall-related injuries to the limbs were evaluated at pre-injury baseline and post-injury at eight weeks, five months and one year. Mean depression levels of all patients remained stable until five months post-injury but then increased between five months and one year. Physical functioning decreased between baseline and eight weeks post-injury, increased between eight weeks and five months, but did not improve thereafter. Both disability and depression were higher one year post-injury than at baseline. Thus, "depressive reactions did not occur as long as patients experienced improvements in physical functioning but became manifest as recovery appeared to stagnate."

Balance, flexibility and falls

Exercise has an important role in both balance and flexibility in older people. Here, balance (postural stability) implies little or no risk of a person losing balance while standing or falling during a physical activity.[31] Although balance is only one of many risk factors for falls, improvement may directly lead to a significant reduction in falls in some older people. Flexibility refers to the range of motion of single or multiple joints and the ability to successfully carry out various tasks. The range of motion depends mainly on the structure and function of muscle, bone and connective tissue.[31] Age, however, affects these tissues such that flexibility is progressively reduced in both women and men after about 30 years. However, exercise can improve muscle and connective tissue properties and also improve flexibility.

As noted previously, postural stability can be improved by exercise participation (i.e. walking, jogging, Tai Chi and strength exercises). Province *et al.*[131] studied the effects of short-term exercise on falls and fall-related injuries in ambulatory and cognitively intact persons aged 60 to 75 years. Training was performed in one or more areas of endurance, flexibility, balance, Tai Chi and resistance. From their data, the authors concluded that "treatments including exercise for elderly adults reduce the risk of falls." Others[132] examined the possibility that weight-bearing exercises, with added resistance from weighted vests, might improve dynamic balance, muscle strength and power and bone mass in postmenopausal women, and thereby reduce the risk of falls and hip fractures. Indeed, significant improvements were seen for indices of lateral stability, lower-body strength, muscular power and leg lean mass. However, there was no significant improvement for femoral neck bone mass. Although these results demonstrated that fall risk elements were favorably altered by the training, a decreased risk of hip fracture remained uncertain. Other studies[133–135] have also shown significant improvements in the flexibility of various joints, including shoulder, neck, wrist, hip, knee and ankle of elderly people who were involved in regular exercise programs.

Guidelines for the prevention of falls were recently released by the American Geriatric Society, British Geriatric Society and the American Academy of Orthopedic Surgeons.[136] The major general considerations included the following: (1) physicians should ask patients and caregivers about falls during routine office visits; (2) involvement in exercise training programs; (3) patients on multiple medications should be carefully assessed as to their possible contribution to falls and modified if appropriate to reduce the risks; (4) referral for home assessments to identify possible environmental hazards; (5) consideration of assistive devices; and (6) involvement in behavioral and education programs. Other potential considerations include bone strengthening medications, cardiovascular intervention, visual evaluation and improved footwear.

Osteoporosis, Bone Fractures and Osteoarthritis

Osteoporosis

An estimated ten million people in the US have osteoporosis and an additional 18 million have decreased bone mass, both of which greatly increase the risk of fractures with increasing age.[137] Importantly, these fractures are not limited to women; about 20% will involve men. Thus, about one-half of women and one in eight men will suffer a bone fracture as a result of osteoporosis during their lifetime. The probability of a future hip fracture for 50-year-old white women is 14%; 6% for African American women, 5–6% for white males and 3% for African American males. In addition, the estimated annual direct medical costs of osteoporotic fractures (hip and vertebral column) is US$10–15 billion; estimated indirect costs are significantly greater. Approximately 28% of patients with hip fractures enter nursing homes within the year following the fracture and 20% die within one year.[137]

Bone-mineral density (BMD) in later life is the strongest predictor of a future fracture. Up to the age of 70 years, BMD is primarily influenced by the peak value achieved during skeletal growth.[138] Up to 85% of the population variance in peak BMD has been attributed to genetic factors, while smoking, body weight, exercise and calcium intake contribute most of the remaining portion.[139] Hence, the prevention or delay of osteoporosis must be through healthy lifestyles and possible medications to prevent bone loss. Indeed, after a two-year study of a group of young male college basketball players, Klesges *et al.*[140] concluded that bone loss is calcium-related and that exercise is positively related to bone mineral content provided calcium intake is adequate to replace its loss. Similarly, de Jong and associates[141] carried out a 17-week randomized trial involving 143 frail elderly persons (aged 78.6 ± 5.6 years). The participants were separated into four groups: (1) supplementation with enriched foods, (2) exercise, (3) both, and (4) neither. The foods were enriched with multiple micronutrients while exercise focused on strength endurance, coordination and flexibility. The authors concluded that foods containing a physiologic dose of micronutrients increased bone density, bone mass and calcium whereas moderately intense exercise preserved lean body mass.

Nutritional factors, primarily an inadequate intake of calcium and vitamin D, contribute significantly to bone loss. The current

recommended calcium intake guidelines are as follows:[142]
(1) 1000 mg/day for postmenopausal women under 65 years who are
on supplemental estrogen; (2) 1500 mg/day for postmenopausal
women under 65 years not on supplemental estrogens; (3) 1000 mg/day
for men 65 years and under; and (4) 1500 mg/day for all individuals
over age 65 years regardless of hormone intake.

The overall role of exercise in the prevention and treatment of
osteoporosis remains somewhat unclear although there is strong
evidence that moderate levels of weight-bearing exercise is positively related to bone mineral content and that (1) disuse results in
the loss of BMD, (2) sedentary people usually have less bone mass
than those who regularly exercise, (3) exercise may produce a
modest increase in BMD, and (4) exercise cannot compensate for
estrogen loss.[143] As such, it is reasonable to highly recommend the
avoidance of a sedentary lifestyle and participate in moderate physical activity. There are, of course, many reasons to exercise regularly other than to prevent or delay osteoporosis. For example, Bravo
et al.[144] studied the effects of a 12-month exercise program in a
group of postmenopausal women between 50 and 70 years of age
with low BMD. They found that spinal BMD stabilized in the exercisers but decreased significantly in the control group; however,
there was no change in femoral BMD in either group. In addition,
the exercising osteopenic women had increased levels of functional
fitness, well-being and self-perceived health.

Other studies have also shown that exercise is important in the prevention of osteoporosis. For example, a multiple linear regression
analysis study of 352 premenopausal women, aged 40 to 54 years,
showed that moderate physical activity had beneficial effects on
BMD.[145] In this report, women who were using estrogen replacement therapy, had smoked within the past five years, or were pregnant were ineligible to participate, as were women with a history of
several diseases/disorders (i.e. type 1 diabetes, inflammatory bowel
disease, parathyroid disease, liver or kidney disease). Others[146] evaluated the effects of brisk walking on BMD in 165 postmenopausal
women who had suffered an upper limb fracture. The women were

divided into two groups: intervention (self-paced brisk walking) or placebo (upper limb exercises). Both groups were assessed at three-month intervals. After two years, among those completing the trial, BMD at the femoral neck had decreased significantly in the placebo group compared with the brisk walking group; lumbar spine BMD increased to a similar extent in both groups. These studies support an earlier report[147] that exercise offers protection against bone loss in premenopausal women. Moreover, men who jog at least nine times per month reportedly develop bone density that is at least 5% greater than those who jog eight or fewer times each month.[148] Compared with sedentary men, the bone density of joggers was about 8% better. Furthermore, those who jogged only one to eight times each month still had significantly higher bone density than the non-joggers.

As noted earlier in this chapter, weight-bearing exercises with added resistance from weighted vests results in significant improvements in lateral stability, lower-body strength, muscular power and leg lean mass.[138] This research group later studied the effects of long-term exercise using weighted vests on hip bone loss in postmenopausal women age 64.1 ± 1.6 years at baseline.[149] Half of the women engaged in weighted vest plus jumping exercise three times per week for 32 weeks of the year for five years. The control group was active but not engaged in the exercise program. BMD of the proximal femur was assessed by dual energy X-ray absorptiometry at baseline and after five years in both groups. After five years, the exercise group maintained hip BMD by preventing significant bone loss while the BMD in all members of the control group decreased significantly. Importantly, the program also appeared to promote long-term adherence and compliance to regular exercise.

Hannan *et al.*[150] recently examined the major risk factors for bone loss in 800 men and women aged 75 ± 4.5 years at baseline (Framingham Osteoporosis Study) and measured a four-year longitudinal change in BMD at the hip, radius and spine. They examined the relation of the following factors at baseline to percent of BMD loss: age, weight, weight change, height, smoking, caffeine and alcohol intake, physical activity, serum 25-OH vitamin D level, calcium intake and current estrogen replacement in women. After multivariant analysis, they found the following: (1) women who gained weight also gained BMD or had insignificant BMD changes; (2) current estrogen users had less bone mass than non-users; (3) men with lower baseline weight and weight loss also lost BMD; (4) men who smoked cigarettes at baseline lost more BMD at the trochanter site than non-smokers; and (5) caffeine, physical activity, serum 25-OH vitamin D level or calcium intake did not affect bone loss. Thus, the major risk factors for osteoporosis were female sex, thinness and weight loss while weight gain protected against bone loss in both sexes. This latter point was recently emphasized by Salamone *et al.*[151] who examined the effect of lifestyle interventions aimed at lowering dietary fat intake and increasing physical activity to produce modest weight loss or prevent weight gain on BMD in premenopausal women. The intervention group experienced a mean weight loss of 3.2 ± 4.7 kg (7.04 ± 10.34 pounds) over an 18-month period; the control group gained 0.42 ± 3.6 kg (0.9 ± 7.92 pounds). The annualized rate of hip BMD loss was two-fold higher in the intervention group. A similar, but non-significant loss was observed in spine BMD. Although increased physical activity attenuated spine BMD loss, it had no significant effect on the loss of BMD at the hip. This data readily explains why those with a low BMI (≤ 19 kg/m^2) or an eating disorder (i.e. anorexia nervosa) are at increased risk for osteoporosis and fractures.

The benefits of exercise on BMD may be mediated through both the indirect effects on lean muscle mass and direct effects on the skeleton. Increased lean mass produces an additional direct loading effect on the skeleton with a compensatory increase in BMD. Increased muscle activity and strain also add to the bone load.

Fractures

An estimated 1.3 million osteoporotic fractures in women reportedly occur annually in the US; for 16% of women, the most serious is hip fracture[152] which is most often related to accidental falls. Femoral neck fractures are also very common in other countries. For example, in 1991–1992 there were an estimated 56,613 such fractures in the UK; the estimate for 2001 was 69,000 at a cost of about £288 million.[153] The total US costs are significantly greater due to a much larger population. Importantly, after adjusting for age and sex, the risk for hip fracture was found to be 10.5 times greater for those living in institutions compared with those living in private homes.[154] These authors suggested that fall prevention programs, particularly those aimed to increase physical activity, would significantly decrease the risk of fractures and would be very cost-effective.

At least 21 published studies[155] have examined the association between physical activity and hip fractures, including several recent ones. For example, Gregg *et al.*[152] sought to determine whether higher levels of physical activity were related to a lower incidence of hip, wrist and vertebral fractures in 9704 non-black women aged 65 years or older. Their results revealed that those involved in higher levels of leisure time sports activity and household chores and fewer hours of daily sitting, had a significantly reduced risk for hip fracture (study was adjusted for age, diet, falls at a baseline and health status). After 7.6 years of follow-up, the most active women had a 36% reduction in hip fractures compared with those who were least active. The intensity of physical activity was also related to fracture risk; compared with inactive women, moderate to vigorous physical activity led to reductions of 42% and 33% in risk for hip and vertebral fractures, respectively.

How much physical activity is needed to significantly decrease the risk of hip fracture in postmenopausal women? To answer this question, Feskanich and associates[156] recently reported the results of a 12-year prospective study involving 61,200 postmenopausal women aged 40 to 77 years (Nurses' Health Study). After controlling for various confounders (i.e. age, BMI, use of postmenopausal hormones and smoking), the risk of hip fracture was lowered by 6% for each one hour per week walking at an average pace. Among women who did no other exercise, the risk of hip fracture decreased by 41% for those who walked for at least four hours per week. Moreover, the risk of hip fracture decreased linearly with increasing level of physical activity among women not taking postmenopausal hormones but not among those taking hormones.

Other studies are also supportive of the role of exercise in preventing osteoporotic fractures. In a randomized controlled trial, 98 healthy sedentary premenopausal women aged 35 to 45 years, were randomly assigned to either a training or control group.[157] The training group was involved in progressive high-impact exercises three times each week for 18 months. BMD was measured in specific axial and lower-limb sites at baseline and after 12 and 18 months. Maximum isometric strength, muscular and cardiovascular performance and dynamic balance were also evaluated. The findings showed that femoral neck BMD increased significantly more in the training group compared with the controls. By contrast, at non-weightbearing sites (e.g. distal radius), there was no difference between the two groups. However, the training group also showed improvement in vertical jump and oxygen consumption per minute at maximum exercise compared with the controls. Similarly, others[155] studied the association between hip fracture risk and recreational physical activity at various ages, changes in activity during adult life, occupational physical activity and how risks vary by adult weight change in postmenopausal women aged 50 to 81 years. The participants consisted of 1327 women with prior hip fractures and 3662 randomly selected controls. Information was gathered on leisure activity before ages 18, 18 to 30 years and during recent years. Compared with sedentary women, there was a significant inverse association between the degree of exercise and the incidence of fractures. In addition, the protective effect was most pronounced in women who had lost weight after age 18. There was no relation between occupational activity and fracture risk.

High-intensity strength training exercises were studied for one year in a group of sedentary estrogen-depleted postmenopausal women aged 50 to 70 years.[158] The participants were divided into two groups; one involved in high-intensity strength training exercises for two days each week using five different exercises (double leg press, knee extension, lateral pull-down, back extension and abdominal flexion) and a non-exercising control group. The strength-training group showed significantly increased femoral neck mineral density and lumbar spine BMD; there was a mild decrease in both areas in the controls. Moreover, total body bone mineral content was preserved in the strength-trained group but it tended to decrease in the controls. In addition, muscle mass, muscle strength and dynamic balance increased in the strength-trained group and decreased in the controls.

Appropriate exercise also reportedly benefits those recovering from a hip fracture.[159] In this report, 148 community-living participants 65 years and older who underwent repair of a fractured hip, participated in a six-month home-based rehabilitation program. The program consisted of a physical therapy component designed to identify and ameliorate impairments in balance, strength, transfers, gait and stair-climbing; a second function component was designed to identify and improve unsafe and/or inefficient performance of specific daily living activities. Of those that were able to complete the program (70%), 94% and 96% progressed in upper and lower extremity conditioning respectively; 33% progressed to the highest level in the graduated resisted exercise program. All participants progressed in the competency-based graded balance program (55% progressed to the most difficult level). Similarly, the majority progressed in transfer maneuvers, stair climbing and outdoor gait. In addition, there was general improvement in elbow and knee extension, gait deviations and performance of various daily living activities. The study results strongly suggest that similar home-based protocols be instituted for those recovering from a hip fracture. In a recent literature review of physical activity, falls and fractures among older persons, the authors concluded that epidemiologic studies support a positive relationship between higher levels of leisure-time physical activity and reduced incidence of hip fractures.[160] More specifically, they found consistent evidence that increased physical activity was associated with a 20% to 40% reduced risk of hip fracture compared with sedentary individuals. In addition, randomized control trials indicated that certain exercise programs, such as lower extremity strength training and balance, reduce the risk of falling.

Interestingly, two recent studies[161,162] suggest that the lipid-lowering statin drugs [3-hydroxy-3-methylglutaryl coenzyme A (HMG-CoA) reductase inhibitors] may stimulate bone formation and reduce the risk of a hip fracture in persons aged 50 years and older. Both reports, however, emphasized that additional prospective controlled trials are needed to exclude the possibility of undetermined confounders.

Arthritis/chronic joint symptoms

Arthritis and other rheumatic conditions comprise the leading cause of adult disability in the US;[163] the cost of this health burden is expected to significantly increase as the population ages. In 2001, the estimated prevalence of arthritis and chronic joint symptoms among American adults was 33.0%, affecting about 69.9 million adults [22.4 million (10.6%) with physician diagnosed arthritis, 20.9 million (10.0%)] with chronic joint symptoms only and 26.6 million (12.4%) with both conditions.[164] The prevalence increased with age and was more common in women than men. In addition, the prevalence was higher among non-Hispanic whites and non-Hispanic blacks than Hispanics. Other important risk factors included not completing high school, being physically inactive and overweight/obese (BMI $\geq$ 25 kg/m^2). The lowest prevalence was in Hawaii (17.8%) and the highest in West Virginia (42.6%).

About 20% of people aged 70 years and older have difficulty performing essential activities of daily living (difficulty transferring from a bed to a chair, eating, dressing, bathing and using the toilet).[165] However, the prevention of activities of daily living may prolong the autonomy of older persons. To evaluate activities of daily living in older persons with knee osteoarthritis, Penninx and associates[166] carried out a randomized controlled trial of a group of persons aged 60 years and older over an 18-month period. The participants were assigned to an aerobic exercise program, a resistance exercise program or an attention control group. The cumulative incidence of activities of daily living disability was lower in the exercise group (37.1%) compared with the control group (52.5%). After adjustment for demographics and physical function at baseline, both exercise programs prevented activities of daily living disability; the relative risks were 0.60 for resistance exercise and 0.53 for aerobic exercise compared with the attention control group. In a similar study, Ettinger et al.[167] determined the effects of structured exercise programs on self-reported disability in 439 community-dwelling adults aged 60 years and older with knee osteoarthritis. The three exercise programs involved aerobic exercise resistance exercise, and health education. Compared with the health education group, their results showed the following: (1) participants in the aerobic exercise group had a 10% lower adjusted mean score, a 12% lower score on knee pain and performed better on the six-minute walk test, time to climb and descend stairs, time to lift and carry ten pounds, and mean time to get in and out of a car; while (2) the resistance exercise group had an 8% lower pain score, greater distance on the six-minute walk, faster times on the lifting and carrying task, and the car task. There were no differences in X-ray scores between either the exercise group or the health education group. This study adds further support for exercise as part of the treatment for knee osteoarthritis.

Occupational physical activities may also be important risk factors for some people. Coggon et al.[168] compared 518 osteoarthritic patients scheduled for surgical knee treatment with a similar number of control participants matched for sex and age. After adjustment for BMI, history of knee injury and the presence of Heberden's nodes, risk for knee osteoarthritis was significantly increased in those who reported kneeling or squatting, walking two miles or more each day and regularly lifting weights of at least 25 kg (55 pounds) in the course of their work. The risks associated with kneeling and squatting were greater in those who were also involved in occupational lifting. Obesity was also a highly important risk factor. Those with a BMI of 30 kg/m^2 or higher, whose work had entailed prolonged kneeling or squatting, had an odds ratio of 14.7 compared with an odds ratio of 1.9 for the non-obese workers involved in kneeling and squatting.

In contrast to this latter report that suggested an increase in knee osteoarthritis in workers who walked two miles or more each day, early studies showed that moderate amounts of physical stress are beneficial to articular cartilage by helping to maintain its functional integrity.[169,170] Excess physical stress may, however, lead to accelerated joint degeneration, although there is some controversy on this topic. For example, Lane and associates[171] determined the five-year longitudinal effects of running and aging on the development of clinical and radiographic osteoarthritis in runners with a mean age of 63 years. They compared the results with a similar group of controls matched for age, years of education and occupation. All participants underwent rheumatologic examinations, completed questionnaires and radiographs were taken of the hands, lateral lumbar spine and knees at baseline and after five years. The authors concluded that running did not accelerate the development of clinical or radiographic osteoarthritis of the knees or spine. With aging, however, 13% of all participants developed osteoarthritis of the hands and 12% developed osteoarthritis of the knees.

Hip osteoarthritis is a major public health problem. Radiographic evidence of this disease is reportedly present in about 10% of people aged 65 years and older and about half of them are symptomatic.[172] These authors reported that the major risk factors for hip osteoarthritis in two UK health districts were obesity, previous hip injury and the presence of Heberden's nodes. There was also a negative association between cigarette smoking and osteoarthritis in men and a weak association with prolonged regular sporting activity. Hip osteoarthritis may also be part of the polyarticular involvement present in generalized osteoarthritis.

An appropriate exercise program has also been shown to be effective in older individuals with rheumatoid arthritis (RA).[173] This study involved 64 RA patients with a mean age of 60 years and mean disease duration of eight years who were admitted to the hospital because of active disease. The patients were randomly assigned to an intensive exercise program or to a conservative exercise program with a mean duration of 30 days. Intensive exercise consisted of knee and shoulder dynamic and isometric muscle strengthening exercises against resistance five times each week and conditioning bicycle training three times each week and was supplemented by the conservative exercise program which consisted of range, motion and isometric exercises. Indices of disease were activity, pain, muscle strength and functional ability; they were assessed at baseline, three, six, 12 and 24 weeks. Medical treatment during the study was the same for all participants. The results showed that both groups improved similarly in disease activity. However, both physical functioning and muscle strength improved significantly for patients in the intensive exercise program compared with the conservative program.

Hypertension

Hypertension is an extremely common medical problem and one of the most important modifiable risk factors for cardiovascular and cerebrovascular diseases, the number one and three leading causes of death in the US. Burt *et al.*[174] reported their survey findings on the prevalence of hypertension in the American adult population, 1988–1991. They found that about 24% of the American adult population, representing 43,186,000 persons, were hypertensive (i.e. mean systolic pressure ≥ 140 mm Hg, or mean diastolic pressure ≥ 90 mm Hg, or current treatment for hypertension). The age-adjusted prevalence in the non-Hispanic black, non-Hispanic white and Mexican American populations was 32.4%, 23.3% and 22.6%, respectively. However, only 69% of the hypertensive population were aware that they had hypertension and only 53% were taking prescribed medication. The authors suggested that these figures may be low since almost 13 million additional adults, classified as normotensive, reported a history of hypertension. Although these numbers are very high, they are significantly lower than the 1976–1980 National Health and Nutrition Examination Survey.[174]

The incidence of hypertension increases with age. Between ages 60 and 74 years, the prevalence is reportedly almost twice that in the American population as a whole. Moreover, among older patients seen by primary care physicians, about 50% of whites and Mexican Americans and 75% of blacks are hypertensive.[174] There is, on average, a 20 mm Hg systolic and 10 mm Hg disastolic increment increase in blood pressure from age 30 to 65 years.[175] In addition, hypertension accelerates atherogenesis and imparts a two- to three-fold increased risk of severe events, including CHD. Increased blood pressure is also a major risk factor for numerous other serious diseases including myocardial infarction, stroke, end-stage kidney disease and peripheral vascular disease;[174] it is also the most common risk factor for congestive heart failure.[176]

Midlife systolic blood pressure is a significant predictor of reduced cognitive function in later life.[177] In this study, 4678 Japanese-American men, average age 78 years and enrolled in the Honolulu Heart Program, were examined a fourth time from 1991 to 1993 and given a cognitive test. When controlled for age and education, the risk for intermediate and poor cognitive function increased progressively with increasing level of midlife systolic blood pressure. For every 10 mm Hg increase in systolic pressure, there was a 7% increase in risk for intermediate cognitive function; for poor cognitive function, the risk was 9%. The level of cognitive function was not, however, associated with midlife diastolic blood pressure.

Hypertension risk factors

The major risk factors for hypertension are varied and include age, family history, race (blacks greater than whites and Mexican Americans), BMI, physical inactivity, excess salt and alcohol intake and psychological stress. The recommended initial treatment for mild to moderate hypertension is aerobic exercise, weight reduction and reduced salt and alcohol intake. If these modifiable factors are not successful, a diuretic or beta-blocker, if necessary and not otherwise contraindicated, should follow.[178]

Exercise

Weight loss and aerobic exercise, along with salt restriction and alcohol reduction, are the most important modifiable factors for blood pressure control. Various types of exercise have been studied, including walking, running, callisthenics, resistive exercises and exercising on a cycle ergometer; all have been successful in long term, post-exercise blood pressure lowering, which suggests that exercise is independently associated with blood pressure lowering.[179] In a recent report, Blumenthal *et al.*[180] studied 133 sedentary overweight men and women with mild unmedicated hypertension (i.e. high normal or stage 1 to 2 hypertension). The participants were randomly assigned to aerobic exercise only, a behavioral weight management program, including exercise, or a waiting list control group. Their results showed that all participants in both active treatment groups had significant blood pressure reductions relative to the control group. In addition, those in weight management plus exercise had slightly larger reductions in both systolic and diastolic pressure than those involved in exercise alone; the mean blood pressure did not change in the control group. Those in both treatment groups also displayed reduced peripheral resistance and increased cardiac output compared with the controls. Thus, although exercise alone was effective in reducing blood pressure, it was more effective when combined with weight management.

In a similar report,[181] the effects of exercise and weight loss on cardiovascular responses during mental stress in mildly to moderately obese hypertensive men and women was carried out. The subjects had high normal or unmedicated stages 1 to 2 hypertension (i.e. systolic blood pressure 130–179 mm Hg, diastolic blood pressure 85–109 mm Hg) and underwent a battery of mental stress tests before and after a six-month treatment program. The participants were randomly assigned to one of three treatments: aerobic exercise, weight management combined with aerobic exercise and a waiting list control group. After six months, compared with the control group, those in both active treatment groups had lower levels of systolic and diastolic blood pressure, total peripheral resistance and heart rate at rest and during mental stress. Both treatment groups also had a greater resting stroke volume and cardiac output than the controls. The diastolic blood pressure was lower for the weight management group than for the exercise-only group during all mental stress tasks. Again, the combination of exercise and weight management was more successful than either alone.

Others[182] sought to determine whether blood pressure reduction in obese (32 ± 4% body fat) sedentary male hypertensives (stages 1 and 2) after acute exercise persist for more than two to three hours, as reported in controlled laboratory settings. Ambulatory blood pressures were taken one day after 45 minutes of 70% VO_2max treadmill exercise and on another day not preceded by exercise. The mean systolic blood pressure was lower by 6–13 mm Hg for the first 16 hours following exercise compared to the day without prior exercise. In addition, 24-hour day and night average systolic blood pressures were also significantly lower on the day following exercise. The diastolic blood pressures were also significantly lower for 12 of the first 16 hours after acute exercise compared with the day without prior exercise, as were the 24-hour day and night diastolic pressures.

In addition to the positive effects of aerobic exercise on blood pressure, progressive resistance exercise has been shown to be effective. In a meta-analysis of a wide variety of publications reporting on the effects of resistance exercise, Kelley and Kelley concluded that this technique is "efficacious" for reducing blood pressure.[183]

Exercise recommendations to control blood pressure

The American College of Sports Medicine's position statement confirms that most studies clearly show that regular aerobic exercise is beneficial in controlling mild to moderate hypertension.[184] They recommended a training intensity of 40% to 65% of maximal heart rate, performed five days per week for 30 to 40 minutes. In addition, treadmill or walking exercise is recommended over either bicycle or arm ergonometry. In agreement with this, Young *et al.*[185] compared the effects on blood pressure of a 12-week moderate intensity aerobic exercise program and a Tai Chi program of light physical intensity in both black and white men and women aged 60 years and older. They measured blood pressure during three screening visits and every two weeks during the exercise period. Mean baseline systolic and diastolic blood pressures were 139.9 mm Hg and 76 mm Hg, respectively. The adjusted mean systolic pressure changes during the 12-week period were −8.4 mm Hg and −7.0 mm Hg in the aerobic exercise and Tai Chi groups, respectively.

For diastolic pressure, the corresponding changes were −3.2 mm Hg in the aerobic group and −2.4 mm Hg in the Tai Chi group. They concluded that programs of moderate intensity aerobic exercise and light exercise have similar effects on blood pressure.

These studies demonstrate that regular exercise lowers blood pressure in patients with mild-moderate hypertension. However, studies of its effects on patients with severe hypertension are scarce. Kokkinos and associates[186] recently examined the effects of regular aerobic exercise on blood pressure and left ventricular hypertophy in African American men aged 35 to 76 years with severe hypertension. They randomly assigned them to an exercise program plus antihypertensive medication, or to antihypertensive medication alone. The exercise group participated in two 16-week phases of aerobic exercise that consisted of stationary cycling for a mean of 44 ± 9 minutes at 60% to 80% of the predicted maximum heart rate, three times per week. After 16 weeks, mean diastolic pressure decreased an average of 5 mm Hg in the exercise group but increased slightly (2.0 mm Hg) in those who did not exercise. Importantly, the diastolic pressure remained significantly lower after 32 weeks of exercise, even with substantial reductions in the dose of antihypertensive medicine. Moreover, the thickness of the left ventricular mass had decreased significantly after 16 weeks in those who exercised; there was no significant change in the non-exercisers.

Wareham *et al.*[187] reported that most methods used to assess physical activity have been imprecise and subjective. With the advent of more accurate methods, they measured the energy expenditure in 775 participants aged 45 to 70 years. Energy was assessed by four days of heart rate monitoring with individual calibration of the relationship between heart rate and energy expenditure. Cardiorespiratory fitness was evaluated in a sub-maximal test. Their results showed a significant inverse linear trend in blood pressure reduction with increasing physical activity. The differences in mean systolic/diastolic blood pressure between the top and bottom quintiles was 6.4/4.0 mm Hg in men and 10.7/5.9 mm Hg in women. The authors concluded that there is a strong correlation between usual energy expenditure and blood pressure.

Hence, it is appropriate to recommend increasing the overall energy expenditure in the prevention and/or treatment of hypertension.

Syndrome X

As a group, hypertensives may have the so-called syndrome X, a metabolic cluster of multiple interrelated abnormalities in lipid and glucose metabolism, gout and a prothrombotic condition that increases the risk of CHD.[186] Insulin resistance, defined as a sub-optimal response of insulin-sensitive tissues to normal or elevated insulin levels, is thought to be the cornerstone of this syndrome.[188] It has also been proposed that this cluster of risk factors for CHD in patients with hypertension explains why interventions directed at reducing the blood pressure has had little effect on CHD risk.[189] Jeppesen and associates[190] tested the hypothesis that the blood pressure level would be less predictive of CHD risk in those with high triglyceride and low high-density lipoprotein cholesterol (HDL-C) levels (the usual syndrome X dyslipidemia characteristics) than in those without abnormal levels. Indeed, their results showed that the blood pressure did not predict the risk of CHD in those with elevated triglyceride and low HDL-C serum levels. Hence, these findings may explain why blood pressure lowering alone in patients with this metabolic syndrome does not produce the expected reduction in CHD.

The basal metabolic rate (BMR) decreases with increasing age. However, as shown by Williamson and Kirwan[191] in a study of healthy men aged 59 to 77 years, resistance exercise significantly increases BMR 48 hours after a single-leg knee extension exercise and bench press lifts. Dengel *et al.*[192] suggested that syndrome X may be the result of a decrease in cardiovascular fitness and the accumulation of body fat with aging. To examine this hypothesis, they studied the effects of a six-month program of aerobic exercise training plus weight loss on VO_2max, body composition, blood pressure, glucose and insulin responses during an oral glucose tolerance test (OGTT), glucose infusion rates (GIR) during three-dose hyperinsulinemic-euglycemic clamps at increasing insulin infusion rates and plasma lipoprotein levels. Compared with a similar group of non-obese sedentary middle-aged men, the obese, hypertensive sedentary group initially had a larger waist girth and waist-to-hip ratio, were more hyperinsulinemic and insulin-resistant and had higher triglyceride and lower HDL-C levels. The aerobic training intervention reduced mean body weight by 9%, body fat by 21%, waist girth by 9% and waist-to-hip ratio by 3%, and increased VO_2max by 16% (P < 0.01 for all). The systolic blood pressure was decreased by 14 ± 3 mm Hg; the corresponding diastolic pressure decreased 10 ± 2 mm Hg. There were also significant changes in the GIR at the low (+42%) and intermediate (+39%) insulin infusion rates and in blood glucose (−21%) and insulin (−51%) responses during OGTT. Moreover, the exercise and weight loss program resulted in lower total cholesterol (14%) and triglyceride levels (34%) and raised the HDL-C level two-fold. This extensive study suggests that hypertension and the various metabolic risk factors for CHD can be significantly improved by appropriate exercise and weight loss in middle-aged men with this metabolic syndrome. As noted by Hazzard,[193] "... sedentary behavior begets central adiposity begets insulin resistance begets hyper-triglyceridemia, hyperglycemia, increased low-density lipoprotein concentrations, decreased high-density lipoprotein concentrations and hypertension ("syndrome X") ...."

Serum Lipids and Exercise

Despite significant progress in recent decades, CHD is still the leading cause of death in the US in both men and women.[194] During this same time period, numerous studies have clearly shown that an increased plasma level of total cholesterol (TC) is a significant independent risk factor for CHD. Moreover, most of the increased risk of an elevated plasma TC is due to an elevated level (>130 mg/dL) of low-density lipoprotein cholesterol (LDL-C). In addition, albeit somewhat late, the Adult Treatment Panel (ATP II) of the National Cholesterol Education Program (NCEP) has given more attention to the well-established importance of low plasma levels (<35 mg/dL) of HDL-C as a major risk factor for CHD.[195] Of additional importance is the well-established value of the TC/HDL-C ratio, first recognized in the Framingham Study by Castelli and Anderson (target ratio ≤ 4.5).[196] These topics have been recently reviewed.[197]

Primarily over the past two decades, increased physical activity has been shown to be significantly associated with reduced risk for CHD. As a result, the ATP II recommended increased emphasis on physical activity and weight loss as important additions to dietary therapy in lowering plasma lipid levels.[195] Increased physical activity is protective against CHD in at least two ways: controlling and/or reducing excess body weight and improving plasma lipid levels (Table 3.4). Denke *et al.*[198] reported that excess body weight was a commonly under-recognized contributor to increased plasma cholesterol levels in white American males. More specifically, they found that in men of all ages, an elevated BMI was associated with higher plasma triglyceride, TC and non-HDL-C levels, as well as lower HDL-C concentrations. However, in young men the higher TC level was primarily reflected by LDL-C whereas in middle-aged and older men, higher TC levels were mainly reflected in the non-HDL-C fraction.[198] These authors followed up this report with a similar study of white American women.[199] They found that for premenopausal women, excess body weight was significantly associated with higher TC, non-HDL-C, LDL-C and triglyceride levels and lower HDL-C levels. In older women, similar differences in triglyceride and HDL-C levels were observed. However, excess body weight was associated with smaller differences in TC, non-HDL-C and LDL-C. Although lower HDL-C concentrations associated with excess body weight were age-dependent, the TC/HDL-C ratios were highest in obese postmenopausal women.

Table 3.4: Physical Activity and Serum Lipids

Increases HDL-Cholesterol
Decreases TC/HDL-C ratio
Decreases TC
Decreases LDL-C
Decreases triglycerides

In an early Healthy Women Study,[200] 507 women were evaluated at baseline and after three years; weekly physical activity was determined on every woman at each examination. During the three-year period weight, blood pressure, levels of TC, LDL-C and triglycerides all increased significantly while the level of HDL-C decreased. However, women engaged in higher levels of physical activity at baseline had less weight gain while those that increased their activity during the three-year period had the smallest increase in weight and smallest decrease in plasma HDL-C. Others[201] studied 102 sedentary premenopausal women to determine whether the quantity and quality of walking needed to decrease the risk of CHD differed significantly from that required to improve cardiorespiratory fitness. The women were randomized to one of four groups: aerobic walkers (8.0 km/h), brisk walkers (6.4 km/h), strollers (4.8 km/h) and sedentary controls. The three intervention groups walked five days each week. Compared with the sedentary group, maximum oxygen uptake increased significantly and in a dose-response manner (i.e. aerobic walkers > brisk walkers > strollers). However, plasma HDL-C levels were not dose-related, but increased significantly and essentially to the same extent in all intervention groups. Kokkinos *et al.*[186] reported that in African American men with severe systemic hypertension, low to moderate aerobic exercise was not overall adequate to favorably modify plasma lipid profiles. However, there was a substantial increase in plasma HDL-C concentrations in those who exercised at intensities 75% and above of age-predicted maximum heart rate, suggesting an exercise intensity threshold. In addition, several recent studies, as described below, also suggest that plasma lipid levels correlate with the level of physical activity.

The official guidelines from the CDC[202] indicate that the majority of health benefits from physical activity can be achieved by briskly walking two miles (3.2 km) most days of the week [energy equivalent of running 8 to 12 km (five to 7.5 miles) per week].[203] However, the guidelines also state that "the recommendation presented ... is intended to complement, not supersede, previous exercise recommendations," and "people who already meet the recommendation are also likely to derive some additional health and fitness benefits from becoming more physically active." Williams,[204] in a cross-sectional survey involving 1837 female recreational runners, found significant increases in plasma HDL-C concentrations in those who exercised at levels greater than the current minimum guidelines. More specifically, plasma HDL-C levels increased by an average of 0.133 mg/dL for every additional kilometer run per week. In an earlier National Runners' Health Study, he also found that in men there are substantial additional benefits if their level of physical activity exceeds the minimum guidelines.[205] Specifically, he reported the benefits of exercise, which include higher HDL-C levels, decreased body weight, triglyceride levels, TC/HDL-C ratio and estimated ten-year risk for CHD, increased with distances run up to 80 km (50 miles) per week.

Other studies have also suggested a dose-response relationship between the level of physical activity and plasma lipid levels. For example, Thune *et al.*[206] studied 5220 men and 5869 women aged 20 to 49 years at entry. After seven years, men reporting sustained very hard exercising compared with the sedentary group had lower plasma TC levels [5.65 mmol/L versus 6.21 mmol/L (218 mg/dL versus 240 mg/dL)], triglyceride levels [1.34 mmol/L versus 1.85 mmol/L (118 mg/dL versus 164 mg/dL)], TC/HDL-C ratios by 19% and higher HDL-C levels [1.52 mmol/L versus 1.36 mmol/L (59 mg/dL versus 52 mg/dL)]. Significant, but slightly lower, figures were found in exercising women compared with sedentary women. Kokkinos and associates[207] added further support for a dose-related response between exercise and increased plasma HDL-C levels in 2906 healthy non-smoking men aged 43 ± 4 years. The group was stratified depending on the number of miles run per week into six groups (zero, five, nine, 12, 17 and 31 miles per week). Their findings showed a gradual increase in plasma HDL-C levels with increased miles run (0.31 mg/dL per mile). Major changes were associated with distances of seven to 14 miles per week at mild to moderate intensities. Moreover, levels of LDL-C, triglycerides and TC/HDL-C ratio also improved with increasing weekly mileage.

A recent eight-month randomized trial involving different amounts and intensities of exercise among overweight men and women with dyslipidemia further demonstrated a dose response between exercise and plasma lipid levels. Here, Kraus *et al.*[208] found that low amounts of exercise at moderate to high intensity (the equivalent of walking or jogging 12 miles per week, respectively) was associated with potentially beneficial improvement. However, exercise equivalent to jogging 20 miles per week resulted in significantly greater improvements in the plasma lipoprotein profile. Moreover, this activity level was required to produce a significant increase in the plasma HDL-C. As suggested by Thompson, this graded response of plasma lipoprotein concentrations to increasing exercise levels may help explain the progressive decrease in cardiovascular risk associated with increasing amounts of exercise.[209]

Stefanick *et al.*[210] studied plasma lipid levels in 180 postmenopausal women 45 to 64 years of age and 197 men 30 to 64 years of age who had low plasma levels of HDL-C and moderately elevated levels of LDL-C. The subjects were randomly assigned to aerobic exercise, the National Cholesterol Education Program (NCEP) Step 2 diet (moderately low in fat and cholesterol), diet plus exercise and a control group. During this one-year study, the plasma LDL-C was significantly reduced among both men and women in the diet plus exercise group compared with the control group. The reduction in LDL-C in men in the Step 2 diet plus exercise group was also significant as compared with men in the exercise group. However, LDL-C changes were not significant among men or women in the diet only group. The authors concluded that the NCEP Step 2 diet failed to lower LDL-C levels in both men and women with high plasma lipid levels who did not engage in aerobic exercise, thereby further highlighting the importance of physical activity in people with plasma lipid abnormalities. These investigators previously demonstrated that physical activity prevented the lowering of HDL-C levels that usually results from a low-fat diet in overweight women and men.[211]

Others[212] studied the effects of exercise on plasma HDL-C levels in a group of elderly persons aged 60 to 80+ years, who were regularly involved in regular non-vigorous physical activity and compared them with a similar group of frail elderly people. They found that plasma HDL-C, adjusted for age, BMI and waist-to-hip ratio was higher in both men and women who engaged in physical activity at least once per week. Although TC levels were higher among the active women, there was a significant trend towards a lower TC/HDL-C ratio. It was suggested that the increased TC level in women was probably due to increased concentrations of HDL-C.

Interestingly, Ginsberg *et al.*[213] studied the effects of a single bout of ultraendurance exercise on plasma lipid levels and oxidative lipid susceptibility in highly trained athletes (26 men, 13 women mean age 38 ± years) who competed in and completed the Hawaii Ironman World Championship Triathlon (2.4-mile swim, 112-mile bike ride and 26.2-mile run). The mean exercise duration was 753 ± 128 minutes (approximately 12.5 ± 2 hours). Their results showed the following data after the intense exercise period, compared with pre-exercise data and corrected for plasma volume: decreased plasma levels of triglycerides (39%), TC (9%) and LDL-C (11%); HDL-C increased mildly, but was not statistically significant. In addition, serum iron, a potential prooxidant, decreased by 45%. With regards to this latter point, a major theory of atherogenesis involves oxidative modification of LDL by various reactive oxygen species.[214] Recognizing this, Vasankari *et al.*[215] studied the effect of a ten-month exercise program on LDL oxidation and other lipid risk factors in a group of overweight/obese elderly men and women (average BMI: men, 29.6 kg/m^2; women, 28.6 kg/m^2). At the end of the ten-month period, serum levels of HDL increased, LDL and TC/HDL ratio decreased, and there was a significant decrease in the level of oxidized LDL.

These studies clearly indicate a significant inverse relationship between "good cholesterol" (i.e. HDL-C) and physical activity. Moreover, the exercise-induced HDL-C changes are most likely the result of the interaction between exercise intensity, frequency, duration of each exercise session and length of the exercise training period.[215] As noted above, there is also substantial evidence for a dose-response relationship. Favorable plasma HDL-C changes appear to occur incrementally and reach statistical significance at about seven to ten miles per week (caloric expenditure 1200–1600 kcal).[216] These authors suggested a practical approach in prescribing exercise is a moderate intensity program (70–80% of predicted maximum heart rate) carried out three to five times per week, for a total of seven to 14 miles. Other modes of physical activity are also recommended as long as they meet the minimum caloric expenditure requirement (i.e. 1200–1600 kcal/week).

Type 2 Diabetes Mellitus

Type 2 diabetes mellitus (non-insulin dependent diabetes mellitus; NIDDM; late-onset diabetes) comprises 90% or more of all cases of diabetes mellitus. A 1992 report estimated that about 12 million Americans had type 2 diabetes, but only half of them were aware they had the disease.[217] A subsequent study estimated the prevalence of diagnosed diabetes in 1988–1994 at about 5.1% of American adults 20 years of age and older.[218] When extrapolated to the 1997 American population, the total was 10.2 million diabetics; there was an estimated 5.4 million additional undiagnosed cases. More recently, the estimated prevalence of diabetes rose from 4.9% in 1990 to 6.5% in 1998, an increase of 33% in eight years.[219] This translates into about 13 million diabetics in 1998 and presumably more than the 5.4 million undiagnosed cases noted above. Unfortunately, the onset of NIDDM begins at least four to seven years prior to clinical diagnosis.[217] Moreover, approximately 50% of men and women aged 65 to 74 years reportedly demonstrate abnormal glucose tolerance (i.e. increased plasma glucose levels but below that required for diagnosis), and about 20% have type 2 diabetes.[220,221] Although not fully understood, insulin resistance is also a very early finding in the pathogenesis of NIDDM.[222] The result of these reports is that overt NIDDM is only the "tip of the iceberg" of disordered glucose metabolism. In addition to the medical problems of diabetes itself, NIDDM is a major risk factor for CHD, stroke, renal failure and blindness among others.

In 1986, the total annual medical cost of NIDDM was conservatively estimated to be US$11.6 billion.[223] By 1992 it had escalated to US$45.2 billion,[224] which was almost 15% of the national health care expenditures.[225] NIDDM expenditures increased to US$77.7 billion in 1997[226] and are currently about US$100 billion per year.[227] These figures represent the direct costs of type 2 diabetes and do not include work absence or lost productivity. Importantly, both personal medical and economic costs will continue to dramatically increase unless vigorous measures are taken to decrease the incidence of this epidemic. Indeed, NIDDM can be prevented in most people by weight control and adequate physical activity.[228,229]

Exercise and type 2 diabetes

Numerous studies have shown that increased physical activity is very successful in preventing NIDDM, and that those with the greatest risk (i.e. increasing age, positive family history, overweight and physically inactive) are helped the most. Helmrich and associates[230] confirmed this by showing that increased physical activity has a protective effect on those with hypertension, are overweight, sedentary and have a family history of diabetes. They emphasized that exercise not only increases muscle mass, retards fat accumulation, lowers both systolic and diastolic blood pressure, but increases tissue insulin sensitivity and lowers both plasma insulin and glucose levels.

In a later study, 110,660 Chinese men and women were screened for impaired glucose tolerance (IGT) and type 2 diabetes, of which 577 had IGT (World Health Organization criteria).[231] The subjects were then randomized into a control group and one of three active treatment groups: diet only, exercise only and diet plus exercise. Regular follow-up examinations were conducted over a period of six years to identify those who developed type 2 diabetes. Compared with the control group, and after adjusting for differences in baseline BMI and fasting glucose levels, the diet, exercise and diet plus exercise interventions were associated with 31%, 46% and 42% reductions in the risk of developing diabetes, respectively.

How much physical activity is needed to prevent type 2 diabetes, or at least delay its onset? The potential benefit of moderate intensity physical activity on NIDDM risk has been somewhat unclear. A prospective Physicians' Health Study, with a five-year follow-up of 21,271 men aged 40 to 84 years and free of cancer, myocardial infarction, cerebrovascular disease or diabetes at baseline, correlated physical activity with the development of NIDDM.[232] Men who exercised at least once per week had a significant reduction in relative risk for NIDDM compared with those who were essentially sedentary. The findings persisted after adjustment for both age and BMI. Similarly, an early study of 87,253 female nurses (Nurses' Health Study) aged 34 to 59 years at baseline and free of cancer, diabetes and cardiovascular disease, were monitored for eight years.[233] The data also showed that women who exercised vigorously at least once per week had a significantly reduced relative risk for type 2 diabetes when compared with the non-exercising women. Multivariate analysis, which included age, family history of diabetes and BMI did not alter the positive effects of physical activity.

Although insulin sensitivity is associated with exercise training, the effects of habitual non-vigorous activity is less well understood. To determine whether habitual, non-vigorous physical activity, as well as vigorous and overall activity is associated with improved insulin sensitivity, Mayer-Davis *et al.*[234] studied 1467 African American, Hispanic and non-Hispanic white men and women aged 40 to 69 years ranging from normal glucose tolerance to mild NIDDM. Their results showed that increased participation in vigorous, non-vigorous and overall physical activity were all significantly associated with improved insulin sensitivity. The findings were similar for sub-groups of sex, ethnicity and those with NIDDM. Others have also recently studied the effects of moderate intensity physical activity on fasting insulin levels in African American, Native American and Caucasian women.[235] The participants were involved in two consecutive, four-day periods of physical activity, one month apart. After adjusting for race, ethnicity, age and education level, they found that an increase of 30 minutes of moderate intensity physical activity was associated with a 6.6% decrease in fasting insulin levels which were independent of race, ethnicities, centrally lean or obese, and those with low and high cardiorespiratory fitness levels.

In a randomized controlled trial, the effects of equivalent diet- or exercise-induced weight loss and exercise without weight loss on various measures of body composition and insulin sensitivity in obese men were evaluated.[236] The results showed that weight loss induced by increased daily physical activity without caloric restriction significantly reduced both obesity (mainly abdominal) and insulin resistance in men. DiPietro and associates[237] also studied the effects of physical training-related improvements in glucose and insulin responses to an oral glucose tolerance test (OGTT) to determine if they are independent of changes in abdominal obesity. Adiposity and OGTT responses were determined before and after a four-month randomized, controlled aerobic training program in healthy elderly men and women whose average age was 73 years. Their results showed a 16% increase in VO_2max and a 24% decrease in serum free fatty acids in the aerobic training group, although there was no effect on abdominal fat. In addition, the glucose response curve shifted to the left, and the area under the OGTT curve decreased by 25% in the training group. However, the improvement in glucose response occurred only in those with IGT at baseline, and without any change in insulin response. There were no changes in any of the variables in the control group.

Hu *et al.*[238] examined the relationship of total physical activity and incidence of NIDDM in women (Nurses' Health Study) and compared the benefits of walking versus vigorous physical activity as predictors of subsequent risk for NIDDM. The study consisted of 70,102 female participants aged 40 to 65 years. During eight years of follow-up, and after adjusting for age, smoking, alcohol use, history of hypertension and increased TC level, the authors concluded that both walking and vigorous physical activity are associated with significant reductions of risk for NIDDM. Moreover, when the total energy expenditures were similar, comparable magnitudes of risk reduction were produced by walking and vigorous physical activity. More recently, these authors updated and expanded their study of the effects of diet and lifestyle with the risk of type 2 diabetes in 84,941 women followed for 16 years (1980–1996).[229] They reported that overweight or obesity was the single most important risk factor for type 2 diabetes. Furthermore, lack of exercise was the second most important risk factor and was independent of body weight. A poor diet and current smoking were also independent risk factors. Importantly, 91% of the 3300 cases of diabetes was attributed to lifestyle.

The results of another recent study involving a diverse group of overweight men and women with IGT was recently published.[239] This three-year study involved 3234 participants aged 25 to 85 years, 45% of whom were minorities. Compared with the control group, those who lost just ten to 15 pounds (5–7% of their body weight) and walked briskly for 30 minutes five days per week decreased their risk by 58%. Persons 60 years and older decreased their risk by 71%.

Although these studies clearly showed that consistent moderate physical activity significantly decreases the risk for type 2 diabetes, others[240] compared the association between cardiorespiratory fitness and impaired fasting glucose levels and NIDDM in men. After six years of follow-up, and age, smoking, alcohol consumption and parental diabetes were adjusted for, the least cardiorespiratory fitness group had a 1.9-fold risk for impaired fasting glucose and a 3.7-fold risk for NIDDM compared with the high-fitness group. The risk for impaired fasting glucose was also increased in older men and those with increased BMI. Thus, low cardiovascular fitness was significantly correlated with an increased risk for both IGT and NIDDM. The value of vigorous physical activity in elderly people was supported in a study by Cononie *et al.*[241] who assessed the effects of seven consecutive days of exercise for 50 minutes at 70% VO_2max on glucose and insulin responses to an oral glucose challenge in sedentary elderly persons. The major results showed that fasting plasma insulin levels and plasma insulin responses to an oral glucose load were reduced by 15% and 20% respectively, but resulted in no change in body weight or body composition. Thus, hyperinsulinemia associated with aging was significantly reduced by repeated episodes of intense exercise in sedentary elderly people, independent of any body changes.

An important additional recent report[242] regarding the effects of exercise on glycemic control and BMI in patients with type 2 diabetes should be included here. In a meta-analysis of controlled clinical trials, these researchers reviewed and quantified the effects of exercise on glycosylated hemoglobin (HbA_{1c}) levels and BMI in patients with type 2 diabetes. The selected studies included only those that evaluated the effects of exercise interventions that lasted at least eight weeks. Thus, 12 aerobic and two resistance training studies were included. The authors concluded that exercise training significantly reduces HbA_{1c} levels "by an amount that should decrease the risk of diabetic complications ... ."

From the studies referenced in this section, as well as others, insulin resistance is a major risk factor for type 2 diabetes and presumably precedes the disease. Furthermore, overweight/obesity and physical inactivity are major independent risk factors for type 2 diabetes. To better understand the possible relation between these two factors, Kriska *et al.*[243] studied two differerent ethnic groups of men and women; Pima Indians who tend to be overweight and Mauritians who are generally leaner. Their findings showed that blood insulin levels in both groups were inversely associated with physical activity. Thus, the beneficial role of physical activity on insulin sensitivity is probably independent of body mass and fat distribution. A subsequent study of a native Canadian population by this group of investigators showed similar results in men but not women.[244] The authors suggested that this lack of relation between physical activity and insulin levels in women is probably due to the fact that women in this population are physically less active than the men and have "a narrower range of activity/fitness values."

Modest physical activity has also been shown to decrease mortality in adults with diabetes. Gregg *et al.*[245] carried out a prospective cohort study of 2896 American men and women 18 years and older and determined all-cause and cardiovascular mortality over an eight-year period. After controlling for sex, age, BMI, smoking and comorbid conditions, those who walked at least two hours per week had a 39% lower all-cause mortality rate and a 34% lower cardiovascular mortality rate compared with individuals who were inactive. Thus, one death per year may be preventable for every 61 people who could be persuaded to walk at least two hours each week.

These and other studies clearly demonstrate that type 2 diabetes is, for the most part, a preventable disorder. That is, weight control and moderate regular exercise greatly reduce the risk of type 2 diabetes. Although moderately vigorous physical activity is almost invariably more effective, regular modest intensity activity is also very effective and should be strongly encouraged, especially for the sedentary, those beginning a physical activity program and the elderly. In any event, it is extremely important in both medical and financial terms that more intense action be taken to better control this rapidly escalating serious disorder. In addition to local education programs, more attention on the national level is extremely important. Furthermore, physicians must become more involved with their at-risk patients well before insulin resistance and glucose intolerance develop.

Physical Activity and Other Endocrine Disorders

The decline in physiological function with aging is associated with a decrease in composition and increase the fat-free mass in elderly men. In addition, increased physical fitness is accompanied by an increase in the production of growth hormone (GH). In a recent report, Hurel and others[246] compared GH production in men running over 40 miles per week with a similar group of age-matched sedentary controls (controls 57.7 ± 2.8 versus runners 60.5 ± 3.4 years of age). Those involved in regular intense exercise were clearly associated with higher GH and testosterone levels, suggesting that exercise may have an important role in counteracting the "normal" decrease in GH with aging.

Dehydroepiandrosterone (DHEA) and its sulfate ester (DHEAS) are the steroids secreted most abundantly by the adrenal glands. Plasma levels of DHEAS decline with age in both men and women,[247–249] at a rate of about 10% per decade from the third to the tenth decade.[246] Abbasi and coworkers[250] recently demonstrated that several factors, including body leaness, physical fitness, higher levels of total and free testosterone levels and a more favorable blood lipid profile were all associated with higher serum levels of DHEAS in older men.

These reports indicate that more studies comparing the effects of exercise on the endocrine system are needed to fully evaluate the importance of physical activity on hormone production, many of which begin to decrease with increasing age.

Coronary Heart Disease

CHD is clearly the most common cause of death in both men and women in the industrialized world. In 1998, there were 724,269 cardiac deaths compared with 538,947 cancer deaths in the US.[194] Since the pathogenesis of cerebrovascular disease, the third most common cause of death in the US (158,060), is the same as for CHD (i.e. atherosclerosis), the total combined deaths due to arteriosclerotic vascular disease was 882,329. Thus, arteriosclerosis accounts for more annual deaths than the other eight major diseases/disorders combined.

Cardiovascular function and age

The loss of physical endurance or cardiovascular capacity is a common observation with aging and results in several costly public health problems, as well as loss of quality of life, increased dependency and decreased life expectancy. The maximal oxygen consumption (VO_2max), an index of maximal cardiovascular function, decreases 5% to 15% per decade after the age of 25 years.[251] In addition, decreases in maximal cardiac output and maximal arteriovenous oxygen difference contribute to the age-related reduction in VO_2max.[31] Moreover, the maximal heart rate decreases six to ten beats per minute per decade of life and is responsible for some of the age-associated decrease in maximal cardiac output.[31] Nevertheless, some of the cardiovascular-associated aging problems can be greatly improved by increasing one's physical activity, regardless of age. That is, it has been clearly shown that older people elicit the same 10–30% increases in VO$_2$max with prolonged endurance physical training as with young adults.[252–254] In addition, the magnitude of the VO$_2$max increase in the elderly is a function of exercise intensity, just as it is with younger adults; however, light-intensity training elicits little or no change.[253,255]

Kasch *et al.*[256] serially measured cardiovascular function in a group of healthy men, aged 44 to 79 years at intervals after baseline of ten, 15, 20 and 25 years. Over this period of time, data from their daily physical activity was evaluated monthly, including mode, frequency, intensity and duration. The investigators found that the groups' mean cardiovascular function remained at 60% greater than the average of ten previously reported cardiovascular studies in similar aging men. In a more recent study,[257] a group of healthy older men (aged 61 to 74 years), compared with a healthy group of younger men (aged 21 to 39 years), underwent invasive central and peripheral measurements of cardiovascular responses during an upright, staged cycle exercise test before and after a three-month exercise training period with cycle ergometry. At baseline, cardiac output and arterio-venous oxygen difference during exercise were significantly lower in older subjects compared with the younger group. With training, the older and younger groups increased maximal oxygen consumption by 17.8% and 20.2% respectively, although peak cardiac output remained the same in both groups. Systemic arterio-venous oxygen difference increased 14.4% in the elderly men and 14.3% in the younger men. Peak leg blood flow increased by 50% in the older group but remained the same in the younger group. The authors concluded that the age-related decline in maximal oxygen consumption results from a reversible deconditioning effect on the distribution of cardiac output to exercising muscle and an age-associated reduction in cardiac output reserve.

McGuire and associates recently reported two 30-year follow-up studies on the effect of age on cardiovascular response to exercise[258] and the effect of age on the cardiovascular adaptation to exercise training.[259] In the first report,[258] the authors found that cardiovascular capacity declined over the 30-year period mainly due to decreased efficiency of maximum peripheral oxygen extraction. However, the maximal cardiac output was maintained even though there was a 6% decline in the maximal heart rate; it was compensated for by an increased maximal stroke volume. Importantly, they found that three weeks of bedrest at age 20 years (in 1966) had a more profound effect on work capacity than did the subsequent 30 years of aging. In the second study,[259] they found that the age-related decline in aerobic power that occurred over the 30-year period was completely reversed by a six-month endurance training program. However, the improved post-training aerobic power was mainly "the result of peripheral adaptation with no effective improvement in maximal oxygen delivery."

Fleg and coworkers[260] also studied the cardiovascular responses to exhaustive upright cycle exercise in highly trained older athletes (63 ± 7 years) and compared the results with untrained sedentary men of similar age. Their aim was to determine whether the markedly enhanced aerobic exercise of older highly trained men, relative to their sedentary peers, is primarily mediated by central or peripheral cardiovascular mechanisms. Their results clearly showed that the higher aerobic capacity of the trained athletes during exhaustive upright cycle ergometry is similarly achieved through central and peripheral mechanisms. In addition, the authors[261] of a 20-year follow-up study of Finnish men, aged 45 to 64 years at baseline, concluded that a relative increase of physical activity between middle and old age is associated with a maintained high level of physical ability.

Coronary Heart Disease and Physical Activity

From 1953 to 1987, about 40 epidemiologic studies evaluated the association between exercise and CHD[262] 30 of which showed a protective effect of physical activity, varying in magnitude from 10% to 50%. Of those that did not find a protective effect, all were earlier studies with probable alternative explanations (i.e. misclassification of activity levels, use of surrogate exercise indicators, inadequate correction of confounding factors, etc.). In 1996, the NIH Consensus Development Panel on Physical Activity and Cardiovascular Health made the following recommendations to improve cardiovascular health.[263]

(1) All Americans should be involved in regular physical activity at a level "appropriate to their capacity, needs and interest."
(2) Children and adults should accumulate a minimum of 30 minutes of moderate-intensity physical activity on most days, but preferably every day of the week.
(3) Intermittent or shorter bouts of activity (at least ten minutes), including occupational and daily living activities, also have significant cardiovascular benefits if performed at moderate intensity. These include brisk walking, swimming, cycling, yard work, etc. as long as the accumulation is at least 30 minutes per day.
(4) Those who currently meet the minimum recommended standards may derive additional fitness and health benefits by increasing either their physical activity or the intensity of activity.
(5) For those with known CHD, cardiac rehabilitation programs that combine physical activity with a reduction of other risk factors (i.e. elevated lipid levels, being overweight or obese, increased blood pressure, etc.) should be used.

However, as noted earlier in this chapter, the Institute of Medicine Committee recently recommended at least one hour of moderate physical activity each day.[29]

Recent studies also suggest that intensive lifestyle changes can lead to regression of coronary atherosclerosis. For example, Ornish and associates[264] randomized older patients with moderate to severe CHD to an intensive lifestyle change (10% fat whole foods vegetarian diet, aerobic exercise, stress management training, smoking cessation and group psychosocial support) or to a "usual-care" control group. The participants were followed for five years. After one year, the experimental group had an average decrease in diameter artery stenosis of 1.75 absolute percentage points (a 4.5% relative decrease) and a 3.1 absolute percentage point decrease after five years (a 7.9% relative improvement). Conversely, the average percent diameter stenosis in the control group increased by 2.3 percentage points after one year (a 5.4% relative worsening) and by 11.8 percentage points after five years (a 27.7% relative worsening). Moreover, during the five-year period the number of cardiac events in the control group was more than double that of the experimental group.

Both weight loss and aerobic exercise are highly effective in reducing the risk for CHD; importantly, both are more effective than either alone. However, which of these is most effective is somewhat controversial. For example, Katzel *et al.*[265] recently compared the effects of weight loss versus aerobic exercise training on risk factors for CHD in healthy, obese middle-aged and older (61 ± 1 years) men. The results suggested that weight loss is the preferred treatment to improve CHD risk. Conversely, diet and exercise are reportedly equally effective in reducing the risk of CHD.[266]

As noted by Myers and associates,[267] most reports regarding physical activity and CHD involved long-term follow-up studies in relatively healthy people; very few focused on more clinically relevant populations. Therefore, they studied 6213 consecutive men referred for treadmill exercise testing for clinical reasons. The participants were divided into two groups: those with an abnormal exercise-test result or a history of CHD or both, and those with a normal exercise-test result and no history of cardiovascular disease. Their results showed that men who died during the study period were older and had a lower maximal heart rate, lower maximal systolic and diastolic blood pressure and lower exercise capacity. After adjusting for age, the peak exercise capacity measured in metabolic equivalents was the strongest predictor of death among both groups. Thus, for each metabolic equivalent increase in exercise capacity there was a 12% improvement in survival.

Coronary heart disease, physical activity and the elderly

Recent evidence suggests that the classic risk factors for CHD among middle-aged persons are equally valid in older people. Importantly, studies have also shown that these risk factors remain equally low in older people who maintain a physically active lifestyle. For example, in a 20-year follow-up study of older track athletes aged 60 to 92 years, Mengelhoch *et al.*[268] concluded that the risk factors remained low and usually stable in older athletes who maintain regular exercise training. In addition, the Zutphen Elderly Study[269] recently reported their ten-year follow-up findings of CHD and all-cause mortality in older persons aged 64 to 84 years. Not only was time spent in more intense physical activity strongly and inversely associated with risks of all-cause mortality, but walking or cycling at least three times per week for 20 minutes was associated with reduced mortality from CHD. Furthermore, they reported that time spent in more intense activity was generally more effective than equivalent time in less intense activities. Similarly, others[270] reported that maintaining or starting a light to moderate physical activity program significantly reduces mortality and "heart attacks" in elderly men with and without diagnosed CHD, compared to those who remain sedentary.

Dose-response: physical activity and coronary heart disease risk

From the studies described above, it is clear that physical activity is of significant benefit in reducing the risk of CHD. In addition, two recent clinical trials support the idea that the incorporation of moderate-intensity activities into one's lifestyle have CHD risk benefits comparable to those derived from structured exercise programs.[271,272] However, the necessary quantity and intensity of physical activity for the primary prevention of CHD remains somewhat controversial. However, as noted above in the Zutphen Elderly Study,[269] along with other recent reports to be discussed, there is good evidence for a graded inverse dose-response relationship between the level of physical activity and risk for CHD.

Several publications indicate that walking is protective against CHD. For example, a cohort of men and women aged 65 years and older, were evaluated regarding their physical activity at baseline and after four to five years (mean 4.2 years).[273] The major outcomes of the study were hospitalizations due to cardiovascular disease and death. Their data showed that walking more than four hours per week was associated with a reduced risk for both CHD hospitalization and death in men and women compared with those who walked less than one hour per week. However, the authors noted that reduced risk for death may be mediated by effects of walking on other risk factors. The effects of walking on CHD in elderly men was also evaluated in the Honolulu Heart Program.[274] The findings, observed after two to four years, indicated that men aged 71 to 93 years who walked less than 0.25 miles per day had a two-fold increased risk of CHD compared with those who walked more than 1.5 miles per day. Moreover, those who walked 0.25 to 1.5 miles per day were also at a significantly higher risk for CHD than those who walked longer distances.

Lakka *et al.*[275] studied the independent associations of leisure-time physical activity and maximal oxygen uptake (a measure of cardio-respiratory fitness) with the risk of acute myocardial infarction (AMI). Their data showed that higher levels of both leisure-time physical activity and cardiorespiratory fitness had a strong, graded, inverse correlation with the risk of AMI. The authors concluded that lower levels of physical activity and cardiorespiratory fitness are independent risk factors for CHD in men. On the other hand, data from a prospective study of 72,488 female nurses aged 40 to 65 years at baseline and followed for eight years, revealed that brisk walking and more vigorous exercise were similarly associated with substantial reductions in the incidence of CHD.[276] It may be that the level of exercise and risk of CHD is different in men and women. The association between physical activity intensity and CHD in women was recently reported.[277] This cohort of 39,372 healthy female health professionals aged 45 and older at baseline, were studied between 1992 and 1995 with a follow-up in 1999. After adjusting for potential confounders, the relative risks for CHD for less than 200, 200–599, 600–1499 and 1500 or more kcal/week expended on all activities were 1.00 (referent), 0.79, 0.55 and 0.75, respectively. Although vigorous activities were associated with lower risk for CHD, walking also predicted a lower risk among women not involved in vigorous activities. Thus, at least one hour walking/week predicted a lower CHD risk. The benefits of physical activity also included women who were overweight, had increased cholesterol levels or were smokers.

More recently, Manson and associates[278] prospectively studied 73,743 postmenopausal women aged 50 to 79 years who were free of cardio-vascular disease and cancer at baseline. They found an inverse asso-ciation between an increasing physical-activity score and risk for both coronary events and total cardiovascular events in both white and black women. Thus, increasing quintiles of energy expenditure had an age-adjusted relative risk of coronary events of 1.00, 0.73, 0.69, 0.68 and 0.47, respectively. Moreover, walking and vigorous exer-cise were associated with similar risk reductions, which did not vary significantly according to race, age or BMI. Conversely, they noted that "prolonged sitting predicts increased cardiovascular risk."

Williams[279] examined the dose-response relationship between CHD risk factors in vigorously active older men. He noted that although older runners ran more slowly than younger runners, those 60 years and older who ran farther had significantly higher plasma levels of HDL-C and lower ratios of TC to HDL-C, plasma triglycerides, sys-tolic and diastolic blood pressure, BMI and waist circumference. Moreover, a recent Harvard Alumni Health Study[280] involving 12,516 middle-aged and older men (39 to 88 years of age) who were fol-lowed for 16 years, found that total physical activity and vigorous activities were associated with the strongest reductions in CHD risk. They noted that although moderate to light activities may be less accurately measured, their data indicated a non-signifcant inverse correlation between CHD risk in this group. They also noted that the association between reduced risk for CHD and physical activity extended to men with multiple coronary risk factors. In a related study, Lee *et al.*[281] prospectively followed 7307 older men, mean age 66.1 years, to determine whether longer exercise periods were more predictive of decreased CHD risk compared with shorter sessions if the same amount of energy was expended. After adjustment for age and other potential confounders, they concluded that as long as the total energy expended was similar, shorter exercise sessions were equally as protective as longer sessions.

An extensive recent report from the Health Professionals' Follow-up Study involving 44,452 American men found that total physical activity, running, weight training and rowing were each inversely associated with CHD risk.[282] The relative ratios corresponding to quintiles of metabolic equivalent tasks (METs) for total physical activity were 1.0, 0.90, 0.87, 0.83 and 0.70. Men who ran an hour or more per week had a 42% risk reduction compared with men who did not run. Men involved in weight training for 30 minutes or more per week had a 23% risk reduction compared with those who did not train with weights, and rowing for one hour or more per week had an 18% risk reduction compared with men not engaged in rowing. In addition, average exercise intensity was associated with reduced CHD risk independent of the total physical activity. Brisk walking for 30 minutes per day was associated with an 18% risk reduction; walking pace was also associated with reduced CHD risk independent of the number of hours walked. Similarly, Wagner *et al.*[283] evaluated the met energy expenditure (EE) as the result of physical activity in 9758 individuals from Northern Ireland and France who were aged 50 to 59 years and free of CHD at baseline. The subjects were categorized as to their high-intensity leisure-time physical activities, or walked or cycled to work. After multivariate adjustment, leisure-time physical activity EE was associated with a significantly lower risk of myocardial infarction and coronary death whereas walking or cycling to work was not independently related to these cardiovascular events. The authors suggested that the greater level of leisure time activities in France may, in part, explain the higher risk of myocardial infarction and CHD death noted in Northern Ireland compared with France.

It is also of interest that aptitude for different sports may be important in CHD protection. Kujala and coauthors[284] investigated the association between natural selection to sports, continuity of physical activity and occurrence of CHD in former male athletes participating at a young age (1920–1965) in different types of sports (endurance, power speed, "other" and healthy controls). In 1985, all former athletes were significantly more active than controls. Moreover, former endurance athletes participated more often in vigorous activity compared with power speed athletes and had significantly less CHD (odds ratio, 0.34). In 1985 and 1995, both endurance and "other" athletes had less CHD than the controls. The authors concluded that both a previous aptitude for endurance athletic events and continuity of vigorous activity were associated with less CHD. However, a power speed aptitude did not give CHD protection.

Physical fitness and coronary heart disease mortality

Physical fitness studies based on point estimates suggest they are reliable long-term predictors of cardiovascular and all-cause mortality in healthy people. Erikssen *et al.*[285] studied the sequential periods 1972–1975 and 1982. All participants received a physical examination, various blood tests, spirometry, chest radiograph, height and weight measurements and an exercise electrocardiographic test at both time periods. The results indicated a graded inverse relation between changes in physical fitness and mortality irrespective of physical fitness status at the initial survey indicating that a change in physical fitness is a strong mortality predictor. Similarly, Blair and coworkers[286] quantified the relation of cardiorespiratory fitness to CHD and all-cause mortality within strata of various personal characteristics associated with CHD and early mortality (i.e. smoking, cholesterol level, blood pressure and health status). The major outcome measures of the 25,341 men and 7,080 women participants was CHD mortality and all-cause mortality. The results showed that low fitness is an important risk of mortality. In addition, the protective effect of physical fitness held for both smokers and non-smokers, those with and without increased plasma cholesterol levels, elevated blood pressure and those who were both healthy and unhealthy. The authors concluded that moderate physical fitness protects against the influence of these other mortality risk factors. Others[287] noted there were about 75,000 yearly instances of acute myocardial infarction (AMI) in the US that occur after heavy physical exertion; of these, there were 25,000 deaths. However, they reported that those regularly involved in physical exertion were protected against the triggering of an AMI under similar conditions.

Additionally, Wei *et al.*[288] compared the relationship between low cardiorespiratory fitness and mortality in overweight and obese men with those of normal weight. The study involved 25,714 adult men (43.8 ± 10.1 years) who received a medical examination during 1970 to 1993 with a mortality follow-up to 1994. Using normal-weight men without CHD as the reference group, the strongest predictor of CHD death in obese men was baseline CHD (relative risk, 14.0). The relative risks for obese men with diabetes, elevated blood cholesterol, hypertension, smoking and low cardiorespiratory fitness were similar (relative risks 4.4 for smoking to 5.0 for low fitness). The relative risk for all-cause mortality in obese men with low fitness was 3.1 compared with the normal weight group. However, low fitness was an independent mortality risk factor in all BMI groups. The authors concluded that cardiorespiratory fitness was "a strong and independent predictor" for both CHD and all-cause mortality; it was as important as diabetes and the other major risk factors.

Although regular physical activity is very effective in decreasing the risk of CHD, there are some contraindications to exercise regardless of age or sex.[31] These include recent electrocardiograph (ECG) changes and myocardial infarction, congestive heart failure, unstable angina, uncontrolled arrythythmias and third-degree heart block. Relative contraindications include uncontrolled hypertension, cardiomyopathy, complex ventricular ectopy and uncontrolled metabolic disturbances.

Exercise and pathogenesis of atherosclerosis

Atherosclerosis is primarily a disorder of lipid and lipoprotein metabolism. Moreover, oxidative modification of low-density lipoproteins is a widely accepted pathogenetic mechanism.[214] As previously indicated in this chapter, regular exercise improves several of the commonly recognized independent CHD risk factors (overweight/obese, hypertension, type 2 diabetes, blood lipid levels, etc.). In addition, physical activity has a positive effect on other established, but less well-known risk factors, including increased plasma fibrinogen[289–292] and factor VII[289] levels, coronary endothelial function,[293] blood mononuclear cells,[294] blood viscosity[295] and oxidative stress.[296,297] Physical activity also lowers the risk for CHD by other, albeit poorly understood, mechanisms. For example, CHD has been associated with chronic inflammation,[298] which is also associated with increased oxidative stress.[214] Moreover, an elevated plasma C-reactive protein (C-RP) level is associated with a two- to five-fold increased risk of coronary events.[299,300] Importantly, recent cross-sectional associations between physical fitness and plasma C-RP were recently studied among a tri-ethnic sample (i.e. African American, Native American and Caucasian) of women aged 55 ± 11 years.[301] The results showed that enhanced physical fitness was associated with significnatly decreased plasma C-RP levels in all three ethnic groups. These findings are not surprising since moderately intense exercise stimulates the immune system (see later section, "Physical Activity and the Immune System").

It has also become recently apparent that there are vascular adaptations to exercise training. Over 100 studies have focused on the role of nitric oxide (NO), a free radical that causes vascular dilatation (endothelium relaxing factor) and therefore has a cardioprotective function in cardiac ischemia and preconditioning.[302] NO is synthesized by three different nitric oxide synthase (NOS) enzymes [inducible (i) NOS, endothelial (e) NOS and neuronal (n) NOS]. Importantly, chronic exercise has been shown to increase both iNOS and eNOS gene expression in endothelial cells of the rat aorta.[303] Moreover, NO not only stimulates vascular dilatation, it inhibits platelet aggregation and has antioxidant, anti-proliferative and anti-apoptotic properties.[304] As a result, long-term NOS inhibition accelerates atherogenesis.[305]

Physical Activity and Stroke

Cerebrovascular disease is the third most common cause of death in the US (158,060 deaths in 1998).[194] The pathogenesis of stroke, as with AMI, is most often the result of atherosclerosis. As noted in the preceding section, physical activity is significantly and inversely associated with CHD. However, the role of physical activity in stroke prevention is less well studied, and early results from epidemiologic studies have been somewhat inconsistent. Although a couple of earlier reports did not show an inverse relationship between stroke and physical activity,[306,307] more recent longitudinal studies did.

In the Framingham Study,[308] two separate analyses were performed; the first was during midlife in both men and women (mean ages 49.7 and 49.9 years, respectively) and a later one when the cohort was older (mean ages 63.0 and 63.7 years, respectively). Physical activity was divided into tertiles; median and high levels were compared with a low level (referent group). In men, the data revealed that increased levels of physical activity were protective against stroke. However, high levels of physical activity did not confer an additional protective effect over medium levels. Interestingly, increased physical activity did not have a protective effect in women. Conversely, the National Health and Nutrition Examination Survey I (NHANES 1) studied 7895 white and black men and women aged 45 to 74 years at baseline.[309] The average follow-up period was 11.6 years. The baseline risk factors of age, smoking, history of diabetes and CHD, education level, systolic blood pressure, total serum cholesterol, BMI and hemoglobin concentration for both men and women were adjusted. In addition, a higher resting pulse rate was associated with an increased risk of stroke in blacks but not in whites. Similarly, the Northern Manhattan Stroke Study, which included white, black and Hispanic men and women, compared leisure-time activity with ischemic stroke risk.[310] Their results showed that leisure-time physical activity was significantly protective of stroke in all groups after adjustment for cardiac disease, peripheral vascular disease, hypertension, diabetes, smoking, alcohol use, obesity, education level and season of enrollment. In addition, the authors reported a dose-response relationship for both intensity (i.e. light to moderate activity versus vigorous activity) and exercise duration (i.e. less than two hours per week, two to less than five hours per week and five or more hours per week).

Other studies were limited to either women or men. In a recent publication, Hu *et al.*[311] reported their findings of the effects of physical activity on risk of stroke in 72,488 female nurses aged 40 to 65 years at baseline (Nurses' Health Study). The follow-up period was eight years. Their data indicated that physical activity, including moderate-intensity exercise (e.g. walking), was associated with a significant reduction in risk of total and ischemic stroke in a dose-response manner. That is, a brisk or striding walking pace was associated with a lower stroke risk compared with an average (i.e. casual) pace.

Three major studies have examined the relation between physical activity and stroke in men. Abbott and associates[312] evaluated the risk of stroke in 7530 men over a 22-year period (the Honolulu Heart Program), and compared the risk in younger (aged 45–54 years) middle-aged men with an older group (aged 55–68 years). The older group consisted of those who were sedentary or mildly active. After exclusion of those with hypertension, diabetes and left ventricular hypertrophy, the relative risk of stroke for inactive men was 3.7 compared with active men. In non-smoking older men, the relative risk of thromboembolic stroke among sedentary men versus active men was 2.8. When partially active older men were compared with those who were physically active, the relative risk was 2.4. However, increased physical activity did not reduce the incidence of thromboembolic stroke in men who smoked cigarettes.

A recent prospective cohort study of 11,130 Harvard University male alumni (the Harvard Alumni Health Study), mean aged 58 years at baseline, compared physical activity and the incidence of stroke after 13 years follow-up.[313] After adjusting for age, smoking, alcohol intake and early parental death, the relative risks of stroke was inversely associated with the level of activity as follows: <1000, 1000–1999, 2000–2999, 3000–3999 and ≥4000 kcal/week of energy expenditure at baseline were 1.00, 0.76, 0.54, 0.78 and 0.82, respectively. Walking ≥20 km/week was associated with a significantly lower risk which was independent of other physical activity components. As noted from the data, the lowest incidence of stroke was associated with an energy expenditure of 2000 to 2999 kcal/week; the incidence increased with either higher or lower activity levels. Similarly, Lee *et al.*[314] reported their findings in a study of exercise and stroke risk in male physicians

(Physicians' Health Study). After adjustment for treatment assignment, age, smoking, alcohol intake, history of angina and parental history of myocardial infarction, the relative risks of stroke associated with vigorous (sweat producing) exercise (i.e. less than once, two to four times and five or more times per week) at baseline were 1.00 (referent), 0.79, 0.80 and 0.79, respectively. In subgroup analyses, the inverse association was stronger for hemorrhagic than ischemic stroke. When further adjustments were made for BMI, history of hypertension, increased serum cholesterol levels and diabetes mellitus, the corresponding relative risks for total stroke were 1.00 (referent), 0.81, 0.88 and 0.86, respectively. Thus, vigorous exercise was again shown to be associated with a decreased risk of stroke in men. The authors suggested that the inverse relationship was mediated by the beneficial effects of exercise on body weight, blood pressure, serum cholesterol and glucose tolerance.

Cancer and Physical Activity

An estimated 1,284,900 new cancer cases will be diagnosed in the US in the year 2002;[315] it is second only to cardiovascular disease as a cause of death (about 555,500 in 2002). Epidemiologic studies consistently indicate that cancer is largely an avoidable disease since more than two-thirds of cancer deaths might be prevented through lifestyle changes.[316,317] In addition to genetic factors, smoking, obesity, poor diet and various environmental toxins are all major risk factors. For example, evidence is now firm that overweight and obesity are important risk factors for cancers of the colon, endometrium, ovary, kidney, breast and lower esophagus. In addition to not smoking and staying lean, physical activity provides the greatest potential for minimizing cancer risk. Indeed, numerous studies have provided considerable support for an inverse relationship between increased physical activity, as measured directly (i.e. subjective recall, former athletic status and job classification) or indirectly (i.e. physical fitness), and decreased incidence and/or mortality rates for various cancers (Table 3.5). However, it is often difficult to ascertain whether physical activity is independently

Table 3.5: Physical Activity and Decreased Cancer Risk

Colon
Estrogen-linked cancers
  Breast
  Ovary
  Endometrium
Prostate
Lung
Pancreas

associated with a decreased incidence of some cancers or whether this is associated with an impaired lifestyle and various other confounding variables. It is somewhat surprising that in 1922 Cherry theorized that increased physical activity prevents cancer.[318] This hypothesis came from his astute observations that primitive societies have significantly lower cancer rates than more civilized cultures and that the amount of job activity was inversely associated with cancer mortality. Several recent reviews on the relationship of physical activity and cancer have been published.[319-321]

The American Cancer Society recommended the following physical activity guidelines for cancer prevention.[322]

(1) Individual Guidelines
  (a) Adults: at least moderate activity for 30 minutes or more on five or more days per week; 45 minutes or more of moderate-to-vigorous activity on five or more days per week may further enhance risk reductions of colon and breast cancers.
  (b) Children and Adolescents: at least 60 minutes per day of moderate-to-vigorous physical activity at least five days per week.
(2) Community Guidelines
  Public, private and community organizations should work to create social and physical environments that support the adoption and maintenance of healthful physical activity behaviors.

Physical activity and colorectal cancer

Cancer of the colon and rectum is one of the most common malignant disorders in both men and women. For year 2002, there were an estimated 107,300 and 41,000 new cases of colon and rectal cancer, respectively (colon: men 50,000, women 57,000, rectum: men 22,600, women 18,400). The estimated number of deaths were 48,100 and 8500 for colon and rectal cancer, respectively.[315] Although epidemiologic studies have not consistently identified strong risk factors for these malignancies, there is increasing evidence that dietary fat increases the risk (discussed in Chapter 4). In addition, the relationship between physical activity and colorectal cancer has been extensively studied over the past two decades. The totality of evidence suggests that inactive people, compared with active persons, have a 1.2- to 3.6-fold increased risk of developing colon cancer.[323,324]

Vena *et al.*[325] studied a group of white male patients aged 30 to 79 years during an eight-year period and compared the amount of lifetime occupational physical activity and incidence of colon and rectal cancer and compared them with a control group with non-neoplastic, non-digestive diseases. Occupational categories were coded into one of five physical activity levels according to Department of Labor ratings. Their findings showed an increased risk of colon cancer associated with sedentary or light occupational physical activity. However, a strong consistent association between physical activity and rectal cancer was not present. Others have also shown an inverse relationship between occupational physical activity and colon cancer. Using the Missouri Cancer Registry, Brownson *et al.*[326] studied the incidence of colon cancer in specific occupations and industries and the levels of occupational physical activity. They concluded that increased colon cancer risks were identified for printing machine operators, workers in food manufacturing, communications and petroleum products. They also reported excess risk among males employed in sedentary jobs and an inverse linear trend in risk according to the level of occupational physical activity.

Similarly, others[327] evaluated the relationship between colon cancer, physical activity and occupation in a case-control study. They found a decreased risk in persons with physically active occupations (i.e. agriculture, forestry and saw millworkers) and an increased risk for railway employees. More recently, Tavani and coworkers[328] investigated the relationship between colon and rectal cancers and occupational physical activity in women and men below 75 years of age. Compared with the lowest level of occupational activity at ages 30 to 39 years, the odds ratios for colon cancer were 0.64 and 0.49 for men and women, respectively. This inverse association for both sexes was similar at ages 15 to 19 and 50 to 59 years. Again, however, rectal cancer risk was not associated with any measure of physical activity.

Several recent studies have compared leisure-time physical activity and risk of colorectal cancer in both men and women. White and associates[329] found that for middle-aged men and women combined, moderate or high intensity recreational activity (i.e. two or more activities per week versus none) was associated with a decreased risk of colon cancer. The relationship was stronger for men than women. Others[330] studied five lifestyle patterns for both men and women. The first consisted of dietary patterns including "Western," "moderation," "calcium/low-fat dairy," "meat and mutagens" and "nibblers, smoking, coffee." The second group consisted of lifestyle patterns labeled "body size," "medication and supplementation," "alcohol" and "physical activity." Among both men and women, an increased level of physical activity was the most marked lifestyle pattern associated with colon cancer (odds ratios 0.42 and 0.52 for men and women, respectively).

Two recent studies on physical activity and colon cancer outside the US have also been reported. Tang *et al.*[331] noted that the mortality rate of colorectal cancer has been increasing in Taiwan over the past 20 years, placing it as the third leading cause of cancer mortality in that country. They studied a cohort of subjects aged 30 to 80 years of age. After evaluating dietary intake, physical activity and other lifestyle activities, they found the odds ratio among men with active leisure-time physical activity was 0.19 times that of sedentary men. However, physical activity was not associated with colon cancer risk in women. Interestingly, they reported a strong inverse dose-response relationship between increased water intake and rectal cancer in men. A similar but statistically non-significant trend was reported for women. Thune and Lund[332] examined occupational and recreational physical activity and the risk of colorectal cancer in a population-based Norwegian cohort. The follow-up periods were 16.3 years for men and 15.5 years for women. Their results showed that physical activity at a level equivalent to walking or cycling for at least four hours per week during leisure-time was associated with a significant decreased risk of colon cancer among both females and males. Moreover, in both sexes there was a stronger preventive effect for physical activity in the proximal compared with the distal colon. They also reported a borderline significant decrease in colon cancer risk for occupational physical activity in men aged 45 years and older compared with the sedentary group. However, no effect was noted for occupational physical activity in women.

Recent large-scale studies limited to either women or men have also been carried out. In multivariate analyses, the Nurses' Health Study compared BMI and leisure-time physical activity with colon cancer risk.[333] They found that women whose energy expenditure exceeded 21 metabolic equivalent task (MET)-hours* per week of leisure-time physical activity had a relative colon cancer risk of 0.54 compared with women who expended less than 21 MET-hours per week. Moreover, women with a BMI greater than 29 kg/m² (obese) had a relative risk for colon cancer of 1.45 compared with women whose BMI was less than 21 kg/m². Others studied the effects of physical activity on colon cancer risks in men. For example, Lee and Paffenbarger[334] reported that men who were highly active physically had 0.19 to 0.56 times the colon cancer risk compared with those who were inactive. However, as with other studies, the level of physical activity was not significantly associated with the risk for rectal cancer. Conversely, in a more recent Physicians' Health Study, essentially the same research group reported that their data did not support the hypothesis that physical activity reduces the risk of colon cancer in men.[335] The authors suggested that "plausible alternate explanations for the null finding include misclassification of physical activity and the potential for increased surveillance for colon cancer (screening effect) among those physically active." These results are, of course, in opposition to the numerous studies cited above, among others.

Several of the studies reported in this section suggested a dose-response relationship between the level of physical activity and colon cancer risk. In addition, Slattery *et al.*[336] presented evidence that vigorous leisure-time activity performed over two decades was significant in reducing the risk for colon cancer. Moreover, the greatest inverse association was observed in those whose physical activity sessions were for longer time periods. They also estimated that 13% of all colon cancers could be attributed to lack of vigorous leisure-time activity.

Giovannucci and coworkers[337] studied the relationship between physical activity, BMI and pattern of fat distribution and risk of colorectal adenomas in women. After controlling for various factors (i.e. age, prior endoscopy, family history of colorectal cancer, smoking, aspirin and intakes of animal fat, dietary fiber, folate and alcohol), physical activity was inversely associated with risk of large (i.e. ≥ 1 cm) distal colon adenomas. The relative risk was 0.57 when comparing high and low quintiles of average leisure-time energy expenditure. They noted that "much of the benefit" came from moderate intensity physical activity such as brisk walking. BMI was also a significant independent risk for large distal colon adenomas, although waist circumference and waist-to-hip ratio were not. In an earlier study, these investigators reported essentially the same results in men.[338] Other published reports are in essential agreement.[339,340]

As a final note, it is of considerable importance that individuals who regularly use aspirin and other non-steroidal anti-inflammatory drugs (NSAIDs) for pain/discomfort, may also have a sigificantly reduced risk of colon cancer.[341-343]

Physical activity and estrogen-linked cancers

Breast

Breast cancer is the most common non-skin malignancy in American women; there were about 180,200 new cases in 1997.[344] In 2002, there were an estimated 205,000 new cases and 38,600 deaths.[315]

Approximately one in nine women will develop breast cancer and about one-fourth will die of the disease. After lung cancer, it is the second most common cause of female cancer deaths. The etiology of breast cancer is varied with only 5% to 10% of cases being due to autosomal dominant genes.[345] Other risk factors include female sex, age (i.e. postmenopausal), high fat diet, obesity, being nulliparous and having the first child after age 30 years.[346] A sedentary lifestyle has also been hypothesized as an important risk factor. Several mechanisms have been proposed to explain the prevention of estrogen-linked cancers by physical activity:[347] (1) maintenance of low body fat and moderation of extraglandular estrogen; (2) reduction in number of ovulatory cycles and subsequent diminution of lifetime exposure to endogenous estrogen; (3) enhancement of natural immune function; and (4) the association of other healthy lifestyle habits. Early observations that led to this hypothesis are the negative effects of early age at menarche and late age of menopause on breast cancer risk.[348] That is, early menarche is associated with a more rapid onset of a regular ovulatory menstrual cycle than late menarche, with resultant longer exposure to estrogen. In addition, regardless of when the age menarche begins, the rapidity with which regular cycling is established is associated with breast cancer risk. However, the relationship between increased physical activity and breast cancer risk is controversial. Some studies clearly suggest that increased physical activity has a protective effect against breast cancer while others have found no association. In any event, the support for increased physical activity as a preventive measure of breast cancer is not as strong as for colon cancer.

Most studies, however, as described in several recent literature reviews, agree that a sedentary lifestyle is a risk factor for this malignancy.[347,349,350] For example, Friedenreich and associates[349] examined 21 studies published before 1997 that evaluated physical activity in relation to breast cancer risk. Of these, 15 found that increased physical activity reduced the risk of breast cancer, while four studies reported no association and two found an increased risk in those who were more physically active. Similarly, Gammon *et al.*[350] reported that seven of nine studies suggested that increased occupational physical activity may be associated with a decreased risk of breast cancer, at least in a subgroup of women. Eleven of 16 studies on recreational activity reported a 12% to 60% decrease in risk among both premenopausal and postmenopausal women. However, a dose-response effect was not noted in most of the reports. In addition, they found the risk reduction associated with exercise was observed more often in case-control studies than in cohort studies. Several specific studies published over the past decade will be presented.

Bernstein *et al.*[351] reported a relative risk of 0.42 for women with a lifetime average of 3.8 hours or more of physical activity per week compared with those who were sedentary. Moreover, they found that over the course of the child-bearing years, four hours of exercise per week resulted in a 58% lower risk of breast cancer compared with sedentary women during this time period. Several more recent studies are also supportive of an inverse association between physical activity and breast cancer. Thune and associates[352] studied 25,624 women, 20 to 54 years of age at baseline, and followed them for a median of 13.7 years. After adjustments for age, BMI, height and parity, women engaged in leisure-time regular exercise, compared with sedentary women, had a relative risk of 0.63. The reduced risk in regularly exercising women was greater in premenopausal than postmenopausal women. It was also greater in women less than 45 years of age at entry compared with older women at entry (aged 45 years or older). These workers also reported that increased occupational physical activity decreased the risk compared to those with little or no activity at work. Data from the Nurses' Health Study involving women aged 30 to 55 years at baseline and followed for 16 years has been analyzed.[353] Here, women engaged in moderate to vigorous physical activity for seven or more hours each week had a relative risk of 0.82 for breast cancer compared to women who were physically active for one hour or less per week. In addition, the authors reported a dose-response trend.

Carpenter *et al.*[354] reported the following odds ratios (OR) for women with relatively stable adult body weights who (1) consistently exercised throughout their lifetime (OR, 0.42); (2) exercised more than four hours per week for at least 12 years (OR, 0.59); and (3) exercised vigorously during the most recent ten years (OR, 0.52). However, physical activity was not found to be protective for women who gained over 17% body weight during adulthood.

Physical activity has also been reported to decrease the risk of breast cancer in women from other countries. For example, Ueji *et al.*[355] found that after adjustment for possible confounding factors (i.e. BMI, height, family history of breast cancer, education level, age at menarche, age at first birth and menopausal status), recreational physical activity was associated with a significant reduction of cancer risk in Japanese women. The odds ratio among women who played a regular sport or who exercised more than 15.3 METs per week was 0.35 compared to those who played no sport or did not participate in regular physical activity. Similarly, a case-control Swiss study reported that physical activity is "a favorable indicator of breast cancer risk."[356]

In addition to the few studies referred to in the review articles quoted above,[347,349,350] two additional recent reports also do not support a role for physical activity in reducing the risk of breast cancer.[357,358] Although most studies clearly agree that increased physical activity significantly decreases the risk of breast cancer, a few do not, for reasons that are not entirely clear. As a result, well-designed studies are sorely needed to clarify the specific reasons for these differences. In addition, the exercise or physical activity dosage needed to provide optimal protection from cancer is unclear. Certainly, case-control studies that quantify the degree of physical activity over time are more reliable than those based on self-reported activities.

Ovary

In 2002, there were an estimated 23,300 new cases of ovarian carcinoma in the US, resulting in 13,900 deaths.[315] In two early studies, Frisch and others[359,360] reported a reduced prevalence of cancers of the breast, ovary and endometrium in college women athletes who continued to be physically active throughout their lifetimes (73.5% of the women athletes from years 1921 to 1981 remained physically active compared with 57.0% of non-athletes). After controlling for age, family history of cancer, age at menarche, number of pregnancies, use of oral contraceptives or estrogen replacement therapy, smoking and leanness, the study found strong evidence for an inverse association between the college female athletes engaged in lifetime physical activity and the risk for these estrogen-linked cancers compared with non-athletic women who engaged in little or no physical activity during the same period of their lives. In Shanghai, occupational activity was evaluated in Chinese women with estrogen-dependent cancers.[361] Here, a postiive association was also found between low occupational physical activity and cancers of the ovary, breast and endometrium. The authors also reported a protective effect in women retired from physically active jobs, suggesting that the benefits of lifelong occupational activity persists after retirement.

More recently, Cottreau and associates[362] reported that increased leisure-time physical activity was significantly associated with a decreased occurrence of ovarian cancer in women studied from 1994 to 1998. After adjustment for age, parity, oral contraceptive use, family history of ovarian cancer, race and BMI, women with the highest level of physical activity had an odds ratio of 0.73 for ovarian cancer compared with women in the lowest level of physical activity. Others,[363] however, reported that increased physical activity was not associated with decreased ovarian cancer and that those with "moderate" or "high" activity levels actually had an increased risk compared with physically inactive women. This latter study is clearly contrary to the hypothesized mechanism(s) outlined above whereby physical activity is thought to decrease the risk of ovarian cancer.

Uterine corpus

Endometrial cancer is the most common malignancy of the female reproductive tract. In 1996, there were an estimated 30,000 cancer cases of the uterine corpus in the US and 6000 deaths;[364] in 2002, the estimated number of new cases increased to 39,300 with 6600 deaths.[315] Established risk factors of endometrial cancer include estrogen replacement therapy, middle-aged obesity, diabetes mellitus and low parity; the effects of diet, weight change, alcohol intake and genetic factors are uncertain.[365] Physical inactivity is also a possible risk factor for endometrial cancer. Over the last decade, several studies have been published on the association between physical activity and endometrial carcinoma.

In 1993, Levi and associates[366] reported a risk of 1.3 to 2.3 for endometrial cancer in Swiss and Italian women whose physical activity level was "moderately low" and over 2.5 for those whose activity was "very low." After adjustment for various potential distorting factors including BMI, the inverse trends in risk remained statistically significant. During this same year, two other studies also found an inverse association between physical activity and endometrial cancer.[367,368] In the latter report,[368] the association remained unchanged after adjustments for caloric intake and BMI.

In a nation-wide Swedish cohort study, increased occupational physical activity was also found to decrease the risk of endometrial cancer.[369] However, the protective effect of physical activity was confined to women aged 50 to 69 years among whom sedentary work was associated with a 60% higher risk compared with the most active women. Conversely, others found no relationship between occupational physical activity and decreased risk of endometrial cancer.[370] They did, however, report an overall "modest" cancer risk reduction in women who were physically active compared with sedentary women. More recently, a cohort study from the Swedish Twin Registry examined the association of physical activity, weight and weight change, fruit, vegetable and alcohol consumption, socioeconomic status, parity and presence of diabetes mellitus with the incidence of endometrial cancer.[365] The data showed that increasing physical activity markedly decreased the risk of endometrial cancer independent of weight and parity; the risk in the highest quartile was 0.2 compared with the sedentary group. Additional independent risk factors included very low fruit and vegetable intake, and increased weight in middle age and early adulthood. There was no evidence of a genetic component.

In summary, most studies support an inverse relationship between the level of both leisure-time and occupational physical activity and estrogen-dependent cancers. However, an inherent problem in most of these studies is controlling for confounding factors, especially BMI. If in fact physically active women are at decreased risk for these malignancies, a major question yet to be answered is whether it is due to increased physical activity or to less body fat because of a physically active lifestyle.

Prostate

Prostate cancer is the most common malignancy in men; in 2002, there were an estimated 189,000 new cases.[315] Of these, there were about 30,200 deaths, making it the third most common cause of cancer death in American men. After colon cancer, prostate cancer is the most studied malignancy with respect to the effect of physical activity.

Kiningham[321] reviewed the literature regarding the association between prostate cancer and physical activity before 1996. Of the five studies that evaluated occupational physical activity and prostate cancer, three found a significant inverse association between prostate cancer and physical activity; one reported no significant trend towards decreased cancer risk and one reported no association between prostate cancer and physical activity. On the other hand, all four studies that compared leisure-time physical activity reported a decreased risk with increasing activity; the relative risks for the most active group, compared with the least active group, ranged from 0.12 to 0.77. Although one study compared total physical activity and found no significant relationship, another one evaluated overall physical fitness and reported a highly significant inverse association between prostate cancer and cardiorespiratory fitness. Another review article, published one year later, evaluated 17 studies that assessed the effect of physical activity on prostate cancer development.[371] Of these, nine indicated that exercise is beneficial in decreasing the risk of prostate cancer, five found no conclusive evidence for this inverse association and three suggested that physical activity actually increased the risk of prostate cancer.

In addition to these early reports, several additional studies on this topic have appeared in the literature since 1996. Of these, one indicated that leisure-time physical activity was beneficial in reducing prostate cancer,[372] one reported a decreased cancer risk for those men involved in physically active occupations[373] and one showed a significantly reduced incidence in men who had high levels of cardiorespiratory fitness.[374] In addition, a recent study reported that increased physical activity reduced the incidence of benign prostatic hypertrophy.[375] Conversely, two studies found no correlation between prostate cancer and physical activity[376,377] and two suggested an increased risk of prostate cancer in men who were physically active.[378,379]

It is important to note here that a recent laboratory study presented evidence of an inhibitory effect of diet and exercise on prostate cancer cell growth *in vitro*.[380] More specifically, a low fat, high fiber diet and exercise intervention in overweight men resulted in serum changes that significantly reduced the growth of androgen-responsive prostate cancer cells. Thus, although most studies suggest that increased physical activity is associated with a reduced risk of prostate cancer, clearly all do not. As a result, further research directed at clarifying these discrepancies is urgently needed in order that reliable physical activity guidelines are available to reduce the risk of this malignancy.

Lung and bronchus

In the year 2002, there were an estimated 169,400 new cancer cases of the lung and bronchus; 90,200 in men and 79,200 in women.[315] Of these, there were an estimated 154,900 deaths (men, 89,200; women 65,700). This malignancy is clearly the most common cause of death due to cancer in men (89,200 lung versus 30,200 prostate). In addition, since 1987 lung cancer has exceeded breast cancer as the leading cause of cancer deaths in women (i.e. about 65,700 versus 39,600 in 2002); it now accounts for about 25% of all female cancer deaths.[315]

The single most important risk factor, which accounts for at least 85% of cases of lung cancer, is tobacco smoking in general and cigarette smoking in particular.[381] Although relatively uncommon, occupational risks include the uranium miners, asbestos workers and probably others.

Several studies have been published comparing the effect of physical activity on lung cancer risk. For example, 17,607 college male alumni aged 30 to 79 years and followed for at least 22 years, were studied to determine if physical activity (i.e. stair-climbing, walking, sports participation and recreational activity) was associated with lung cancer risk.[382] The authors found that highly active men had a significantly decreased risk for both colon and lung cancer, having an average of 0.19 and 0.39 times respectively, compared with their inactive colleagues. There was no association between physical activity and risks of rectal, prostatic or pancreatic cancers. Thune and Lund[383] studied the effects of leisure-time and work activity with the risk of lung cancer in both men (53,242) and women (28,274). They reported that leisure-time activity, but not work activity, was inversely related to lung cancer risk in men after adjustment for age, smoking habits, BMI, and geographical residence. Men who exercised at least four hours per week had a relative risk of 0.71 compared with men who did not exercise. Interestingly, this reduced association was particularly strong for both small cell carcinoma and adenocarcinoma; there was no correlation with squamous cell carcinoma. Moreover, they found no association between physical activity and lung cancer in women. Similarly, Lee *et al.*[384] reported an inverse dose-response relationship between physical activity and lung cancer in men. The relative cancer risks were 1.00 (referent), 0.87, 0.76 and 0.61 for energy expenditures of <4200, 4200–8399, 8400–12,599 and ≥12,600 kj/week, respectively (12,600 kj per week compares with about six to eight hours per week of moderate intensity physical activity).

Pancreas

Pancreatic carcinoma represented the fifth leading cause of cancer-related deaths in 2002 (30,300 cases; 29,700 deaths)[315] Other than cigarette smoke, few environmental factors have been associated with the risk of pancreatic cancer.[385] However, in a recent report consisting of two cohort studies, the Health Professionals Follow-up Study and the Nurses' Health Study involving 46,648 men and 117,041 women respectively, Michaud *et al.*[386] reported their findings on the relationship between pancreatic cancer, overweight/obesity and physical activity. Their results showed that in individuals with a BMI of 30 kg/m^2 or more had an increased risk of pancreatic cancer compared to those whose BMI was 23 kg/m^2 or less (risk ratio, 1.72). In addition, they reported an inverse relationship between pancreatic cancer and moderate physical activity (multivariable risk ratio, 0.45 for the highest versus the lowest categories). The authors emphasized that increased physical activity was particularly effective in reducing the risk of pancreatic cancer in those who were overweight/obese. This study was the first to recognize the relationship between physical activity and pancreatic cancer. Others, referring to this study, emphasized the following two points.[387] First, reduced risk is primarily associated with sustained exercise at a moderate intensity level such as walking or hiking rather than vigorous short-term activity. Second, physical activity is clearly more effective in obese individuals (BMI $\geq$ 30 kg/m^2) compared with those who are overweight (BMI 25–29.9 kg/m^2).

Physical Activity and Other Medical Disorders

Gallbladder disease

Gallbladder disease varies widely among countries. An early study of 26 countries showed a variation from 0% in Accra, Ghana to 37.1% in Malmo, Sweden.[388] Gallstones reportedly affect 10% to 15% of American adults and result in an estimated 500,000 annual cholecystectomies at an estimated hospitalization cost in 1993 of US$5 billion.[389] Although gallstones are twice as common in women than in men, the significant geographical variation also suggests that differences in lifestyle may be important etiologic factors. Indeed, obesity is a major risk factor for gallstones and these individuals are strongly encouraged to lose weight.[390] Several recent studies also suggest that physical inactivity may be an important independent risk factor for gallbladder disease.

The association of anthropometric measurements, lifestyle factors and various serum tests was investigated in a prospective study of 7831 Japanese American men in Hawaii.[391] A progressively higher risk of gallbladder disease was associated with increased BMI, height, pack-years of cigarette smoking and diastolic blood pressure. After controlling for the effect of these variables, the authors demonstrated a significant inverse association between the presence of gallstones and level of physical activity. More recently, the association between physical activity and gallstones was investigated in 45,813 American male health professionals (Health Professionals Follow-up Study) aged 40 to 75 years.[392] After controlling for multiple confounders (i.e. age, body weight, dietary and alcohol intake, smoking habits and medication use), their data showed an inverse relation between physical activity and gallbladder disease. Men who watched television more than 40 hours per week had a relative risk of gallstones of 3.32 compared with men who viewed television less than six hours per week. The authors concluded that 34% of cases of symptomatic gallstone disease could be prevented by 30 minutes of endurance-type exercise training five times each week.

Leitzmann *et al.*[393] sought to determine if physical activity may also be an important risk factor for gallstones in women, both as an independent factor and as a result of its role in controlling body weight. This prospective ten-year study involved 60,290 women aged 40 to 65 years in 1986 (Nurses' Health Study). As with the male studies, recreational physical activity was inversely related to the risk of cholecystectomy; the multivariate relative risk for women in the highest physical activity quintile compared with the lowest was 0.69. In addition, sedentary women were independently associated with an increased risk of cholecystectomy.

Gastrointestinal hemorrhage

Gastrointestinal hemorrhage (GIH) in persons aged 65 years and older occurs approximately five times as often as in middle-aged adults.[394]

Moreover, as the elderly population has increased, there has been a proportional increase in the number of deaths due to GIH. Important risk factors for GIH include age, gender, gastric ulcers, chronic liver disease, neoplasms, coagulopathies and NSAIDS. In addition, after adjustment for various confounding factors (i.e. comorbid conditions, oral medications and various demographic characteristics), physical disability has been shown to be an independent risk factor for GIH.[368]

To assess whether physical activity is associated with GIH, Pahor and associates[395] studied a cohort of 8205 persons aged 68 years and older with a three-year follow-up. After adjusting for potential confounders (i.e. age, gender, BMI, blood pressure, chronic medical disorders, medications and recent hospital admissions), the relative risks for severe GIH associated with regular walking, gardening and vigorous physical activity were 0.6, 0.8 and 0.7 respectively, compared with the less active control group.

Fibromyalgia

Widespread musculoskeletal pain is a common disorder and reportedly affects 11% to 13% of adults in the UK.[396,397] Fibromyalgia, a severe form of musculoskeletal pain, affects about 1% of adults.[398] People with fibromyalgia are generally treated with analgesics, NSAIDs and anti-depressants, all of which are relatively ineffective and produce only temporary relief. However, several randomized controlled studies have generally shown that exercise therapy is beneficial in reducing pain and discomfort.[399-401] In a recent study, Richards and Scott[402] showed that prescribed graded aerobic exercise, primarily walking on treadmills and cycling on exercise bicycles, significantly decreased the pain compared with relaxation exercise. The authors concluded that graded aerobic exercise "is a simple, cheap, effective and potential widely available treatment for fibromyalgia."

Psychological disorders and physical activity

Several important areas of concern in the elderly include depression, cognitive function and self-efficacy or self control. The financial and personal costs of these disorders can be considerable. Numerous publications suggest that psychological function is significantly improved in most people, both young and old, who become physically active.

Depression

Depression is one of the most frequently studied mental health disorders since it is a significant cause and consequence in older persons of disability, presence of chronic diseases and increased mortality risk. The prevalence of mood disorders in the US reportedly ranges from 5% to 10% of older community dwellers to 18% of nursing home residents.[403,404] Moreover, research has long reported that depression is also very common among physicians and that the physician suicide rate is higher than that of the general public. Although anti-depressant medications are commonly prescribed for these individuals, a significant number do not respond. In addition, unwanted side effects may impair a person's quality of life and lead to reduced compliance.

There is an extensive literature on the association between physical activity and depression. A recent review of the subject[405] concluded that "sufficient evidence now exists for the effectiveness of exercise in the treatment of clinical depression." In addition, the author noted that increased physical activity has a moderate reducing effect on anxiety and improves physical self-perceptions, as well as self-esteem in some cases. Although a few studies have not found a positive association between physical activity and depression,[31,406] most studies support a positive effect of physical activity in depressed persons. The results of several of these will be reviewed here.

Relatively few studies on physical activity and well-being in children and adolescents have been published. Recently, however, Steptoe and Butler[407] collected data from a cohort of adolescents, mean age 16.3 years (2223 boys; 2838 girls). They found that those actively involved in sport and vigorous recreational activities were positively associated with emotional well-being, independently of sex, social class, health status and use of hospital services. Conversely, adolescents who regularly participated in non-vigorous activities were, as a group, associated with "high psychological and somatic symptoms." Two subsequent "Letters To The Editor" were strongly supportive of the psychological benefits of exercise in young people (*Lancet* 1996;348:477).

In an early controlled study, Martinsen *et al.*[408] reported their findings of a group of men and women aged 17 to 60 years who were randomly allocated to either a training or control group. The training group underwent a nine-week program consisting of one hour of instructor-controlled systematic aerobic exercise at 50% to 70% maximum aerobic capacity three times per week. The control group attended occupational therapy during the time the training group exercised. The results showed that for those in the training group with a small increase in maximum oxygen uptake (<15%), the anti-depressive effect (assessed with the Beck Depression Inventory) was similar to the control group. However, the anti-depressive effects for those with a moderate (15–30%) or large (>30%) increase in maximum oxygen uptake were significantly greater than the control group. Similarly, in the Alameda County Study,[409] the risk of depression was evaluated using three waves of data from subjects who were not depressed at baseline. The final results showed that persons with a low physical activity level at baseline were at a significantly greater risk for depression at follow-up compared with subjects who were highly active at baseline. Importantly, adjustments for physical health, socioeconomic status, life events, social supports and other health habits had little effect on the association.

McNeil and associates[410] studied a group of moderately depressed elderly subjects, mean age 72.5 years, who were randomly assigned to one of three interventions: experimenter-accompanied exercise (i.e. walking), a social contact control condition and a wait-list control. Both exercise and social contact resulted in significant reductions in both the total and psychological subscale of the Beck Depression Inventory. However, unlike the control conditions, the exercise condition resulted in decreased somatic symptoms. Thus, exercise had a broader effect in reducing depressive symptoms compared with control conditions in the moderately depressed elderly. More recently, others studied the effects of exercise training in older persons with major depression.[411] Here, men and women 50 years and older with a major depressive disorder (MDD) were randomly assigned to a program of aerobic exercise, anti-depressent medication (sertraline hydrochloride), or combined exercise and medication. All individuals underwent comprehensive evaluations of depression (Hamilton Rating Scale and Beck Depression Inventory) scores before and after treatment. Secondary outcome measures included aerobic capacity, life satisfaction, self-esteem, anxiety and dysfunctional cognitions. After 16 weeks of treatment, the groups did not differ statistically. The authors concluded that although anti-depressent medication may facilitate a more rapid therapeutic response, exercise was equally effective in reducing depression among patients with MDD. In addition, two meta-analyses[412,413] suggest that exercise may be as effective as psychotherapy and more effective than other behavioral interventions[414] for treating depression. Furthermore, a recent study[415] involving both men and women (mean age 49) found that simply walking on a treadmill for 30 minutes each day for ten days resulted in "substantial improvement in mood in patients with major depressive disorders ...."

Two large groups (800 in each) of independently living elderly people aged 65 to 84 years (born in 1904–1913 and in 1914–1923) were studied for physical activity and psychological well-being.[416] The epidemiological results, according to log-linear and regression analysis, showed an increased prevalence of depression in those who were sedentary. Conversely, meaningfulness of life and better subjective health were significantly related to regular and intensive physical exercise, especially among the younger cohort (i.e. aged 65 to 74 years). More recently, these workers studied 32 subjects aged 71.5 ± 1.2 years, in a 20-week randomized controlled trial with a 26-month follow-up.[417] These community-dwelling patients had a major or minor depression or dysthymia. The exercisers engaged in ten weeks of supervised weight-lifting exercise followed by ten weeks of unsupervised exercise; the control group attended lectures for ten weeks. Their results showed that patients randomized to exercise had a significantly reduced Beck Depression Inventory after both 20 weeks and 26 months. Moreover, at 26 months of follow-up, 33% of the exercisers were still regularly lifting weights compared with 0% of the controls.

In addition to the positive effects of physical activity on psychological well-being, it appears to enhance both mood and creativity. For example, Steinberg *et al.*[418] studied 63 participants who were assigned to either an exercise (aerobic workout or aerobic dance) or a "neutral" video watching condition. Mood was measured using an adjective list and creative thinking was evaluated by three measures of the Torrance test. Their results showed that both mood and creativity were improved by physical exercise; moreover, these two effects were independent of each other.

As a final note, it is well documented that alcoholic addiction is often associated with high levels of depression and anxiety. In an early study, Palmer and associates[419] examined the usefulness of physical exercise as a treatment intervention to decrease anxiety and depression in chronic alcoholics. Their findings, following a 28-day in-patient exercise treatment program, indicated that regular physical exercise (walking or jogging three days per week consistent with the 1980 American College of Sports Medicine guidelines) resulted in significantly less state anxiety, trait anxiety and depression compared with the non-exercising control group. However, there were no changes in self-concept or aerobic capacity.

Cognitive function

Numerous studies have documented a positive effect of aerobic fitness on various markers of cognitive function (e.g. attention, memory, reaction time, and fluid and crystallized intelligence). The underlying presumption about this relationship is that the age-related decrease in cardiovascular function leads to decreased cerebral blood flow resulting in brain hypoxia. If true, aerobic exercise may slow or retard the decline in cognition. Indeed, as recently reviewed,[31] early studies consistently found better performance by physically active individuals on simple and choice reaction times, short-term recall, reasoning, fluid intelligence and memory. In this regard, Rogers and associates[420] studied a group of older volunteers approaching retirement. This four-year longitudinal prospective study examined the effects of various levels of physical activity on cerebral perfusion and cognition. The participants were assigned to one of three groups: (1) those who continued to work; (2) those who retired but participated in regular, planned physical activities; and (3) those who retired but did not become involved in any type of regular physical activity. After four years of follow-up, the retirees who remained physically inactive exhibited significant declines in cerebral blood flow throughout the study period. However, those who continued to work, as well as the retirees who elected regular involvement in physical activities, sustained more constant cerebral blood flow. Moreover, these latter two groups scored better on cognitive testing after the fourth year compared to the sedentary group.

More recently, in a randomized controlled six-month trial, a cohort of elderly Japanese men and women, mean age 79 years (range 75–87 years), were randomly assigned to one of two groups, exercise or control.[421] The physically active group exercised for 60 minutes, two days each week for six months. The control group received no instructions regarding exercise. At baseline and at six-month follow-up, the subjects were evaluated using six different neurobehavioral function measurements (i.e. Mini-Mental State Exam, Hasegawa Dementia Scale Revised, Visuospatial Cognitive Performance Test, Button score, Up & Go test and Functional Reach). The results demonstrated that the exercise group showed significant interactions between group and time difference in the Up & Go test and Functional Reach but showed no significant interactions in the other measurements.

Dementia, a common and very costly age-related disorder, is primarily due to Alzheimer's and cerebrovascular diseases. Since little attention has been paid to possible modifiable lifestyle habits for its prevention, Laurin and associates[422] recently studied the association between physical activity and the risk of both cognitive impairment and dementia in a large group of randomly selected men and women aged 65 years and older (Canadian Study of Health and Aging). After five years follow-up, their findings showed that compared with no exercise, physical activity was associated with significantly lower risks of cognitive impairment, Alzheimer's disease and dementia of any type. More specifically, the odds ratios for high levels of physical activity were 0.58, 0.50 and 0.63 for cognitive impairment, Alzheimer's disease and dementia of any type, respectively.

Kramer *et al.*[423] recently re-emphasized that neural areas and cognitive processes do not deteriorate uniformly during the aging process. That is, executive control processes (i.e. planning, scheduling, inhibition and working memory), and the prefrontal and frontal brain regions that support them, show large and disproportionate changes with age. To further understand this association, they further investigated the relationship between aerobic fitness and executive control processes. Over a six-month period, they studied a group of 124 previously sedentary adults aged 60 to 75 years. The participants were randomly assigned to either aerobic (walking) or anaerobic (stretching and toning) exercise. From their results, they concluded that the aerobic-trained group showed "substantial improvements in performance on tasks requiring executive control compared with the anaerobically trained subjects." They further suggested that the selective nature of executive control improvements, which are supported by the frontal and prefrontal brain regions, might explain the ambiguity of previous studies[424] relating to aerobic fitness with improved neurocognitive function.

In a distinctly different area of study, Grealy and coworkers[425] assessed the impact of exercise and virtual reality on the cognitive rehabilitation of persons with traumatic brain injury. Here, a consecutive sample of 13 traumatic brain-injured adults were compared with a control group (n = 25) of similar age, and who had previous traumatic brain injury. The measurements consisted of tests of attention, information gathering, learning and memory. After four weeks of exercise intervention, these patients performed significantly better than the control group on digit symbol, verbal and visual learning tasks. The exercise group also showed greater improvement than the controls in reaction and movement times following a single bout of exercise in a virtual environment.

Although most human studies support a positive correlation between physical activity and cognition, clearly some do not. For example, Dustman et al.[424] reviewed 12 longitudinal studies in which physical fitness improvements ranged from 8% to 47%, suggesting that there were modest or mixed improvements in neuropyschological function. It is apparent, therefore, that more carefully controlled trials are needed that include larger sample sizes, more critical fitness assessment and improved study design to more fully understand the possible relationship between cognition and physical activity. However, on a more basic note, experiments using adult animals have shown that both metabolic[426] and neurochemical[427] (i.e. increased levels of brain-derived neurotrophic factor; BDNF) functions improve with aerobic fitness. Oliff and others[428] also reported that voluntary running in rats upregulates BDNF mRNA expression in the hippocampus. Moreover, there was a strong positive correlation between the distance run and BDNF mRNA expression. On the basis of their studies, the authors suggested that BDNF upregulation induced by exercise may increase the brain's resistance to damage and neurodegeneration that occurs with aging. Similarly, voluntary exercise has been shown to increase cell proliferation and neurogenesis in the adult mouse dentate gyrus, an important brain structure for memory function.[429] Running also enhanced learning and long-term potentiation in mice.[430]

Basic studies support a role for exercise in improving cognitive functions in humans.[431] Recognizing that the human brain gradually loses tissue beginning in the third decade of life, Colcombe et al.[432] studied the high resolution magnetic resonance imaging scans from 55 older persons. As with prior studies, they found a significant decline in tissue densities as a function of age. However, these losses were substantially reduced as a function of cardiovascular fitness, even after controlling for other variables. The authors concluded that these findings "extend the scope of beneficial effects of aerobic exercise beyond cardiovascular health, and they suggest a strong solid biological basis for the benefits of exercise on the brain health of older adults."

Sleep quality

Complaints regarding sleep quality is a well-recognized common problem in middle-aged and older adults. Although the elderly (i.e. aged 65 years or older) currently constitute only 12% to 13% of the American population, they reportedly receive 35% to 40% of the prescribed sedatives-hypnotics, most of which are for long-term use.[433]

In an early vigorously controlled study to test the effect of exercise on sleep in a group of older volunteers without sleep complaints, Vitiello *et al.*[434] found that aerobic exercise had a positive effect on polysomnographically defined sleep. However, an attention-control stretching intervention had no effect. In a subsequent study,[431] the effects of moderate intensity exercise training (four 30- to 40-minute sessions of low-impact aerobics and brisk walking) on self-reported sleep quality among healthy sedentary adults aged 50 to 76 years who reported moderate sleep complaints was carried out. The participants were randomized to 16 weeks of community-based exercise or to a waitlisted control condition. Their results showed that, compared with the controls, the exercise training group showed significant improvement in the Pittsburgh Subjective Sleep Quality Index (PSQI) global sleep score at 16 weeks, as well as in the sleep parameters of rated sleep quality, sleep-onset latency and sleep duration. Similarly, Singh and coinvestigators[435] tested the hypothesis that exercise improves subjective sleep quality and activity in depressed persons aged 60 years and older. This randomized controlled trial covered a ten-week period and consisted of 32 subjects aged 60 to 84 years with major or minor depression or dysthymia. The interventions consisted of a group who participated in a supervised weight-training program three times per week or an attention-control group. There were seven major outcome measurements (e.g. PSQI and six others). The results showed that exercise significantly improved all subjective sleep quality and depression measures. The depression measures were reduced by about twice that of the controls. In addition, quality of life scales were also significantly improved.

Although most people would probably not be surprised that exercise (e.g. recreational and physical labor) greatly improves sleep quality, Buchner[436] pointed to two examples that illustrate how little is apparently known about exercise and sleep quality in the elderly. He noted that a major geriatrics textbook did not list exercise as a non-pharmacologic approach to insomnia nor did the 1996 surgeon general's report on physical activity list or discuss improved sleep as a possible health benefit of physical activity. Unfortunately, sleep complaints are probably too often treated with sedatives or hypnotics with their well-recognized side effects.

Physical Activity for the Very Old and Frail

Physical frailty and fall-related injuries are major threats to quality of life and functioning, especially in the very old (i.e. aged 80 years or older). Physical frailty, which includes impaired strength, mobility, balance and endurance, results in many serious problems in everyday living. Thus, the impact that the future aging population will have on the health care system and society in general will be related in large part to the level of functioning, loss of independence and need for long-term care for the longest-living people. In 1985, about 45% of elderly nursing home residents were 85 years and older.[437] The number has undoubtedly increased significantly since then, both in those over 85 years old and the total number of older residents. As a result, estimated costs of nursing home care could rise to between US$84 and $139 billion a year, in 1985 dollars, of which Medicaid reimburses about 40% of this amount.[437]

Many of the very elderly could be more independent and care for themselves for a much longer time period if they were in better physical and mental health. Importantly, numerous studies have shown that aging *per se* is not a deterrent to increasing the level of physical activity of older people. Moreover, it would markedly reduce the nursing home and other health care costs. Indeed, over the past ten to

15 years, abundant evidence dispels myths of futility and provides reassurance of the safety and benefits of exercise in the oldest old.

Muscle weakness, which is prevalent and morbid in the very old, is closely linked to frailty, functional decline, immobility, falls and injuries. The decrease in muscle mass and strength associated with aging is multifactorial and has been attributed to (1) biological age-related changes; (2) the presence of acute and chronic diseases; (3) a sedentary lifestyle; and (4) various nutritional deficiencies.[438] With adequate counseling and education, the latter two can significantly retard or even prevent the loss of muscle mass, its accompanying physical weakness and the subsequent related problems.

Surveys in the US have shown that after 74 years of age, 28% of men and 66% of women are unable to lift objects weighing over 4.5 kg (about ten pounds).[439] Certainly, much of this decline in strength is due to a significant reduction in muscle mass. To evaluate this effect further, Frontera and associates[440] studied a group of healthy, untrained volunteers, aged 60 to 72 years, over a 12-week strength-training period (eight repetitions per set; three sets per day; three days per week) at 80% of the one repetition maximum for extensors and flexors of both knee joints. Each person was evaluated at baseline, and after six and 12 weeks of training. After 12 weeks, extensor and flexor strength had increased 107.4% and 226.7%, respectively. In addition, midthigh composition, determined from computerized tomographic scans, showed significant increases in total thigh area (4.8%), total muscle area (11.4%) and quadriceps area (9.3%). Moreover, muscle biopsies of the vastus lateralis showed increases in both type I and type II fiber areas (33.5% and 27.6%, respectively).

Fiatarone *et al.*[441] conducted a randomized placebo-controlled study comparing progressive resistance exercise training, multinutrient supplementation, both interventions and neither in 100 frail men and women, mean age 87.1 years, over a ten-week period. Compared with the non-exercising groups, the exercisers showed the following: (1) 113% increased muscle strength (non-exercisers 3%); (2) increased gait velocity by 11.8% (non-exercisers decreased 1%); and (3) increased stair-climbing power by 28% (non-exercisers 3.6%). They also found that the level of spontaneous activity increased significantly in the exercising groups. Nutritional supplementation had no additional effects. These authors also studied a group of frail institutionalized very old, ambulatory but not acutely ill men aged 90 ± 1 years who underwent an eight-week program of high-intensity resistance training.[442] At baseline, quadriceps strength was negatively correlated with walking time. Both fat-free and regional muscle masses correlated directly with muscle strength. Those who completed the program experienced a 174% average gain in strength. In addition, the midthigh muscle area increased an average of 9.0% and the mean tandem gait speed improved 48%.

More recently, Gill and associates[443] randomly assigned 188 physically frail persons 75 years and older who lived at home to undergo a six-month home-based physical therapy intervention program. The program focused either on improving impairment of balance, muscle strength, ability to move from one position to another and mobility or an educational program (i.e. the control group). Compared with the control group, the intervention group had significantly less functional decline after both seven and 12 months. Although the benefit of intervention was significant among those with moderate frailty, it was not effective in those with severe frailty. Thus, except for individuals with severe frailty, a home-based exercise program can result in a significant reduction in the progression of functional decline among most physically frail persons.

These and other reports clearly indicate that exercise training in the very old and even frail elderly, that increases strength and mobility is more dependent on the intensity of the physical activity than age, health status or nutritional deficiencies. Thus, a meaningful exercise program for the very old, as with middle-aged and young adults, will result in improvements in gait, velocity, balance, stair-climbing power, aerobic capacity, disability, morale and depressive symptoms.

Physical Activity and the Immune System

In about 300 BC, Aristotle reportedly stated that "A man falls into ill health as a result of not caring for exercise."[444] Scientific studies on the association between physical activity and immunity have been reported since early in the 20th century. In a 1984 literature review, Simon[445] attempted to answer part of the "athlete's lore" that physical conditioning increases the resistance to infection. He concluded, however, that "further studies will be needed before it can be concluded that exercise affects the host response to infection in any clinically meaningful way." Since then, studies on this topic have markedly intensified. Although there have been about 400 published reports on the effects of exercise on the immune system since 1990,[446] significant confusion and controversy still exist. These conflicting results are primarily related to exercise intensity and duration, as well as the mode of exercise. Indeed, these contradictory studies have led to the "inverted J theory," which suggests that moderate regular exercise improves immune function and thereby decreases disease susceptibility (Fig. 3.1).[447]

However, as the intensity and duration of exercise increases, the susceptibility to disease increases while the immune functions decrease.

Intense exercise and immunity

A wide variety of studies indicate that strenuous, prolonged exercise impairs upper airway antimicrobial defenses and makes elite athletes more susceptible to upper respiratory tract infections (URTI). That

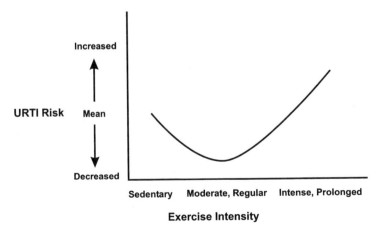

Figure 3.1: "Inverted J theory." Effect of exercise intensity on upper respiratory tract infections.

is, marathon runners or others engaged in comparable intense prolonged training are at increased risk of URTI. The following reports are representative examples of this phenomenon.

Peters and Bateman[448] prospectively studied the incidence of URTI in 150 randomly selected runners who ran the 1982 Cape Town, South Africa Marathon and compared the findings with the incidence in individually matched controls who did not participate in the race. Pertinent information including training background, running experience and state of health was obtained from both groups before the race and two weeks after the race. The results showed that respiratory tract symptoms occurred in 33.3% of the marathoners compared with 15.3% of controls and were more frequent in the marathoners who ran a faster race compared with the slower runners. Moreover, the incidence of upper respiratory symptoms in slow runners did not differ from the controls. In a later study, Peters[349] not only confirmed these findings, but also found that altitude did not further increase the susceptibility of ultramarathoners to post-race URTI.

In what is the largest epidemiological report on the effects of intense exercise and URTI, Nieman and coworkers[450] studied the incidence of URTI in 2311 competing runners in the 1987 Los Angeles Marathon race and compared the findings with a control group of less intense runners who did not compete in the race. The authors collected demographic, training and URTI episodes and symptom data for the two-month period before the race. During the pre-race training period, 40% of the marathon runners had at least one URTI episode. In addition, during the two-week period following the race, 12.9% of the marathoners reported an URTI compared with 2.2% of the control group. The authors concluded that runners training ≥ 96 km/week (~60 miles/week) had twice the risk for sickness compared with those running ≤ 32 km/week (~20 miles/week).

Linde[451] compared the incidence of URTI in a group of 44 elite orienteers (i.e. participants in Scandinavian mountain races who use maps and compass to reach the finish line) with 44 non-athletes of comparable age, sex and occupational distribution. Using daily personal logs, both groups recorded all illness symptoms during a one-year period. The data showed that the orienteers experienced significantly more URTI episodes during the year than the control group. While only 10% of the athletes reported no URTI episodes, about 33% of the controls reported no URTI problems. Moreover, the average duration of symptoms in the control group was 6.4 days compared with 7.9 days in the orienteers. In another report,[452] a cohort of 530 male and female runners [average age about 40 years; average running 32 km/week (~nine miles/week)] recorded any daily upper respiratory symptoms for one year. On average, each person experienced 1.2 URTI per year. However, after controlling for various confounders, the odds ratio for URTI was more than twice as high for those running ≥27 km/week (~17 miles/week) compared with those running <16 km/week (~ten miles/week).

Various intervention studies have been based on the theory that prolonged intense exercise results in an increased production of oxygen-derived free radicals which may negatively affect the immune system. In this regard, it is widely accepted that ascorbate (vitamin C) is the predominant water-soluble antioxidant in blood and interstitial fluids and that one of its major targets in promoting immunocompetence is phagocytes and primarily the neutrophil.[453] With this in mind, Peters *et al.*[454] studied the effect of daily vitamin C supplementation (600 mg) on the incidence of URTI in marathon runners following a competitive ultramarathon race (i.e. >42 km; >26 miles). Here, age-matched ultramarathon runners were randomly separated into vitamin C-supplemented and placebo groups. Symptoms of URTI were monitored for two weeks after the race. The findings showed that 68% of the placebo-supplemented group developed upper respiratory tract symptoms compared with 33% of the ascorbate-supplemented group. In addition, the duration and severity of symptoms was significantly less in those supplemented with vitamin C. The results of this and other studies led to the hypothesis that exercise-induced stimulation of the neutrophil oxidative burst increases the rate of release of reactive oxygen species which are then neutralized by increased plasma ascorbate levels.[455]

Vitamin E, a well-established potent lipid-soluble antioxidant, has also been studied with respect to its possible effects on exercise and the immune system. For example, Cannon *et al.*[456] reported their results of vitamin E supplementation on post-exercise neutrophilia and the acute phase response in a group of young (22–29 years) and older (55–74 years) men after a running exercise of 45 minutes. Although vitamin E was not effective in the prevention of post-exercise neutrophilia in the younger group, it suppressed the effect in the older group. Decreased concentrations of various other essential nutrients, such as trace metals, have been reported in blood and tissues after intense training and competition. Konig *et al.*[457] recently reported a literature review of the association of zinc, iron and magnesium on the regulation of exercise-induced stress and immune function and concluded that "there is evidence they are related to exercise-induced stress and immune function."

The exact mechanisms of decreased immune functions following prolonged intense physical activity is complex. The major changes that take place during and following intense, prolonged exercise are as follows: (1) increased neutrophil concentration both during exercise and in the post-exercise period; (2) increased lymphocyte concentration (i.e. lymphocyte sub-populations including CD4+ T-cells, CD8+ T-cells, CD19+ B-cells and CD16+ natural killer cells); and (3) suppressed functions of natural killer (NK) cells and B-cells. Several literature reviews of immune function losses associated with prolonged intense exercise have been published.[458–461]

Moderate intensity exercise and immunity

Although intense exercise, such as running a marathon or cross-country skiing, significantly depresses the immune system and may lead to an increased incidence of URTI, moderate exercise training appears to be associated with a reduction in URTI (Fig. 3.1). Although the number of studies comparing moderate intensity exercise and immunity are few, and no large retrospective or prospective studies comparable to those reported in the preceding section have been reported, there is some epidemiologic and experimental evidence that support the view that moderate exercise is protective against URTI.[462]

Nieman *et al.*[463] carried out a randomized controlled 15-week exercise study (i.e. five 45-minute weekly sessions of brisk walking at 60% heart rate reserve) in a group of mildly obese sedentary women to investigate the relationship between cardiorespiratory fitness, changes in NK cell number and activity and URTI. Although the number of NK cells did not increase, there was a significant increase in NK cell activity, especially during the initial six-week period. In addition, the exercise group had significantly fewer upper respiratory symptom days than the non-exercise group (3.6 versus 7.0 days, respectively). Moreover, cardiovascular improvement also correlated with a reduction in respiratory tract symptoms. More recently, Mathews and associates[464] carried out an observational exercise study of 547 healthy men (51%) and women (49%) aged 20 to 70 years. The number of URTI was determined at 90-day intervals over a 12-month period. Their results showed that men and women engaged in moderate physical activity reduced their risk of URTI by 20% to 30%, thereby adding further support for the inverted J theory.

Aging, exercise and immunity

The aging process is associated with a decline in immune function leading to an increased risk of infections, occurrence of auto-antibodies and various lymphoproliferative disorders (i.e. multiple myeloma, non-Hodgkin's lymphoma and chronic lymphocytic leukemia). Although some immune functions decline with age, others (e.g. NK cells) retain or even increase their activity.[465] T-cells, which have a central role in cell-mediated immunity, show the largest age-related changes in both distribution and function. However, some of the age-related decline is probably not due to aging *per se* but rather to a sedentary lifestyle, as well as to various nutritional deficiencies as discussed in Chapter 4.

In a cross-sectional study, Shinkai *et al.*[466] examined resting immune functions in an elderly group of male runners (mean age 63.8 $\pm$ 3.3 years) and compared the results with an age-matched sedentary group (mean age 65.8 $\pm$ 3.5 years). They found that the elderly runners with an aerobic power 33% greater than the control group retained superior T-cell function (lymphocyte response to both phytohem-agglutinin and pokeweed mitogen), as well as increased cytokine production of interleukin-2, interleukin-4 and interferon-gamma. However, there were no differences in circulating lymphocyte subset counts, NK cell activity, lymphocyte responsiveness to allogenic antigens, or interleukin-1 beta. Two later reports,[467,468] however, suggested that habitual physical activity by elderly people may enhance NK cell activity, thereby retaining some aspects of the age-associated decline in T-cell function. Similarly, Nieman and associates[469] studied a group of physically active elderly women aged 65 to 84 years with a 67% greater aerobic power than an age-matched sedentary control group. The physically fit group demonstrated a 56% greater lymphocyte response to phytohemagglutinin and a 54% greater NK cell activity than the sedentary group. Moreover, the active women experienced a "cold" incidence during the study period of 21% compared with 50% for the controls. However, the authors noted no differences in total leukocyte or lymphocyte subset counts, suggesting that the functional activities per cell were greater in the physically fit group. Thus, endurance training in later life is associated with a lesser age-related decline in certain aspects of circulating T-cell functions related to cytokine production.

A recent literature review[470] of this topic noted that three general approaches have been undertaken to study the effect of exercise training on the immune system in the elderly: (1) cross-sectional studies, (2) longitudinal studies and (3) animal studies. The authors noted that although both cross-sectional and animal studies have generally supported the association between exercise and improved immune function, prospective studies have been inconsistent. However, it was noted that these studies usually involved small numbers of participants over a short time period. Moreover, two recent studies[471,472] found that increased physical activity was associated with lower blood inflammation levels (i.e. reduced C-reactive protein), which may partly explain the association between CHD and inflammation, as well as an improved immune system.

Life Expectancy of Elite Athletes

Although numerous studies, as discussed above, indicate that individuals involved in intense, prolonged physical activity have an increase in URTI, early studies suggested that elite athletes may have an increased average life expectancy.[473,474] Subsequent reports indicated that moderate physical activity is also associated with increased longevity,[475,476] especially due to decreased CHD[468] and possibly cancer.

As noted earlier in this chapter, Sarna *et al.*[54] studied the life expectancy in 2613 Finnish world-class male athletes involved in track and field, cross-country skiing, ice hockey, basketball, boxing, wrestling, weight-lifting and shooting. The reference group consisted of 1712 men from the Finnish Defence Forces matched for age and area of residence. The average life expectancies, adjusted for occupation, marital status and age at entry to the cohort was as follows: (1) endurance sports (long-distance runners and cross-country skiers), 75.6 years; (2) team games (soccer, ice hockey, etc.), 73.9 years; and (3) power sports (boxing, weight-lifting, etc.), 69.9 years. The mortality odds ratio, compared with the referents, were 0.49 for endurance sports and 0.61 for team sports. The authors noted that the decreased mortality was primarily due to decreased CHD and cancer. Athletes involved in power sports, however, had the same life expectancy as the reference cohort (i.e. 69.9 years). Thus, life expectancy was highest for endurance athletes and next highest for team athletes, both of which were significantly greater than the power athletes and reference group.

Very recently, Kujala and associates[478] reported their mortality findings, due to several major diseases, in elite male athletes compared with the general population. The following standardized mortality ratios in highly trained athletes, compared with the general population, were as follows: (1) all-cause mortality: endurance sports 0.57, mixed sports 0.68 and power sports 0.90; (2) CHD: endurance sports 0.56, mixed sports 0.60 and power sports 0.95; (3) hypertension: endurance sports 0.73, mixed sports 0.34 and power sports 2.63;

(4) chronic lung diseases: endurance sports 0.00, mixed sports, 0.27 and power sports 0.58; and (5) lung cancer: endurance sports 0.14, mixed sports 0.37 and power sports 0.46. The investigators suggested that differences in biological characteristics between athletes involved in endurance and power sports may explain their involvement in certain sports, as well as accounting for the difference in risk of developing CHD.

Oxidants, Antioxidants and Exercise

Although oxygen is critical for life, many essential intracellular reactions in which it is required result in the formation of highly reactive and potentially destructive chemical species known as free radicals. A free radical is an atom, molecule or compound with one or more unpaired electrons in its outer orbital(s). For stability, all elements require two electrons in each orbital (spinning in opposite directions). To satisfy this requirement, free radicals attack sites of increased electron density. Hence, all compounds with a nitrogen atom become a target since nitrogen has two unpaired electrons (the 2 S electrons). Compounds with carbon-carbon double bonds are also electron-rich. Thus, DNA, RNA, enzymes and other proteins are free radical targets, as are polyunsaturated fatty acids and phospholipids, of which bilipid cell membranes are composed (lipid peroxidation). As a result, free radicals are very important in aging and numerous diseases/disorders (e.g. coronary heart and cerebrovascular diseases, cancer, immune deficiencies, ischemia/reperfusion injury, cataracts, neurodegenerative disorders, etc.)[214] A more detailed discussion of free radicals and oxidative stress is presented in Chapter 4.

Strenuous physical activity dramatically increases oxygen consumption and possible increased oxidative stress. There are several mechanisms by which reactive oxygen species (ROS), particularly the superoxide anion radical ($O_2^{-\cdot}$), may be increased as a result of exercise.[479]

(1) Electrons "leaked" from the mitochondrial electron transport chain react with oxygen (O_2 + electron $\rightarrow O_2^{-\cdot}$).

(2) Ischemia-reperfusion injury (xanthine + $O_2 \xrightarrow{XO}$ uric acid + O_2^{-}).
(3) Auto-oxidation of catecholamines.

Superoxide, in the presence of superoxide dismutase (SOD), of which two major metalloenzymes exist (mitochondrial Mn-SOD; cytoplasmic Cu-Zn-SOD), is converted to hydrogen peroxide ($2\,O_2^{-} + 2\,H^+ \xrightarrow{SOD} H_2O_2 + O_2$). This may then lead to the production of the highly reactive hydoxyl radical (HO·) by a transition metal ion (Fenton and Haber-Weiss Reactions) such as Fe^{2+} or Cu^+ ($H_2O_2 + Fe^{2+} \rightarrow HO· + OH^- + Fe^{3+}$). In addition to the hydroxyl radical, other ROS include hydrogen peroxide, singlet oxygen and the superoxide anion. There are also several important reactive nitrogen species [e.g. nitric oxide, other oxides of nitrogen, the thiyl radical (RS·), etc.].

As clearly demonstrated in this chapter, exercise is extremely important in health promotion and disease prevention. It delays age-associated cell deterioration, the likelihood of obesity and improves cardiac, respiratory and muscle functions. It also decreases the risk of several malignancies. Yet, oxygen uptake and free radical production increase during exercise. As a result, oxidative damage may occur in various organs and tissues (e.g. muscle, liver, blood, etc.) depending on a variety of variables including duration and intensity of exercise, antioxidant supplementation and the body's ability to adapt to increased oxidative stress. How then does exercise protect against diseases/disorders known to be related to oxidative stress?

Effects of exercise on antioxidant systems

Under physiologic conditions, there are generally adequate antioxidant reserves to cope with the production of excess ROS. This protective system can be divided into two categories; enzymatic and non-enzymatic antioxidants.

Enzymatic antioxidants and exercise

The major enzyme antioxidants include catalase, glutathione peroxidase and two superoxide dismutases (Mn-SOD and Cu/Zn-SOd, mitochondrial and cytoplasmic respectively). These enzymes are supported by several auxiliary enzymes such as glutathione reductase, glucose-6-phosphate dehydrogenase and glutathione sulfur-transferase.

Numerous studies have shown that exercise stimulates an increased production of various antioxidant enzymes. Several examples will be cited. Cesquini *et al.*[480] evaluated the levels of reduced glutathione (GSH) and several antioxidant enzymes in the blood of non-exercised and exercised rats (adapted to swimming endurance training). They found that the concentration of GSH, an antioxidant tripeptide required by glutathione peroxidase (GPx) to inactivate hydrogen peroxide, was about 30% higher in the exercised rats than in the resting controls. In addition, GPx, glutathione reductase and SOD activities were all significantly higher in the exercised rats compared with the sedentary control group. Catalase, however, was similar in the exercised and control animals. Furthermore, although lipid peroxidation is well known to increase following exercise in inactive individuals, there was no significant difference between the exercised and control rats.

Others,[481] using two age groups of rats (young, four weeks; middle-aged, 14 months), studied the effects of long-term swimming training on the oxidative status of DNA, proteins and phospholipids. They found that the concentration of thiobarbituric acid reactive substances and 4-hydroxynonenal protein adducts, both of which are products of lipid peroxidation, did not differ in the gastrocnemius muscle between exercised and non-exercised animals in the two age groups. Moreover, the extent of protein carbonylation and the amount of 8-hydroxy-deoxyguanosine in nuclear DNA (the product of hydroxyl radical reacting with guanosine) were lower in the exercised animals than in the sedentary rats. Furthermore, the activities of DT-diaphorase, a major proteolytic enzyme for oxidatively modified proteins, and proteasome, a large cytosomal protein complex responsible for degrading proteins, were significantly higher in the exercised rats in both age groups compared with the sedentary animals. The authors concluded that moderate endurance exercise stimulates an adaptive response against oxidative stress.

Selman and associates[482] investigated whether long-term cold exposure, which increases the metabolic rate and ROS production similar to exercise, increases the activities of catalase, GPx and SOD in liver, heart, skeletal muscle, kidney and duodenum of short-tailed field voles born and maintained at either 8 ± 3°C or 22 ± 3°C. Their findings showed that, compared with the animals maintained at 22 ± 3°C, catalase activity increased significantly in those maintained at 8 ± 3°C in skeletal muscle and kidney while both catalase and GPx activities were significantly increased in the heart. Total SOD activity, however, did not differ between the two groups in any tissue. Several additional recent studies also showed that exercise increases the anti-oxidative capacity in laboratory animals.[483–485] Similar reports from recent human studies have also been published,[486–489] along with two literature reviews of the relationship between exercise, aging and oxidative stress.[490,491]

Regular exercise stimulates the release of catecholamines which results in increased oxidative stress; however, it is protective from acute cardiac events. Noting this, Mehta and Li[492] examined the effect of epinephrine on the free radical release and endogenous SOD gene and protein expression in human coronary artery endothelial cells (HCAECs). HCAECs were incubated with epinephrine, alone or with trolox (water-soluble analog of vitamin E), the lipid-soluble vitamin E, or a $beta_1$-adrenergic blocker (atenolol). After one and 24 hours incubation with epinephrine, superoxide generation increased by 102% and 81% in the HCAECs. There was also a significant increase in both MnSOD and Cu/ZnSOD mRNA and protein. Furthermore, both MnSOD and Cu/ZnSOD activities were increased. However, pretreatment of HCAECs with trolox and vitamin E decreased superoxide generation and blocked the upregulation of SOD mRNA and protein. Treatment of the cells with atenolol also blocked SOD upregulaton. The authors concluded that epinephrine, via $beta_1$-adrenoceptor activation, causes the generation of superoxide which then upregulates SOD. They suggested that these findings may explain the long-term benefits of exercise.

Non-enzymatic antioxidants and exercise

The non-enzymatic antioxidants include vitamins C and E, beta-carotene and other carotenoids (e.g. lycopene, lutein, etc.), thiols (mainly reduced GSH), flavonoids (e.g. quercetin, rutin, etc.) and a variety of low molecular weight compounds such as uric acid, bilirubin, ubiquinone and lipoic acid. An important feature of most of these antioxidants is that their cellular concentrations are heavily dependent on various nutritional factors.

Although reports on the effects of antioxidant supplementation and physical performance have been mixed, there is considerable evidence that antioxidants may prevent some exercise-induced damage, at least over the long term. As noted by Packer,[479] several studies have given little support that antioxidant supplementation improves athletic performance. However, there is considerable evidence that antioxidants reduce oxidative damage to skeletal muscle and other tissues caused by vigorous exercise and increase endurance. Several examples demonstrating these latter positive effects will be briefly reviewed.

In an early study, Sumida *et al.*[493] found that individuals who ingested 300 mg alpha-tocopherol daily for four weeks exhibited a lower exercise-induced increase in lipid peroxidation after supplementation compared with vitamin E pretreatment. In addition, vitamin E supplementation decreased enzyme leakage (i.e. beta-glucuronidase and mitochondrial glutamic-oxaloacetic transaminase), possibly by decreasing exercise-induced oxidative damage of the mitochondrial membranes. Others[494] reported that mountain climbers, supplemented with vitamin E, did not exhibit the deterioration in physical performance observed in non-supplemented climbers. Moreover, the vitamin E-supplemented climbers had decreased breath pentane levels compared with non-supplemented climbers. Similarly, Novelli *et al.*[495] studied the effect of trapping free radicals on endurance to swimming in mice. Following intraperitoneal injection of each of three free radical spin-trappers, each mouse was submitted to a swimming test to control resistance to exhaustion (1) without any treatment,

(2) after administration of each spin-trapper in a random order and (3) after saline. Control experiments were performed with both saline and vitamin E supplementation. Their results showed that endurance was greatly prolonged by pretreatment with all three spin-trappers and with vitamin E. The authors concluded that since saline alone did not enhance time to exhaustion, increased endurance was not due to the effect of training. Rather, the increased time to exhaustion was due to free radical scavenger supplementation (i.e. vitamin E and spin-trappers).

Hartmann and associates[496] studied DNA damage in human peripheral leukocytes after a single bout of exhaustive exercise (treadmill run to exhaustion) and the effect of vitamin E supplementation. Blood leukocytes were examined for DNA strand breakage before and 24 hours after exercise. Their results showed a significant increase in DNA strand breakage after 24 hours compared with the pre-exercise sample. However, in subjects supplemented with vitamin E for 14 days prior to a run (1200 mg/day), exercise-induced DNA damage was significantly reduced. More specifically, vitamin E supplementation completely prevented exercise-induced DNA damage in four of five subjects. Reznick and coworkers[497] also demonstrated that vitamin E supplementation markedly decreased oxidative damage to gastrocnemius muscle protein of exercised rats. Thus, following intense exercise in rats fed a normal diet, the muscle protein carbonyl content increased by 17.23% compared to an increase of 5.78% to 8.27% in vitamin E-supplemented rats. Other antioxidants have also been shown to be effective in reducing the effects of exercise-induced oxidative stress.[498,499]

In summary, numerous studies clearly show that exercise stimulates the upregulation of various antioxidant enzymes and thereby decreases the potential negative effects of exercise-induced ROS. Furthermore, although antioxidant supplementation may not increase performance, it clearly improves endurance and decreases or even prevents the negative effects of exercise-induced oxidative stress.

Chapter Summary

A sedentary lifestyle is clearly a very important risk factor for numerous diseases and disorders such as cancer, coronary and cerebrovascular diseases, hypertension, type 2 diabetes, osteoporosis, decreased immunity, falls/fractures and various psychological disorders, among others (Table 3.1). It is also associated with increased all-cause mortality and appears to accelerate the aging process. Therefore, people of all ages should be strongly encouraged to increase their level of physical activity. Importantly, the majority of health benefits from physical activity can be achieved by briskly walking for two miles (3.2 km) most days of the week (CDC and Prevention and the American College of Sports Medicine).[202] As the report noted, however, "people who already meet the recommendation are also likely to derive some additional health and fitness benefits from becoming more physically active."

References

1. Murray CJL, Lopez AD. Evidence-based health policy — lessons from the Global Burden of Disease Study. *Science* 1996;274:740–743.
2. CDC. State-specific prevalence of participation in physical activity — 1994. *MMWR* 1996;45:673–675.
3. Casperson CJ, Merritt RK. Physical activity trends among 26 states, 1986–1990. *Med Sci Sports Exerc* 1995;27:713–720.
4. Ransdell LB, Wells CL. Physical activity in urban white, African-American, and Mexican-American women. *Med Sci Sports Exerc* 1997;30:1608–1615.
5. Durham J, Owen P, Bender B, *et al*. State-specific changes in physical inactivity among persons ≥65 years — United States, 1987–1992. *MMWR* 1995;44:663–673.
6. Francis KT. Status of the year 2000 health goals for physical activity and fitness. *Phys Ther* 1999;79:405–414.
7. US Department of Health and Human Services. *Healthy People 2010: Understanding and Improving Health*, 2nd Ed. Government Printing Office, Washington, DC, US, November 2000.
8. Gordon-Larsen P, McMurray RG, Popkin BM. Determinants of adolescent physical activity and inactivity patterns. *Pediatrics* 2000;105:1227–1228.

9. Kimm SYS, Glynn NW, Kriska AM, *et al.* Decline in physical activity in black girls and white girls during adolescence. *N Engl J Med* 2002;347:709–715.

10. The National Institute of Child Health and Human Development Study of Early Child Care and Youth Development Network. Frequency and intensity of activity of third-grade children in physical education. *Arch Pediatr Adolesc Med* 2003;157:185–190.

11. Andersen RE, Crespo CJ, Bartlett SJ, *et al.* Relationship of physical activity and television watching with body weight and level of fatness among children. *JAMA* 1998;279:938–942.

12. Strauss RS, Rodzilsky D, Burack G, Colin M. Psychosocial correlates of physical activity in healthy children. *Arch Pediatr Adolesc Med* 2001;155:897–902.

13. CDC. Missed opportunities in preventive counseling for cardiovascular disease — United States, 1995. *JAMA* 1998;279: 741–742.

14. Frolkis JP, Zyzanski SJ, Schwartz JM, Suhan PS. Physician noncompliance with the 1993 National Cholesterol Education Program (NCEP-ATPH) guidelines. *Circulation* 1998;98:85:851–855.

15. Wells KB, Lewis CE, Leake B, *et al.* Do physicians preach what they practice? A study of physicians' health habits and counseling practices. *JAMA* 1984;252:2846–2848.

16. Orleans CT, George LK, Houpt JL, *et al.* Health promotion in primary care: a survey of US family practitioners. *Prevent Med* 1985;14: 636–647.

17. Mann KV, Putnam RW. Physicians' perceptions of their role in cardiovascular risk reduction. *Prevent Med* 1989;18:45–58.

18. Wee CC, McCarthy EP, Davis RB, Phillips RS. Physician counseling about exercise. *JAMA* 1999;282:1583–1587.

19. Albright CL, Cohen S, Gibbons L, *et al.* Incorporating physical activity advice into primary care: physician-delivered advice within the activity counseling trial. *Am J Prev Med* 2000;18:225–234.

20. Sennott-Miller L, Kligman EW. Healthier lifestyles: how to motivate older patients to change. *Geriatrics* 1992;47:52–59.

21. Strauss E, Durand E, Blaustein A. Keeping in shape: exercise fundamentals for the midlife patient. *Geriatrics* 1997;52:62–79.

22. Gunnarsson OT, Judge JO. Exercise at midlife: how and why to prescribe it for sedentary patients. *Geriatrics* 1997;52:71–80.

23. Estabrooks PA, Glasgow RE, Dzewaltowski DA. Physical activity promotion through primary care. *JAMA* 2003;289:2913–2916.

24. CDC. Prevalence of health-care providers asking older adults about their physical activity level — United States, 1998. *MMWR* 2002; 51:412–414.
25. Deitrick RW. Exercise prescription and counseling. *Fed Pract* 1998;53–60(September).
26. Stewart AL, Verboncoeur CJ, McLellan BY, *et al.* Physical activity outcomes of CHAMPS II: a physical activity promotion program for older adults. *J Gerontol Med Sci* 2001;56A:M465–M470.
27. Elley CR, Kerse N, Arroll B, Robinson E. Effectiveness of counseling patients on physical activity in general practice: cluster randomised controlled trial. *BMJ* 2003;326:793–796.
28. Pate RR, Pratt M, Blair SN, *et al.* Physical activity and public health. *JAMA* 1995;273:402–407.
29. Schmid RE. Exercise — do it for diet. *Associated Press, Salt Lake Desert News*, 6 September 2002.
30. Allen C, Glasziou P, Del Mar C. Bed rest: a potentially harmful treatment needing more careful evaluation. *Lancet* 1999;354:1229–1233.
31. American College of Sports Medicine: Position Stand. Exercise and physical activity for older adults. *Med Sci Sports Exerc* 1998;30: 992–1008.
32. Dutta C, Ory M, Buchner D, *et al. Exercise: A Guide From the National Institute on Aging.* National Institute on Aging, Bethesda, MD, 2000.
33. Gill TM, DiPietro L, Krumholz HM. Role of exercise stress testing and safety monitoring for older persons starting an exercise program. *JAMA* 2000;284:342–349.
34. Butler RN, Davis R, Lewis CB, *et al.* Physical fitness: how to help older patients live stronger and longer. *Geriatrics* 1998;53:26–40.
35. Blair SN. Evidence for success of exercise in weight loss and control *Ann Intern Med* 1993;119:702–706.
36. Blair SN, Kohl HW III, Barlow CE, *et al.* Changes in physical fitness and all-cause mortality: a prospective study of healthy and unhealthy men. *JAMA* 1995;273:1093–1098.
37. Asikainen T, Miilunpalo S, Oja P, *et al.* Walking trials in postmeno-pausal women: effect of one versus two daily bouts on aerobic fitness. *Scand J Med Sci Sports* 2002;12:99–105.
38. Williamson DF, Madans J, Anda RF, *et al.* Recreational physical activity and ten-year weight change in a US national cohort. *Int J Obesity* 1993;17:279–286.

39. Anderson RE, Wadden TA, Bartlett SJ, *et al.* Effects of lifestyle activity versus structured aerobic exercise in obese women. *JAMA* 1999;281:335–340.

40. Coakley EH, Kawachi I, Manson JE, *et al.* Lower levels of physical function are associated with higher body weight among middle-aged and older women. *Int J Obes Relat Metab Disord* 1998;22:958–965.

41. Harger BS, Miller JB, Thomas JC. The caloric cost of running: its impact on weight reduction. *JAMA* 1974;228:482–483.

42. Fogelholm M, Kukkonen-Harjula K, Nenonen A, Pasanen M. Effects of walking training on weight maintenance after a very-low-energy diet in premenopausal obese women. *Arch Intern Med* 2000;160:2177–2184.

43. Martinez-Gonzalez MA, Martinez JA, Hu FB, *et al.* Physical inactivity, sedentary lifestyle and obesity in the European Union. *Int J Obes Relat Metab Disord* 1999;23:1192–1201.

44. Donnelly JE, Jacobsen DJ, Heelan KS, *et al.* The effects of 18 months of intermittent versus continuous exercise on aerobic capacity, body weight and composition, and metabolic fitness in previously sedentary, moderately obese females. *Int J Obes Relat Metab Disord* 2000;24:566–572.

45. Astrup A. Physical activity and weight gain and fat distribution changes with menopause: current evidence and research issues. *Med Sci Sports Exerc* 1999;31(Suppl 11):S564–S567.

46. Rissanen A, Fogelholm M. Physical activity in the prevention and treatment of other morbid conditions and impairments associated with obesity: current evidence and research issues. *Med Sci Sports Exerc* 1999;31(Suppl 11):S635–S645.

47. Lawlor DA, Taylor M, Bedford C, Ebrahim S. Is housework good for health? Levels of physical activity and factors associated with activity in elderly women. Results from the British Women's Heart and Health Study. *J Epidemiol Community Health* 2002;56:473–478.

48. Jakicic JM, Winters C, Lang W, Wing RR. Effects of intermittent exercise and use of home exercise equipment on adherence, weight loss, and fitness in overweight women: a randomized trial. *JAMA* 1999;282:1554–1560.

49. Irwin ML, Yasui Y, Ulrich CM, *et al.* Effect of exercise on total and intra-abdominal body fat in postmenopausal women: a randomized controlled trial. *JAMA* 2003;289:323–330.

50. Paffenbarger RS Jr., Hyde RT, Wing AL, *et al.* The association of changes in physical-activity level and other lifestyle characteristics with mortality among men. *N Engl J Med* 1993;328:538–545.

51. Blair SN, Kohl HW III, Barlow CE, *et al.* Changes in physical fitness and all-cause mortality: a prospective study of healthy and unhealthy men. *JAMA* 1995;273:1093–1098.

52. Lee I-M, Hsieh C-C, Paffenbarger RS. Exercise intensity and longevity in men: the Harvard Alumni Health Study. *JAMA* 1995;273:1179–1184.

53. Lee IM, Paffenbarger RS Jr. Associations of light, moderate and vigorous intensity physical activity with longevity: the Harvard Alumni Health Study. *Am J Epidemiol* 2000;151:293–299.

54. Sarna S, Sahi T, Koskenvuo M, Kaprio J. Increased life expectancy in world class male athletes. *Med Sci Sports Exerc* 1993;25:237–244.

55. Kushi LH, Fee RM, Folsom AR, *et al.* Physical activity and mortality in postmenopausal women. *JAMA* 1997;277:1287–1292.

56. Pereira MA, Kriska AM, Day RD, *et al.* A randomized walking trial in postmenopausal women: effects on physical activity and health 10 years later. *Arch Intern Med* 1998;158:1695–1701.

57. Gregg EW, Cauley JA, Stone K, *et al.* Relationship of changes in physical activity and mortality among older women. *JAMA* 2003;289:2379–2386.

58. Kujala UM, Kaprio J, Sarna S, Koskenvuo M. Relationship of leisure-time physical activity and mortality. *JAMA* 1998;279:440–444.

59. Bijnen FCH, Casperson CJ, Feskens EJM, *et al.* Physical activity and 10-year mortality from cardiovascular diseases and all causes: the Zutphen Elderly Study. *Arch Intern Med* 1998;158:1499–1505.

60. Hakim AA, Petrovitch H, Burchfiel CM, *et al.* Effects of walking on mortality among nonsmoking retired men. *N Engl J Med* 1998;338:94–99.

61. Weller I, Corey P. The impact of excluding non-leisure energy expenditure on the relation between physical activity and mortality in women. *Epidemiology* 1998;9:632–635.

62. Villeneuve PJ, Morrison HI, Craig CL, Schaubel DE. Physical activity, physical fitness and risk of dying. *Epidemiology* 1998;9:626–631.

63. Andersen LB, Schnohr P, Schroll M, Hein HO. All-cause mortality associated with physical activity during leisure time, work, sports and cycling to work. *Arch Intern Med* 2000;160:1621–1628.

64. Stessman J, Maaravi Y, Hammerman-Rozenberg R, Cohen A. The effects of physical activity on mortality in the Jerusalem 70-year-old Longitudinal Study. *J Am Geriatr Soc* 2000;48:499–504.

65. Lee I-M, Paffenbarger RS. Do physical activity and physical fitness avert premature mortality? In: *Exercise and Sport Sciences Reviews*. JO Holloszy (ed.) 1996;24:135–171.

66. Katzmarzyk PT, Craig CL. Musculoskeletal fitness and risk of mortality. *Med Sci Sports Exerc* 2002;34:740–744.

67. Mundal R, Kjeldsen SE, Sandvik L, *et al.* Exercise blood pressure predicts cardiovascular mortality in middle-aged men. *Hypertension* 1994;24:56–62.

68. Cole CR, Foody JA, Blackstone EH, *et al.* Heart rate recovery after submaximal exercise testing as a predictor of mortality in a cardiovascularly healthy cohort. *Ann Intern Med* 2000;132:552–555.

69. Cole CR, Blackstone EH, Pashkow FJ, *et al.* Heart-rate recovery immediately after exercise as a predictor of mortality. *N Engl J Med* 1999;341:1351–1357.

70. Erikssen G, Liestol K, Bjornholt JV, *et al.* Changes in physical fitness and changes in mortality. *Lancet* 1998;352:759–762.

71. Myers J, Prakash M, Froelicher V, *et al.* Exercise capacity and mortality among men referred for exercise testing. *N Engl J Med* 2002;346:793–801.

72. Kujala UM, Sarna S, Kaprio J, Koskenvuo M. Hospital care in later life among former world-class Finnish athletes. *JAMA* 1996;276:216–220.

73. Bortz WM II. Effect of exercise on aging — effect of aging on exercise. *J Am Geriatr Soc* 1980; 28:49–51.

74. Norman A, Bellocco R, Vaida F, Wolk A. Total physical activity in relation to age, body mass, health and other factors in a cohort of Swedish men. *Int J Obes* 2002;26:670–675.

75. Gregg EW, Cauley JA, Seeley DG, *et al.* Physical activity and osteoporotic fracture risk in older women. *Ann Intern Med* 1998;129:81–88.

76. Heath GW, Hagberg JM, Ehsani AA, *et al.* A physiologic comparison of young and old endurance athletes. *J Appl Physiol* 1981;51:634–640.

77. Satariano WA, Haight TJ, Tager IB. Reasons given by older people for limitation or avoidance of leisure time physical activity. *J Am Geriatr Soc* 2000;48:505–512.

78. Bortz WM II. The disuse syndrome. *West J Med* 1984;141:691–694.

79. Bortz WM. Disuse and aging. *JAMA* 1982;248:1203–1208.

80. Hodgson J. *Age and Aerobic Capacity of Urban Midwestern Males.* Thesis, University of Minnesota, Minneapolis, MN, 1971.

81. de Vries H. Physiological effects of an exercise training regimen upon men aged 52–88. *J Gerontol* 1970;25:325–336.

82. Dehn M, Bruce R. Longitudinal variations in maximal oxygen intake with age and activity. *J Appl Physiol* 1972;33:805–807.

83. Buchner DM, Wagner EH. Preventing frail health. *Clin Geriatr Med* 1992;8:1–17.

84. Kasch F, Phillips W, Carter J, *et al.* Cardiovascular changes in middle-aged men during two years of training. *J Appl Physiol* 1973;34:53–57.

85. Tzankoff SP, Norris AH. Longitudinal changes in basal metabolic rate in men. *J Appl Physiol* 1978;33:536–539.
86. Imamura K, Ashida H, Ishikawa T, Fujii M. Human major psoas muscle and sarcospinalis muscle in relation to age: a study by computed tomography. *J Gerontol* 1983;38:678–681.
87. Poehlman ET, Toth MJ, Gardner AW. Changes in energy balance and body composition at menopause: a controlled longitudinal study. *Ann Intern Med* 1995;123:673–675.
88. Feigenbaum MS, Pollock ML. Prescription of resistance training for health and disease. *Med Sci Sports Exerc* 1999;31:38–45.
89. Jette AM, Branch LG. The Framingham Disability Study: II. Physical disability among the aging. *Am J Public Health* 1981;71:1211–1216.
90. de Jong N, Paw MJ, de Groot LC, *et al.* Dietary supplements and physical exercise affecting bone and body composition in frail elderly persons. *Am J Public Health* 2000;90:947–954.
91. Binder EF, Schechtman KB, Ehsani AA, *et al.* Effects of exercise training on frailty in community-dwelling older adults: results of a randomized, controlled trial. *J Am Geriatr Soc* 2002;50:1921–1928.
92. Larsson L, Grimby G, Karlsson J. Muscle strength and speed of movement in relation to age and muscle morphology. *J Appl Physiol* 1979;46:451–456.
93. Dutta C, Hadley EC. The significance of sarcopenia in old age. *J Gerontol* 1995;50:Spec No:1–4.
94. Volpi E, Sheffield-Moore M, Rasmussen BB, Wolfe RR. Basal muscle amino acid kinetics and protein synthesis in healthy young and older men. *JAMA* 2001;286:1206–1212.
95. Campbell WW, Crim MC, Dallal GE, *et al.* Increased protein requirements in the elderly: new data and retrospective reassessments. *Am J Clin Nutr* 1994;60:167–175.
96. Freedman VA, Martin LG, Schoeni RF. Recent trends in disability and functioning among older adults in the United States: a systematic review. *JAMA* 2002;288;3137–3146.
97. Cohen RA, van Nostrand JF. Trends in the health of older Americans: United States 1994. *Vital Health Stat* 1995;3:3–7.
98. Trupin L, Rice DP, Max W. *Medical Expenditures for People With Disabilities in the United States, 1987*. Washington DC: US Department of Education, National Institute on Disability and Rehabilatation Research, 1995.
99. Congressional Budget Office. *Projections for Long-term Care Services for the Elderly*, March 1999. Available at *http://www.cbo.gov*.

100. Davis JW, Ross PD, Preston SD, *et al.* Strength, physical activity and body mass index: relationship to performance-based measures and activities of daily living among older Japanese women in Hawaii. *J Am Geriatr Soc* 1998;46:274–279.

101. MacRae PG, Asplund LA, Schnelle JF, *et al.* A walking program for nursing home residents: effects on walk endurance, physical activity, mobility and quality of life. *J Am Geriatr Soc* 1996;44:175–180.

102. Fries JF, Singh G, Morfield D, *et al.* Running and development of disability with age. *Ann Intern Med* 1994;121:502–509.

103. Wang BWE, Ramey DR, Schettler JD, *et al.* Postponed development of disability in elderly runners: a 13-year longitudinal study. *Arch Intern Med* 2002;162:2285–2294.

104. Hunter GR, Treuth MS, Weinsier RL, *et al.* The effects of strength conditioning on older women's ability to perform daily tasks. *J Am Geriatr Soc* 1995;43:756–760.

105. Graves JE, Pollock MK, Carroll JF. Exercise, age and skeletal muscle function. *South Med J* 1994;87:S17–S22.

106. Bassey EJ, Bendall MJ, Pearson M. Muscle strength in the triceps surae and objectively measured customary walking activity in men and women over 65 years of age. *Clin Sci* 1988;74:85–89.

107. Fiatarone MA, Marks EC, Ryan ND, *et al.* High-intensity strength training in nonagenarians: effects on skeletal muscle. *JAMA* 1990;263:3029–3034.

108. Fiatarone MA, O'Neill EF, Ryan ND, *et al.* Exercise training and nutritional supplementation for physical frailty in very elderly people. *N Engl J Med* 1994;330:1769–1775.

109. McMurdo MET, Rennie L. A controlled trial of exercise by residents of old people's homes. *Age Ageing* 1993;22:11–15.

110. Morey MC, Pieper CF, Sullivan RJ, *et al.* Five-year performance trends for older exercisers: a hierarchical model of endurance, strength and flexibility. *J Am Geriatr Soc* 1996;44:1226–1231.

111. Gill TM, Allore H, Guo Z. Restricted activity and functional decline among community-living older persons. *Arch Intern Med* 2003; 163:1317–1322.

112. Brooke-Wavell K, Athersmith LE, Jones PRM, Masud T. Brisk walking and postural stability: a cross-sectional study in postmenopausal women. *Gerontology* 1998;44:288–292.

113. Lord SR, Ward JA, Williams P, Strudwick M. The effect of a 12-month exercise trial on balance, strength and falls in older women: a randomized controlled trial. *J Am Geriatr Soc* 1995;43:1198–1206.

114. Wolfson L, Whipple R, Derby C, *et al.* Balance and strength training in older adults: intervention gains and Tai Chi maintenance. *J Am Geriatr Soc* 1996;44:498–506.

115. Wolf SL, Barnhart HX, Kutner NG, *et al.* Reducing frailty and falls in older persons: an investigation of Tai Chi and computerized balance training. *J Am Geriatr Soc* 1996;44:489–497.

116. Ooi WL, Barrett S, Hossain M, *et al.* Patterns of orthostatic blood pressure change and their clinical correlates in a frail, elderly population. *JAMA* 1997;277:1299–1304.

117. Hawryluk M. Fall-related injuries cost Medicare billions. *Am Med News* 2002;16:5,8.

118. Tinetti ME, Speechley M, Ginter SF. Risk factors for falls among elderly persons. *N Engl J Med* 1988;319:1701–1707.

119. Perry BC. Falls among the elderly. *J Am Geriatr Soc* 1982;30:367–371.

120. Baker SP, Harvey AH. Fall injuries in the elderly. *Clin Geriatr Med* 1985;1:501–512.

121. Kannus P, Parkkari J, Koskinen S, *et al.* Fall-induced injuries and deaths among older adults. *JAMA* 1999;281:1895–1899.

122. Rivara FP, Grossman DC, Cummings P. Injury prevention: first of two parts. *N Engl J Med* 1997;337:543–547.

123. Tinetti ME, Speechley M. Prevention of falls among the elderly. *N Engl J Med* 1989;320:1055–1059.

124. Tideiksaar R. Preventing falls: how to identify risk factors, reduce complications. *Geriatrics* 1996;51:43–53.

125. Nevitt MC, Cummings SR, Kidd S, Black D. Risk factors for recurrent nonsyncopal falls. *JAMA* 1989;261:2663–2668.

126. Rivara FP, Grossman DC, Cummings P. Injury prevention: second of two parts. *N Engl J Med* 1997;337:613–617.

127. Thapa PB, Gideon P, Cost TW, *et al.* Antidepressants and the risk of falls among nursing home residents. *N Engl J Med* 1998;339:875–882.

128. Tinetti ME, Doucette J, Claus E, Marottoli R. Risk factors for serious injury during falls by older persons in the community. *J Am Geriatr Soc* 1995;43:1214–1221.

129. Luukinen H, Koski K, Laippala P, Kivela S-L. Factors predicting fractures during falling impacts among home-dwelling older adults. *J Am Geriatr Soc* 1997;45:1302–1309.

130. Scaf-Klamp W, Sanderman R, Ormel J, Kempen GIJM. Depression in older people after fall-related injuries: a prospective study. *Age Ageing* 2003;32:88–94.

131. Province MA, Hadley EC, Hornbrook MC, *et al.* The effects of exercise on falls in elderly patients: a preplanned meta-analysis of the FICSIT trial. *JAMA* 1995;273:1341–1347.

132. Shaw JM, Snow CM. Weighted vest exercise improves indices of fall risk in older women. *J Gerontol MEDSCI* 1998;53:M53–M58.

133. Hubley-Kozey CL, Wall JC, Hogan DB. Effects of a general exercise program on passive hip, knee and ankle range of motion of older women. *Top Geriatr Rehabil* 1995;10:33–44.

134. Leslie DK, Frekang GA. Effects of an exercise program on selected flexibility measures of senior citizens. *Gerontologist* 1975;4:182–183.

135. Lesser M. The effects of rhythmic exercise on the range of motion in older adults. *Am Correct Ther J* 1978;32:118–122.

136. American Geriatrics Society, British Geriatrics Society, American Academy of Orthopaedic Surgeons Panel on Falls Prevention. Guidelines for the prevention of falls in older persons. *J Am Geriatr Soc* 2001;49:664–672.

137. Marwick C. Consensus panel considers osteoporosis. *JAMA* 2000;283:2093–2095.

138. Marshall D, Johnell O, Wedel H. Meta-analysis of how well measures of bone mineral density predict occurrence of osteoporotic fractures. *BMJ* 1996;312:1254–1259.

139. Ralston SH. Science, medicine and the future: osteoporosis. *BMJ* 1997;315:469–472.

140. Klesges RC, Ward KD, Shelton ML, *et al.* Changes in bone mineral content in male athletes. *JAMA* 1996;276:226–230.

141. de Jong N, Paw MJMC, de Groot LCPGM, *et al.* Dietary supplements and physical exercise affecting bone and body composition in frail elderly persons. *Am J Public Health* 2000;90:947–954.

142. NIH Consensus Development Panel on Optimal Calcium Intake. Optimal calcium intake. *JAMA* 1994;272:1942–1948.

143. Chesnut CH. Bone mass and exercise. *Am J Med* 1993;95(Suppl 5A):34S–36S.

144. Bravo G, Gauthier P, Roy P-M, *et al.* Impact of 12-month exercise program on the physical and psychological health of osteopenic women. *J Am Geriatr Soc* 1996;44:756–762.

145. Zhang J, Feldblum PJ, Fortney JA. Moderate physical activity and bone density among perimenopausal women. *Am J Public Health* 1992;82:736–738.

146. Ebrahim S, Thompson PW, Baskaran V, Evans K. Randomized placebo-controlled trial of brisk walking in the prevention of postmenopausal osteoporosis. *Age Ageing* 1997;26:253–260.

147. Reid IR, Legge M, Stapleton JP, *et al.* Regular exercise dissociates fat mass and bone density in premenopausal women. *J Clin Endocrinol Metab* 1995;80:1764–1768.

148. Mussolino ME, Looker AC, Orwoll ES. Jogging and bone mineral density in men: results from NHANES III. *Am J Public Health* 2001;91:1056–1059.

149. Snow CM, Shaw JM, Winters KM, Witzke KA. Long-term exercise using weighted vests prevents hip bone loss in postmenopausal women. *J Gerontol Med Sci* 2000;55A:M489–M491.

150. Hannan MT, Felson DT, Dawson-Hughes B, *et al.* Risk factors for longitudinal bone loss in elderly men and women: the Framingham Osteoporosis Study. *J Bone Min Res* 2000;15:710–720.

151. Salamone LM, Cauley JA, Black DM, *et al.* Effect of a lifestyle intervention on bone mineral density in premenopausal women: a randomized trail. *Am J Clin Nutr* 1999;70:97–103.

152. Gregg EW, Cauley JA, Seeley DG, *et al.* Physical activity and osteoporotic fracture risk in older women. *Ann Intern Med* 1998;129:81–88.

153. Hollingworth W, Todd CJ, Parker MJ. The cost of treating hip fractures in the twenty-first century. *J Public Health* 1995;17:269–276.

154. Butler MEG, Norton R, Lee-Joe T, *et al.* The risks of hip fracture in older people from private homes and institutions. *Age Ageing* 1996;25:381–385.

155. Farahmand BY, Persson P-G, Michaelsson K, *et al.* Physical activity and hip fracture: a population-based case-control study. *Int J Epidemiol* 2000;29:308–314.

156. Feskanich D, Willett W, Colditz G. Walking and leisure-time activity and risk of hip fracture in postmenopausal women. *JAMA* 2002;288:2300–2306.

157. Heinonen A, Kannus P, Sievanen H, *et al.* Randomised controlled trial of effect of high-impact exercise on selected risk factors for osteoporotic fractures. *Lancet* 1996;348:1343–1347.

158. Nelson ME, Fiatarone MA, Morganti CM, *et al.* Effects of high-intensity strength training on multiple risk factors for osteoporotic fractures. *JAMA* 1994;272:1909–1914.

159. Tinetti ME, Baker DI, Gottschalk M, *et al.* Systematic home-based physical and functional therapy for older persons after hip fracture. *Arch Phys Med Rahabil* 1997;78:1237–1247.

160. Gregg EW, Pereira MA, Caspersen CJ. Physical activity, falls and fractures among older adults: a review of the epidemiologic evidence. *J Am Geriatr Soc* 2000;48:883–893.

161. Meier CR, Schlienger RG, Kraenzlin ME, *et al.* HMG-CoA reductase inhibitors and the risk of fractures. *JAMA* 2000;283:3205–3210.
162. Wang PS, Solomon DH, Mogun H, Avorn J. HMG-CoA reductase inhibitors and the risk of hip fractures in elderly patients. *JAMA* 2000;283:3211–3216.
163. CDC. Prevalence of disabilities and associated health conditions among adults — United States, 1999. *MMWR* 2001;50:120–125.
164. CDC. Prevalence of self-reported arthritis or chronic joint symptoms among adults — United States, 2001. *MMWR* 2002;51:948–950.
165. Kramarow E, Lentzner H, Rooks R, *et al. Health and Aging Chartbook: Health, United States, 1999.* National Center for Health Statistics, Hyattsville, Md, 1999.
166. Penninx BWJH, Messier SP, Rejeski J, *et al.* Physical exercise and the prevention of disability in activities of daily living in older persons with osteoarthritis. *Arch Intern Med* 2001;161:2309–2316.
167. Ettinger WH, Burns R, Messier SP, *et al.* A randomized trial comparing aerobic exercise and resistance exercise with a health education program in older adults with knee osteoarthritis: the Fitness Arthritis and Seniors Trial (FAST). *JAMA* 1997;277:25–31.
168. Coggon D, Croft P, Kellingray S, *et al.* Occupational physical activities and osteoarthritis of the knee. *Arth Rheum* 2000;43:1443–1449.
169. Koplan JP, Siscovick DS, Goldbaum GM. The risks of exercise: a public health view of injuries and hazards. *Public Health Rep* 1985;100:188–195.
170. Salter RB, Field P. The effects of continuous compression on living articular cartilage. *J Bone Joint Surg* 1960;42A:31–49.
171. Lane NE, Michel B, Bjorkengren A, *et al.* The risk of osteoarthritis with running and aging: a 5-year longitudinal study. *J Rheumatol* 1993;20:461–468.
172. Cooper C, Inskip H, Croft P, *et al.* Individual risk factors for hip osteoarthritis: obesity, hip injury and physical activity. *Am J Epidemiol* 1998;147:516–522.
173. van den Ende CHM, Breedveld FC, le Cessie S, *et al.* Effect of intensive exercise on patients with active rheumatoid arthritis: a randomised clinical trial. *Ann Rheum Dis* 2000;59:615–621.
174. Burt VL, Whelton P, Roccella EJ, *et al.* Prevalence of hypertension in the US adult population: results from the Third National Health and Nutrition Examination Survey, 1988–1991. *Hypertension* 1995;25:305–313.
175. Kannel WB. Blood pressure as a cardiovascular risk factor: prevention and treatment. *JAMA* 1996;275:1571–1576.

176. Levy D, Larson MG, Vasan RS, *et al.* The progression from hypertension to congestive heart failure. *JAMA* 1996;275:1557–1562.
177. Launer LJ, Masaki K, Petrovitch H, *et al.* The association between midlife blood pressure level and late-life cognitive function: the Honolulu-Asia Aging Study. *JAMA* 1995;274:1846–1851.
178. Kaplan NM, Gifford RW. Choices of initial therapy for hypertension. *JAMA* 1996;275:1577–1580.
179. Arroll B, Beaglehole R. Exercise for hypertension. *Lancet* 1993; 341:1248–1249.
180. Blumenthal JA, Sherwood A, Gullette ECD, *et al.* Exercise and weight loss reduce blood pressure in men and women with mild hypertension. *Arch Intern Med* 2000;160:1947–1958.
181. Georgiades A, Sherwood A, Gullette ECD, *et al.* Effects of exercise and weight loss on mental stress-enduced cardiovascular responses in individuals with high blood pressure. *Hypertension* 2000;36:171–176.
182. Taylor-Tolbert NS, Dengel DR, Brown MD, *et al.* Ambulatory blood pressure after acute exercise in older men with essential hypertension. *Am J Hypertens* 2000;13:44–51.
183. Kelley GA, Kelley KS. Progressive resistance exercise and resting blood pressure: a meta-analysis of randomized controlled trials. *Hyperten Balt* 2000;35:838–843.
184. American College of Sports Medicine. Physical activity, physical fitness and hypertension: position stand. *Med Sci Sports Exerc* 1993;25(10):i–x.
185. Young DR, Appel LJ, Jee SJ, Miller ER III. The effects of aerobic exercise and Tai Chi on blood pressure in older people: results of a randomized trial. *J Am Geriatr Soc* 1999;47:277–284.
186. Kokkinos PF, Narayan P, Colleran JA, *et al.* Effects of regular exercise on blood pressure and left ventricular hypertrophy in African-American men with severe hypertension. *N Engl J Med* 1995;333:1462–1467.
187. Wareham NJ, Wong M-Y, Hennings S, *et al.* Quantifying the association between habitual energy expenditure and blood pressure. *Int J Epidemiol* 2000;29:655–660.
188. Reaven GM, Lithell H, Landsberg L. Hypertension and associated metabolic abnormalities — the role of insulin resistance and the sympathoadrenal system. *N Engl J Med* 1996;334:374–384.
189. Reaven GM. Are insulin resistance and/or compensatory hyperinsulinemia involved in the etiology and clinical course of patients with hypertension. *Int J Obes* 1995;19(Suppl 1):2–5.

190. Jeppesen J, Hein HO, Suadicani P, Gyntelberg F. High triglycerides and low HDL cholesterol and blood pressure and risk of ischemic heart disease. *Hypertension* 2000;36:226–232.

191. Williamson DL, Kirwan JP. A single bout of concentric resistance exercise increases basal metabolic rate 48 hours after exercise in healthy 59- to 77-year-old men. *J Gerontol Med Sci* 1997;52A:M352–M355.

192. Dengel DR, Hagberg JM, Pratley RE, *et al.* Improvements in blood pressure, glucose metabolism and lipoprotein lipids after aerobic exercise plus weight loss in obese, hypertensive middle-aged men. *Metabolism* 1998;47:1075–1082.

193. Hazzard WR. Weight control and exercise: cardinal features of successful preventive gerontology. *JAMA* 1995;274:1964–1965.

194. Guyer B, Hoyert DL, Martin JA, *et al.* Annual summary of vital statistics — 1998. *Pediatrics* 1999;104:1229–1246.

195. Expert Panel on Detection, Evaluation and Treatment of High Blood Cholesterol in Adults. Summary of the second report of the National Cholesterol Education Program (NCEP) expert panel on detection, evaluation and treatment of high blood cholesterol in adults (Adult Treatment Panel II). *JAMA* 1993;269:3015–3023.

196. Castelli WP, Anderson K. A population at risk: prevalence of high cholesterol levels in hypertensive patients in the Framingham Study. *Am J Med* 1986;80(Suppl 2A):23–32.

197. Knight JA. *Laboratory Medicine and the Aging Process.* ASCP Press, Chicago, IL, 1996, pp. 111–143.

198. Denke MA, Sempos CT, Grundy SM. Excess body weight: an unrecognized contributor to high blood cholesterol levels in white American men. *Arch Intern Med* 1993;153:1093–1103.

199. Denke MA, Sempos CT, Grundy SM. Excess body weight: an underrecognized contributor to dyslipidemia in white American women. *Arch Intern Med* 1994;154:401–407.

200. Owen JF, Mathews KA, Wing RR, Kuller LH. Can physical activity mitigate the effects of aging in middle-aged women? *Circulation* 1992;85:1265–1270.

201. Duncan JJ, Gordon NF, Scott CB. Women walking for health and fitness: how much is enough? *JAMA* 1991;266:3295–3299.

202. Pate RR, Pratt M, Blair SN, *et al.* Physical activity and public health: a recommendation from the Centers for Disease Control and Prevention and the American College of Sports Medicine. *JAMA* 1995;273:402–407.

203. American College of Sports Medicine. *Guidelines for exercise testing and prescription*, 4th Ed. Lea & Febiger, Philadelphia, 1991.

204. Williams PT. High-density lipoprotein cholesterol and other risk factors for coronary heart disease in female runners. *N Engl J Med* 1996;334:1298–1303.
205. Williams PT. Lipoproteins and adiposity show improvement at substantially higher exercise levels than those currently recommended. *Circulation* 1994;90:I–471 (Abstract).
206. Thune I, Njolstad I, Lochen M-L, *et al.* Physical activity improves the metabolic risk profiles in men and women. *Arch Intern Med* 1998;158:1633–1640.
207. Kokkinos PF, Holland JC, Narayan P, *et al.* Miles run per week and high-density lipoprotein cholesterol levels in healthy, middle-aged men. *Arch Intern Med* 1995;155:415–420.
208. Kraus WE, Houmard MA, Duscha BD, *et al.* Effects of the amount and intensity of exercise on plasma lipoproteins. *N Engl J Med* 2002;347:1483–1492.
209. Thompson PD. Additional steps for cardiovascular health. *N Engl J Med* 2002;347:755–756.
210. Stefanick ML, Mackey S, Sheehan M, *et al.* Effects of diet and exercise in men and postmenopausal women with low levels of HDL cholesterol and high levels of LDL cholesterol. *N Engl J Med* 1998;339:12–20.
211. Wood PD, Stefanick ML, Williams PT, Haskell WL. The effects on plasma lipoprotein of a prudent weight-reducing diet, with and without exercise, in overweight men and women. *N Engl J Med* 1991;325:461–466.
212. Knight S, Bermingham MA, Mahajan D. Regular non-vigorous physical activity and cholesterol levels in the elderly. *Gerontology* 1999; 45:213–219.
213. Ginsberg GS, Agil A, O'Toole M, *et al.* Effects of a single bout of ultraendurance exercise on lipid levels and susceptibility of lipids to peroxidation in triathletes. *JAMA* 1996;276:221–225.
214. Knight JA. *Free Radicals, Antioxidants, Aging and Disease.* AACC Press, Washington, DC, 1999.
215. Vasankari TJ, Kujala UM, Vasankari TM, Ahotupa M. Reduced oxidized LDL levels after a 10-month exercise program. *Med Sci Sports Exer* 1998;30:1496–1501.
216. Kokkinos PF, Fernhall B. Physical activity and high density lipoprotein cholesterol levels: what is the relationship? *Sports Med* 1999;28:307–314.

217. Harris MI, Klein R, Welborn TA, Knuiman MW. Onset of NIDDM occurs at least 4–7 years before clinical diagnosis. *Diabetes Care* 1992;15:815–819.

218. Harris MI, Flegal KM, Cowie CC, *et al.* Prevalence of diabetes, impaired fasting glucose and impaired glucose tolerance in US adults: the Third National Health and Nutrition Examination Survey, 1988–1994. *Diabetes Care* 1998;21:518–524.

219. Mokdad AH, Ford ES, Bowman BA, *et al.* Diabetes trends in the US: 1990–1998. *Diabetes Care* 2000;23:1278–1283.

220. Cefalu WT, Ettinger WH, Bell-Farrow AD, Rushing JT. Serum fructosamine as a screening test for diabetes in the elderly: a pilot study. *J Am Geriatr Soc* 1993;41:1090–1094.

221. Broughton DL, Taylor R. Deterioration of glucose tolerance with age: the role of insulin resistance. *Age Ageing* 1991;20:221–225.

222. Yki-Jarvinen H. Pathogenesis of non-insulin-dependent diabetes mellitus. *Lancet* 1994;343:91–95.

223. Huse DM, Oster G, Killen AR, *et al.* The economic costs of non-insulin dependent diabetes mellitus. *JAMA* 1989;262–2713.

224. Ray N, Willis S, Thamer M. *Direct and Indirect Costs of Diabetes in the United States in 1992.* American Diabetes Association, Alexandria, VA, 1993.

225. Rubin RJ, Altman WM, Mendelson DN. Health care expenditures for people with diabetes mellitus, 1992. *J Clin Endocrinol Metab* 1994;78:809A–809F.

226. American Diabetes Association. Economic consequences of diabetes mellitus in the US in 1997. *Diabetes Care* 1998;21:296–309.

227. Brancati FL, Kao WHL, Folsom AR, *et al.* Incident type 2 diabetes mellitus in African American and white adults. *JAMA* 2000; 283:2253–2259.

228. Erickson K-F, Lindgarde F. Prevention of type 2 (non-insulin-dependent) diabetes mellitus by diet and physical exercise. *Diabetologia* 1991;34:891–898.

229. Hu FB, Manson JE, Stampfer MJ, *et al.* Diet, lifestyle and the risk of type 2 diabetes mellitus in women. *N Engl J Med* 2001;345:790–797.

230. Helmrich SP, Ragland Dr, Leung RW, Paffenbarger RS Jr. Physical activity and reduced occurrence on non-insulin-dependent diabetes mellitus. *N Engl J Med* 1991;325:147–152.

231. Pan X-R, Li G-W, Hu Y-H, *et al.* Effects of diet and exercise in preventing NIDDM in people with impaired glucose tolerance. *Diabetes Care* 1997;20:537–544.

232. Manson JE, Nathan DM, Krolewski AS, *et al.* A prospective study of exercise and incidence of diabetes among US male physicians. *JAMA* 1992;268:63–67.

233. Manson JE, Rimm EB, Stampfer MJ, *et al.* Physical activity and incidence of non-insulin-dependent diabetes mellitus in women. *Lancet* 1991;338:774–778.

234. Mayer-Davis EJ, D'Agostino R, Karter AJ, *et al.* Intensity and amount of physical activity in relation to insulin sensitivity. *JAMA* 1998;279:669–674.

235. Irwin ML, Mayer-Davis EJ, Addy CL, *et al.* Moderate intensity physical activity and fasting insulin levels in women. *Diabetes Care* 2000;23:449–454.

236. Ross R, Dagone D, Jones PJH, *et al.* Reduction in obesity and related comorbid conditions after diet-induced weight loss or exercise-induced weight loss in men. *Ann Intern Med* 2000;133:92–103.

237. DiPietro L, Seeman TE, Stachenfeld NS, *et al.* Moderate-intensity aerobic training improves glucose tolerance in aging independent of abdominal obesity. *J Am Geriatr Soc* 1998;46:875–879.

238. Hu FB, Sigal RJ, Rich-Edwards JW, *et al.* Walking compared with vigorous physical activity and risk of type 2 diabetes in women. *JAMA* 1999;282:1433–1439.

239. Landers SJ. Diet and exercise best medicine in preventing diabetes. *Am Med News* 2001;44(32):28–30.

240. Wei M, Gibbons LW, Mitchell TL, *et al.* The association between cardiorespiratory fitness and impaired fasting glucose and type 2 diabetes mellitus. *Ann Intern Med* 1999;130:89–96.

241. Cononie CC, Goldberg AP, Rogus E, Hagberg JM. Seven consecutive days of exercise lowers plasma insulin responses to an oral glucose challenge in sedentary elderly. *J Am Geriatr Soc* 1994;42:394–398.

242. Boule NG, Haddad E, Kenny GP, *et al.* Effects of exercise on glycemic control and body mass in type 2 diabetes mellitus: a meta-analysis of controlled clinical trials. *JAMA* 2001;286:1218–1227.

243. Kriska AM, Pereira MA, Hanson RL, *et al.* Association of physical activity and serum insulin concentrations in two populations at high risk for type 2 diabetes but differing by BMI. *Diabetes Care* 2001;24:1175–1180.

244. Kriska AM, Hanley AJG, Harris SB, Zinman B. Physical activity, physical fitness and insulin and glucose concentrations in an isolated native Canadian population experiencing rapid lifestyle change. *Diabetes Care* 2001;24:1787–1792.

245. Gregg EW, Gerzoff RB, Caspersen CJ, *et al.* Relationship of walking to mortality among US adults with diabetes. *Arch Intern Med* 2003;163:1440–1447.

246. Hurel SJ, Koppiker N, Newkirk J, *et al.* Relationship of physical exercise and ageing to growth hormone production. *Clin Endocrinol (Oxf)* 1999;51:687–691.

247. Smith MR, Rudd BT, Shirley A, *et al.* A radioimmunoassay for the estimation of serum dehydroepiandrosterone sulphate in normal and pathological sera. *Clin Chim Acta* 1975;65:5–13.

248. Orentreich N, Brind JL, Vogelman JH, *et al.* Long-term longitudinal measurements of plasma dehydroepiandrosterone sulfate in normal men. *J Clin Endocrinol Metab* 1992;75:1002–1004.

249. Birkenhager-Gillesse EG, Derksen J, Lagaay AM. Dehydroepiandrosterone sulfate (DHEAS) in the oldest old, aged 85 and over. *Ann NY Acad Sci* 1994;719:543–552.

250. Abbasi A, Duthie EH Jr., Sheldahl L, *et al.* Association of dehydroepiandrosterone sulfate, body composition, and physical fitness in independent community-dwelling older men and women. *J Am Geriatr Soc* 1998;46:263–273.

251. Heath G, Hagberg J, Ehsani A, Holloszy J. A physiological comparison of young and older endurance athletes. *J Appl Physiol* 1981; 51:634–640.

252. Hagberg J, Graves J, Limacher M, *et al.* Cardiovascular responses of 70- to 79-year-old men and women to exercise training. *J Appl Physiol* 1989;66:2589–2594.

253. Hagberg J, Montain S, Martin W, Ehsani A. Effect of exercise training on 60- to 69-year-old persons with essential hypertension. *Am J Cardiol* 1989;64:348–353.

254. Kohrt W, Malley M, Coggan A, *et al.* Effects of gender, age and fitness level on response of VO2max to training in 60- to 71-year olds. *J Appl Physiol* 1991;71:2004–2011.

255. Seals D, Reiling M. Effect of regular exercise on 24-hour arterial pressure in older hypertensive humans. *Hypertension* 1991;18: 583–592.

256. Kasch FW, Boyer JL, van Camp SP, *et al.* Effect of exercise on cardiovascular ageing. *Age Ageing* 1993;22:5–10.

257. Beere PA, Russell SD, Morey MC, *et al.* Aerobic exercise training can reverse age-related peripheral circulatory changes in healthy older men. *Circulation* 1999;100:1085–1094.

258. McGuire DK, Levine BD, Williamson JW, *et al.* A 30-year follow-up of the Dallas Bed Rest and Training Study. I. Effect of age on the cardiovascular response to exercise. *Circulation* 2001;104:1350–1357.

259. McGuire DK, Levine BD, Williamson JW, *et al.* A 30-year follow-up of the Dallas Bed Rest and Training Study. II. Effect of age on cardiovascular adaptation to exercise training. *Circulation* 2001; 104:1358–1366.

260. Fleg JL, Schulman SP, O'Connor FC, *et al.* Cardiovascular responses to exhaustive upright cycle exercise in highly trained older men. *J Appl Physiol* 1994;77:1500–1508.

261. Marti B, Pekkanen J, Nissinen A, *et al.* Association of physical activity with coronary risk factors and physical ability. Twenty-year follow-up of a cohort of Finnish men. *Age Ageing* 1989;18:103–109.

262. Powell KE, Thompson PD, Caspersen CI, Kendrick JS. Physical activity and the incidence of coronary heart disease. *Am Rev Public Health* 1987;8:253–287.

263. NIH Consensus Development Panel on Physical Activity and Cardiovascular Health. Physical activity and cardiovascular health. *JAMA* 1996;276:241–246.

264. Ornish D, Scherwitz LW, Billings JH, *et al.* Intensive lifestyle changes for reversal of coronary heart disease. *JAMA* 1998;280:2001–2007.

265. Katzel LI, Bleecker ER, Colman EG, *et al.* Effects of weight loss versus aerobic exercise training on risk factors for coronary disease in healthy, obese, middle-aged and older men. *JAMA* 1995;274:1915–1921.

266. Hellenius M-L, de Faire U, Berglund B, *et al.* Diet and exercise are equally effective in reducing risk for cardiovascular disease. Results of a randomized controlled study in men with slightly to moderately raised cardiovascular risk factors. *Atherosclerosis* 1993;103:81–91.

267. Myers J, Prakash M, Froelicher V, *et al.* Exercise capacity and mortality among men referred for exercise testing. *N Engl J Med* 2002; 346:793–801.

268. Mengelkoch LJ, Pollock ML, Limacher MC, *et al.* Effects of age, physical training and physical fitness on coronary heart disease risk factors in older track athletes at twenty-year follow-up. *J Am Geriatr Soc* 1997;45:1446–1453.

269. Bijnen FCH, Caspersen CJ, Feskens EJM, *et al.* Physical activity and 10-year mortality from cardiovascular diseases and all causes. *Arch Intern Med* 1998;158:1499–1505.

270. Wannamethee SG, Shaper AG, Walker M. Changes in physical activity, mortality and incidence of coronary heart disease in older men. *Lancet* 1998;351:1603–1608.

271. Dunn AL, Marcus BH, Kampert JB, *et al.* Comparison of lifestyle and structured interventions to increase physical activity and cardiorespiratory fitness. *JAMA* 1999;281:327–334.

272. Andersen RE, Wadden TA, Bartlett SJ, *et al.* Effects of lifestyle activity versus structured aerobic exercise in obese women: a randomized trial. *JAMA* 1999;281:335–340.

273. LaCroix AZ, Leveille SG, Hecht JA, *et al.* Does walking decrease the risk of cardiovascular disease hospitalizations and death in older adults? *J Am Geriatr Soc* 1996;44:113–120.

274. Hakim AA, Curb JD, Petrovitch H, *et al.* Effects of walking on coronary heart disease in elderly men: the Honolulu Heart Program. *Circulation* 1999;100:9–13.

275. Lakka TA, Venalainen JM, Rauramaa R, *et al.* Relation of leisure-time physical activity and cardiorespiratory fitness to the risk of acute myocardial infarction in men. *N Engl J Med* 1994;330:1549–1554.

276. Manson JE, Hu FB, Rich-Edwards JW, *et al.* A prospective study of walking compared with vigorous exercise in the prevention of coronary heart disease in women. *N Engl J Med* 1999;341:650–658.

277. Lee I-M, Rexrode KM, Cook NR, *et al.* Physical activity and coronary heart disease in women: is "no pain, no gain" passe? *JAMA* 2001;285:1447–1454.

278. Manson JE, Greenland P, LaCroix AZ, *et al.* Walking compared with vigorous exercise for the prevention of cardiovascular events in women. *N Engl J Med* 2002;347:716–725.

279. Williams PT. Coronary heart disease risk factors of vigorously active sexagenarians and septuagenarians. *J Am Geriatr Soc* 1998;46:134–142.

280. Sesso HD, Paffenbarger RS Jr, Lee I-M. Physical activity and coronary heart disease in men: the Harvard Alumni Health Study. *Circulation* 2000;102:975–980.

281. Lee I-M, Sesso HD, Paffenbarger RS. Physical activity and coronary heart disease risk in men: does the duration of exercise episodes predict risk? *Circulation* 2000;102:981–986.

282. Tanasescu M, Leitzmann MF, Rimm EB, *et al.* Exercise type and intensity in relation to coronary heart disease in men. *JAMA* 2002;288:1994–2000.

283. Wagner A, Simon C, Evans A, *et al.* Physical activity and coronary event incidence in Northern Ireland and France: the Prospective Epidemiological Study of Myocardial Infarction (PRIME). *Circulation* 2002;105:2247–2252.

284. Kujala UM, Sarna S, Kaprio J, *et al.* Natural selection of sports, later physical activity habits and coronary heart disease. *Br J Sports Med* 2000;34:445–449.

285. Erikksen G, Liestol K, Bjornhott J, *et al.* Changes in physical fitness and changes in mortality. *Lancet* 1998;352:759–762.

286. Blair SN, Kampert JB, Kohl HW III, *et al.* Influences of cardiorespiratory fitness and other precursors on cardiovascular disease and all-cause mortality in men and women. *JAMA* 1996;276:205–210.

287. Mittleman MA, Maclure M, Tofler GH, *et al.* Triggering of acute myocardial infarction by heavy physical exertion: protection against triggering by regular exertion. *N Engl J Med* 1993;329:1677–1683.

288. Wei M, Kampert JB, Barlow CE, *et al.* Relationship between low cardiorespiratory fitness and mortality in normal-weight, overweight and obese men. *JAMA* 1999;282:1547–1553.

289. Connelly JB, Cooper JA, Meade TW. Strenuous exercise, plasma fibrinogen and factor VII activity. *Br Heart J* 1992;67:351–354.

290. Ernst E. The role of fibrinogen as a cardiovascular risk factor. *Atherosclerosis* 1993;100:1–12.

291. MacAuley D, McCrum EE, Stott G, *et al.* Physical activity, physical fitness, blood pressure and fibrinogen in the Northern Ireland health and activity survey. *J Epidemiol Comm Health* 1996;50:258–263.

292. Levenson J, Giral P, Megnien JL, *et al.* Fibrinogen and its relations to subclinical extracoronary and coronary atherosclerosis in hypercholesterolemic men. *Arterioscler Thromb Vasc Biol* 1997;17:45–50.

293. Hambrecht R, Wolf A, Gielen S, *et al.* Effect of exercise on coronary endothelial function in patients with coronary artery disease. *N Engl J Med* 2000;342:454–460.

294. Smith JK, Dykes R, Douglas JE, *et al.* Long-term exercise and atherogenic activity of blood mononuclear cells in persons at risk of developing ischemic heart disease. *JAMA* 1999;281:1722–1727.

295. Koenig W, Sund M, Doring A, Ernst E. Leisure-time physical activity but not work-related physical activity is associated with decreased plasma viscosity: results from a large population sample. *Circulation* 1997;95:335–341.

296. Deskur E, Przywarska I, Dylewicz P, *et al.* Exercise-induced increase in hydrogen peroxide plasma levels is diminished by endurance training after myocardial infarction. *Int J Cardiol* 1998;67:219–224.

297. Higashi Y, Sasaki S, Kurisu S, *et al.* Regular aerobic exercise augments endothelium-dependent vascular relaxation in normotensive

as well as hypertensive subjects: role of endothelium-derived nitric oxide. *Circulation* 1999;100:1194–1202.

298. Muhlestein JB. Chronic infection and coronary artery disease. *Sci Med* 1998;November/December:16–25.

299. Muhlestein JB, Horne BD, Carlquist JF, *et al.* Cytomegalovirus seropositivity and C-reactive protein have independent and combined predictive value for mortality in patients with angiographically demonstrated coronary artery disease. *Circulation* 2000;102:1917–1923.

300. Ridker PM, Hennekens CH, Buring JE, *et al.* C-reactive protein and other markers of inflammation in prediction of cardiovascular disease in women. *N Engl J Med* 2000;342:836–843.

301. LaMonte MJ, Durstine JL, Yanowitz FG, *et al.* Cardiorespiratory fitness and C-reactive protein among a tri-ethnic sample of women. *Circulation* 2002;106:403–406.

302. Bolli R. Cardioprotective function of inducible nitric oxide synthase and role of nitric oxide in myocardial ischemia and preconditioning: an overview of a decade of research. *J Mol Cell Cardiol* 2001; 33:1897–1918.

303. Yang AL, Tsai SJ, Jiang MJ, *et al.* Chronic exercise increases both inducible and endothelial nitric oxide synthase gene expression in endothelial cells of rat aorta. *J Biomed Sci* 2002;9:149–155.

304. Kojda G, Harrison DG. Interactions between NO and reactive oxygen species: pathophysiological importance in atherosclerosis, hypertension, diabetes, and heart failure. *Cardiovasc Res* 1999;43:562–571.

305. Naruse K, Shimuzu K, Muramatsu M, *et al.* Long-term inhibition of NO synthesis promotes atherosclerosis in the hypercholesterolemic rabbit thoracic aorta: PGH2 does not contribute to impaired endothelium-dependent relaxation. *Arterioscler Thromb* 1994;14:746–752.

306. Menotti A, Keys A, Blackburn H, *et al.* Twenty-year stroke mortality and prediction in twelve cohorts of the Seven Countries Study. *Int J Epidemiol* 1990;19:295–301.

307. Lindsted KD, Tonstad S, Kuzma JW. Self-report of physical activity and patterns of mortality in Seventh-Day Adventist men. *J Clin Epidemiol* 1991;44:355–364.

308. Kiely DK, Wolf PA, Cupples LA, *et al.* Physical activity and stroke risk: the Framingham Study. *Am J Epidemiol* 1994;140:608–620.

309. Gillum RF, Mussolino ME, Ingram DD. Physical activity and stroke incidence in women and men. The NHANES I epidemiologic follow-up study. *Am J Epidemiol* 1996;143:860–869.

310. Sacco RL, Gan R, Boden-Albala B, *et al.* Leisure-time physical activity and ischemic stroke risk: the Northern Manhattan Stroke Study. *Stroke* 1998;29:380–387.

311. Hu FB, Stampfer MJ, Colditz GA, *et al.* Physical activity and risk of stroke in women. *JAMA* 2000;283:2961–2967.

312. Abbott RD, Rodriquez BL, Burchfiel CM, Curb JD. Physical activity in older middle-aged men and reduced risk of stroke: the Honolulu Heart Program. *Am J Epidemiol* 1994;139:881–893.

313. Lee I-M, Paffenbarger RS. Physical activity and stroke incidence: the Harvard Alumni Health Study. *Stroke* 1998;29:2049–2054.

314. Lee I-M, Hennekins CH, Berger K, *et al.* Exercise and risk of stroke in male physicians. *Stroke* 1999;30:1–6.

315. Jemal A, Thomas A, Murray T, Thun M. Cancer statistics, 2002. *CA Cancer J Clin* 2002;52:23–47.

316. Doll R, Peto R. The causes of cancer: quantitative estimates of avoidable risks of cancer in the United States today. *J Natl Acad Sci* 1981; 66:1191–1308.

317. Harvard Report on Cancer Prevention, Volume 1: Causes of Cancer. *Cancer Causes Control* 1996;7:S5–58.

318. Cherry T. A theory of cancer. *Med J Aust* 1922;1:425–438.

319. Woods JA. Exercise and resistance to neoplasia. *Can J Physiol Pharmacol* 1998;76:581–588.

320. Shepherd RJ, Shek PN. Association between physical activity and susceptibility to cancer: possible mechanisms. *Sports Med* 1998; 26:293–315.

321. Kiningham RB. Physical activity and the primary prevention of cancer. *Primary Care* 1998;25:515–536.

322. Byers T, Nestle M, McTierman A, *et al.* American Cancer Society guidelines on nutrition and physical activity for cancer prevention: reducing the risk of cancer with healthy food choices and physical activity. *CA Cancer J Clin* 2002;52:92–119.

323. Lee I-M. Physical activity, fitness and cancer. In: *Physical Activity, Fitness and Health. International Proceedings and Consensus Statement.* C Bouchard, RJ Shepherd and T Stephens (eds.) Human Kinetics, Champaign, IL, 1994, pp. 814–831.

324. US Department of Health and Human Services. *Physical Activity and Health: A Report of the Surgeon General.* Centers for Disease Control and Prevention, National Center for Chronic Disease Prevention and Health Promotion, Atlanta, GA, 1996.

325. Vena JE, Graham S, Zielezny M, *et al.* Occupational exercise and risk of cancer. *Am J Clin Nutr* 1987;45:318–327.

326. Brownson RC, Zahm SH, Chang JC, Blair A. Occupational risk of colon cancer. *Am J Epidemiol* 1989;130:675–687.

327. Fredriksson M, Bengtsson N-O, Hardell L, Axelson O. Colon cancer, physical activity and occupational exposure: a case-control study. *Cancer* 1989;63:1838–1842.

328. Tavani A, Braga C, LaVecchia C, *et al.* Physical activity and risks of cancers of colon and rectum: an Italian case-control study. *Br J Cancer* 1999;79:1912–1916.

329. White E, Jacobs EJ, Daling JR. Physical activity in relation to colon cancer in middle-aged men and women. *Am J Epidemiol* 1996;144:42–50.

330. Slattery ML, Edwards SL, Boucher KM, *et al.* Lifestyle and colon cancer: an assessment of factors associated with risk. *Am J Epidemiol* 1999;150:869–877.

331. Tang R, Wang JY, Lo SK, Hsieh LL. Physical activity, water intake and risk of colorectal cancer in Taiwan: a hospital-based case-control study. *Int J Cancer* 1999;82:484–489.

332. Thune I, Lund E. Physical activity and risk of colorectal cancer in men and women. *Br J Cancer* 1996;73:2234–2240.

333. Martinez ME, Giovannucci E, Spiegelman D, *et al.* Leisure-time physical activity, body size and colon cancer in women: Nurses' Health Study Research Group. *J Natl Cancer Inst* 1997;89:948–955.

334. Lee IM, Paffenbarger RS Jr. Physical activity and its relation to cancer risk: a prospective study of college alumni. *Med Sci Sports Exerc* 1994;26:831–837.

335. Lee IM, Manson JE, Ajani U, *et al.* Physical activity and risk of colon cancer: the Physicians' Health Study (United States). *Cancer Causes Control* 1997;8:568–574.

336. Slattery ML, Edwards SL, Ma KN, *et al.* Physical activity and colon cancer: a public health perspective. *Ann Epidemiol* 1997;7:137–145.

337. Giovannucci E, Colditz GA, Stampfer MJ, Willett WC. Physical activity, obesity and risk of colorectal adenoma in women (United States). *Cancer Causes Control* 1996;7:253–263.

338. Giovannucci E, Ascherio A, Rimm EB, *et al.* Physical activity, obesity and risk of colon cancer and adenoma in men. *Ann Intern Med* 1995;122:327–334.

339. Neugut AI, Terry MB, Hocking G, *et al.* Leisure and occupational physical activity and risk of colorectal adenomatous polyps. *Int J Cancer* 1996;68:744–748.

340. Enger SM, Longnecker MP, Lee ER, *et al.* Recent and past physical activity and prevalence of colorectal adenomas. *Br J Cancer* 1997;75:740–745.

341. Giovannucci E, Rimm EB, Stampfer MJ, *et al.* Aspirin use and the risk for colorectal cancer and adenoma in male health professionals. *Ann Intern Med* 1994;121:241–246.

342. La Vecchia C, Negri E, Franceschi S, *et al.* Aspirin and colorectal cancer. *Br J Cancer* 1997;76:675–677.

343. Sandler RS. Aspirin and other non-steroidal anti-inflammatory agents in the prevention of colorectal cancer. *Important Adv Oncol* 1996; 123–137.

344. Parker SL, Tong T, Bolden S, Wingo PA. Cancer statistics, 1997. *CA Cancer J Clin* 1997;47:5–27.

345. Arver B, Du Q, Chen J, *et al.* Hereditary breast cancer: a review. *Semin Cancer Biol* 2000;10:271–288.

346. Statland BE. Nutrition and cancer. *Clin Chem* 1992;38:1587–1594.

347. Kramer MM, Wells CL. Does physical activity reduce risk of estrogen-dependent cancer in women? *Med Sci Sports Exerc* 1996;28:322–334.

348. Henderson BE, Pike MC, Casagrande JT. Breast cancer and the oestrogen window hypothesis. *Lancet* 1981;2:363–364.

349. Friedenreich CM, Thune I, Brinton LA, Albanes D. Epidemiologic issues related to the association between physical activity and breast cancer. *Cancer* 1998;83:600–610.

350. Gammon MD, John EM, Britton JA. Recreational and occupational physical activities and risk of breast cancer. *J Natl Cancer Inst* 1998;90:100–117.

351. Bernstein L, Henderson BE, Hanisch R, *et al.* Physical exercise and reduced risk of breast cancer in young women. *J Natl Cancer Inst* 1994;86:1403–1408.

352. Thune I, Brenn T, Lund E, Gaard M. Physical activity and the risk of breast cancer. *N Engl J Med* 1997;336:1269–1275.

353. Rockhill B, Willett WC, Hunter DJ, *et al.* A prospective study of recreational physical activity and breast cancer risk. *Arch Intern Med* 1999;159:2290–2296.

354. Carpenter CL, Ross RK, Paganini-Hill A, Bernstein L. Lifetime exercise activity and breast cancer risk among post-menopausal women. *Br J Cancer* 1999;80:1852–1858.

355. Ueji M, Ueno E, Osei-Hyiaman D, *et al.* Physical activity and the risk of breast cancer: a case control study of Japanese women. *J Epidemiol* 1998;8:116–122.

356. Levi F, Pasche C, Lucchini F, LaVecchia C. Occupational and leisure time physical activity and the risk of breast cancer. *Eur J Cancer* 1999;35:775–778.

357. Gammon MD, Schoenberg JB, Britton JA, *et al.* Recreational physical activity and breast cancer risk among women under age 45 years. *Am J Epidemiol* 1998;147:273–280.

358. Rockhill B, Willett WC, Hunter DJ, *et al.* Physical activity and breast cancer risk in a cohort of young women. *J Natl Cancer Inst* 1998;90:1155–1160.

359. Frisch RE, Wyshak G, Albright NL, *et al.* Lower prevalence of breast cancer and cancers of the reproductive system among former college athletes compared to non-athletes. *Br J Cancer* 1985;52:885–891.

360. Frisch RE, Wyshak G, Albright NL, *et al.* Lower lifetime occurrence of breast cancer and cancers of the reproductive system among former college athletes. *Am J Clin Nutr* 1987;45:328–335.

361. Zheng W, Shu XO, McLaughlin JK, *et al.* Occupational physical activity and the incidence of cancer of the breast, corpus uteri and ovary in Shanghai. *Cancer* 1993;71:3620–3624.

362. Cottreau CM, Ness RB, Kriska AM. Physical activity and reduced risk of ovarian cancer. *Obstet Gynecol* 2000;96:609–614.

363. Mink PJ, Folsom AR, Sellers TA, Kushi LH. Physical activity, waist-to-hip ratio and other risk factors for ovarian cancer: a follow-up study of older women. *Epidemiology* 1996;7:38–48.

364. Hill HA, Austin H. Nutrition and endometrial cancer. *Cancer Cause Control* 1996;7:19–32.

365. Terry P, Baron JA, Weiderpass E, *et al.* Lifestyle and endometrial cancer risk: a cohort study from the Swedish Twin Registry. *Int J Cancer* 1999;82:38–42.

366. Levi F, La Vecchia C, Negri E, Franceschi S. Selected physical activities and the risk of endometrial cancer. *Br J Cancer* 1993;67:846–851.

367. Sturgeon SR, Brinton LA, Berman ML, *et al.* Past and present physical activity and endometrial cancer risk. *Br J Cancer* 1993; 68:584–589.

368. Shu XO, Hatch MC, Zheng W, *et al.* Physical activity and risk of endometrial cancer. *Epidemiology* 1993;4:342–349.

369. Moradi T, Nyren O, Bergstrom R, *et al.* Risk of endometrial cancer in relation to occupational physical activity: a nationwide cohort study in Sweden. *Int J Cancer* 1998;76:665–670.

370. Olson SH, Vena JE, Dorn JP, *et al.* Exercise, occupational activity and risk of endometrial cancer. *Ann Epidemiol* 1997;7:46–53.

371. Oliveria SA, Lee IM. Is exercise beneficial in the prevention of prostate cancer? *Sports Med* 1997;23:271–278.
372. Hartman TJ, Albanes D, Rautaiahti M, *et al.* Physical activity and prostate cancer in the Alpha-Tocopherol, Beta-Carotene (ATBC) Cancer Prevention Study (Finland). *Cancer Causes Control* 1998;9:11–18.
373. Sharma-Wagner S, Chokkalingam AP, Malker HS, *et al.* Occupation and prostate cancer risk in Sweden. *J Occup Environ Med* 2000; 42:517–525.
374. Oliveria SA, Kohl HW III, Trichopoulos D, Blair SN. The association between cardiorespiratory fitness and prostate cancer. *Med Sci Sports Exerc* 1996;28:97–104.
375. Platz EA, Kawachi I, Rimm EB, *et al.* Physical activity and benign prostatic hyperplasia. *Arch Intern Med* 1998;158:2349–2356.
376. Giovannucci E, Leitzmann M, Spiegelman D, *et al.* A prospective study of physical activity and prostate cancer in male health professionals. *Cancer Res* 1998;58:5117–5122.
377. Liu S, Lee IM, Linson P, *et al.* A prospective study of physical activity and risk of prostate cancer in US physicians. *Int J Epidemiol* 2000;29:29–35.
378. Cerhan JR, Torner JC, Lynch CF, *et al.* Association of smoking, body mass and physical activity with risk of prostate cancer in the Iowa 65+ Rural Health Study (United States). *Cancer Causes Control* 1997;8:229–238.
379. Pu YS. Prostate cancer in Taiwan: epidemiology and risk factors. *Int J Androl* 2000;23(Suppl 2):34–36.
380. Tymchuk CN, Barnard RJ, Heber D, Aronson WJ. Evidence of an inhibitory effect of diet and exercise on prostate cancer growth. *J Urology* 2001;166:1185–1189.
381. Hecht SS. Tobacco and cancer: approaches using carcinogen biomarkers and chemoprevention. *Ann N Y Acad Sci* 1997;833:91–111
382. Lee IM, Paffenbarger RS Jr. Physical activity and its relation to cancer risk: a prospective study of college alumni. *Med Sci Sports Exerc* 1994;26:831–837.
383. Thune J, Lund E. The influence of physical activity on lung-cancer risk: a prospective study of 81,516 men and women. *Int J Cancer* 1997;70:57–62.
384. Lee IM, Sesso HD, Paffenbarger RS Jr. Physical activity and risk of lung cancer. *Int J Epidemiol* 1999;28:620–625.
385. Ahlgren JD. Epidemiology and risk factors in pancreatic cancer. *Semin Oncol* 1996;23:241–250.

386. Michaud DS, Giovannucci E, Willett WC, *et al.* Physical activity, obesity, height and the risk of pancreatic cancer. *JAMA* 2001;286:921–929.

387. Gapstur SM, Gann P. Is pancreatic cancer a preventable disease? *JAMA* 2001;286:967–968.

388. Brett M, Barker DJP. The world distribution of gallstones. *Int J Epidemiol* 1976;5:335–341.

389. National Institutes of Health Consensus Development Conference statement on gallstones and laparoscopic cholecystectomy. *Am J Surg* 1993;165:390–398.

390. Hofmann AF. Primary and secondary prevention of gallstone disease: implications for patient management and research priorities. *Am J Surg* 1993;165:541–548.

391. Kato I, Nomura A, Stemmermann GN, Chyou P-H. Prospective study of clinical gallbladder disease and its association with obesity, physical activity and other factors. *Dig Dis Sci* 1992;37:784–790.

392. Leitzmann MF, Giovannucci EL, Rimm EB, *et al.* The relation of physical activity to risk for symptomatic gallstone disease in men. *Ann Intern Med* 1998;128:417–425.

393. Leitzmann MF, Rimm EB, Willett WC, *et al.* Recreational physical activity and the risk of cholecystectomy in women. *N Engl J Med* 1999;341:777–784.

394. Pahor M, Guralnik JM, Salive ME, *et al.* Physical activity and risk of severe gastrointestinal hemorrhage in older persons. *JAMA* 1994; 272:595–599.

395. Pahor M, Guralnik JM, Salive ME, *et al.* Disability and severe gastrointestinal hemorrhage: a prospective study of community dwelling older persons. *J Am Geriatr Soc* 1994;42:1–10.

396. Macfarlane GJ, Morris S, Hunt IM, *et al.* Chronic widespread pain in the community: the influence of psychological symptoms and mental disorder on healthcare seeking behavior. *J Rheumatol* 1999; 26:413–419.

397. Croft P, Rigby AS, Boswell R, *et al.* The prevalence of chronic widespread pain in the general population. *J Rheumatol* 1993;20: 710–713.

398. Lawrence RC, Helmick CG, Arnett FC, *et al.* Estimates of the prevalence of arthritis and selected musculoskeletal disorders in the United States. *Arthritis Rheum* 1998;41:778–799.

399. McCain GA. Role of physical fitness training in the fibrositis/fibromyalgia syndrome. *Am J Med* 1986;81:73–77.

400. Burckhardt CS, Mannerkorpi K, Hedenberg L, Bjelle A. A randomized, controlled clinical trial of education and physical training for women with fibromyalgia. *J Rheumatol* 1994;21:714–720.
401. Gowans SE, deHerck A, Voss S, Richardson M. A randomized, controlled trial of exercise and education for individuals with fibromyalgia. *Arthritis Care Res* 1999;12:120–128.
402. Richards SCM, Scott DL. Prescribed exercise in people with fibromyalgia: parallel group randomised controlled trial. *BMJ* 2002;325:185–187.
403. Weissman MM, Myers JK. Affective disorders in a US urban community. *Arch Gen Psychiatry* 1978;35:1304–1311.
404. Borson S, Barnes RA, Kukull WA, *et al.* Symptomatic depression in elderly medical outpatients. *J Am Geriatr Soc* 1986;34:341–347.
405. Fox KR. The influence of physical activity on mental wellbeing. *Public Health Nutr* 1999;2:411–418.
406. Cooper-Patrick L, Ford DE, Mead LA, *et al.* Exercise and depression in midlife: a prospective study. *Am J Public Health* 1997;87:670–673.
407. Steptoe A, Butler N. Sports participation and emotional wellbeing in adolescents. *Lancet* 1996;347:1789–1792.
408. Martinsen EW, Medhus A, Sandvik L. Effects of aerobic exercise on depression: a controlled study. *BMJ* 1985;291:109.
409. Camacho TC, Roberts RE, Lazarus NB, *et al.* Physical activity and depression: evidence from the Alameda County Study. *Am J Epidemiol* 1991;134:220–231.
410. McNeil JK, LeBlanc EM, Joyner M. The effect of exercise on depressive symptoms in the moderately depressed elderly. *Psychol Aging* 1991;6:487–488.
411. Blumenthal JA, Babyak MA, Moore KA, *et al.* Effects of exercise training on older patients with major depression. *Arch Intern Med* 1999;159:2349–2356.
412. North TC, McCullagh P, Tran ZV. Effect of exercise on depression. *Exerc Sport Sci Rev* 1990;18:379–415.
413. Craft LL, Landers DM. The effect of exercise on clinical depression and depression resulting from mental illness: a meta-analysis. *J Sport Exerc Psch* 1998;20:339–357.
414. Singh NA, Clements KM, Fiatarone MA. A randomized controlled trial of progressive resistance training in depressed elders. *J Gerontol A Biol Sci Med Sci* 1997;52:M27–M35.
415. Dimeo F, Bauer M, Varahram I, *et al.* Benefits from aerobic exercise in patients with major depression: a pilot study. *Br J Sports Med* 2001;35:114–117.

416. Ruuskanen JM, Ruoppila I. Physical activity and psychological well-being among people aged 65 to 84 years. *Age Ageing* 1995;24:292–296.

417. Singh NA, Clements KM, Singh MAF. The efficacy of exercise as a long-term antidepressant in elderly subjects: a randomized, controlled trial. *J Gerontol Med Sci* 2001;56A:M497–M504.

418. Steinberg H, Sykes EA, Moss T, *et al.* Exercise enhances creativity independently of mood. *Br J Sports Med* 1997;31:240–245.

419. Palmer J, Vacc N, Epstein J. Adult inpatient alcoholics: physical exercise as a treatment intervention. *J Studies Alcohol* 1988;49:418–421.

420. Rogers RL, Meyer JS, Mortel KF. After reaching retirement age physical activity sustains cerebral perfusion and cognition. *J Am Geriatr Soc* 1990;38:123–128.

421. Okumiya K, Matsubayashi K, Wada T, *et al.* Effects of exercise on neurobehavioral function in community-dwelling older people more than 75 years of age. *J Am Geriatr Soc* 1996;44:569–572.

422. Laurin D, Verreault R, Lindsay J, *et al.* Physical activity and the risk of cognitive impairment and dementia in elderly persons. *Arch Neurol* 2001;58:498–504.

423. Kramer AF, Hahn S, Cohen NJ, *et al.* Ageing, fitness and neurocognitive function. *Nature* 1999;400;418–419.

424. Dustman RE, Emmerson R, Shearer D. Physical activity, age and cognitive-neurophychological function. *J Aging Phys Act* 1994;2:143–181.

425. Grealy MA, Johnson DA, Rushton SK. Improving cognitive function after brain injury: the use of exercise and virtual reality. *Arch Phys Med Rehabil* 1999;80:661–667.

426. Black JE, Isaacs KR, Anderson BJ, *et al.* Learning causes synaptogenesis, whereas motor activity causes angiogenesis, in cerebellar cortex of adult rats. *Proc Natl Acad Sci USA* 1990;87:5568–5572.

427. Neeper SA, Gomez-Pinilla F, Choi J, Cotman C. Exercise and brain neurotrophins. *Nature* 1995;373:109.

428. Oliff HS, Berchtold NC, Isackson P, Cotman CW. Exercise-induced regulation of brain-derived neurotrophic factor (BDNF) transcripts in the rat hippocampus. *Brain Res Mol Brain Res* 1998;30:147–153.

429. van Praag H, Kempermann G, Gage FH. Running increases cell proliferation and neurogenesis in the adult mouse dentate gyrus. *Nature Neurosci* 1999;2:266–270.

430. van Praag H, Christie BR, Sejnowski TJ, Gage FH. Running enhances neurogenesis, learning, and long-term potentiation in mice. *Proc Natl Acad Sci* 1999;96:13427–13431.

431. Nakamura Y, Nishimoto K, Akamatu M, *et al.* The effect of jogging on P300 event related potentials. *Electromyogr Clin Neurophysiol* 1999;39:71–74.
432. Colcombe SJ, Erickson KI, Raz N, *et al.* Aerobic fitness reduces brain tissue loss in aging humans. *J Gerontol Med Sci* 2003;58A:178–180.
433. King AC, Oman RF, Brassington GS, *et al.* Moderate-intensity exercise and self-rated quality of sleep in older persons: a randomized controlled trial. *JAMA* 1997;277:32–37.
434. Vitiello MV, Prinz PN, Schwartz RS. Slow wave sleep but not overall sleep quality of healthy older men and women is improved by increased aerobic fitness. *Sleep Res* 1994;23:149 (Abstract).
435. Singh NA, Clements KM, Fiatarone MA. A randomized controlled trial of the effect of exercise on sleep. *Sleep* 1997;20:95–101.
436. Buchner DM. Physical activity and quality of life in older adults. *JAMA* 1997;277:64–66 (Editorial).
437. Schneider EL, Guralnik JM. The aging of America: impact on health care costs. *JAMA* 1990;263:2335–2340.
438. Fiatarone MA, Evans WJ. The etiology and reversibility of muscle dysfunction in the aged. *J Gerontology* 1993;48(Special Issue):77–83.
439. Jette AM, Branch LG. The Framingham Disability Study: II. Physical disability among the aging. *Am J Public Health* 1981;71:1211–1216.
440. Frontera WR, Meredith CN, O'Reilly KP, *et al.* Strength training in older men: skeletal muscle hypertrophy and impaired function. *J Appl Physiol* 1988;64:1038–1044.
441. Fiatarone MA, O'Neill EF, Ryan ND, *et al.* Exercise training and nutritional supplementation for physical frailty in very elderly people. *N Engl J Med* 1994;330:1769–1775.
442. Fiatarone MA, Marks EC, Ryan ND, *et al.* High intensity strength training in nonagenarians: effects on skeletal muscle. *JAMA* 1990;263:3029–3044.
443. Gill TM, Baker DI, Gottschalk M, *et al.* A program to prevent functional decline in physically frail, elderly persons who live at home. *N Engl J Med* 2002;347:1068–1074.
444. Mackinnon LT. Current challenges and future expectations in exercise immunology: back to the future. *Med Sci Sports Exerc* 1994;26:191–194.
445. Simon HB. The immunology of exercise: a brief review. *JAMA* 1984;252:2735–2738.
446. Nieman DC. Exercise immunology: practical applications. *Int J Sports Med* 1997;18:S91–S100.

447. Nieman DC. Exercise and resistance to infection. *Can J Physiol Pharmacol* 1998;76:573–580.

448. Peters EM, Bateman ED. Respiratory tract infections: an epidemiological survey. *S Afr Med J* 1983;64:582–584.

449. Peters EM. Altitude fails to increase susceptibility of ultramarathon runners to post-race upper respiratory tract infections. *S Afr J Sports Med* 1990;5:4–8.

450. Nieman DC, Johanssen LM, Lee JW, *et al.* Infectious episodes in runners before and after the Los Angeles Marathon. *J Sports Med Phys Fit* 1990;30:316–328.

451. Linde R. Running and upper respiratory tract infections. *Scand J Sports Sci* 1987;9:21–23.

452. Heath GW, Ford ES, Craven TE, *et al.* Exercise and the incidence of upper respiratory tract infections. *Med Sci Sports Exerc* 1991;23:152–157.

453. Anderson R, Lukey PT. A biological role for ascorbate in the selective neutralization of extracellular phagocyte-derived oxidants. *Ann NY Acad Sci* 1987;498:229–247.

454. Peters EM, Goetzsche JM, Grobbelaar B, Noakes TD. Vitamin C supplementation reduces the incidence of postrace symptoms of upper respiratory tract infection in ultramarathon runners. *Am J Clin Nutr* 1993;57:170–174.

455. Peters EM. Exercise, immunology and upper respiratory tract infections. *Int J Sports Med* 1997;18(Suppl 1):S69–S77.

456. Cannon JG, Orencole SF, Fielding RA, *et al.* Acute phase response in exercise: interaction of age and vitamin E on neutrophils and muscle enzyme release. *Am J Physiol* 1990;259:R1214–R1219.

457. Konig D, Weinstock C, Keul J, *et al.* Zinc, iron, and magnesium status in athletes — influence on the regulation of exercise-induced stress and immune function. *Exerc Immunol Rev* 1998;4:2–21.

458. Nieman DC. Immune response to heavy exertion. *J Appl Physiol* 1997;82:1385–1394.

459. Pedersen BK, Ostrowski K, Rohde T, Bruunsgaard H. Nutrition, exercise and the immune system. *Proc Nutr Soc* 1998;57:43–47.

460. Hoffman-Goetz L. Influence of physical activity and exercise on innate immunity. *Nutr Rev* 1998;56:S126–S130.

461. Woods JA, Davis M, Smith JA, Nieman DC. Exercise and cellular innate immune function. *Med Sci Sports Exerc* 1999;31:57–66.

462. Nieman DC, Pedersen BK. Exercise and immune function: recent developments. *Sports Med* 1999;27:73–80.

463. Nieman DC, Nehlsen-Cannarella SL, Markoff PA, *et al.* The effects of moderate exercise training on natural killer cells and acute upper respiratory tract infections. *Int J Sports Med* 1990;11:467–473.
464. Mathews CE, Ockene IS, Freedson PS, *et al.* Moderate to vigorous physical activity and risk of upper-respiratory tract infection. *Med Sci Sports Exerc* 2002;34:1242–1248.
465. Sansoni P, Cossarizza A, Brianti V, *et al.* Lymphocyte subsets and natural killer cell activity in healthy old people and centenarians. *Blood* 1993;82:2767–2773.
466. Shinkai S, Kohno H, Kimura K, *et al.* Physical activity and immune senescence in men. *Med Sci Sports Exerc* 1995;27:1516–1526.
467. Shinkai S, Konishi M, Shepherd RJ. Aging and immune response to exercise. *Can J Physiol Pharmacol* 1998;76:562–572.
468. Venjatraman JT, Fernandes G. Exercise, immunity and aging. *Aging Milano* 1997;9:42–56.
469. Nieman DC, Henson DA, Gusewitch G, *et al.* Physical activity and immune function in elderly women. *Med Sci Sports Exerc* 1993;25:823–831.
470. Woods JA, Lowder TW, Keylock KT. Can exercise training improve immune function in the aged? *Ann NY Acad Sci* 2002;959:117–127.
471. Abramson JL, Vaccarino V. Relationship between physical activity and inflammation among apparently healthy middle-aged and older US adults. *Arch Intern Med* 2002;162:1286–1292.
472. Ford ES. Does exercise reduce inflammation? Physical activity and C-reactive protein among US adults. *Epidemiology* 2002;13:561–568.
473. Karvonen MJ. Endurance sports, longevity and health. *Ann NY Acad Sci* 1977;301:653–655.
474. Yamaji K, Shepherd RJ. Longevity and causes of death of athletes. *J Human Ergology* 1977;6:15–27.
475. Paffenbarger RS, Hyde RT, Wing AL, Hsieh CC. Physical activity, all-cause mortality and longevity of college alumni. *N Engl J Med* 1986;314:605–613.
476. Pekkanen J, Marti B, Nissinen A, *et al.* Reduction of premature mortality by high physical activity: a 20-year follow-up of middle-aged Finnish men. *Lancet* 1987;1:1473–1477.
477. Powell KE, Thompson PD, Caspersen CJ, Kendrick JS. Physical activity and the incidence of coronary heart disease. *Annu Rev Public Health* 1987;8:253–287.
478. Kujala UM, Tikkanen HO. Disease-specific mortality among elite athletes. *JAMA* 2001;285:44–45.

479. Packer L. Oxidants, antioxidant nutrients and the athlete. *J Sports Sci* 1997;15:353–363.

480. Cesquini M, Torsoni MA, Ogo SH. Adaptive response to swimming exercise: antioxidant systems and lipid peroxidation. *J Anti-Aging Med* 1999;2:357–364.

481. Radak Z, Kaneko T, Tahara S, *et al.* The effect of exercise training on oxidative damage of lipids, proteins and DNA in rat skeletal muscle: evidence for beneficial outcomes. *Free Rad Biol Med* 1999;27:69–74.

482. Selman C, McLaren JS, Himanka MJ, Speakman JR. Effect of long-term cold exposure on antioxidant enzyme activities in a small mammal. *Free Rad Biol Med* 2000;28:1279–1285.

483. Itoh H, Ohkuwa T, Yamamoto T, *et al.* Effects of endurance physical training on hydroxyl radical generation in rat tissues. *Life Sci* 1998; 63:1921–1929.

484. Navarro-Arevalo A, Sanchez-del-Pino MJ. Age and exercise-related changes in lipid peroxidation and superoxide dismutase activity in liver and soleus muscle tissues of rats. *Mech Ageing Dev* 1998;104:91–102.

485. Navarro-Arevalo A, Canavate C, Sanchez-del-Pino MJ. Myocardial and skeletal muscle aging and changes in oxidative stress in relationship to rigorous exercise training. *Mech Ageing Dev* 1999;108:207–217.

486. Pilger A, Germadnik D, Formanek D, *et al.* Habitual long-distance running does not enhance urinary excretion of 8-hydroxy-deoxyguanosine. *Eur J Appl Physiol* 1997;75:467–469.

487. Brites FD, Evelson PA, Christiansen MG, *et al.* Soccer players under regular training show oxidative stress but an improved plasma antioxidant status. *Clin Sci Colch* 1999;96:381–385.

488. Hernandez R, Mahedero G, Caballero MJ, *et al.* Effects of physical exercise in pre- and postmenopausal women on lipid peroxidation and antioxidant systems. *Endocr Res* 1999;25:153–161.

489. Leaf DA, Kleinman MT, Hamilton M, Deitrick RW. The exercise-induced oxidative stress paradox: the effects of physical exercise training. *Am J Med Sci* 1999;317:295–300.

490. Ji LL. Exercise and oxidative stress: role of the cellular antioxidant systems. *Exerc Sports Sci Rev* 1995;23:135–166.

491. Ji LL, Leeuwenburgh C, Leichtweis S, *et al.* Oxidative stress and aging: role of exercise and its influences on antioxidant systems. *Ann N Y Acad Sci* 1998;854:102–117.

492. Mehta J, Li D. Epinephrine upregulates superoxide dismutase in human coronary artery endothelial cells. *Free Rad Biol Med* 2001; 30:148–153.

493. Sumida S, Tanaka K, Kitao H, Nakadomo F. Exercise-induced lipid peroxidation and leakage of enzymes before and after vitamin E supplementation. *Int J Biochem* 1989;21:835–838.
494. Simon-Schnass I, Pabst H. Influence of vitamin E on physical performance. *Int J Vit Nutr Res* 1988;58:49–54.
495. Novelli GP, Bracciotti G, Falsini S. Spin-trappers and vitamin E prolong endurance to muscle fatigue in mice. *Free Rad Biol Med* 1990;8:9–14.
496. Hartmann A, Nieb AM, Grunert-Fuchs M, *et al.* Vitamin E prevents exercise-induced DNA damage. *Mut Res* 1995;346:195–202.
497. Reznick A, Witt EH, Matsumoto M, Packer L. Vitamin E inhibits protein oxidation in skeletal muscle of resting and exercised rats. *Biochem Biophys Res Comm* 1992;189:801–806.
498. Sen CK, Rankinen T, Vaisanen S, Rauramaa R. Oxidative stress after human exercise: effect of N-acetylcysteine supplementation. *J Appl Physiol* 1994;76:2570–2577.
499. Leeuwenburgh C, Ji LL. Glutathione and glutathione ethyl ester supplementation alter glutathione homeostasis during exercise. *J Nutr* 1998;128:2420–2426.

4

Nutrition: Its Role in Aging, Health and Disease

Introduction

Numerous clinical and epidemiological studies have repeatedly confirmed the close relationship between health and nutrition. Indeed, malnutrition is well recognized as an enormous problem in many disadvantaged countries. Although significantly less of a problem in the industrialized nations, poor nutrition is still common and a major risk factor for numerous diseases/disorders. Poor nutrition not only includes excess caloric intake with its numerous health-related disorders (Chapter 2), but an inadequate intake of protein, fiber, various micronutrients (i.e. vitamins and minerals), n-3 fatty acids and excess saturated fat. Thus, inadequate nutrition includes (1) undernutrition due to insufficient caloric intake; (2) overnutrition due to excessive caloric intake; (3) deficiencies of protein and various micronutrients; and (4) dietary imbalance due to disproportionate food intake.[1] The major nutrition-associated diseases/disorders are listed in Table 4.1.

Dietary Guidelines

Although the elderly are the largest population segment in Western societies at risk for protein calorie malnutrition, poor nutrition

Table 4.1: Nutrition-Associated Diseases and Clinical Disorders

Nutritional Problem	Diseases/Disorders
Caloric (energy) deficit	Marasmus, increased morbidity/mortality, others
Protein deficit	Decreased immune function (lymphopenia, anergy), increased mortality, dementia, others
Excessive caloric intake	Obesity, type 2 diabetes, various cancers, hypertension, accelerated aging, coronary heart disease, cerebrovascular disease, depression
Deficient folic acid, vitamins B_6, B_{12}	Anemia, dementia, coronary heart disease, peripheral vascular disease, neural tube defects
Deficient vitamins A, C, D, E, carotenoids, flavonoids	Various cancers, coronary heart disease, cerebrovascular disease, decreased immune functions, cataracts, macular degeneration, neurodegenerative disorders, osteoporosis, others
Deficient trace metals (Zn, Mg, Se, Ca, Cu, etc.)	Decreased immune function, various cancers, coronary heart/cerebrovascular diseases, osteoporosis
Low fiber intake	Colon cancer, diverticulitis, constipation

characterized by excessive caloric and fat intake and vitamin/ mineral deficiencies are common not only in the elderly but in young adults, adolescents and children (Chapter 2). In general, a nutritious diet is best recognized and defined by the widely distributed Food Guide Pyramid (Fig. 4.1).[2] This guide calls for eating a variety of foods to supply critical nutrients, as well as the appropriate number of calories to maintain a healthy weight. The daily recommended adult servings are as follows: (1) bread, cereal, rice and pasta group, six to 11 servings; (2) fruit group, two to four servings; (3) vegetable group, three to five servings; (4) meat, poultry, fish, dry beans, eggs and nuts group, two to three servings; (5) milk, yogurt and cheese group, two to three servings; and (6) fats, oils and sweets group should be used sparingly.

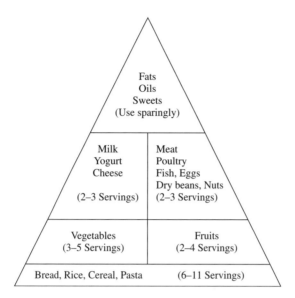

Figure 4.1: The Food Guide Pyramid.[2]

A serving size for each group is listed in Table 4.2. The specific number of servings beyond the indicated minimum varies, however, for each person depending on their body characteristics, metabolic rate and level of physical activity. Unfortunately, as Truswell recently reported,[3] these guides show food groups (e.g. meats, cereals, etc.) but do not emphasize the low-fat foods within the groups. For example, if someone eats six to 11 servings of bread or cereal, that person may well consume as much energy from fat as margarine or butter placed on the bread as from carbohydrate. Furthermore, these guides do not make it clear that predominately unsaturated fats (oils) should replace those rich in saturated fats.

Russell and associates[4] developed a narrower food pyramid for those aged 70 years and older (Fig. 4.2). Since the elderly are frequently dehydrated, their pyramid base consists of eight or more glasses of water each day. Although older people require the same nutrients as younger adults, they generally do not need as many calories. As a result, recommended servings are indicated with added servings (designated ≥) depending on the individual's needs [lifestyle (i.e. activity

Table 4.2: Examples: Single Food Group Servings

Group 1 (Bread, Cereal, Rice, Pasta)
1 slice bread
1/2 bagel or English muffin
1 ounce of ready-to-eat cereal
1/2 cup cooked rice or pasta

Group 2 (Fruits)
Medium-sized apple, orange, banana
3/4 cup of 100% fruit juice
1/2 cup chopped, cooked, or canned fruit

Group 3 (Vegetables)
1 cup raw leafy vegetables
3/4 cup vegetable juice
1/2 cup cooked, chopped or raw vegetables

Group 4 (Meat, Poultry, Fish, Eggs, Dry Beans, Nuts)
2–3 ounces cooked lean meat, poultry, fish
(average hamburger meat or half medium chicken breast is about 3 ounces)
1/2 cup tuna
1 cup cooked beans or peas
2 eggs

Group 5 (Milk, Yogurt, Cheese)
2 ounces of processed cheese
1 cup of milk or yogurt
1 1/2 ounces of natural cheese
2 cups cottage cheese

level), body composition (height, etc.)]. This modified pyramid indicates ≥ 6 servings of bread, cereal, rice and pasta; $\geq$ two servings of fruit; $\geq$ three servings of vegetables; $\geq$ two servings of meat, poultry, fish, dry beans, eggs and nuts; three servings of milk (low fat), cheese and yogurt. As with the standard food pyramid, fats, oils and sweets should be used sparingly. The flag is added at the pyramid peak as a reminder that many older people need vitamin and mineral supplements (e.g. calcium, vitamins D and B_{12}, and others) since aging metabolic changes may impede the absorption of some micronutrients from foods. In addition, small symbols (i.e. dots, triangles and an f +)

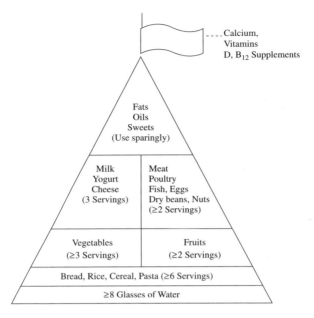

Figure 4.2: Modified Food Guide Pyramid for the elderly (after Russell *et al.*[4]).

floating throughout the pyramid, although not shown in Figure 4.2, respectively represent naturally occurring and added fats, sugars and a reminder to consume more fiber.

The food guide pyramid (Fig. 4.1), introduced in 1992, recommended that people should avoid fats and eat more carbohydrate-rich foods (e.g. bread, cereal, rice and pasta) in order to reduce serum cholesterol levels. Recent research studies, however, have shown that a high intake of refined carbohydrates (e.g. white bread and white rice) negatively affect the body's insulin and glucose levels. Hence, replacing these unhealthy carbohydrates with healthy fats (e.g. monounsaturated and polyunsaturated) decreases the risk of heart disease. As a result, a "new" food pyramid has been recently recommended (Fig. 4.3).[5]

The Nutrition Committee of the American Heart Association recently published dietary guidelines to prevent coronary heart disease (CHD).[6] The guidelines, designed to assist individuals in establishing and maintaining healthy lifestyles to decrease the risk of CHD, include the following general recommendations.

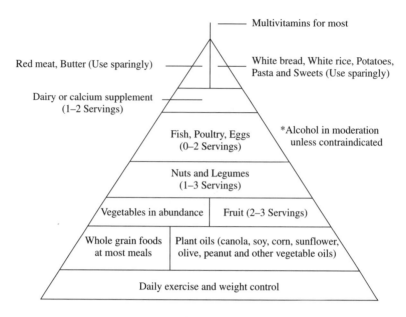

Figure 4.3: "New" Food Pyramid (after Willet and Stampfer[5]).

(1) Establish a healthy eating pattern including foods from all major food groups. These include a variety of fruits, vegetables, grains and fat-free and low-fat dairy products, fish, legumes, poultry and lean meats.

(2) Maintain a healthy body weight by matching caloric intake with overall energy needs. This includes limiting consumption of foods with high caloric density and/or low nutritional quality including a high sugar content. In addition, maintain a level of physical activity that achieves fitness and balances energy expenditure with energy intake.

(3) Maintain a desirable blood cholesterol and lipoprotein profile by limiting the intake of foods with a high content of saturated fatty acids and cholesterol. Emphasis should be directed to the use of grains and unsaturated fatty acids from vegetables, fish, legumes and nuts.

(4) Maintain a desirable blood pressure by (i) limiting the intake of sodium chloride to less than six grams a day; (ii) limiting alcohol consumption (no more than one drink a day for women and two

drinks a day for men); and (iii) maintaining a healthy body weight and a dietary pattern that emphasizes vegetables, fruits and a low-fat or fat-free diet.

Since these guidelines are discussed in detail, the publication is highly recommended for those professionals interested in the prevention of CHD, the number one cause of death in the United States and other industrialized countries.

Essential Vitamins and Minerals

Medical teaching has generally been that a healthy person can obtain adequate nutritional needs from diet alone. However, some studies suggest that these recommendations may not be adequate for optimal health. For example, several observational studies have found that periconceptual folic acid supplementation is associated with significant risk reduction of neural tube defects. In an early randomized trial, a high-dose folic acid supplement reduced the incidence of recurrent neural tube defects by 70%.[7] In addition, a randomized trial of a daily multivitamin that included 800 ug of folic acid in pregnant women without a history of affected pregnancy was stopped early because of a clear benefit in the prevention of a neural tube defect.[8] Furthermore, as the general population responds to nutritional advice to reduce total fat intake and increase the proportion of unsaturated fat from the diet, total vitamin E intake may fall while the requirement for vitamin E will increase. Future research, much of which is currently underway, will add critical information as to what constitutes a truly "healthy" diet and whether the current daily Dietary Reference Intakes (DRI) for vitamins and minerals is fully adequate to promote optimal health. The DRI now replaces the Recommended Dietary Allowances (RDA) which have been published since 1941. "The DRI are reference values that are quantitative estimates of nutrient intakes to be used for planning and assessing diets for healthy people."[9] The daily DRI for the major vitamins and minerals for several age groups are presented in Table 4.3.

Table 4.3: Vitamins/Minerals: Daily Dietary Reference Intakes*[9]

Micronutrient	Women	Men	Children (9–13 years)	Children (4–8 years)
Vitamin A (ug)	700	900	600	400
Vitamin C (mg)	75	90	45	25
Vitamin D (ug)	5–15	5–15	5	5
Vitamin E (mg)	15	15	11	7
Vitamin K (ug)	90	120	60	55
Thiamin (mg)	1.1	1.2	0.9	0.6
Riboflavin (mg)	1.1	1.3	0.9	0.6
Niacin (mg)	14	16	12	8
Vitamin B_6 (mg)	1.3–1.5	1.3–1.7	1.0	0.6
Folic acid (ug)	400	400	300	200
Vitamin B_{12} (ug)	2.4	2.4	1.8	1.2
Pantothenic acid (mg)	5	5	4	3
Biotin (ug)	30	30	20	12
Choline (mg)	425	550	375	250
Calcium (mg)	1000–1200	1000–1200	1300	800
Chromium (ug)	20–25	30–35	25	15
Copper (ug)	900	900	700	440
Fluoride (mg)	3	4	2	1
Iodine (ug)	150	150	120	90
Iron (mg)	8–18	8	8	10
Magnesium (mg)	320	420	240	130
Manganese (mg)	1.8	2.3	1.9	1.5
Molybdenum (ug)	45	45	34	22
Phosphorus (mg)	700	700	1250	500
Selenium (ug)	55	55	40	30
Zinc (mg)	8	11	8	5

*Interested readers are referred to Ref. No. 8 for more specific information regarding recommendations for other groups (i.e. other ages, infants, pregnancy and lactation).

Aging and Malnutrition

Nutritional well-being is a critical component of the health, independence and quality of life in older persons. Unfortunately, they represent the largest population segment at risk for malnutrition and dehydration in the US. Lowenstein[10] suggested a reference value of 1500 kcal/day as a minimum daily energy level for elderly people.

Wier, however, recommended 1800 kcal/day "particularly for those with selective protein rejection."[11]

About 85% of elderly persons living in their urban homes reportedly have one or more chronic disorders that could be improved with proper nutrition.[12] This interesting report used a revised Nutrition Screening Initiative Checklist of ten yes or no items to evaluate a person's nutritional status (Table 4.4). The nutrition score is as follows: (1) 0–2 points is rated good and should be rechecked in six months; (2) 3–5 points indicates moderate nutritional risk, and should be rechecked in three months; and (3) ≥ 6 points indicate high nutritional risk and immediate need for professional assistance (physician, dietitian or other qualified health or social service professional).

Nelson *et al.*[13] studied a group of older adults in an urban county clinic and hospital to determine the prevalence of hunger. About equal numbers of clinic and hospital patients were evaluated. The authors found that 12% did not have enough food, 13% had not eaten for an entire day, and 14% reported going hungry but not eating because they could not afford food. About 40% of the patients received food

Table 4.4: Nutrition Self-Test[12]

Condition	Points If "Yes"
1. Current disorder/illness led to changed kind and/or food amount	2
2. Eats two or less full meals/day	3
3. Eats few fruits, vegetables, milk products	2
4. Three or more drinks of beer, wine or liquor most days	2
5. Tooth/mouth problems make it hard to eat	2
6. Occasional inadequate money to buy food	4
7. Eats alone most of the time	1
8. Takes three or more prescription/over-the counter drugs/day	1
9. Lost or gained ten or more pounds in past six months without trying	2
10. Physically unable to always shop, cook, or feed self	2

stamps in the previous year, but half of them recently experienced either a reduction or complete loss of food stamps.

Unfortunately, nutritional deficits are too often labeled "biologic" when, in fact, they are "pathologic" since they affect overall well-being, cognitive functions, hospitalization outcomes, and the course of various medical conditions. The signs of malnutrition in older persons are often masked by concurrent disease, acute infections, or non-specific mental or functional changes. In addition, the recognition of malnutrition is often missed since changes in body composition are also common in the elderly (i.e. increased body fat, decreased skeletal muscle mass and bone density). For example, Wendland *et al.*[14] recently described the "iatrogenic component." In this study, they retrospectively analyzed the nutrient intake and delivery data obtained from 21 consecutive days in older residents of long-term care facilities in a geriatric teaching facility. They found that even if the diets (i.e. unrestricted and lactose-free) were completely consumed (about 2000 kcal/day), neither supplied sufficient quantities of vitamins and minerals needed to meet recommended intakes "making these deficiencies iatrogenic in nature." Moreover, as the caloric intake levels decreased to ranges commonly observed (i.e. 1000–1500 kcal/day), the number and severity of risk nutrient deficiencies increased. This problem is presumably also a common one among community-dwelling older people.

Total caloric malnutrition

Nutritional deficiency commonly increases with advancing age.[15] Numerous studies have shown that being underweight is significantly more common in the elderly than being overweight. Undernutrition is frequently associated with frailty and a deterioration of functional status; it is also a more significant risk factor for death. Indeed, about 16% of Americans over 65 years of age reportedly ingest fewer than 1000 calories/day, a level incompatible with an adequate intake of critical vitamins and minerals.[16] These underweight individuals are significantly depleted of muscle mass and fat stores (marasmus-like syndrome).

Approximately 60% of older people in long-term care facilities are reportedly malnourished.[17] Similarly, Saletti and associates[18] reported that 33% of elderly Swedish subjects living in assisted accommodations and 71% living in nursing homes were malnourished. Others[19] found that 40% of older patients were undernourished [Body Mass Index (BMI) <20 kg/m^2] at the time of hospital admission. These findings were substantiated in a later report in which 43% of patients were undernourished at the time of hospitalization as determined by low BMI and decreased serum albumin levels.[20] In this study, the outcomes of 353 elderly patients, mean age 81.8 years, were evaluated upon discharge after six months from an acute geriatric ward.[21] The major variables predicting mortality within six months of discharge were a Barthel Index on admission less than 65 years of age, malnutrition, presence of pressure sores and polypharmacy (many were taking five or more drugs).

The reasons of the nutritional decline in the elderly are complex and multifactorial. They include various diseases/disorders, psychological and social problems, relative immobility, malabsorption, decline in senses of taste and smell, chewing difficulties and medications, as well as social and financial problems (Table 4.5).[22–24]

Although the causes of caloric malnutrition are multiple, often complex and not readily reversible or treatable, some are and should be vigorously pursued since they are not secondary to aging or disease *per se* (i.e. excess alcohol intake, cognitive decline due to protein and vitamin/mineral deficiencies, physical inactivity and dentition problems among others). A few examples will be presented. Goodwin[22] recently reviewed the negative effects of ethanol, cognition and institutionalization on the nutritional status of the elderly. He emphasized the association between low blood levels of vitamins C, B$_{12}$, folate and riboflavin and poor scores on tests of cognitive function. The adverse effects of alcohol abuse on nutrition reportedly results from the following: (1) alcohol substitution for more nutritious calorie sources; (2) alcohol-depressed central nervous system (CNS) functioning; (3) alcohol-related dysfunction of the liver, pancreas, gut and other organs; and (4) possible increased

Table 4.5: Causes of Malnutrition in Older Persons

Adverse drug-nutrient interactions
Alcoholism
Anorexia (tardive or nervosa)
Chewing problems (e.g. dentures, loss of teeth, etc.)
Decreased social activity
Physical inactivity
Malabsorption syndromes
Medical disorders
    Cancer
    Cardiopulmonary disease
    Diabetes mellitus
    Hepatic disorders
    Hyperparthyroidism
    Hyperthyroidism
    Renal disease
Medications (e.g. digoxin, psychotropic drugs, etc.)
Neurological/psychological factors
    Bereavement
    Cognitive function
    Dementia
    Depression
    Isolation
    Paranoia
Physiologic disorders
    Atrophic gastritis
    Constipation
    Decreased senses of taste and smell
    Lactose intolerance
    Swallowing difficulties
Relative poverty
Shopping and food preparation difficulties
Unappealing foods (i.e. low salt, low fat, etc.)

metabolic requirements for various important nutrients. His review of prior published studies regarding the relationship between institutionalization and poor nutrition is in agreement with the observations noted above.

With respect to chewing difficulties, Mojon *et al.*[17] studied 324 institutionalized frail older adults, mean age 85 years, 50% of whom were malnourished (BMI <21 kg/m^2 and/or serum albumin <3.3 g/dL). Among the edentulous, wearing dentures with defective bases or not wearing them at all were the factors most often associated with malnutrition. Other chewing problems included the number of occluding pairs of teeth, number of retaining roots and the presence of loose teeth. Using these criteria, 31% of the group were orally compromised. Similarly, Krail and associates[25] studied the effects of the number of teeth, denture type and masticatory function on nutrient intake in elderly men in Veterans' Administration Hospitals. They found that dietary intake of fiber, zinc, magnesium and calcium, as well as various vitamins, protein and fiber, did not meet the minimum recommended standards. Moreover, nutrient intakes progressively decreased with impaired dentition independent of age, smoking status and alcohol intake. In addition, the dietary deficiencies were inversely related with masticatory function. The authors suggested that prevention of tooth loss and replacement of missing teeth may improve the diets of elderly people.

Protein-energy malnutrition

Protein-energy malnutrition is also very common in the elderly. Indeed, numerous reports indicate that 30% to 55% of hospitalized patients are protein undernourished.[26] The US minimum recommended daily allowance (RDA) for protein intake is shown in Table 4.6.[27] Many older people selectively reject protein while eating more tasty foods (snack foods and sweets). For example, one study of a group of underweight elderly people found that most of them rejected about half of the total calories and consumed only 10 to 30 grams of protein a day.[11] In two studies, about 60% of older patients were found to be protein-energy undernourished at the time of hospital admission or developed serious nutritional deficits prior to discharge.[28,29] These nutritional deficits are often associated with an increased risk of various morbid events.[30] In addition to muscle wasting, prolonged protein and micronutrient deficiency impairs immune competence and threatens survival during an acute illness. For example, Potter *et al.*[31] found that elderly malnourished hospitalized patients were much more likely to develop sepsis, which significantly increased their length of hospital stay. In

Table 4.6: Minimum Daily Allowance of Dietary Protein (g/day)[27]

Age (Years)	Males	Females
11–14	45.0	46.0
15–18	59.0	44.0
19–50	60.0	46.0
50+	63.0	50.0

addition, Weir[11] reported that "many of our patients showed apathy and indifference, loss of interest in former activities and hobbies, mental confusion, forgetfulness, sometimes incontinence and even full-blown senility."

Sullivan and associates[32] referred to several prior studies that reported (1) protein-energy undernutrition is often not diagnosed during hospitalization and the risk for further nutritional deterioration is frequently not recognized; (2) elderly hospitalized patients commonly subsist on very low nutrient intakes for days; and (3) even when nutritional deficiencies are recognized, adequate nutrition support is uncommonly provided. To further examine this problem, these authors[32] prospectively studied protein-energy malnutrition in elderly hospitalized patients. They found that 21% had an average daily nutrient intake of less than 50% of their calculated maintenance requirement. Severity of illness, length of stay and admission serum albumin and prealbumin levels of this group did not differ significantly from the other patients studied. Upon discharge, the undernutrition group had significantly lower blood levels of cholesterol, albumin and prealbumin. They also had high rates of in-hospital mortality and 90-day mortality. The authors stressed that their findings are not unique to their hospital. Rather, they referenced several earlier studies that also reported that hospitalized patients too often receive less than optimal nutritional care.

Others[33] set out to determine the extent to which patients with objective signs of protein-energy undernutrition had been diagnosed and whether the diagnosis was documented in the patients' medical record. This cross-sectional study involved 121 non-critically ill patients, aged 70 years and older. The results showed the following: (1) nine patients had weight/height ratios below 60% of normal, 16 patients between 60% and 75% of normal and 41 patients between 74% to 90% of normal; (2) of these 66 patients, only 24 were recognized as being undernourished on admission and only five received nutritional support while in the hospital; and (3) none of the patients were diagnosed as having malnutrition on discharge. It has also been reported that protein-energy undernutrition is a strong independent risk factor for mortality within one year of discharge.[34] This study involved 350 randomly selected patients (99% male; 75% were white), 322 of whom were discharged alive; the mean age was 76 years. Within one year of discharge, 20% died. The variable most strongly associated with mortality was the discharge weight (BMI ≤ 18 kg/m^2 and ≥ 35 kg/m^2), self-dressing ability and a discharge diagnosis of cardiac arrhythmia (most often atrial fibrillation). When these four factors were included in their analysis model, the differentiation of survivors from those who died before one year had a sensitivity of 69%, specificity of 69% and overall predictive value of 69%.

Protein-calorie malnutrition is not limited to hospitalized patients. Rudman and Feller[35] reviewed the literature prior to 1989 and reported that the prevalence of protein-calorie undernutrition was 30% to 60% in nursing home populations; the annual mortality rate was 10% to 40%. These latter people were older, more dependent and had lower serum levels of albumin and cholesterol, lower BMI, smaller triceps skin fold and lower blood hematocrit and hemoglobin levels than those more likely to survive.

Measurement of Nutritional Status

The presence of malnutrition based solely on weight is often not reliable since some patients are dehydrated while others may be protein malnourished but not calorically deficient (selective protein rejection), edematous, or cannot be easily or accurately weighted due to illness or immobilization. As a result, several more objective measures of poor nutrition and increased morbidity have been studied. These include various anthropometric and laboratory measurements (Table 4.7); several of these will be briefly discussed.

Table 4.7: Measurements for Protein-Calorie Malnutrition

Anthropometric Measurements
Percentage of ideal body weight
Body mass index (BMI)
Triceps skinfold thickness
Mid-arm muscle circumference
Corrected arm muscle area
Creatinine/height index

Laboratory Measurements
Hemoglobin/hematocrit
Plasma amino acids
Serum albumin
Serum cholesterol
Total lymphocyte count (% lymphocytes X WBC)
Transferrin
Transthyretin (prealbumin)

Antropometric measurements

BMI is perhaps the most commonly used measure to evaluate one's nutritional status. It is calculated by the formula, BMI = weight (kg)/ height $\times$ height (m^2). The generally accepted target BMI is 20.0–24.9 kg/m^2 while 25.0–29.9 kg/m^2 is considered overweight, and $\geq$30 kg/m^2 is obese. Undernutrition is present when BMI is <20 kg/m^2 (see Chapter 2 for a more detailed discussion).

Friendman *et al.*[36] described the use of a corrected arm muscle area (CAMA) as a measure of malnutrition. The CAMA (cm^2) = AMA (cm^2) $-$ 10 for men and AMA (cm^2) $-$ 6.5 for women; AMA (cm^2) = mid-arm circumference (cm)/4 pi, where pi = 3.1416. The mid-arm circumference was measured at the halfway point between the acromion and the olecranon. Using these measurements, severe wasting malnutrition was defined as CAMA $\leq$16.0 cm^2 for men and 16.9 cm^2 for women. They found that the malnourished subjects had a significantly higher 90-day mortality (50%) than the non-malnourished subjects (6.2%).

Laboratory tests for protein-energy malnutrition

Albumin

Serum albumin is the major protein synthesized in the liver; its half-life is about 20 days. Albumin has many physiologic functions including maintenance of oncotic pressure and the transportation of various substances (e.g. calcium and other ions, various hormones, drugs, etc.) through the vascular system to organs and tissues. As a result, the measurement of serum albumin is a very useful measure of chronic protein energy malnutrition, especially in the absence of liver disease or a chronic inflammatory disorder (i.e. rheumatoid arthritis, systemic lupus erythematosus, tuberculosis, sarcoidosis, etc.), all of which are associated with a decreased concentration. Indeed, numerous studies have shown that a decreased serum albumin level is a risk factor not only for CHD,[37] but for overall mortality in various settings.

Phillips *et al.*[38] prospectively studied 7735 middle-aged men over a 9.2-year period. They found a "marked increase in mortality rate with decreasing serum albumin concentrations ..." This increase persisted after adjustment for age, social class, town of residence, cigarette smoking, blood pressure and serum cholesterol. More specifically, serum albumin levels less than 4.0 g/dL showed a mortality rate of 23/1000/year compared with 4/1000/year for a concentration of 4.8 g/dL or higher. A later study was undertaken "to identify variables that could explain the association between low albumin and a nine- to 12-year mortality follow-up" among community-dwelling and institutionalized people 60 years and older.[39] After controlling for age, blood urea nitrogen, triglycerides, history of various diseases and inability to shop owing to medical conditions, the risk of mortality for those in the community-dwelling group with albumin levels of 40 g/L (4.0 g/dL) or higher was about half the risk (0.46) of those with albumin values less than 40 g/L. Serum albumin was also inversely associated with mortality among the institutionalized subjects after controlling for various confounders. Interestingly, the authors concluded that serum albumin is a long-term predictor of mortality in community-dwelling individuals, but a short-term predictor for those who are institutionalized. Others[40] studied the serum albumin level in 15,511 patients 40 years of age and older within 48 hours of hospitalization for acute illness to predict in-hospital death, length of stay and readmission. Here, patients with albumin levels less than 3.4 g/dL were more likely to die, were hospitalized longer and readmitted sooner, more often than those with normal albumin levels. The in-hospital mortality rate was 14% among those with low albumin levels compared with 4% among patients with normal levels. Importantly, the serum albumin concentration was a significantly stronger predictor of death, length of stay and readmission than age.

More recently, Sullivan and Walls[41] evaluated protein-energy undernutrition as a risk factor for mortality beyond one year after hospital discharge in a group of elderly patients (mean age 76 years, 99% men, 75% white). The 322 patients were followed for an average of six years. Upon admission and at discharge, each patient completed a comprehensive medical, functional, neuro-psychological, socioeconomic and nutritional assessment. The authors also created a "nutrition risk" indicator which included serum albumin and other nutrition indicators in the data set. The patients were divided into three nutrition groups: (1) "high-risk" — serum albumin <3.0 g/dL or BMI <19 kg/m^2; (2) "low-risk" — serum albumin ≥3.5 g/dL and BMI ≥22 kg/m^2; and (3) "moderate-risk" — including all others. Within the six-year period following hospital discharge, 237 patients died (74%). The variable most strongly associated with mortality at discharge was the "nutrition-risk." Other, albeit less important risk factors, were a diagnosis of congestive heart failure, discharge location (home versus institution), age and marital status. Similarly, a two-year follow-up study of elderly male patients on a geriatric rehabilitation unit found that serum albumin level 3.5 g/dL or less on admission was a stronger predictor of two-year post-hospitalization mortality than infection, Nutritional Status Score of moderate or severe compromise and discharge to a place other than home.[42]

Albumin levels and mortality have also been studied in patients with various clinical conditions, including hip fractures.[43] Here,

39 consecutive patients with hip fractures were followed for 12 months, ten of whom died during this time. Those who were living in institutions prior to their fracture had significantly lower albumin levels upon hospital admission than those living in private homes (29.8 g/L versus 34.4 g/L). Furthermore, those who died had significantly lower admission levels than those alive after 12 months (29.4 g/L versus 34.2 g/L). Patients with albumin levels of 30 g/L (3.0 g/dL) or lower were particularly at risk for increased mortality. Gibbs *et al.*[44] recently evaluated the preoperative albumin level as a predictor of operative mortality and morbidity in 54,215 patients who underwent non-cardiac surgery in 44 Veterans Affairs medical centers. The authors concluded that serum albumin level is a "better predictor of surgical outcomes than many preoperative patient characteristics." They also concluded that serum albumin "should be used more frequently as a prognostic tool to detect malnutrition and risk of adverse surgical outcomes."

Transferrin

The serum transferrin level has also been used as an indicator of protein-calorie undernutrition (normal level $\geq$ 200 mg/dL).[45] Levels of 150–200 mg/dL, 100–150 mg/dL and <100 mg/dL are indicative of mild, moderate and severe protein depletion, respectively.[46] However, since the half-life of transferrin is less than albumin (i.e. <18 days), nutritional depletion results in decreased serum levels before any changes in serum albumin are noted. Care must also be exercised in interpreting transferrin values since increased concentrations are typical of iron deficiency anemia, whereas decreased levels are common in the anemia of chronic disease.

Cholesterol

Cholesterol is a basic element of cell membranes and is likely to be essential in large tissue repair processes such as sepsis or following trauma. Hypocholesterolemia occurs in a variety of acute and chronic disorders and numerous epidemiologic studies have reported an inverse relationship between low serum cholesterol levels and increased mortality. More specifically, Oster *et al.*[47] showed an increased mortality rate among patients admitted to an acute care hospital with an admission serum cholesterol level below 120 mg/dL. Others[48] studied the clinical characteristics, lipoprotein abnormalities and outcomes of elderly hospitalized patients with hypocholesterolemia. Their results showed that 9% of patients 65 years of age and older whose admission cholesterol level was 160 mg/dL or more, decreased to less than 120 mg/dL during their hospital stay. These patients were more likely than the control group to have undergone surgery and not to have taken food orally for five or more days. They had a longer length of stay, more complications and were more likely to die while hospitalized. Gui and associates[49] reported that 38% of the critically ill surgical patients admitted to the intensive care unit were hypocholesterolemic (<120 mg/dL). This compared with 17% of all patients admitted to the surgical service with levels below 130 mg/dL. They found a U-shaped relationship between cholesterolemia and mortality and noted that the hypocholesterolemic patients were often, although not always, malnourished.

Hypocholesterolemia has also been reported as a predictor of death in nursing home residents.[50] These workers studied the relationship of cholesterol, albumin, hemoglobin and glucose levels and anthropometric variables to the risk of death in 224 nursing home residents. They found a ten-fold increase in relative risk for death with cholesterol levels less than 3.4 mmol/L (<131.5 mg/dL). They also noted that decreased levels of albumin and hemoglobin and elevated glucose were associated with increased mortality. The authors suggested that since hypocholesterolemia also correlated significantly with the presence of decubiti, increased leukocyte count and use of enteral feeding, the association between low cholesterol levels and risk of death was most likely due to increased malnutrition and infection.

Total lymphocyte count

Decreased immune function, a well-known phenomenon of protein-energy malnutrition, is characterized by a decrease in total lympho-cyte count (total white blood cell count times the percentage of lymphocytes). Protein malnutrition may also lead to anergy to various skin tests. A total lymphocyte count less than 1800/uL is a useful nonspecific marker for chronic protein malnutrition; counts less than 800/uL suggest severe malnutrition (reference range 2000–3500/uL). Skin tests for mumps and/or *Candida* antigens with less than 5 mm induration at 24 to 48 hours are also an indication of protein deficiency.[45,51] These individuals are also more susceptible to infections from *Mycobacteria*, *Listeria* and *Salmonella* microorganisms.[51] In addition, protein malnutrition negatively impairs various complement system components including mucosal secretory IgA antibodies, antibody affinity and the ability of phagocytes to kill ingested bacteria and fungi.[52]

Amino acids

The concentration of plasma amino acids depends on several factors including the amount and composition of dietary protein, muscle protein metabolism and the reserve labile protein in various tissues, particularly in the liver. Polge *et al.*[53] compared the plasma amino acid levels between two groups of elderly people, one of which was healthy and the other malnourished. Both groups were of similar age and sex. The study results showed that both essential and non-essential amino acids were significantly decreased in the protein energy malnourished patients compared with the control group. Plasma branched-chain and urea cycle amino acids were significantly decreased as were alanine and glutamic acid plus glutamine levels. The authors concluded that the plasma amino acid pattern reflects the severity of protein energy malnutrition in elderly patients.

Protein Supplementation
in Protein-Energy Malnutrition

A recent study evaluated a nutritional intervention program in elderly nursing home residents.[54] This prospective, randomized, controlled study determined the nutritional status at day 0 and day 60. It consisted of a dietary intake record, anthropometry, hand-grip strength and a mini-nutritional assessment. The subjects were divided into four groups based on their mini-nutritional assessment score as follows: the well nourished group received no supplementation (score 24); those at risk of malnutrition were randomized to oral supplementation or no supplementation (score 17–23.5); and those who were malnourished received oral supplementation (score <17). On day 60, the total energy intake was significantly higher in both supplemented groups. Those at risk of malnutrition who were supplemented significantly improved their mini-nutritional assessment score and increased their weight (1.4 ± 0.5 kg; about 3.1 pounds) compared with the non-supplemented at risk group. Supplementation of the malnourished group also significantly increased their mini-nutritional assessment score and weight grain (1.5 ± 0.4 kg; about 3.3 pounds).

Bos *et al.*[55] studied the metabolic response to short-term nutritional supplementation [1.67 MJ (about 400 kcal) and 30 g of protein each day for ten days] in moderately malnourished elderly people and compared the results with a group of healthy young adults. A control group of malnourished elderly patients received no supplementation. The supplemented malnourished elderly group had a significantly greater fat-free mass gain than the elderly malnourished unsupplemented group. They also had a significantly greater increase in fasting rate of protein synthesis than the healthy young supplemented adults. The authors concluded there was an anabolic protein metabolic response to short-term dietary supplementation in malnourished elderly people and that it likely improves both muscle strength and functional capacity.

Economic Costs of Hospitalized Malnourished Patients

An increased prevalence of medical complications and mortality rate are reportedly associated with malnutrition in hospitalized patients.[56] However, several early studies suggested that providing nutritional support to these patients reduces both medical complications and mortality.[57-59] It also presumably reduces the length of stay and financial costs.

To evaluate and quantify these two latter questions, Reilly and associates[56] retrospectively reviewed the hospital records of 771 patients in two acute care hospitals using generally accepted criteria for malnutrition (i.e. serum albumin ≤ 3.5 g/dL, total lymphocyte count ≤ 1500/uL, height/weight ratio $<80\%$ of normal, subjective/historical notes in hospital records from health professionals). The study found the likelihood of malnutrition (LOM) was present in 59% and 48% of medical and surgical patients, respectively. Moreover, LOM patients were respectively 2.6 and 3.4 times as likely to suffer a minor or major complication and 3.8 times as likely to die compared to patients without LOM. The increased length of stay ranged from 1.1 to 12.8 excessive days. In terms of 1985 dollars, the LOM status increased excess costs and charges by US$1738 and US$3557 per patient, respectively. When complications occurred, the excess costs and charges per patient were US$2996 and US$6157. Importantly, they found that serum albumin was the strongest predictor of cost. The authors concluded that very few patients with LOM received early nutrition support. They also concluded that early detection and aggressive treatment of patients with LOM is very cost-effective.

Similarly, Robinson *et al.*[60] prospectively audited 100 admissions to a general medical service to study the association of initial patient nutritional status to actual length of stay (LOS) and hospital charges. This information was then compared with the allowed LOS and estimated reimbursement under the diagnosis-related groups (DRGs) payment system. They found that 45% of the malnourished group were hospitalized longer than allowed under DRGs compared with 30% of normal patients and 37% of those who were borderline malnourished. The average LOS for the malnourished group was 15.6 ± 2.2 days compared to about 10 days in the other two groups. Although the estimated 1987 DRG reimbursement was similar for all three groups (US$4352 to US$5124), the actual hospital charges were significantly greater in the malnourished and borderline malnourished group (US$16,691 ± US$4389 and US$14,118 ± US$4962, respectively) compared to the normal patients (US$7692 ± US$687). As a result, the DRG system has a severe adverse financial impact in the care of poorly nourished patients. The authors recommended early recognition and aggressive treatment of malnourished patients in order to decrease the LOS and cost deficit incurred by poorly nourished patients.

In a later study, Bernstein *et al.*[26] projected cost reductions and revenue potential for their community hospital in 1988 dollars at 1%, 5% and 10% reduction in LOS by identifying malnourished patients and vigorously managing their nutritional status. The estimated cost reductions were approximately US$500,000, US$2 million and US$5 million dollars respectively, while the corresponding projected revenue potentials were approximately US$1 million, US$5.5 million and US$11 million, respectively. The authors indicated that even a minimum level of timely nutritional support for selected patients could save US acute-care hospitals at least US$6 billion (1988 dollars) annually by reducing the average length of stay. These latter authors recently published practice guidelines for a malnutrition treatment program in a community hospital.[61] The importance of nutritional care management was recently reviewed.[62]

Nutrition Counseling

In Western societies, undernutrition has been replaced not only by an increased consumption of high-fat foods, but of total caloric excess. As a result, nutritional counseling is a very important part of health promotion. As with other health matters, primary care physicians are the most frequently consulted professional group for nutritional advice.[63] Yet, an early national survey reported that about 75% of American adults who thought they were not getting enough exercise indicated that they had never received exercise advise from their doctors and only 15% of dieters and 8% of ex-smokers reported that their physicians' recommendation had motivated them to diet or stop smoking.[64] Indeed, fewer than half of Massachusetts primary care physicians polled in 1981 reported even asking their patients about diet, exercise or stress.[65] Unfortunately, a more recent survey by the same researchers found that even fewer Massachusetts physicians counseled their patients regarding these matters than they did 13 years previously.[66] Of the physicians surveyed, 73% practiced internal medicine, 18% family practice and 9% general practice. The results of this latter study were as follows: (1) 55% agreed people should "avoid foods high in saturated fats"; (2) 63% for "moderation in alcohol drinking"; (3) 52% for "avoid excess calories"; (4) 49% for "moderate daily physical activity"; (5) 47% for "eat a balanced diet"; (6) 13% for "decrease salt consumption"; and (7) 6% for "minimize sugar intake."

A nutrition study involving Dutch consumers found that physicians were perceived to have a very high level of expertise and were consulted more often about nutritional needs than any other professional group.[67] Although most of these physicians expressed interest in the role of nutrition in health, they indicated that there are several major barriers to involving themselves in nutrition issues with their patients. The major ones, as with most other physicians, are (1) lack of professional training in nutrition, (2) lack of time to give nutritional advice even if they feel qualified, and (3) an impression that most patients lack the motivation to change their dietary patterns or lifestyles. Nevertheless, other studies indicate that most people are very concerned about their lifestyle and would welcome more appropriate counseling.[68] Moreover, they felt that physicians should be more concerned about patient lifestyles and disease prevention.

National objectives and guidelines clearly call upon physicians to help reduce the number of chronic diseases by advising patients to consume fewer calories and exercise more. Unfortunately, physicians are most likely to provide behavioral recommendations to those who already have a disease or disorder (e.g. obesity, CHD, cancer, diabetes, hypertension, etc.). In order to understand the various factors that influence physicians' advising decisions, Kreuter *et al.*[69] studied 915 adult patients and 27 physicians from four community-based family medicine clinics. They found that a high BMI was the strongest predictor of receiving advice to increase physical activity, while an elevated blood cholesterol level was the strongest predictor of receiving advice to eat less. However, neither the actual content of the patients' diet nor their level of physical activity was guided by "quick but fallible heuristics (i.e. learning by self-teaching) that systematically exclude patients whose needs are not easily visible."

Is physician counseling effective? A study of 12,835 obese (BMI $\geq$30 kg/m^2) adults 18 years and older who had visited their physicians for a routine examination during the previous 12 months was recently published.[70] Here, less than half (42%) of the participants were counseled to lose weight. The authors found that those most likely to be counseled were female, middle-aged, more educated, lived in the northeast, reported poorer perceived health, were more obese and had type 2 diabetes. Importantly, those who were advised to lose weight were significantly more likely to try than those who were not counseled to do so. The authors stressed that barriers to counseling must be identified and addressed. Another recent study measured the effect of brief behavioral counseling in general medical practice on the consumption of fruits and vegetables among 217 patients aged 18 to 70 years from a low income population.[71] The participants were randomly assigned to either of two counseling groups: brief individual behavioral counseling or nutrition education counseling. Again, behavioral counseling was very effective. The consumption of fruits and vegetables increased from baseline to 12 months by 1.5 and 0.9 portions, respectively; those eating five or more portions each day increased by 42% and 27%, respectively. Certainly, the ultimate benefits of appropriate counseling can be enormous: increased life expectancy and quality of life, as well as decreased medical costs.

A major reason for the lack of appropriate counseling is that medical students and residents are taught to diagnose and treat disease. Hence, physicians focus on the "chief complaint," past medical history, physical examination and laboratory tests to confirm or rule out possible diseases/disorders that may already be present. Medical schools generally teach very few, if any, courses in nutrition, health promotion and behavioral counseling. Unfortunately, improving physician counseling will not be easy. It will require some changes in medical school curricula, as well as appropriate financial compensation for practicing professionals for the significant amount of time required. In addition, there must be more patient referrals to other professionals including dieticians and sports medicine specialists. Furthermore, readily available and reliable information must be available for the general population. As with the current anti-smoking campaigns, the public must be equally informed as to the health benefits of a desirable diet, as well as the many diseases associated with poor nutrition.

Free Radicals and Antioxidants

Many of the benefits of a quality diet are that it contains various antioxidants (e.g. vitamins C, E, carotenoids, flavonoids, selenium, etc.). These micronutrients neutralize (i.e. scavenge) highly toxic and reactive oxygen-derived chemical species known as free radicals, as well as other reactive oxygen species (ROS) which are normally produced in abundance in all body cells. Thus, micronutrients may be protective of numerous diseases/disorders that have been associated with free radical reactions. In addition to aging, over 100 medical conditions have been linked to oxidative stress although their importance is not fully understood. The major medical conditions and organs that are associated with increased ROS are listed in Table 4.8.[72] A brief review of free radicals, other ROS and natural antioxidant mechanisms will be presented. Failure to appreciate these phenomena makes it difficult to understand the role of antioxidants in the aging process, as well as in disease prevention. An extensive review of free radicals and their importance in aging and disease has been recently published.[72] The air we breathe is truly a "double-edged sword." We obviously need it for life; yet,

Table 4.8: Major Diseases/Disorders Associated with ROS[72]

Aging
Coronary heart disease
Cerebrovascular disease
Cancer (various types)
Cataracts and macular degeneration
Neurodegenerative disorders (i.e. Parkinson's disease, Alzheimer's disease, etc.)
Immune system deficiencies
Respiratory disorders (e.g. emphysema, respiratory distress syndrome, etc.)
Kidney, liver disorders
Chemical toxicity (transition metals, ozone, tobacco smoke, etc.)

many intracellular reactions in which it is involved result in the formation of oxygen-derived free radicals. Although most radicals are potentially harmful, others are essential in many metabolic pathways; they are also critical for phagocytic cells to kill ingested microorganisms.

What is a free radical? It is an atom, molecule or compound with one or more unpaired electrons in its outer orbital. For stability, however, chemical substances require two electrons in each outer orbital (they rotate in opposite directions, i.e. they are "paired"). Oxygen itself is a free radical since it contains an electron in each of two outer orbitals. However, their rotations are parallel, hence oxygen is a biradical. Since free radicals need an additional electron for stabilization, they attack sites of increased electron density such as nitrogen, which is electron-rich (i.e. contains two unpaired electrons). As a result, free radicals attack and inactivate proteins, including enzymes. The hydroxyl radical also reacts with the nitrogen-rich DNA and RNA purine bases (e.g. guanosine to form 8-hydroxyguanosine).[73] Furthermore, subsequent studies have shown that oxyradicals react with DNA to produce over 30 different adducts excluding protein and lipid addition products, as well as inter- and intra-strand cross-links.[74] These reactions may then cause gene mutations, rearrangements and deletions which can lead to various malignancies.[75]

Furthermore, polyunsaturated fatty acids and phospholipids contain multiple carbon-carbon double bonds (C=C), hence they are also electron-rich. Since all cell membranes are composed of a polyunsaturated bilipid layer, they are disrupted by ROS, as are other unsaturated fatty acids, including low-density lipoproteins (LDL). This process, known as lipid peroxidation, is an autocatalytic free radical reaction whereby polyunsaturated fatty acids and phospholipids undergo degradation by a chain reaction to form lipid hydroperoxides, as well as a lipid free radical, in cell membranes, body fluids, etc.[72] Since the reaction is autocatalytic (i.e. once started it continues until neutralized), a single radical may result in the formation of thousands of hydroperoxides before it is stopped; cell death may be the end result. However, lipid perioxidation can be stopped by appropriate lipid soluble antioxidants such as vitamin E and lipoic acid.

Free radical formation

Superoxide ($O_2^{-\cdot}$) is a free radical anion produced in abundance in all cells; its production is particularly high in mitochondria where oxygen is abundant and electrons are transferred along the respiratory chain [a free radical is indicated by an elevated dot ($\cdot$) indicating a single electron in the outer orbital].

$$O_2 + electron \rightarrow O_2^{-\cdot}$$

Superoxide is also produced in several enzyme-catalyzed oxidation reactions, including xanthine oxidase (XO) and monoamine oxidase (MAO).

$$Xanthine + H_2O + O_2 - XO \rightarrow Uric\ acid + 2O_2^{-\cdot} + 2H^+$$

In addition, about 3% of oxyhemoglobin ($HbFe^{2+}$) is non-enzymatically oxidized to methemaglobin ($HbFe^{3+}$) daily with the production of superoxide.

$$HbFe2^+ + O_2 \rightarrow HbFe^{3+} + O_2^{-\cdot}$$

Antioxidant enzymes

There are numerous enzymes that either inactivate or prevent the formation of free radicals. Superoxide is converted to hydrogen perioxide (H_2O_2) by either of two superoxide dismutases (SOD; cytoplasmic SOD requires zinc and copper; mitochondrial SOD requires manganese).

$$2O_2^{-\cdot} + 2H^+ - SOD \rightarrow H_2O_2 + O_2$$

Two major enzymes, catalase and glutathione peroxidase (GPx), rapidly inactivate most of the hydrogen peroxide thus formed (GPx requires selenium).

$$2H_2O_2 - Catalase \rightarrow 2H_2O + O_2$$

$$H_2O_2 + 2GSH - GPx \rightarrow GSSG + 2H_2O$$

It is apparent from this latter reaction that glutathione (GSH) is a critical antioxidant. Indeed, GSH has been referred to as the "master antioxidant." This simple tripeptide (L-gamma-glutamyl-L-cysteinyl-glycine) is ubiquitously distributed in essentially all cells. In addition to its role as an antioxidant, it is important in amino acid transport, biosynthesis and activity of proteins, enzymes and hormones, and defense against various toxic compounds. Importantly, glutathione reductase (GR) reduces oxidized glutathione (GSSG) back to GSH, thereby further assuring the removal of hydrogen peroxide.

$$GSSG + 2H^+ - GR \rightarrow 2GSH$$

Miscellaneous antioxidant pathways

Although hydrogen peroxide and other peroxides (e.g. ROOH) are not highly reactive, they are readily converted to free radicals in the presence of various transition metal ions (e.g. iron, copper, manganese, nickel, cadmium, etc.) by the Fenton Reaction.

$$H_2O_2 + Fe^{2+} \rightarrow HO^\cdot + OH^- + Fe^{3+}$$

The hydroxyl radical (HO·) is the most potent of all naturally occurring radicals. Other natural radicals include R· (alkyl), RO· (alkoxyl) and HOO· (peroxyl).

Importantly, numerous metal-binding proteins are normally produced to prevent the formation of free radicals. That is, transferrin, ferritin, hemoglobin and myoglobin among others, bind iron; ceruloplasmin binds copper while metallotheinin binds various other transition metal ions (e.g. Ni, Cd, etc.). However, in spite of these protective mechanisms, abundant free radicals are still produced although many of them can be neutralized by an adequate dietary intake of free radical "scavengers" (i.e. exogenous antioxidants such as vitamins C, E, carotenoids, flavonoids, etc.). It should also be noted that there are numerous natural endogenous free radical scavengers (e.g. uric acid, bilirubin, melatonin, various proteins, etc.). Unfortunately, these mechanisms are not completely adequate. For example, Ames *et al.*[76] estimated that in every rat cell there are 100,000 free radical "hits/day" (in every human cell there are about 10,000 "hits/day").

Other radicals, including nitric oxide (NO·), also known as endothelium relaxing factor, and other nitrogen- and sulfur-centered radicals are normally produced. Although nitric oxide is critical for normal vascular function, and not toxic itself, under certain conditions excess amounts react with superoxide ($O_2^{-\cdot}$) to produce the highly reactive peroxynitrite anion ($ONOO^-$).

$$NO^\cdot + O_2^{-\cdot} \rightarrow ONOO^-$$

Peroxynitrite may then react with various compounds, including the amino acid tyrosine to form nitrotyrosine.

Aging, caloric restriction and antioxidants

The free radical theory of aging was first proposed by Harman in 1956;[77,78] an excellent extensive review of this theory was recently published.[79] As such, it is reasonably presumed that diet is very important in aging and that appropriate antioxidants may slow the aging process. However, the only method repeatedly shown to increase the lifespan of laboratory animals is caloric restriction. In 1935, McKay *et al.*[80] first reported that by restricting total food intake in young rats, but with an adequate supply of protein and critical micronutrients, longevity can be significantly increased. That is, reducing the caloric intake to 60% of the amount consumed by rats allowed food *ad libitum*, their lifespan was increased by 30% to 50%.[81] This study has been repeatedly verified.[82–84] Furthermore, Chung *et al.*[85] studied the effects of caloric restriction on DNA damage in rat cell mitochondria compared with the nuclei. Here, DNA damage in both nuclei and mitochondria was significantly reduced in the caloric-restricted rats compared with those who received food *ad libitum*.

The biological pathways whereby caloric restriction slows the aging process are unknown, although various hypotheses have been proposed (e.g. hormonal alterations, improved immune system and oxidative stress).[86] Considerable evidence supports decreased oxidative stress as the major explanation for this phenomenon. For example, several studies have shown an inverse correlation between caloric restriction and the activity of the antioxidant enzyme catalase.[87,88] Caloric restriction in non-human primates has also shown that sexual and skeletal maturation are delayed and that other aspects so successful in rodents also apply to non-human primates.[89] In addition, energy restriction in rhesus monkeys lowers body temperature and thereby slows the metabolic rate,[90] increases physical activity without exerting a negative influence on behavior,[91] and slows the post-maturational decline in serum dehydroepiandrosterone sulfate levels.[92] It also significantly improves the immune system.[93] Hence, there is little reason not to assume that these factors also apply to human aging. For example, the presence of an increased system oxidant load in older adults has been associated with "unsuccessful" aging.[94] In this report, free living and disabled older adults had lower antioxidant and higher lipid peroxide levels than healthy adults; disabled older people had higher peroxide levels than older free living persons. Moreover, plasma concentrations of vitamins C and E, protein thiols and lipid peroxides were independently associated with either aging or aging with disability. Others[95] reported that healthy centenarians show a particular antioxidant profile in which higher levels of the fat-soluble vitamins A and E appear to correlate with extreme longevity. These latter authors suggested that this centenarian antioxidant profile is "probably linked to not only their antioxidant properties but also to their function in other homeostatic mechanisms such as immunomodulation."

Studies of the association between caloric restriction and increased lifespan have generally involved laboratory animals in their weaning or young adult stages. Can dietary restriction initiated in late adulthood also slow various age-related phenomena? Indeed, several recent studies showed that caloric restriction in late adulthood reverses mitochondrial protein alterations in rats.[96-98] The authors concluded that it is conceivable that dietary restriction "conducted in old age can be beneficial not only to retard age-related functional decline but also to restore functional activity in young rodents."[97]

The subject of oxidative stress, caloric restriction and aging has been reviewed.[89,99,100] In their review, Sohal and Weindruch[99] suggested the following in support for the hypothesis of an imbalance between prooxidants and antioxidants in caloric restriction: (1) antioxidative enzymes that are overexpressed in the fruit fly retard age-related oxidative damage and extends the maximum lifespan; (2) variations in longevity of various animal species inversely correlates with mitochondrial generation rates of the superoxide anion radical (O_2^-); and (3) caloric restriction lowers steady-state levels of oxidative stress and damage, slows age-related changes and extends the maximum lifespan of mammals. Conversely, caloric excess significantly accelerates aging independent of the numerous diseases and disorders associated with being overweight (Chapter 2).

Because of the recent advances in understanding the aging process, numerous entrepreneurs are luring many people of all ages to purchase their anti-aging products which they claim, "based on scientific evidence," slow the aging process. Because of these false claims, 51 well-established scientists who study aging recently issued a public warning that there is "no truth to the fountain of youth."[101] Indeed, no simple anti-aging remedy has been proven to be effective. As these researchers pronounced, "the primary goal of biomedical research and efforts to slow aging should not be the mere extension of life. It should be to prolong the duration of healthy life." Hence, a lifestyle characterized by proper diet, possible vitamin and mineral supplements where appropriate, regular exercise, weight control, not smoking, or drinking alcohol in excess will, for most people, not only increase their life expectancy, but the quality of life.

Diseases/Disorders and Nutrition

In addition to the above-cited basic studies in both laboratory animals and humans, numerous epidemiologic and clinical publications have also generally shown that various nutritional antioxidants are protective against numerous diseases. The most studied antioxidants include, in addition to vitamins A, C and E, various carotenoids (e.g. alpha- and beta-carotene and lycopene), flavonoids and synthetic antioxidants (Table 4.9). According to Packer *et al.*,[102] an "ideal" antioxidant would have the following characteristics: (1) high

Table 4.9: Major Nutritional Antioxidants

Antioxidant	Source(s)
Vitamin A/carotenoids	Orange-colored fruits and vegetables, spinach, peas, broccoli, peppers, tomatoes, etc.
Vitamin C (ascorbic acid)	Citrus fruits, cruciferous vegetables, potatoes, various other fruits and vegetables
Vitamin E (tocopherols, tocotrienols)	Nuts, whole grains, vegetable oils, seeds, butter, egg yolk, sweet potatoes
Flavonoids (polyphenols)	Brightly colored fruits/vegetables, onions, apples, red grapes, tea, chocolate, potatoes
Metal ions (e.g. Zn, Se, Fe, Mn, Cu)	Fruits, vegetables, grains
Probucol, butylated hydroxytoluene	Synthetic antioxidants

specificity for free radical quenching, (2) metal chelation properties, (3) antioxidant interaction, and (4) effects on gene expression. Other important criteria include adequate intestinal absorption and bioavailability, appropriate cellular, extracellular and tissue concentrations, and cellular/aqueous location.

Over 600 carotenoids have been identified, about 40 of which are present in various fruits and vegetables. The major carotenoids are vitamin A, alpha- and beta-carotene, lycopene and lutein. Although vitamin A is of prime importance in vision, it is also involved in the immune system (mainly cell-mediated immunity), fetal development, spermatogenesis and hematopoiesis. Beta-carotene has probably been the most extensively studied antioxidant in this group. It is fat-soluble and has been shown to trap free radicals and quench singlet oxygen.

Vitamin E (tocopherols) was first described in 1922 as being important in the prevention of fetal death and sterility in rats. It was originally called "factor X" and "antisterility factor." It is now recognized as a highly potent lipid-soluble antioxidant. As such, it is particularly important as a free radical "chain breaker" in cell membranes and serum lipids (i.e. prevents lipid peroxidation).[72] Vitamin E may also be important in other biological processes including (1) maintenance of cell membrane integrity, (2) DNA synthesis, (3) stimulation of the immune system, and (4) direct and regulatory interaction with the prostaglandin synthetase complex of enzymes involved in prostaglandin metabolism.

Vitamin C (ascorbic acid) is water soluble and has numerous well-defined biological activities, as well as being a very important antioxidant; it has chain-breaking properties and can directly neutralize various reactive oxygen species (e.g. superoxide, hydroxyl radical and singlet oxygen).[72] Its deficiency was initially recognized as the cause of scurvy, but because of its potent antioxidant properties, it is now recognized as being important in numerous other diseases/disorders. Interestingly, one of its major functions is to regenerate vitamin E after the latter has "trapped" a free radical in a bilipid cell membrane. However, it too then becomes a relatively inactive radical which is either recycled (i.e. by alpha-lipoic acid) or eliminated in the urine.

Several thousand naturally occurring flavonoids have been identified; they are responsible for the brilliant coloring of fall leaves. They are also excellent antioxidants and rich in brightly colored fruits and vegetables (e.g. broccoli, red and purple grapes, tea, chocolate, etc.). There are several flavonoid subgroups (flavonols, flavones flavanols and flavanones) with variable antioxidant properties depending on their structures (Fig. 4.4). More specifically, the flavanols, of which quercetin is a major one, are scavengers of superoxide, singlet oxygen and lipid peroxyradicals.[103] In addition, many of these compounds prevent free radical formation by sequestering metal ions due to chelation by adjacent hydroxyl groups. The most frequently studied flavonoids include quercetin, morin, rutin, catechin, fiscetin and myricetin.

Various transition metal ions are also important antioxidants since they are critical components of various antioxidant enzymes such as glutathione peroxidase (Se), the superoxide dismutases (Cu-Zn; Mn) and catalase (Fe).[72] Moreover, zinc has other important antioxidant roles including protection of protein sulfhydryl groups and inhibition of metal-catalyzed free radical reactions (i.e. prevents Fenton and Haber-Weiss reactions).[104] Furthermore, manganese can prevent cell damage by scavenging electrons from peroxyl radicals.[105]

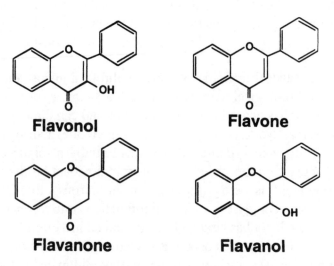

Figure 4.4: The major flavonoid subclasses.

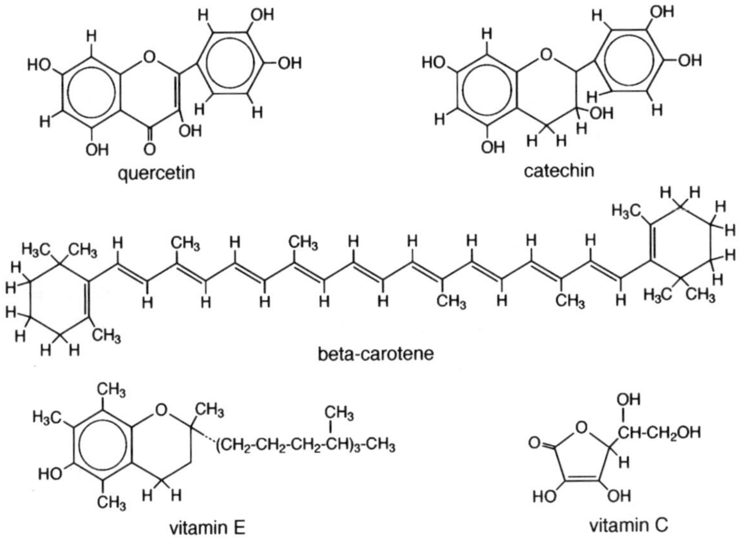

Figure 4.5: Chemical structures of several important dietary antioxidants.

Probucol, butylated hydoxytoluene and various other synthetic antioxidants have been studied in numerous experimental free radical-associated disorders.

The chemical structures of ascorbic acid, beta-carotene, vitamin E and two major flavonoids (quercetin and catechin) are presented in Fig. 4.5.

Aging, Disease and Micronutrients

The average life expectancy of Americans in 1900 was 47 years and the percentage of Americans 65 years and older was 4%. The average life expectancy currently approaches 77 years; those 65 years and older represent 12% to 13% of the population. The 65 and over segment is expected to reach 20% within the next 20 to 30 years. The issue most likely to affect the quality of life of older people is their health needs. Hence, greater emphasis in the areas of aging research, better treatment and disease prevention (health promotion) is critical. With respect to this latter item, the ten major causes of death in the US are, to a significant extent (65–70%), lifestyle-related (Chapter 1). In

addition to weight control, increased physical activity and not smoking or abusing alcohol and other drugs, good nutrition is critical for
successful aging. The maintenance of a healthy mental and physical
state is one of the major public health challenges. Since extensive studies
have now confirmed a close relationship between health and nutrition,
it is important to emphasize this relationship in the elderly, particularly
regarding the link between nutrition and several chronic degenerative
diseases. Nevertheless, many of these age-associated chronic diseases
begin years to decades before they are clinical recognized. As such, to
prevent or delay the onset of these disorders, vigorous preventive
efforts should begin in childhood.

The extensive problems of protein energy malnutrition in older
individuals were discussed earlier, as was the relationship between
caloric restriction and aging. The remainder of this chapter will
focus on the importance of diet, particularly micronutrients
(vitamins and essential minerals) in maintaining health and the prevention of various diseases and other clinical disorders. Indeed, "in
the present state of knowledge, combined supplementation, including Zn, Se, vitamins C and E and carotenoids, may be the best way to
prevent accelerated aging and reduce the risk of several common
age-related diseases."[106]

Common vitamin deficiencies

A recent study of elderly Europeans sought to determine the
minimum requirement of various micronutrients.[107] Vitamin data on
486 men and 519 women aged 74 to 79 years from eight countries
were collected. The report noted that there was an inadequate intake
of at least one micronutrient (i.e. iron, thiamine, riboflavin and pyri-
doxine) in 23.9% of the men and 46.8% of women. In those whose
energy intake was at least 1500 kcal/day, 19% of the men and 26% of
the women still had an inadequate intake of at least one of the micronutrients. Other common vitamin deficiencies in the elderly include
folic acid and vitamins B_6 and B_{12}.[108] Indeed, Naurath and
associates[109] provided strong evidence that even in the presence of
normal serum levels of folic acid and vitamins B_6 and B_{12}, many

elderly were vitamin deficient as determined by metabolite assays before and after supplementation. The authors suggested that these individuals may benefit from vitamin supplements.

Deficiencies of vitamins A, C, E, carotenoids and flavonoids are all commonly found in elderly people. These nutrients will be discussed in some detail under the various section headings (i.e. arteriosclerosis, cancer, immune deficiencies, etc.).

Folic acid

Folic acid deficiency is common not only in the elderly, but in young adults as well. Indeed, about one-third of American women of child-bearing age are folate deficient. The current recommended folic acid intake (0.4 mg/d; 400 ug/d) would decrease the incidence of neural tube defects by 48% (see discussion under "Birth Defects").[110] To increase the possibility that more women take the recommended amount, but prevent an excess in the non-target population, the US Food and Drug Administration (FDA) developed a compromise for the fortification of grain products.[111] By adding 140 ug of folic acid into each 100 g of grain products, the FDA estimated that this level of fortification would not result in an excess intake (>1000 ug/d) in non-target consumers of high amounts of grain products (i.e. the elderly and young men). Importantly, levels greater than 1000 ug/d may mask the anemia associated with vitamin B_{12} deficiency and pernicious anemia.

Vitamin B_{12} (cobalamin)

Vitamin B_{12} deficiency is estimated to affect 10% to 15% of people over 60 years of age.[112] These authors noted that the major reason the elderly are more often vitamin B_{12} deficient than young adults is due to the high prevalence of atrophic gastritis in the elderly and not due to malabsorption. Importantly, the absorption of crystalline vitamin B_{12} remains intact in those with atrophic gastritis. As a result, the elderly are encouraged to obtain vitamin B_{12} from either supplements or fortified foods (e.g. breakfast cereals) to ensure an adequate supply (recommended intake is 2.4 ug/d).

As with folic acid, cobalamin levels are insensitive for screening since patients with low normal levels (201–300 pg/mL) may have markedly elevated metabolites (i.e. methylmalonic acid and homocysteine) which fall to normal with vitamin B_{12} treatment.[113] Others[114] reported that about 90% of older people with serum cobalamin levels less than 150 pmol/L show evidence of tissue vitamin B_{12} deficiency [i.e. neutrophil hypersegmentation, elevated erythrocyte mean cell volume (MCV) and increased homocysteine]. As a result of these and other studies, routine vitamin B_{12} screening has been recommended in older people.[115,116]

In addition to the well-recognized relationship between vitamin B_{12} deficiency due to a lack of gastric intrinsic factor (pernicious anemia), several other clinical disorders have been associated with cobalamin deficiency. In a seminal report, Fata et al.[117] showed a linear relationship between serum vitamin B_{12} levels and antibody levels after vaccination with pneumococcal polysaccharide vaccine. The higher the prevaccination serum cobalamin level, the greater the vaccine antibody response. Importantly, the authors found no correlation between serum folate levels and antibody levels before and after vaccination. Others[118] studied 124 patients over 75 years of age with erythrocyte macrocytosis (MCV >95 fl). Although an elevated MCV was neither sensitive nor specific for any single disorder, it led to a specific diagnosis in 65% of the patients and was even higher (75%) in a subgroup whose MCV was great than 100 fl. In this latter category, vitamin B_{12} or folate deficiency was noted in 37.8% of the patients. Other diagnoses included myelodysplastic syndrome, refractory anemia and sideroblastic anemia. The authors suggested that those with macrocytosis not specifically diagnosable at the time of the study may represent an early sign of the myeloplastic syndrome or leukemia.

Vitamin B_{12} deficiency has been associated with cognitive impairment since pernicious anemia was first described in 1858. However, diagnosing vitamin B_{12} deficiency with primarily neuropsychiatric manifestations can be difficult in older persons. Indeed, a significant variety of signs and symptoms including confusion, memory loss, depression and hallucinations in people with low serum levels of B_{12} have been described in the absence of hematologic abnormalities, neuropathy or spinal cord degeneration. Conversely, low B_{12} levels are not uncommonly found in cognitively normal older people. Furthermore, some cognitively deficient elderly individuals with low B_{12} levels may have ischemic dementia, Alzheimer's disease or some other abnormality. In a longitudinal observational investigation, Crystal *et al.*[119] studied a cohort of 410 non-demented ambulatory people aged 75 to 85 years. Of these, 22 had vitamin B_{12} levels below 150 pg/mL. During the five-year follow-up, three of the 22 B_{12} deficient patients became demented (13.6%) compared with 57 of the 388 subjects (14.7%) with higher levels. There were no hematologic abnormalities in any of the patients with low B_{12} levels. Moreover, none of the three patients with low B_{12} levels who become demented responded to monthly B_{12} injections.

Although often quoted as a cause of reversible dementia, the relationship is thought by some to be generally associated with psychiatric morbidity other than dementia.[120] For example, Penninx and associates[121] measured serum levels of vitamin B_{12}, folate, methylmalonic acid and homocysteine in 700 disabled, non-demented women 65 years of age and older. Depressive symptoms were measured by means of the Geriatric Depression Scale and categorized as no depression, mild depression or severe depression. The authors concluded that metabolically significant cobalamin deficiency is associated with a two-fold risk of severe depression. In addition, Chandra[122] recently reported that cognitive functions improved significantly after one year in a group of elderly men and women placed on a multivitamin/mineral supplement.

Iron

Iron deficiency, the most common nutritional deficiency worldwide, has numerous negative health effects. These include changes in immune function, energy metabolism, work capacity, and motor and mental development.[123,124] Although iron deficiency is primarily a very serious problem in underdeveloped countries, it continues to be relatively common in the US, especially in certain age/sex groups. For example, Looker *et al.*[125] examined 24,894 Americans aged one year and older from 1988 to 1994. Their results showed the following: 9% of toddlers aged one to two years and 9% to 11% of adolescent girls and women of childbearing age were iron deficient; iron deficiency anemia was present in 3% and 2% to 5%, respectively. Thus, about 700,000 American toddlers and 7.8 million adolescent girls and women of childbearing age were iron deficient and 240,000 toddlers and 3.3 million females of childbearing age had iron deficiency anemia. Among persons aged 50 years and older, iron deficiency was estimated to be no greater than 7%.

Trace elements

The major essential trace elements include fluorine (bone and teeth), zinc (metalloenzymes), copper (enzyme cofactor), iodine (thyroid hormone), vanadium (metalloenzymes), selenium (enzymes), manganese (metalloenzymes), molybdenum (enzyme cofactor) and cobalt (vitamin B_{12}). A few examples of the less appreciated essential elements follow.

Selenium plays a key role in protecting cells against free radicals since it is a critical component of glutathione peroxidase, an antioxidant enzyme.[72] As such, low levels have been associated with several diseases, including cancer (discussed in later sections). Selenium also modulates the immune system.[126]

Zinc is a highly important component of numerous proteins, including the cytoplasmic antioxidant enzyme superoxide dismutase (Cu/Zn-SOD).[72] Another essential role, among others, is that it protects protein sulfhydryl groups (-SH) from oxidation by competing with various transition metals (e.g. iron, nickel, cadmium, copper, etc.) that convert hydrogen peroxide to the potent hydroxyl free radical.[106] Other trace elements, including manganese and copper, are important enzyme components although their effects are not fully understood. For example, copper is both an antioxidant [component of cytoplasmic superoxide dismutase (Cu/Zn:SOD)] and prooxidant since the cuprous ion can convert hydrogen perioxide to the hydroxyl radical (Fenton reaction.)[72] Manganese is also an important antioxidant since it is a component of the mitochrondrial superoxide dismutase (Mn:SOD).

In summary, a healthy diet and perhaps a multivitamin and mineral supplement, especially for the elderly, may be the best way to slow the aging process and reduce the risk of the various common age-associated diseases discussed in subsequent sections of this chapter.

Arteriosclerosis: Coronary Heart Disease, Ischemic Stroke and Peripheral Vascular Disease

Although the incidence of coronary heart disease (CHD) has progressively decreased since the 1960s, it clearly remains the leading cause of death in the US and other industrialized nations; cerebrovascular disease (CVD) is the third leading cause of death. Together, they closely approach the total of the other eight major causes of death in the US (Chapter 1, Table 1.1). Moreover, arteriosclerosis, the primary cause of CHD, stroke and peripheral vascular disease is responsible for about 40% of total mortality in Europe, Japan and the US. Furthermore, a recent study found that the lifetime risk of developing CHD at age 40 years is one in two for men and one in four for women.[127] The authors emphasized that this information should promote efforts in education, screening and treatment to prevent CHD in the elderly as well as in young adults. With respect to sex, it is emphasized that CHD is not just a man's disease; it is also clearly the leading cause of death in women. Following menopause, the incidence of CHD in women parallels that of men.

The commonly recognized risk factors for arteriosclerosis are age, sex, obesity, smoking, physical inactivity, increased plasma lipids (total cholesterol, low-density lipoproteins, others) and decreased high-density lipoproteins (HDL). Less appreciated important risk factors include increased hematocrit and plasma levels of fibrinogen, factors VII and VIII, homocysteine, leukocyte count (neutrophil count), uric acid, iron and C-reactive protein, decreased serum albumin and clinical depression (Chapter 1).[37,128,129] Additional risk factors for ischemic stroke include hypertension, asymptomatic carotid artery stenosis, increased alcohol consumption (more than five drinks a day) and atrial fibrillation.[130]

The pathogenesis of arteriosclerosis is still not completely understood, but a highly significant forward step was made in 1979. Here, Goldstein *et al.*[131] postulated that modification of low density lipoproteins (LDL), recognized by the acetyl-LDL cell receptor ("scavenger" receptor), but not the normal LDL receptor, may be required for lipid loading of macrophage-derived foam cells. Subsequent studies showed that LDL is initially minimally modified (MM-LDL) in the arterial subendothelial space.[132] Here, MM-LDL can induce leukocyte-endothelial cell adhesions and promote secretion of both monocyte chemotactic protein-1 and macrophage colony-stimulating factor (MCSF) by endothelial cells. This leads to monocyte binding to endothelial cells and their subsequent migration into the subendothelial space where MCSF stimulates their conversion into macrophages. These macrophages further oxidize MM-LDL to oxidized LDL which is then taken up by the "scavenger" receptor system. Importantly, oxidized LDL is chemotactic for monocytes and T-cells which can result in further recruitment into the developing atheroscleorotic lesion. Furthermore, oxidized LDL is toxic to macrophages and thereby inhibits their motility, preventing their re-entry into the circulation.[133,134] Here they remain and continue to phagocytize oxidized LDL and eventually become microscopically recognized "foam" cells. The recognition that oxidized LDL may account for the presence of foam cells led to the oxidation hypothesis of arteriosclerosis.[135] The following is a brief summary of this widely accepted theory.

(1) Circulating monocytes are recruited by a chemotactic factor produced by endothelial cells due to locally-produced toxic oxidized LDL.

(2) Monocytes attach to the endothelial cells before entering the subendothelial space where they phagocytize and oxidize LDL. However, oxidized LDL is also toxic to the monocytes/macrophages and they are unable to re-enter the circulation.

(3) There is enhanced macrophage uptake of LDL by the acetyl-LDL receptor with the formation of foam cells.

(4) Oxidized LDL cytotoxicity may increase the entry of LDL into the monocytes/macrophages in the early phases with loss of some endothelial functions.

There is considerable basic research, as well as epidemiologic and clinical evidence, that further supports the free radical oxidative theory of atherosclerosis.

(1) Oxidized LDL extracted from atherosclerotic lesions has all of the physical, immunological and biological properties attributed to *in vitro* preparations of oxidized LDL.

(2) Autoantibodies to epitopes of oxidized LDL are bound to atherosclerotic lesions and in the serum of both laboratory animals and humans.

(3) Studies of serum antioxidant reserve and dose-response of free radical trapping by antioxidants correlate with antioxidant levels.

(4) Numerous epidemiologic studies show an inverse relationship between dietary and/or plasma concentrations of antioxidants and ischemic heart disease.

(5) Atherogenesis can be inhibited or slowed in hypercholesterolemic animals and non-human primates by the administration of various antioxidants.

As a final note, a very recent study adds further support for the LDL oxidation theory of atherogenesis.[136] Here, oxidized LDL was measured in 135 patients with acute myocardial infarction (AMI; n = 45), unstable angina pectoris (n = 45), stable angina pectoris (n = 45), and in 46 control subjects. In addition, oxidized LDL was immunohistochemically evaluated in 33 atherectomy specimens obtained from different cohort of patients with unstable angina pectorus (n = 23) and stable angina pectorus (n = 10). The results showed that AMI patients had significantly higher oxidized LDL levels than both groups with angina, as well as the control group. Moreover, in the atherectomy specimens, the oxidized LDL positive macrophages in the surface area were significantly higher in patients with unstable angina than in those with stable angina.

Antioxidants and experimental atherogenesis

In addition to numerous basic publications that support the oxidative stress hypothesis of arteriosclerosis, most albeit not all, studies involving laboratory animals and humans indicate that antioxidants are anti-atherogenic.

Vitamin E (alpha-tocopherol)

As noted above, the initial atherosclerotic event involves the attachment of circulating monocytes to the arterial endothelial surface. These phagocytic cells then enter the subendothelial space and phagocytize the oxidized LDL particles. In this regard, it was recently demonstrated that vitamin E (alpha-tocopherol) has an anti-atherogenic effect on human monocytes.[137] In this study, monocytes from alpha-tocopherol-supplemented humans had a significant decrease in the release of reactive oxygen species (ROS), lipid peroxidation, IL-1 beta secretion and monocyte endothelial cell adhesion compared with the non-supplemented controls. Moreover, when LDL is oxidatively stimulated (i.e. exposure to macrophages and copper ions) a lag phase precedes the oxidation of polyunsaturated fatty acids. During this lag phase, the various antioxidants disappear, alpha-tocopherol being the first and beta-carotene the last.[138] These latter authors noted that the *in vitro* loading of LDL with vitamin E resulted in a linear increase in the oxidative resistance as the vitamin E concentration increased. Jialal *et al.*[139] subsequently reported similar results in human plasma when they showed that the time-course curves of LDL oxidation, lag phase and oxidation rate were dependent on the oral dose of alpha-tocopherol. In addition, humans supplemented with vitamin E have increased LDL alpha-tocopherol levels and LDL oxidative resistance and decreased oxidized LDL cytotoxicity to cultured endothelial cells.[140]

Yoshida and coworkers[141] noted that the increased risk for CHD in patients with type 2 diabetes cannot be completely explained by the presence of conventional risk factors. They compared the lag time of LDL oxidation with the vitamin E/lipid peroxide ratio of LDL in patients with diabetes with two control groups (non-diabetes with hypertriglyceridemia and normotriglyceridemia) and found a significant shortening of the lag time in those with type 2 diabetes (mean 43, 48 and 54 minutes, respectively). After regression analysis, their data suggested that LDL in patients with diabetes is more susceptible to oxidative modification primarily due to reduced vitamin E/lipid peroxide ratios. They suggested that enhanced susceptibility of LDL to ROS may be the major factor underlying the increased incidence of vascular disease in those with type 2 diabetes. In a related study, troglitazone, a novel anti-diabetic drug which has structural similarities with vitamin E, was shown to increase the resistance of LDL to oxidation by over 20%.[142] More specifically, troglitazone therapy was associated with a significant reduction in the amount of preformed LDL hydroperoxides, suggesting that it has significant antioxidant activity and may be of benefit to diabetics.

Prasad and Kalra[143] compared the atherogenic effects of a high cholesterol diet in vitamin E-supplemented rabbits with non-supplemented controls. They measured blood concentrations of total cholesterol, LDL, HDL, triglycerides and malondialdehyde (MDA), a product of lipid perioxidation. The atheomatous lesions in each rabbit aorta were examined by both gross and microscopic techniques (MDA was quantified in both the atheromatous lesions and blood). Their results clearly demonstrated that the vitamin E supplemented rabbits had significantly lower MDA blood and tissue levels and less severe aortic atheromatous changes.

Sun and associates[144] fed male New Zealand white rabbits an atherogenic diet which produced hypercholesterolemia. The rabbits were then divided into three groups according to their antioxidant supplements: (1) intravenous injection of beta-carotene; (2) dietary supplementation with alpha-tocopherol; and (3) a combination of both antioxidants. Their findings showed that intravenous beta-carotene significantly decreased serum total and LDL cholesterol levels, thoracic atherosclerotic lesions and aortic intimal thickness but had no effect on LDL oxidation compared with the controls. Added alpha-tocopherol significantly decreased LDL oxidation, aortic atherosclerotic area and aortic intimal thickness, but had no effect on plasma total or LDL cholesterol levels compared with the controls. The combined antioxidants significantly reduced total and LDL cholesterol levels, susceptibility of LDL to oxidation, atherosclerotic lesion area and aortic intimal thickness. Vitamin E supplementation has also been shown to be effective in reducing experimentally-induced atherosclerosis in primates.[145] Thus, vitamin E supplementation not only prevented atherosclerosis in monkeys, but resulted in regression of established atherosclerotic lesions.

Increased total body iron is a risk factor for atherosclerosis.[146] In addition, iron is capable of oxidizing LDL *in vitro*. However, since it was unknown whether increased dietary iron could alter LDL *in vivo*, these workers sought to determine whether increased dietary iron results in increased LDL-cholesterol oxidation and, if so, whether antioxidants can prevent such changes. Here, three groups of rats received diets differing only in iron content (35, 50 and 300 mg/kg). The results showed that dietary iron not only increased LDL-VLDL lipid perioxidation (MDA and lipid hydroperoxide concentrations), but protein modification (i.e. changed sulfhydryl concentration). Increased iron levels led to an even higher degree of oxidative change and protein modification. However, alpha-tocopherol and beta-carotene supplementation prevented these oxidative changes.

Using data from the Cholesterol Lowering Atherosclerosis Study (CLAS), Asen *et al.*[147] studied a group of non-smoking 40- to 59-year-old men with previous bypass graft surgery. The rate of preintrusive atherosclerosis was determined using high-resolution B-mode ultrasound quantification of the common carotid artery far wall intima-media thickness (IMT). Their results showed that those supplemented with 100 or more IU of vitamin E per day had significantly less carotid IMT progression compared with low vitamin E users. Vitamin C supplementation ($\geq$250 mg/d) had no measurable effect. In a related study, Mezzetti and associates[148] assessed arterial (internal mammary artery) and plasma levels of vitamins C and E and lipid peroxidation products in 48 males (24 smokers, 24 non-smokers) undergoing coronary bypass surgery. They found that vitamins C and E levels were significantly lower and lipid peroxidation products significantly higher in smokers compared with non-smokers. Plasma vitamin C and E levels were strongly related to their tissue content in both smokers and non-smokers. In addition, vitamin E content was significantly associated with that of vitamin C only in the arterial tissue of both groups, suggesting the existence of a functional interaction between these antioxidants. As predicted based on their solubility, lipid peroxidation products were significantly and inversely related to the concentrations of vitamin C in plasma and vitamin E in tissue in both groups. The severity of coronary atherosclerosis was inversely and directly correlated with the arterial levels of vitamin E and lipid peroxidation products respectively in both smokers and non-smokers. However, no correlation was found between the severity of atherosclerosis and the content of vitamins and lipid peroxidation products in plasma.

Vitamin C (ascorbic acid)

Vitamin C forms the first line of antioxidant defense in human plasma exposed to various oxidative insults, including aqueous free radicals, activated neutrophils and cigarette smoke.[149] Vitamin C has also been shown to be a very effective antioxidant in its ability to protect LDL cholesterol against oxidation.[150] Thus, Frei *et al.*[151] demonstrated that vitamin C is the most effective aqueous-phase antioxidant in human plasma. Although ascorbic acid is a water soluble antioxidant and therefore not present in LDL particles, it delays LDL oxidation by sparing fat-soluble antioxidants (e.g. vitamin E) present in LDL particles. This antioxidant-sparing property appears to be somewhat vitamin C-specific since probucol, at an equipotent antioxidant concentration, showed no sparing effect of vitamin E or beta-carotene.[152] However, as might be expected due to its fat insolubility, vitamin C is significantly less effective than vitamin E in the prevention of lipoprotein oxidation *in vitro*.[153] Here, vitamins C and E were orally administered to healthy male and female volunteers. Plasma lipoproteins were isolated before and after vitamin supplementation and incubated with copper. Administration of both vitamins resulted in

57% decrease in lipid peroxidation products (i.e. thiobarbituric acid reactive substances); vitamin E alone resulted in a 52% decrease while vitamin C alone reduced the oxidation products by 15%.

Endothelial dysfunction in coronary and peripheral arteries occurs in atherosclerosis, hypercholesterolemia, smoking and hypertension. This results in loss of endothelium-dependent vasodilatation and is associated with decreased production and/or enhanced degradation of endothelium relaxing factor (i.e. nitric oxide; NO). Several studies have shown that vitamin C, whether infused or chronically ingested, improves the defective vasodilatation associated with these clinical disorders.[154-157] More specifically, Heitzer *et al.*[154] found that in control subjects (non-smokers), vitamin C had no effect on forearm blood flow in response to acetylcholine, an endothelium-dependent vasodilator. However, in chronic smokers the attenuated forearm blood flow response to acetylcholine were markedly improved by concomitant administration of vitamin C. Others[155] demonstrated that vitamin C improves endothelium-dependent vasodilatation in the forearm resistance vessels in hypercholesterolemic patients. Moreover, Gokee and coworkers[156] reported that in patients with coronary artery disease (CAD), long-term "ascorbic acid treatment may benefit patients with CAD."

A more recent publication[157] indicated that vitamin C has a "sustained beneficial effect" on endothelium-derived nitric oxide action and that the prognostic impact of endothelial dysfunction and vascular oxidative stress on cardiovascular events in patients with CAD. Here, endothelium-dependent and independent vasodilation was determined in a group of patients with documented CAD by measuring forearm blood flow responses to the vasodilators, sodium nitroprusside and acetylcholine. The effect of vitamin C coadministration was assessed in a subgroup of patients. Cardiovascular events, including myocardial infarction, ischemic stroke, coronary angioplasty and coronary or peripheral bypass surgery were studied. Their findings showed that patients experiencing cardiovascular events had lower vasodilator responses to both sodium nitroprusside and actelycholine. Conversely, vitamin C administration resulted in greater benefit. The authors suggested that increased vascular oxidative stress, as demonstrated by the positive response to vitamin C, "may represent an important underlying mechanism for endothelial dysfunction and for the pathogenesis of cardiovascular events." The topic of ascorbic acid and its relation to endothelial dysfunction was recently reviewed.[158]

Carotenoids

As with alpha-tocopherol, beta-carotene is lipid soluble. It is not only a vitamin A precursor, but a very effective quencher of singlet oxygen and inhibitor of lipid peroxidation. However, this compound reportedly exhibits effective free radical-trapping activity only at low (physiologic) oxygen tension.[159] Moreover, compared with vitamin E, it is a relatively weak antioxidant. In human LDL particles, beta-carotene is consumed only after alpha-tocopherol has been completely utilized.[160] As a result, Frei[161] suggested that the underlying mechanisms whereby beta-carotene is anti-atherogenic and anti-carcinogenic may be primarily due to factors other than its antioxidant properties.

Miscellaneous antioxidants and atherogenesis

The initial *in vitro* study with probucol, a synthetic antioxidant, indicated that it was an effective LDL oxidation inhibitor.[162] In addition, treatment of receptor-deficient Watanabe heritable hyperlipemic (WHHL) rabbits with probucol was found to inhibit the progression of atherosclerotic lesions.[163] Moreover, Carew *et al.*[164] reported that the rate of LDL degradation in the macrophage-rich fatty streaks of probucol-treated WHHL rabbits was reduced to about one-half that in the rabbits not given probucol. These authors further noted that most of the LDL degradation in the fatty streaks takes place within macrophages. In non-lesioned aortas, where macrophages were scarce, LDL degradation was confined primarily to endothelial and smooth muscle cells.

As noted previously, the flavonoids make up a very large group of multi-ringed phenolic antioxidants that scavenge superoxide, singlet oxygen and lipid peroxy radicals.[165] In addition, those with orthodihydroxy groups can bind metal ions and thereby prevent free radical formation and oxidative stress. Mammalian 15-lipoxygenase has been implicated early in atherogenesis by inducing plasma LDL oxidation in the subendothelial space. However, quercetin and other flavonoids which are rich in brightly colored fruits and vegetables, reportedly inhibit lipoxygenase activity. Luiz da Silva *et al.*[166] compared quercetin and several of its glycosides with ascorbic acid and alpha-tocopherol on rabbit reticulocyte 15-lipoxygenase-induced human LDL peroxidation. Their results demonstrated that although all of the tested antioxidants were somewhat effective in inhibiting lipoxygenase-induced LDL oxidation, quercetin and quercetin glycosides were more efficient than vitamins C and E. Others[167,168] studied the antioxidant effectiveness of *trans*-resveratrol, a flavonoid rich in red grapes. They reported that this compound was not only protective of LDL against copper-catalyzed oxidation, but that it was more effective than vitamin E. In addition, epicatechin and quercetin, also present in red grapes, had about twice the oxidative inhibitory capacity of resveratrol. Similarly, Visioli and Galli[169] showed that preincubation of LDL particles with eleuropein, a major polyphenolic component of olive oil, also effectively inhibits copper-induced LDL oxidation.

Dihydrolipoic acid, the reduced form of alpha-lipoic acid, has been described as "a universal antioxidant" since it is active in cell membranes as well as the aqueous phase.[170] These workers reported that dihydrolipoic acid may act as "a strong direct chain-breaking antioxidant." Thus, lipoic acid enhances the antioxidant potency of other antioxidants, especially vitamins C and E. More recently, alpha-lipoic acid was also found to be comparable to vitamin C in improving nitric oxide-mediated vasodilatation in diabetic patients.[171] Moreover, lipoic acid "normalizes lipid perioxidation and prevents the oxidation of reduced glutathione, possibly through recycling mechanisms, thereby maintaining normal metabolic function."[172]

Antioxidants: basic, epidemiologic and clinical studies

Numerous epidemiologic studies and clinical trials have shown that the overall diet is very important in the pathogenesis of arteriosclerosis. As discussed later, there is an extensive literature on specific nutrients or foods and the risk of CHD. However, relatively little is known about the role of overall eating patterns and CHD. To examine this association further, two major dietary patterns ("prudent" and "Western") were identified in women aged 38 to 63 years from the Nurses' Health Study.[173] The prudent pattern was characterized by a higher intake of fruits, vegetables, legumes, fish, poultry and whole grains while the Western diet was characterized by higher intakes of red and preserved meats, sweets and desserts, French fries and refined grains. After adjusting for confounding coronary risk factors, the prudent diet was associated with relative risk of 0.76 comparing the highest with the lowest quintile. The extreme quintile comparison was 1.46 for the Western diet. For those who were jointly in the highest prudent diet quintile and lowest Western diet quintile, the relative risk was 0.64 compared with those with the opposite profile pattern.

Hu and Willett[174] recently reviewed 147 original and review publications of metabolic and epidemiologic studies and dietary intervention trials of diet and CHD. They concluded that the evidence is substantial that diets using non-hydrogenated unsaturated fats as the major form of dietary fat, whole grains as the major source of carbohydrates, an abundance of fruits and vegetables and adequate omega-3 (n-3) fatty acids "can offer significant protection against CHD." Moreover, these diets plus regular physical exercise, not smoking and not being overweight "may prevent the majority of cardiovascular disease in Western populations." More specifically, the major dietary components correlated with arteriosclerosis include various antioxidants (vitamins C, E and flavonoids), fiber, saturated and unsaturated fats, trans fatty acids, folic acid and vitamin B_6 (Table 4.10). The relation between each of these dietary factors and CHD and ischemic stroke will be presented in some detail. Although few studies have evaluated the effects of

Table 4.10: Dietary Factors and Arteriosclerosis

Vitamins C, E, B$_6$
Folic acid
Flavonoids (polyphenolics)
Dietary fiber (soluble, insoluble)
Fish oils (mainly n-3 fatty acids)
Cholesterol
Total fat and saturated fatty acids
Polyunsaturated fatty acids
Trans fatty acids
Magnesium

multivitamins on heart disease, a prospective study by Rimm *et al.*,[175] showed that the daily use of a multivitamin was associated with a lower risk of CHD in women. Moreover, consistent evidence for the association of low dietary intake of various essential antioxidants (certain vitamins and other micronutrients) and an increased risk of CHD has been demonstrated in numerous epidemiologic and clinical studies.

Mediterranean diet

Although the human genetic profile has not changed significantly over the past 10,000 or so years, major changes have occurred in our food supply, energy expenditure and physical activity. Simopoulus[176] noted that current diets in industrialized countries are characterized by the following: (1) an increase in energy intake but decrease in energy expenditure; (2) an increase in saturated fat, omega-6 (n-6) fatty acids, and trans fatty acids and a decrease in omega-3 (n-3) fatty acids; (3) a decrease in complex fatty acids and fiber; (4) an increase in grains and decrease in fruits and vegetables; (5) a decrease in protein and calcium; and (6) a marked increase in the ratio of n-6 to n-3 fatty acids (about 16 : 1 versus 2 : 1). He concluded that the depletion of n-3 fatty acids in Western diets is the "result of agribusiness, modern agriculture, and aquaculture. The high ratio of n-6 to n-3 fatty acids in the result of excessive production of vegetable oils and the indiscriminate recommendation to substitute saturated fat and butter with oils high in n-6 fatty acids to lower serum cholesterol levels without taking into consideration their adverse effect on overall human metabolism."

The traditional Mediterranean diet, in contrast to American and northern European diets, includes significant amounts of fruits, vegetables, fish, nuts, seeds, olive oil and wine and a decrease in the amount of red meat. Interest in the Mediterranean diet was first noted from the results in the Seven Countries Study by Keys *et al.*[177] in which they demonstrated that the mortality rate from CHD in southern Europe was two- to three-fold lower than in northern Europe or the US. Since then, numerous studies have shown that the traditional Mediterranean diet is associated with a decreased incidence of both CHD and cancer and an increased life expectancy. Several examples will be cited.

Gjonca and Bobak[178] analyzed mortality data from Albania and found a paradox of high adult life expectancy in this very low-income country. They concluded that this was best explained by a diet low in total energy and in meat and milk products, but high in fruits, vegetables and complex carbohydrates. Others carried out a randomized prospective prevention trial in 615 patients recovering from a myocardial infarction in which the Cretan Mediterranean diet was compared with the prescribed diet of the American Heart Association.[179] After a mean follow-up of 27 months, recurrent myocardial infarction, all cardiovascular events and cardiac and total death were decreased by more than 70% in the Mediterranean diet group compared with those on the commonly prescribed diet. Importantly, the dietary protective effects were not related to serum levels of total, LDL or HDL cholesterol. Rather, the protective effects were related to an increase in plasma n-3 fatty acids and oleic acid and a decrease in linoleic acid. Moreover, increased plasma concentrations of vitamins C and E were present in those consuming the Mediterranean diet. Other studies by these investigators showed similar positive effects of the Mediterranean diet in decreasing the incidence of CHD and possibly cancer.[180,181]

Joshipura *et al.*[182] prospectively studied 84,251 women aged 34 to 59 years over a 14-year period and 42,148 men aged 40 to 75 years over an eight-year period (Nurses' Health Study and the Health Professionals' Follow-up Study, respectively). At baseline, all participants were free of diagnosed cancer, diabetes and cardiovascular disease. After adjustment for the standard cardiovascular risk factors, the relative risk for persons in the highest quintile of fruit and vegetables intake was 0.80 compared with the lowest quintile. For a single daily serving increase in fruits and vegetables, there was a 4% lower risk for CHD. (The reader is referred to unsaturated fatty acids under the "Non-Antioxidants and Arteriosclerosis" section.)

More recently, a population-based prospective study of 22,043 Greek adults examined the association of adherence to a Mediterranean diet and longevity.[183] The results showed that a higher adherence to the Mediterranean diet were (1) associated with a reduction in total mortality (adjusted hazard ratio, 0.75); (2) inversely associated with death from CHD (adjusted hazard ratio, 0.67); and (3) inversely associated with death due to cancer (adjusted hazard ratio, 0.76). Unfortunately, a study of people in Olmstead County, Minnesota found that only 16% of people met the standard dietary recommendations for consuming five or more servings of fruits and/or vegetables each day and no more than 35% of calories from fat.[184] Moreover, 51% met neither recommendation.

Vitamin E (tocopherols)

Gey *et al.*[185] reported an inverse relationship between mortality from CHD and plasma vitamin E levels. These researchers recognized that many people dying from CHD could not be explained solely by their blood lipid profiles. This was also true when the blood lipid levels were combined with other risk factors such as smoking and hypertension. In this large cross-cultural European population study, which differed six-fold in age-specific CHD mortality, the authors concluded that the differences were primarily attributable to plasma vitamin E levels. These findings are in agreement with two subsequent American studies, one involving 87,245 female nurses[186] and the other

38,910 male physicians.[187] The ongoing US female nurse study found that the risk of major CHD among those who took 100 IU supplemental vitamin E was 40% lower than women who did not take supplemental vitamin E. The results were similar in the male physician study. Here, in those who consumed at least 100 IU of vitamin E per day, the multivariate relative risk was 0.63 compared with those who consumed no vitamin E supplements.

The Established Populations for Epidemiologic Studies of the Elderly also reported a positive effect for vitamin E on atherosclerosis.[188] Here, over 11,000 subjects participated in a nine-year study in which supplemental vitamin E reduced the relative mortality risk of CHD by 47% and total mortality by 34%. Similarly, Knekt *et al.*[189] found an inverse association between dietary vitamin E intake and coronary mortality in both men and women with relative risks of 0.68 and 0.35 respectively between the highest and lowest tertiles. They also reported similar associations for the dietary intake of vitamin C and carotenoids among women.

More recently, the results of a randomized control trial of vitamin E supplementation in patients with CHD (Cambridge Heart Antioxidant Study) were reported.[190] Here, 2002 patients with angiographically-proven CHD were randomized to take either vitamin E (400 or 800 IU/day) or placebo. Over 90% of the participants had angina, evidence of cardiac ischemia, or both. During a mean follow-up of 17 months, 41 controls and 14 vitamin E recipients suffered a non-fatal myocardial infarction. The authors concluded that vitamin E supplementation in patients with symptomatic CHD significantly reduces the rate of non-fatal heart attacks, with beneficial effects apparent after one year. In a related study, Miwa *et al.*[191] measured plasma vitamin E levels in 29 patients with active variant angina (group 1), 13 patients with inactive stage of variant angina without anginal attacks during the previous six months (group 2), 32 patients with significant coronary artery stenosis and stable angina (group 3) and a control group of 30 patients without CHD (group 4). Their results showed that vitamin E levels were significantly lower in group 1 than in the other three groups. They also noted that plasma vitamin E levels were significantly correlated with those in the LDL fractions. Moreover, patients in group 1 had significantly lower levels of vitamin E in LDL fractions than those in group 4 (controls). The authors further reported that in a sub-population of group 1, still suffering anginal attacks while receiving calcium channel blockers, the addition of vitamin E acetate (300 mg/d) significantly elevated their plasma levels and inhibited the occurrence of angina. Similarly, Riemersma and coworkers[192] studied 100 patients with angina pectoris and compared them with 394 matched individuals without anginal symptoms. They found that plasma levels of vitamins C and E and beta-carotene were significantly and inversely related to the risk of angina; the concentration of vitamin A was not significant. Importantly, smoking was a confounding factor and when corrected for, the effect of beta-carotene disappeared. Although smoking reduced the effect of vitamin C, it was still statistically significant. Vitamin E, however, remained independently and inversely related to anginal risk after adjusting for age, blood pressure, serum lipid levels, weight and smoking.

Of further interest here is the report by Regnstrom and associates.[193] This group evaluated vitamin E levels in both serum and LDL from 64 consecutive male survivors of AMI who were less than 45 years of age. These serum parameters were associated with the severity of CHD as assessed by a semi-quantitative scoring system involving coronary angiograms (global stenosis score). Lipid-adjusted serum and LDL vitamin E levels were significantly lower in the CHD patients than in 35 age-matched controls. However, the absolute serum and LDL vitamin E concentrations did not differ between the two groups. In addition, there was no association between the serum concentration or lipid-adjusted serum vitamin E levels and the stenosis score. Conversely, a significant inverse correlation was present between the LDL vitamin E concentration and the global stenosis score. Of additional interest is the prospective cohort study of 34,486 postmenopausal women (Iowa Women's Health Study)[194] in which those with no apparent CHD were followed for about seven years. After adjusting for various risk factors, increased dietary vitamin E consumption was associated with a decreased risk of death from CHD.

In particular, the findings suggested that in postmenopausal women the intake of increased amounts of vitamin E from food was enough to reduce the incidence of fatal heart disease without the need for vitamin E supplements. By contrast, the dietary intake of vitamins A and C was not associated with a lower risk of dying from CHD.

Since obesity is a well known risk factor for atherosclerosis, Kuno *et al.*[195] determined the antioxidant status of obese girls by measuring the plasma levels of alpha-tocopherol, beta-carotene and LDL. The investigators found that the plasma alpha-tocopherol/lipids ratio was significantly lower in obese girls than in normal weight controls, as were the LDL beta-carotene and LDL alpha-tocopherol levels; however, no differences were observed in the plasma levels. The LDL in obese girls also contained more polyunsaturated fatty acids than normal and their peroxidizability index, a measure of lipid susceptibility to oxidative stress, was significantly higher than the control group. These results suggest that obese girls may be more prone to develop atherosclerosis in later life than non-obese girls.

Two additional studies supporting a positive role for vitamin E in atherogenesis were recently published. In the first, Mazzetti *et al.*[196] assessed whether systemic oxidative stress could predict the risk of an initial myocardial infarction, ischemic stroke and congestive heart failure. This longitudinal study from 1992 to 1997 involved 102 apparently health elderly Italians 80 years and older. Their findings showed the following: (1) subjects with plasma vitamin E levels in the highest quartile had one-sixth the risk of cardiovascular events compared with those in the lowest quartile; (2) subjects with plasma levels of oxidized lipids, measured by a fluorescent technique, in the highest quartile had a seven times greater risk than those with oxidized lipids in the lowest quartile; and (3) there was no association between vitamin C, beta-carotene or total cholesterol levels and risk of cardiovascular events. Moreover, multivariate adjustment for other known risk factors did not alter the results. Others,[197] in a cross-sectional study, evaluated 60 people 75 years and older, 30 of whom had "vascular successful aging" (VASA) and 30 controls with moderate carotid artery atherosclerosis. The VASA group had significantly higher vitamin E/total cholesterol levels both in plasma and in isolated LDLs; their LDLs also had greater resistance to *in vitro* oxidation. Moreover, the level of fluorescent lipid peroxidation products was lower in the VASA group compared with the control group. Multivariate analysis indicated that only plasma vitamin E levels and fluorescent lipid peroxidation products were independently associated with VASA.

The preceding more basic research studies involving both laboratory animals and humans clearly indicate the importance of oxidative stress in atherogenesis. In addition, numerous observational studies have shown a significant inverse correlation between vitamin E and various atherosclerotic disease processes. However, randomized prospective trials focused primarily on individuals with existing CHD, perhaps a more complex situation, the results have been somewhat inconsistent. For example, a recent report by the Heart Outcomes Prevention Evaluation (HOPE) Study,[198] 4761 men and women at high risk for cardiovascular events were randomly assigned according to a two-by-two factorial design to receive either 400 IU of vitamin E daily or matching placebo and either an angiotensin-converting enzyme inhibitor or matching placebo over a mean period of 4.5 years. The major measureable outcome was a composite of myocardial infarction, stroke and death from cardiovascular disease. Their results showed no benefits from vitamin E supplementation. Similarly, the Multiple Risk Factor Intervention Trial, a nested case-control study, found no significant correlation between serum antioxidant (carotenoids, retinol, alpha-, gamma- and total tocopherol) levels by quartiles with the risk of death from CHD or non-fatal myocardial infarction.[199]

Pryor[200] recently reviewed the role of vitamin E and heart disease and wrote "it is possible, or even likely, that each condition for which vitamin E provides benefit will have a unique dose-effect curve." Moreover, he added that "different antioxidants appear to act synergistically, so supplementation with vitamin E may be more effective if combined with other micronutrients." In this regard, Salonen and associates[201] recently studied the efficacy of vitamins C and E supplementation on the progression of carotid artery atherosclerosis. They hypothesized that there might be an "enhanced preventive effect in men and smokers and synergism between vitamins." This randomized study of hypercholesterolemic smoking and non-smoking men and postmenopausal women was a double-masked two-by-two factorial trial, randomization in four groups to receive twice daily either 136 IU d-alpha-tocopherol, 250 mg of slow-release vitamin C, a combination of the two vitamins, or a placebo for three years. Disease progression was determined by ultrasonographic assessment of the common carotid artery mean intima-media thickness. The results showed that the vitamin combination was significantly more effective than either vitamin alone in retarding disease progression. Thus, the proportion of men with carotid atherosclerotic progression was reduced by 74% in those taking both vitamins compared with placebo.

It is important to recognize that science will never be "complete" and at some point the "weight of the scientific evidence must be judged adequate ..."[200] In any event, supplementation with 100–400 IU/day of vitamin E is safe. Furthermore, the evidence suggests that the major effect of vitamin E is at intake levels at or greater than 100 IU/day. Since it is difficult to obtain more than 30 IU/d from a low fat balanced diet, some supplementation is most likely beneficial in reducing the risk of CHD and various other diseases/disorders. Indeed, the American Dietetic Association also indicated that some individuals may require vitamin and/or mineral supplementation in addition to a good diet to ensure adequate nutritional needs.[202] Additionally, Willett and Stampfer[203] recently stated that they "also believe that vitamin E supplements are reasonable for most middle-aged and older Americans who are at increased risk of coronary disease."

Vitamin C (ascorbic acid)

Most of the interest and early clinical evidence that ascorbic acid has a protective role against atherosclerosis comes from a body of evidence that suggests that this disease is lower in populations that have an increased intake of leafy green vegetables and fruit.[204] More specifically, Trout[205] reviewed the literature before 1991 and found that vitamin C deficiency was an important cardiovascular risk factor in the following situations:

(1) The elderly are generally more likely to consume less fruits and vegetables and inadequate amounts of vitamin C compared with younger people.
(2) Sex is an important factor in determining vitamin C status for the elderly. Older men consistently have lower plasma ascorbic acid levels than women of similar age and require three times the amount of dietary vitamin C to achieve comparable levels.
(3) It has long been recognized that smoking is associated with very low plasma ascorbic acid levels. This is undoubtedly due to the formation of more than one billion free radicals with each puff on a cigarette.[206]
(4) Diabetics have lower plasma and leukocyte ascorbic acid concentrations than non-diabetics.

As with vitamin E, studies regarding the correlation of vitamin C intake and arteriosclerosis have been mixed. In a large-scale study involving over 11,000 elderly non-institutionalized American adults, there was a significant correlation between vitamin C intake from food and/or supplements and lower cardiovascular mortality.[207] In addition, after adjustment for smoking, disease history, race and education level, men whose vitamin C intake was $\geq$500 mg/day lived, on average six years longer than those whose intake was <500 mg/day. Harats et al.[208] studied the effects of vitamin C in healthy male students consuming a diet high in saturated fatty acids. After a one-month period, during which each participant consumed about 50 mg ascorbic acid daily (low-C diet), half of the subjects were randomly assigned to 500 mg ascorbic acid/day (high-C diet) for two months while the other half continued to receive 50 mg/day. Mean plasma ascorbate levels increased from 13.5 umol/L for those on the low-C diet to 51.7 umol/L for those on the high-C diet. Importantly, those on the high-C diet had a significant increase in the lag period of *in vitro* LDL oxidation (test measures reserve antioxidant capacity) which correlated with plasma ascorbate levels. Since LDL vitamin E levels were unchanged with the two diets, the authors concluded that this was presumptive evidence for an interaction between aqueous and lipophilic antioxidants in preventing or delaying LDL oxidation (similar to data cited in Ref. No. 148). Nyyssonen *et al.*[209] also reported that vitamin C deficiency, as assessed by decreased fasting plasma ascorbate levels, is an important risk factor for CHD. In this study, using a Cox proportional hazards model adjusted for age, year of examination and season of the year, men who had vitamin C deficiency (plasma levels less than 11.4 umol/L; 2.0 mg/L) had a relative risk for myocardial infarction of 3.5 compared with those who had normal plasma levels.

More recently, Vita and associates[210] investigated the relations between plasma antioxidant status and the degree of atherosclerosis and coronary artery disease activity in 149 patients undergoing cardiac catheterization (65 patients had stable angina, 84 had unstable angina or a myocardial infarction within two weeks). Their results showed that age, diabetes mellitus, male gender and hypercholesterolemia were all independent predictors of the severity of atherosclerosis. However, none of the 12 measured plasma antioxidant/oxidant markers correlated with the extent of atherosclerosis. However, lower plasma ascorbate levels predicted the presence of an unstable coronary syndrome. Moreover, when only patients with significant coronary artery disease were evaluated, plasma ascorbate and total thiol levels both predicted the presence of an unstable coronary syndrome, but did not predict the severity of atherosclerosis. The authors concluded that their data was consistent with a protective role for antioxidants in coronary artery disease by influencing lesion activity rather than reducing the extent of the atherosclerotic process.

Others[211] studied the relationship between dietary and supplemented vitamins C, E and carotenoids and the average carotid artery thickness in 6318 women and 4989 men aged 45 to 64 years. Their findings in both sexes aged 55 years and older showed an inverse relationship between vitamin C intake and average artery wall thickness after adjusting for age, BMI, serum glucose level, blood pressure, HDL and LDL cholesterol, total caloric intake, smoking, race and education level. Interestingly, the authors also reported an inverse relationship between arterial wall thickness and vitamin E intake among women but not men. Conversely, in a study involving only men, supplementary and dietary vitamin E intake was inversely associated with coronary artery lesion progression but no benefit was found for dietary or supplementary vitamin C.[212]

More recently, a group of healthy elderly men and women were subjected to vitamin C supplementation.[213] Lipids, lipid peroxidation, enzymatic and non-enzymatic antioxidant status were evaluated after 30, 60 and 90 days. Prior to supplementation, the activities/levels of enzymatic and non-enzymatic antioxidants were decreased whereas lipid peroxidation was increased. However, vitamin C supplementation decreased the concentrations of lipoperoxides, cholesterol, triacyglycerol and phospholipids, and increased the activities of the enzymatic antioxidants (e.g. superoxide dismutase, catalase, glutathione peroxidase, glutathione reductase and glutathione-S transferase). In addition, the levels of vitamins A, C and E were significantly increased.

As with vitamin E, most clinical studies support a cardioprotective effect of vitamin C, although the results have been inconsistent and somewhat confusing. In contrast to the basic studies whereby the effects of a single variant can be reliably measured and analyzed, clinical studies are more difficult to evaluate due to numerous interacting biological processes. As a result, it is not too surprising that the results of these studies are somewhat inconsistent and may lead to various interpretations.

Vitamin A/carotenoids

Observational epidemiologic studies suggest that those who consume higher dietary levels of fruits and vegetables rich in beta-carotene have a lower risk of CHD.[214] However, the plasma concentration of vitamin A is controlled by a hemostatic mechanism involving retinal-binding protein.[215] As a result, an increase in dietary vitamin A does not result in a long-term increase in circulating and tissue levels since the excess is stored in the liver. As a result, an increase in dietary vitamin A may not have any preventive effect on the incidence of disease that involve free radical mechanisms.[216] However, not all dietary beta-carotene is converted to retinal; some is absorbed and distributed unaltered.[217] Moreover, the concentration of lycopene is slightly higher than that of beta-carotene and is a significantly more efficient quencher of singlet oxygen.[218]

With regards to the effectiveness of the carotenoids in the preventiuon of LDL oxidation, studies have been mixed with some showing that beta-carotene is an effective antioxidant[219,220] while others have not demonstrated a positive antioxidant effect.[221,222] Moreover, the major clinical studies have generally not shown the carotenoids to be protective of atherogenesis. For example, Hennekens *et al.*[223] published data from their 12-year study of 11,036 healthy physicians randomly assigned to receive beta-carotene and 11,035 assigned a placebo. They reported "virtually no early or late differences in the overall incidence" of CHD or in overall mortality. These results are in agreement with two other large clinical studies.[224,225]

Flavonoids

A high intake of dietary saturated fat is well-known to be a very important risk factor for CHD. It is somewhat paradoxical that the French have comparable plasma cholesterol levels and a relatively high dietary intake of fat compared with other Western countries, yet the incidence of CHD is lower (so-called "French Paradox"). This phenomenon has been attributed, at least in part, to their higher dietary intake of flavonoids (Fig. 4.3), which are rich in red/purple grapes (i.e. red wine[226]), olives and green tea,[227] as well as various brightly colored fruits and vegetables.

Hertog *et al.*[165] measured the concentration of certain flavonoids, including quercetin, in various foods. They then assessed the total intake of flavonoids by Dutch men aged 65 to 84 years and followed them for five years. After adjustment for age, BMI, smoking, serum total and HDL cholesterol, blood pressure, physical activity, coffee consumption, vitamins (C, E and beta-carotene) and dietary fiber, a decreased risk for CHD was still significant in those with higher levels of flavonoids. More recently, these authors completed a ten-year follow-up of the Zutphen Elderly Study and re-calculated the relative-risk estimates.[228] They reported that the relative risk of a coronary event among men in the highest tertile compared with the lowest tertile of flavonoid intake was 0.47. They also noted that flavonol intake was inversely associated with all-cause mortality. The authors concluded that their current results strengthened their initial findings and showed a dose-response relationship between flavonol (mainly quercetin) intake and a first myocardial infarction, as well as the risk of CHD mortality.

In agreement with these studies, Knekt and associates[229] reported their findings based on data from 5133 Finnish men and women aged 30 to 69 years and free from heart disease at baseline (years 1967–1972); the cohort was followed until 1992. The primary outcome measures were dietary flavonoid intake, total mortality and mortality from CHD. After adjusting for age, smoking, serum cholesterol level, blood pressure and BMI, they concluded that individuals with a low intake of flavonoids had a significantly higher risk of CHD than those with a high flavonoid intake.

As indicated above, numerous basic studies, along with several clinical trials have shown that flavonoids are excellent antioxidants and are protective of CHD. However, as with vitamins C and E, not all clinical studies are in agreement. For example, Rimm *et al.*[230] reported a prospective cohort study involving 34,789 American male health professionals and compared their dietary intake of flavones and flavonols with the incidence of non-fatal myocardial infarction between 1986 and 1992. They concluded that their data did not support a strong inverse association between flavonoid intake and total CHD. However, this study did not exclude the possibility that these antioxidants have a protective effect in men with previously established cardiovascular disease. Moreover, several more recent reports[231–233] reaffirmed a prior Israeli study[234] which showed that the consumption of red wine (rich in polyphenols) but not white wine, reduced the propensity of plasma LDL to undergo lipid peroxidation in response to copper ion stimulation as determined by the decreases in the concentration of various lipid peroxidation products (e.g. thiobarbituric acid reactive substances, lipid peroxides, conjugated dienes and a significant prolongation of the lag phase before oxidation).

Stein and associates[232] assessed the effect of ingesting purple grape juice on vascular endothelial function and LDL susceptibility to oxidation in patients with coronary artery disease. Here, short-term (i.e. 14 days) ingestion of purple grape juice improved the flow-mediated vasodilatation of the brachial artery and reduced the oxidation of LDL suggesting that flavonoids may prevent cardiovascular events independent of the alcohol content of wine. Furthermore, Folts[235] not only found that red wine and purple grape juice enhances platelet and endothelial production of the vasodilator nitric oxide, but that 5.0 ml/kg of red wine or 5–10 ml/kg of purple grape juice inhibits platelet activity. Others[236–238] have also shown that purple grape juice inhibits platelet aggregation and suppresses platelet-mediated thrombosis, thereby decreasing the risk of cardiovascular events.

A recent meta-analysis of wine consumption showed "evidence of a significant inverse relation between light-to-moderate wine consumption and vascular risk."[233] Here, from 13 studies involving 209,418 persons, the relative risk of vascular disease associated with wine intake was 0.68 relative to non-drinkers. Interestingly, strong evidence from ten studies involving 176,042 persons supported a J-shaped relationship between the amount of red wine intake and vascular risk. Thus, a significant inverse association was found with daily intake up to 150 ml of red wine. Perhaps the failure of a couple of studies to show an inverse relation between red wine consumption and CHD is due to technique differences.[231]

Non-antioxidants and arteriosclerosis

Cholesterol and saturated fatty acids

Cholesterol, normally produced in the liver, is an essential compound; it is needed for the synthesis of some hormones, as well as being a necessary component of cell membranes. An increased plasma cholesterol level is, however, a well-known major risk factor for arteriosclerosis (CHD, ischemic stroke and peripheral vascular disease). About 70% of plasma cholesterol is circulated in the form of low density lipoprotein (LDL-cholesterol; LDL-C), the so-called "bad" cholesterol. A lesser amount of cholesterol circulates with high-density lipoprotein (HDL-C; "good" cholesterol). The total plasma cholesterol target is 200 mg/dL (5.18 mmol/L) or less. Nevertheless, total cholesterol misclassifies a person about 40% of the time. That is, a person can have a plasma cholesterol of 240 mg/dL and be at little risk or a total cholesterol of 200 and be at increased risk. The total cholesterol/HDL-C ratio is a very reliable risk indicator, the higher the ratio, the greater the risk.[239] These authors noted that a ratio of 3.5 or less would approach the "ideal," but recognized this would not be possible for most Americans since an estimated 90% would then require treatment. As a compromise, they recommended a cutoff ratio of 4.5 for all adults. Using these figures, a ratio of 7.1 and 9.6 would double the relative risk for women and men, respectively. Thus, a total cholesterol of 200 mg/d (target level) but an HDL of 20 mg/dL doubles the risk in men and almost triples the risk for women. Importantly, the risk ratio is considerably more meaningful than a mere number. Furthermore, the ratio holds for men, women and the elderly. It should also be recognized that exercise generally increases HDL-C and thereby lowers the ratio (relative risk for Boston marathoners, 3.1; for vegetarians, 2.9[239]). Additionally, the risk for ischemic stroke is significantly increased in those with low HDL-C levels.[240]

Dietary modification is essential in reducing increased cholesterol levels. One should begin with a diet high in fiber and low in cholesterol and other fatty substances, especially saturated fats which are rich in butter, cheese, beef, pork, etc. In a randomized trial, Knopp *et al.*[241] studied 444 men with LDL-C levels above the 75th age-specific percentile. These hypercholesterolemic participants were randomized to diets consisting 30%, 26%, 22% and 18% fat. Mean percent LDL-C reductions were 5.3%, 13.4%, 8.4% and 13.0% Moreover, the corresponding apolipoprotein B levels decreased 8.6%, 10.7%, 4.3% and 5.3%. Thus, moderate dietary fat restriction significantly reduced LDL-C and apoprotein B levels after one year.

Increased dietary intake of trans fatty acids, which raises plasma cholesterol levels, also increases the incidence of CHD. These fatty acids are produced when vegetable oils are hydrogenated to solidify them (i.e. some margarines and other food items). Since the relation between trans fatty acids and CHD was still unclear in the 1990s, Hu *et al.*[242] prospectively studied 80,082 women (Nurses' Health Study) aged 34 to 59 years. Their findings supported prior studies that replacing saturated and trans fatty acids with monounsaturated and polyunsaturated fats was more effective in preventing CHD than reducing overall fat intake. In addition, the recently published Zutphen Elderly Study,[243] which involved 667 men aged 64 to 84 years between 1985 and 1995, reported the average trans fatty acid intake decreased from 4.3% to 1.9% of total energy. After adjustment for age, BMI, smoking and dietary covariates, trans fatty acid intake at baseline was positively associated with the risk of CHD.

The National Cholesterol Education Program (NCEP) recommends beginning with the step 1 diet (30% of calories from total fat, 10% from saturated fat, and <300 mg of cholesterol/day). The step 2 diet (7% of calories from saturated fat and <200 mg of cholesterol/day) is recommended if the step 1 diet fails to adequately reduce the serum cholesterol level. However, for many people these minimal goals may not be achieved. If these and other lifestyle changes (i.e. decreased fat intake, caloric reduction, increased dietary fiber and exercise) are not successful, oral medications should probably be considered.[244-247]

Indeed, diet has been considered by some as relatively ineffective in reducing blood cholesterol levels.[248] To compare the effects of a dietary portfolio of cholesterol-lowering food versus lovastatin, Jenkins and associates[249] carried out a randomized controlled trial involving hyperlipidemic men and women (mean age, 59 years; BMI, 27.6 kg/m^2). The participants were randomly assigned to one of three interventions: control diet very low in saturated fat (e.g. whole-wheat cereals and low-fat dairy foods); the same diet plus lovastatin (20 mg/day); or a portfolio diet high in plant sterols, soy protein, viscous fibers and almonds. Their results showed mean decreases in LDL-C of 8.0%, 30.9% and 28.6% for the control, statin and portfolio diets, respectively. Moreover, the respective reductions in serum C-reactive protein levels were 10.0%, 33.3% and 28.2%. Thus, although a diet low in saturated fat resulted in a mild improvement in serum LDL-C and C-reactive protein, the portfolio diet was as effective as a low saturated-fat diet plus statin medication.

Dietary fiber

Since the minimal goals of the NCEP steps 1 and 2 diets may not be successful, other dietary changes should be recommended. Numerous studies have shown that both water-soluble and -insoluble fibers are hypocholesterolemic agents. Water-soluble fibers are concentrated in fruits, dried beans, legumes, barley psyllium and whole grains while insoluble fibers are rich in whole wheat products, wheat and corn bran, and various fruits and vegetables (e.g. cauliflower, green beans, potatoes, fruit and vegetable skins).

In an early dose-controlled study, 156 adults with LDL-C levels greater than 160 mg/dL (4.14 mmol/L) or between 130 and 160 mg/dL (3.37 to 4.14 mmol/L) were randomized to one of seven groups.[250] Six groups received either oatmeal or oat bran (28 g, 56 g and 84 g). The seventh group received 28 g of farina (beta-glucan, a water-soluble fiber). After six weeks, the groups who were receiving 84 g of oatmeal, 56 g of oat bran and 84 g of oat bran had LDL-C decreases of 10.1%, 15.9% and 11.5%, respectively. Moreover, 56 g of oatmeal, which contains more beta-glucan than oatmeal, resulted in a significantly greater decrease in plasma LDL-C levels than those receiving 56 g of oatmeal, suggesting that beta-glucan is particularly effective in lowering LDL-C levels. In a later observational study, over 40,000 male health professionals followed up to six years, Rimm and coworkers[251] concluded that "fiber, independent of fat intake, is an important dietary component for the prevention of coronary disease." In the same year, dietary fiber was shown to be an independent risk factor for CHD in Finnish men.[252] Here, fiber was particularly effective in preventing death from coronary disease in middle-aged smoking men. Subsequent studies involving women (Nurses' Health Study) also concluded that diets rich in fiber, especially from cereal sources, are protective against CHD.[253,254]

A high cereal fiber diet has also been shown to reduce the risk of CHD in the elderly.[255] In this prospective cohort study, 3588 men and women aged 65 years and older and free of CHD at baseline, were followed from 1989 to 2000. After adjustment for age, sex, education, diabetes, smoking history, daily physical activity, exercise intensity, alcohol intake, and fruit and vegetable fiber consumption, cereal fiber consumption was inversely associated with a 21% lower risk in the highest quintile intake compared with the lowest quintile. Interestingly, neither fruit nor vegetable fiber was associated with incident CHD in similar analyses. Others had previously reported that a high intake of fruits, vegetables and whole grains significantly reduce the risk of stroke in both men[256] and women.[257,258]

The mechanism(s) whereby whole grains, fruits, and vegetables protect against atherogenic diseases is probably multifactorial. In addition to cholesterol lowering, these foods are rich in a wide variety of antioxidants (vitamins C and E, phytic acid, flavonoids, phytoestrogens, selenium, zinc, copper, manganese and others).

Unsaturated fatty acids

Since a low rate of CHD in the Eskimo population exposed to a diet rich in fish oil was first reported,[259] numerous studies support the antiatherogenic, antiarrhythmic and antithrombotic effects of n-3 (omega-3) polyunsaturated fatty acids (PUFA).[260,261] In an early study, 852 men living in Zutphen, a small Dutch village, had been closely monitored for 20 years.[262] The authors reported that those who had eaten, on average, two fish meals/week had an overall reduction in CHD mortality of more the 50% compared with non-fish eaters. Several years later, Burr and coworkers[263] (the Diet and Reinfarction Trial) examined the effects of dietary intervention in the secondary prevention of myocardial infarction (MI). Here, 2033 men who had recovered from an MI were randomly allocated to receive advice or not to receive advice regarding three dietary possibilities: (1) reduction in saturated fat and an increase in the ratio of PUFA to saturated fat; (2) increase in fatty fish intake; and (3) increase in cereal fiber. The trial was prematurely stopped after two years because the fish advice group had a 29% reduction in all-cause mortality and a 33% reduction in deaths from ischemic heart disease. Interestingly, there was no reduction in recurrent non-fatal MI. In a later report, 1822 men aged 40 to 55 years and free of cardiovascular disease at baseline, were studied to examine the relation between baseline fish consumption and the 30-year risk of death from CHD.[264] Again, the data showed an inverse relation between fish consumption and death from CHD, especially from MI.

Several subsequent studies also supported a role for n-3 unsaturated fatty acids in the prevention of CHD. In the Lyon Heart Study,[265] patients who had suffered an MI were advised to eat a Mediterranean diet (rich in fruits, vegetables, bread and canola oil) that emphasized the use of canola oil margarine, which contains alpha-linolenic acid, an n-3 fatty acid precursor to longer-chain n-3 fatty acids. The control group was only advised to eat a "prudent" diet. After five years, overall mortality was reduced by 70% and cardiac death by 81% in those on the Mediterranean diet compared with the control group. A study one year later involved 334 patients with primary cardiac arrest and 493 population-based randomly selected controls free of current or prior heart disease, comorbidity, use of fish oils, and matched for age and sex.[266] The results showed that an average intake of 5.5 g of n-3 fatty acids per month (equivalent of one fatty fish meal per week) was associated with a 50% reduction in the risk of primary cardiac arrest. In addition, compared with a measured erythrocyte cell membrane n-3 PUFA level of 3.3% of total fatty acids (mean of lowest quartile), a red blood cell n-3 PUFA level of 5.0% was associated with a 70% reduction in the risk of primary cardiac arrest. To further investigate the benefits of food rich in n-3 PUFA, the GISSI Prevenzione Investigators[267] recently reported their findings on 11,324 survivors of a recent MI who were randomly assigned supplements of n-3 PUFA (1.0 g/d). The primary end points were death, non-fatal MI, and stroke. Their results showed that n-3 PUFA supplementation significantly decreased the rate of death, non-fatal MI, and ischemic stroke.

Two very important recent studies added further evidence that increased n-3 fatty acid intake significantly decreases the risk of CHD in both men and women. In the first study,[268] dietary consumption and follow-up data from the Nurses' Health Study (84,688 female nurses aged 34–59 years) showed that after adjustment for the usual confounding factors, the relative risks of CHD were 0.79 for fish consumption 1–3 times/month, 0.71 for 2–4 times/week and 0.66 for ≥5 times/week. The second report,[269] the Physicians' Health Study, compared the risk of sudden cardiac death with blood levels of long-chain n-3 fatty acids. The results showed that blood levels of n-3 fatty acids were "strongly associated with reduced risk of sudden death among men without evidence of prior cardiovascular disease."

Fish intake has also been shown to be inversely associated with ischemic stroke in both men and women. In a 12-year Health Professional Follow-up Study, the relative risk for men who ate fish one to three times per month, compared with those who ate fish less than once per month, was 0.57.[270] Similarly, a 14-year prospective cohort study of women aged 34 to 59 years (Nurses' Health Study) showed that increased consumption of fish and omega-3 polyunsaturated fatty acids was associated with a significant decreased risk of thrombotic cerebral infarction.[271] Furthermore, there was a progressive inverse association beween the frequency of fish consumption and risk of thrombotic infarction.

What is the mechanism whereby n-3 PUFA are protective of people with ischemic heart disease and stroke? Goodnight[272] suggested four possible pathways: (1) a reduction in platelet-vascular interactions and thrombosis; (2) an inhibitory effect on atherogenesis; (3) a damping of the vascular response to injury; and (4) a reduction in the rate of sudden cardiac death by decreasing ventricular arrhythmias. Various studies in both experimental animals and humans suggest that dietary fish oil decreases the frequency of arrythmias and sudden death in people with known or covert CHD. In an early experimental study, McLennan *et al.*[273] showed that the administration of tuna fish oil reduced the incidence of arrhythmias and prevented ventricular fibrillation during both occlusion and reperfusion of the coronary artery in rats. Similarly, Billman and coworkers[274] reported that infusion of fish oil completely prevented the acute occurrence of ventricular fibrillation in dogs. Importantly, in a prospective, double-blinded and placebo-controlled human study, 79 patients with moderate- to low-grade ventricular arrhythmias were randomly assigned to fish oil (40 patients) or placebo (39 patients).[275] The results showed that a moderate dose of fish oil (15 ml cod liver oil daily) significantly reduced the frequency of ventricular premature complexes.

To further evaluate the role of n-3 polyunsaturated fatty acids (PUFA) in CHD, Thies *et al.*[276] randomized a group of patients awaiting carotid endarterectomy by allocating patients' control, sunflower oil (n-6 PUFA), or fish oil (n-3 PUFA) capsules until they underwent surgery. The primary outcome was evaluated by plaque morphology indicative of stability or instability, and outcome measures of eicosapentaenoic acid, docosahexaenoic acid and linoleic acid in plaques; plaque morphology, and presence of macrophages in the plaques. Their findings showed that atherosclerotic plaques readily incorporate n-3 PUFA from fish oil supplementation, thereby enhancing plaque stability. Conversely, n-6 PUFA did not affect plaque fatty acid composition or stability. The authors concluded that "stability of plaques could explain reductions in non-fatal and fatal cardiovascular events associated with increased n-3 PUFA intake."

In another important recent study, the association between a fish-rich diet and leptin, a satiety factor and product of the obesity gene which is synthesized and secreted mainly in adipose tissue, was evaluated in two related homogeneous African tribal groups in Tanzania.[277] The results showed that a diet rich in fish resulted in lower plasma leptin levels in both men and women, independent of body fat.

Folic acid, vitamins B$_6$ and B$_{12}$

In 1969, McCully[278] reported that children with homocystinuria, an inherited recessive metabolic disorder, not only had markedly elevated plasma homocysteine levels but severe atherosclerosis. He postulated that increased homocysteine levels are atherogenic and proposed a metabolic pathway.[279] It was subsequently noted that homocystinuria heterozygotes also had increased plasma homocysteine levels and premature atherosclerosis and later studies showed that an increased plasma homocysteine level is a major arteriosclerosis risk factor for all persons. For example, Genest *et al.*[280] studied 170 men (50 ± 7 years old) with premature CHD and compared them with 255 control subjects who were clinically free of disease. The plasma homocysteine mean level of the group with heart disease was 13.66 ± 6.7 umol/L compared with the control group of 10.93 ± 4.9 umol/L. In addition, 28% of the patients with CHD had levels greater than the 90th percentile of the control (i.e. ≥15 umol/L). Similarly, Stampfer and associates[281] reported their findings from a prospective Physicians' Health Study of plasma homocysteine levels and acute MI. The study covered a period of five years and consisted of 14,916 men aged 40 to 84 years with no prior history of heart disease or stroke. Their results also showed that plasma homocysteine levels were significantly higher in those who developed an MI compared with the control group.

Numerous studies have since been published showing that increased plasma homocysteine levels are atherogenic, not only for CHD,[282–287] but also for stroke,[288–290] carotid artery wall thickness[291] and peripheral arterial occlusive disease.[292] With respect to folic acid intake and stroke, Bazzano *et al.*[293] studied 9764 men and women aged 25 to

74 years over an average of 19 years. Here, the relative risk was 0.79 for incident stroke events in the highest quartile of folate intake (median intake, 405 ug/day) compared with those in the lowest quartile (median intake, 99 ug/day).

For most people, homocysteine levels are readily controllable since homocysteine metabolism is dependent on folic acid and vitamins B_6 and B_{12} (Fig. 4.6). To assess the relationship between serum folate levels and the risk of fatal CHD, Morrison and associates[294] restrospectively studied a cohort of 5056 Canadian men and women aged 35 to 79 years who were free of heart disease. After 15 years of follow-up, there was a statistically significant association between serum folate levels and risk of fatal CHD. Furthermore, treatment with homocysteine-lowering therapy with folic acid and vitamins B_6 and B_{12} significantly reduces the incidence of important adverse events after successful angioplasty.[295]

More recent studies have also shown that an increased dietary intake of these nutrients significantly decreased plasma homocysteine levels and risk of the associated diseases.[296-300] Another

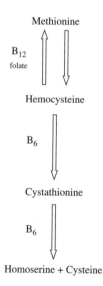

Methionine

B_{12}
folate

Hemocysteine

B_6

Cystathionine

B_6

Homoserine + Cysteine

Figure 4.6: Simplified chemical sequence for homocysteine metabolism.

important aspect of the study by Rimm *et al.*[287] is that daily intakes of 400 ug of folate and 3 mg of vitamin B_6 significantly minimize the morbidity and mortality from cardiovascular disease. Moreover, as with several other nutrients, their results futher support the view that current recommended dietary allowances for various nutrients are too low to provide optimal health benefits.

Although these and other studies support the association between increased homocysteine levels and CHD, some have questioned whether this association is causal.[301] To further evaluate this association, Klerk *et al.*[302] assessed the relation between the MTHFR 677C $\rightarrow$ T polymorphism, a genetic alteration in an enzyme involved in folate metabolism that causes elevated homocysteine levels. Indeed, the results showed that individuals with this genotype had a 16% greater odds of developing CHD, particularly in those individuals with low folic acid levels. Thus, this study further supports the relation between low folic acid intake, increased homocysteine levels and increased risk of CHD.

Magnesium

Magnesium (Mg) is the fourth most abundant cation in the body after sodium, potassium and calcium; it is the second most abundant intracellular cation (second to potassium). The great majority of Mg is in bone (57%) and soft tissues (40%), especially muscle. The remainder is in erythocytes and extracellular fluids. Mg is a cofactor for over 325 enzymes[303] which are involved in various membrane functions (e.g. hormone receptor binding), gating of calcium channels, transmembrane ion flux, regulation of adenylate cyclase and cellular energy production among others. As such, Mg plays a critical role in neuronal activity, neuromuscular transmission, cardiac excitability, blood pressure and vasomotor tone.

Mg deficiency is very common. Epidemiologic studies suggest that dietary Mg intake has progressively declined since 1900 from about 500 mg/day to about 200–250 mg/day. The minimum recommended daily allowance is 350 mg/day for men and 280 mg/day for women;

Table 4.11: Major Causes of Decreased Plasma Magnesium

Inadequate dietary intake	Malabsorption
Total parenteral nutrition	Chronic alcoholism
Diarrhea (chronic)	Medications (e.g. diuretics)
Diabetic ketoacidosis	

the desirable intake is 6–8 mg/day/kg body weight [420–560 mg/day for a 70 kg (150 pound) man].[304] The major causes of decreased plasma Mg levels are listed in Table 4.11.

Although numerous publications have stressed the high frequency of inadequate Mg intake, it is poorly appreciated by the general public as well as the medical profession. Touitou *et al.*[305] measured both serum and red blood cell Mg levels in 381 unselected healthy elderly men and women, most of whom were over 75 years old and were not taking any medication. Their findings showed that 10% had decreased serum Mg levels. Perhaps more importantly, twice this number (i.e. 20%) were hypomagnesemic when red cell levels were determined. Since Mg is primarily an intracellular cation, this latter figure best represents the prevalence of Mg deficiency. In agreement with this, an early study showed that serum Mg was the most frequent abnormal test in patients admitted to the intensive care unit (other routine tests included electrolytes, urea nitrogen, creatinine, calcium and total protein).[306] Here, 20% of the patients were hypomagnesemic while an additional 9% were hypermagnesemic.

Decreased serum Mg levels may result in various cardiac abnormalities. Atrial fibrillation is a common arrhythmia that is frequently treated with digoxin. DeCarli *et al.*[307] studied 45 consecutive patients with symptomatic atrial fibrillation and found that 20% had decreased serum Mg levels. Compared with those with normal serum concentrations, the hypomagnesemic patients required twice the dose of digoxin to control their arrhythmia. Others reported that low postoperative serum Mg levels were common in patients undergoing cardiac surgery.[308] In this placebo-controlled double blind study, the hypomagnesemic patients had significantly increased frequencies of postoperative ventricular dysrhythmias. However, Mg administration not only decreased the dysrhythmic frequency, but increased cardiac stroke volume.

Since a major function of magnesium is to control arterial tone, low serum levels may result in coronary artery spasm and ischemic heart disease. Indeed, several studies have shown a causal relationship between low serum Mg levels and non-occlusive acute myocardial infarction.[309,310] Moreover, the second Leicester Intravenous Magnesium Intervention Trial studied the effect of intravenous $MgSO_4$ in 2316 patients with suspected MI.[311] Here, the long-term outcome showed a 21% decrease in mortality rate from ischemic heart disease and a 16% reduction in all-cause mortality in those treated with intravenous Mg compared with the untreated group. Others have also reported an inverse association between ischemic heart disease and serum magnesium levels.[312,313]

Nut consumption and coronary heart disease

Evidence for the role of various vegetable and fish oils in lowering the risk of CHD has accumulated over the past few decades. More recently, epidemiologic studies indicate that nut consumption also lowers the risk of CHD in different population groups.[314] However, the mechanism whereby nuts are cardioprotective is not well understood, although the favorable fatty acid profile (low in saturated fatty acids and high in unsaturated fatty acids) appears to lower plasma cholesterol levels. The dietary fiber in nuts may also have additional cardioprotective effects.

In an attempt to further understand the mechanism of reduced coronary mortality from nut consumption, Albert *et al.*[315] prospectively studied 21,454 male physicians for an average of 17 years (Physicians' Health Study). They concluded that the inverse association between nut intake and total CHD death is "primarily due to a reduction in the risk of sudden death." Others,[316] reporting on the effects of walnut consumption in plasma fatty acids and lipoproteins, concluded that walnuts beneficially alter lipid distribution among the various lipoprotein subclasses, suggesting an additional mechanism underlying the anti-atherogenic properties of nuts. In addition, pecan consumption has been shown to significantly lower plasma levels of LDL, HDL, and total cholesterol while increasing the levels of insoluble fiber, monounsaturated fatty acids, polyunsaturated fatty acids and magnesium.[317] Finally, Feldman[318] recently reviewed the scientific evidence that walnut consumption reduces the risk of CHD. He reported that five controlled, peer-reviewed intervention trials consistently demonstrated that walnuts lower blood cholesterol levels.

Sodium and congestive heart failure

Congestive heart failure (CHF) is a common medical problem in individuals with chronic CHD, hypertension and various other cardiac disorders. Cross-sectional epidemiologic studies indicate that a higher intake of dietary sodium is associated with an increased risk of left ventricular hypertrophy and associated CHF. To further evaluate this association, Jiang *et al.*[319] followed 5233 normal weight and 5129 overweight healthy men and women. After 19 years of follow-up, the researchers concluded that a high sodium diet (i.e. ≥ 113.6 mmol/day; 2.6 g/day) is a strong independent risk factor for CHF in overweight persons.

Summary

The prevention of atherosclerosis and its associated diseases (CHD, stroke and peripheral vascular disease) is multifactorial. Although diets low in cholesterol and saturated fat but rich in antioxidants, magnesium and n-3 polyunsaturated fatty acids are very important, they are only one aspect to the solution of reducing the incidence of atherosclerosis-related diseases. Other important factors include weight control, physical exercise and abstinence from smoking. Nevertheless, a healthy diet that is rich in fruits, vegetables, grains, fiber, and low in saturated fat and trans fatty acids is extremely important (Figs. 4.1 and 4.2). In addition, multivitamin and mineral supplements are likely to be important in middle-aged and elderly adults where the risk of various free radical-related diseases is high and good nutrition is often absent. Certainly, the benefits of these supplements far outweigh any dangers and most likely significantly decrease the risk of heart disease, stroke, some cancers, and various other diseases/disorders. Indeed, on the basis of recent studies, Fletcher and Fairfield recommend that all adults should take a multivitamin daily; older persons should take additional vitamins B_{12} and D separately.[320]

Cancer

Cancer is the second leading cause of death in the US and other industrialized countries. In 2002, the estimated number of cancer cases and deaths in the US was 1,284,900 and 555,500, respectively.[321] A recent American Cancer Society report indicated that black Americans have about a 33% higher death rate for all cancers than white Americans.[322] The average annual incidence rates per 100,000 persons for all cancer sites for the major racial/ethnic groups were as follows: blacks, 445.3; whites, 401.4; Asian/Pacific Islanders, 283.4; Hispanics, 270.0; and American Indians/Native Alaskans, 202.7. In 1998, 53% of all cancer-related deaths in the US were associated with four sites: lung/bronchus, colon/rectum, prostate and breast.[323]

Cancer is, however, largely a preventable disease. As Sporn[324] wrote, "I start with the assumption, perhaps a prejudice, that cancer is a preventable rather than a treatable disease, and that much of our frustration with the 'cancer problem' stems from our inability to bring this concept to fruition." Indeed, about 65% of all cancers are secondary to cigarette smoking and poor nutrition.[325] With respect to nutrition and cancer, numerous studies suggest that an adequate intake of various antioxidants (e.g. vitamins C and E, carotenoids and flavonoids), folic acid, vitamins B_6 and B_{12} and trace metals (e.g. selenium and zinc) may significantly reduce the risk of various cancers. Indeed, a recent randomized trial suggested that the Mediterranean diet reduces the incidence of several cancers.[181] However, since the etiology of many cancers is not well understood, there are unexplained inconsistencies in various studies, not only with respect to lifestyle differences, but in men and women. For example,

Khaw *et al.*[326] prospectively studied 19,496 men and women aged 45 to 79 years. Their results showed that the plasma ascorbic acid concentration was not only inversely related to mortality from all-causes and from ischemic heart disease in both men and women, but was inversely related to cancer mortality in men but not women.

Although the exact mechanisms whereby these micronutrient deficiencies remains largely unknown, they can mimic radiation or various carcinogens in damaging DNA by causing single- and double-strand breaks, oxidative lesions, or both. Indeed, a causative role for reactive oxygen species as a cancer cause has been hypothesized;[327] a large body of circumstantial evidence now supports this hypothesis.[72] For example, 8-hydroxy-2'-deoxyguanosine (8-OHdG) is a well established biomarker of oxidative damage to DNA. In a randomized crossover study, Chen and associates[328] assessed its responsiveness to diet in a group of non-smoking healthy men and women who consumed two antioxidant-rich liquid formula diets, one of which was rich in vitamin E, a potent antioxidant. Their findings showed a 22% decrease in the 8-OHdG/deoxyguanine ratio and a significant downward trend in leukocyte 8-OHdG among all subjects throughout the nutrient-rich study phases. Thus, a diet rich in antioxidants significantly decreases DNA damage and presumably the risk of various cancers.

Aside from nutrition, other important lifestyle risk factors include overweight/obesity (Chapter 2), physical inactivity (Chapter 3) and smoking, excessive alcohol intake, environmental toxins and long-term sunlight exposure (Chapter 5). In this section, the role of nutrition in the prevention of various cancers will be presented.

Colorectal cancer

Colon cancer is the third most commonly occurring cancer in American men and women. In 2002, there were an estimated 107,300 cases of colon cancer in the US (men, 50,000; women, 57,300) and 48,100 deaths (men, 23,100; women 25,000).[321] Rectal cancer accounted for

an estimated 41,000 cases (men, 22,600; women, 18,400) and 8500
deaths (men, 4700; women, 3800).[321] Unfortunately, the etiology of
colorectal cancer remains largely unknown. Early reported risk
factors other than genetics (about 10–15% of cases), have included
overweight/obesity, physical inactivity, and high fat, low fiber diets.
Other modifiable risk factors that can prevent colon cancer include
adequate folic acid intake, reducing alcohol use and decreasing red
meat consumption, among others. For example, the prospective Health
Professionals Follow-up Study followed 49,927 men aged 40 to
75 years for ten years.[329] They evaluated the following possible risk
factors: obesity, physical inactivity, alcohol consumption early adulthood cigarettes smoking, red meat consumption and low intake of
folic acid from supplements. After adjusting for age and family history of colorectal cancer and comparing the risk for the combined
six modifiable risk factors at or above the 20th , 10th or 5th percentiles versus below, the population attributable risk percent increased
from 39% to 45% to 55%, respectively.

Dietary fiber

Observational studies around the world have consistently found that
the risk of colorectal cancer is lower in populations with high intakes
of fruits and vegetables. Moreover, upon moving from one country
to another and adopting a different diet, the risk may increase. Since
fruits and vegetables are rich in various antioxidants (carotenoids,
vitamin C and flavonoids), folic acid, and other anti-carcinogenic
components such as fermentable fiber, it has been widely accepted
that they are protective against colorectal cancer. However, several
recent studies are not in complete agreement, although the findings
are somewhat inconsistent.

The hypothesis that dietary fiber may decrease the risk of colorectal
cancer was first proposed by Burkitt.[330] Most of the subsequent ana-
lytic epidemiologic reports were from case-control studies. Potter[331]
reviewed 17 studies before 1996 and found that 11 showed an
inverse correlation between dietary fiber intake and colon cancer.
Howe *et al.*[332] reviewed 13 case-control studies from several countries;

the combined data showed a strong overall inverse relationship between dietary fiber intake and colorectal cancer. Similarly, Meyer and White[333] conducted a five-year population-based case-control study in men and women aged 30 to 62 years living in western Washington State. High dietary fiber intake was associated with progressively lower relative risks for colon cancer with odds ratios of 1.0, 0.9, 0.8 and 0.6 across the quartiles of fiber consumption in men; for women, the ratios were 1.0, 0.9, 0.5 and 0.5. More recently, a case-control Italian study involved 1225 cases of colon cancer, 728 cases of rectal cancer and 4154 controls.[334] After allowing for the usual confounding factors, most types of fiber reduced the risk of both cancers. More specifically, when the results of the fourth and first quintiles (i.e. 80th and 20th percentiles) were compared, the odds ratios of colorectal cancer were 0.68 for total fiber, 0.67 for soluble non-cellulose polysaccharides (SNPs), 0.71 for total insoluble fiber, 0.67 for cellulose, 0.82 for insoluble SNPs and 0.88 for lignin. When the fiber sources were classified, the odds ratios were 0.75 for vegetable fiber, 0.85 for fruit fiber and 1.09 for cereal fiber.

More recent reports, however, have not shown an inverse relationship between dietary fiber intake and colorectal cancer. For example, in 1999 Fuchs and associates[335] published their prospective study of 88,757 women 34 to 59 years of age. After 16 years of follow-up, and adjustment for age, various established risk factors and total energy intake, they found no association between dietary fiber and risk for colorectal cancer. The following year, Michels and coworkers[336] published data from both the Nurses' Health Study (88,764 women) and Health Professionals' Follow-up Study (47,325 men); they concluded that frequent consumption of fruits and vegetables "does not appear to confer protection from colon or rectal cancer." Similarly, a recent report found that a low-fat, high-fiber diet rich in fruits and vegetables did not decrease the recurrence risk of colorectal adenomas,[337] nor did a diet supplemented with wheat-bran fiber.[338] Conversely, Terry *et al.*[339] subsequently reported that total fruit and vegetable consumption was inversely associated with colorectal cancer in Swedish women. Here, those who consumed less than 1.5 servings of fruits and vegetables each day had a relative risk for colorectal cancer of 1.65 compared with the women who consumed 2.5 servings each day. A subanalysis of the data indicated that the association was largely due to fruit consumption.

The inconsistencies in these studies is perplexing and may be due, at least in part, to several things such as differential recall of dietary habits by case subjects compared with control subjects, to various dietary habits by case subjects compared with control subjects, or to various dietary micronutrients associated with diets high in fiber. Until recently, most studies have shown an inverse relation between both vegetable and fruit intake and colorectal cancer, including cohort studies.[340] Perhaps, as noted in a study of German vegetarians[341] with reduced overall mortality and incidence of colon cancer, individuals who have a relatively high intake of fruits and vegetables may simply be more health conscious and have a more healthy lifestyle than those whose intake of fruits and vegetables is low. In any event, after reviewing the literature on early detection and prevention of colorectal cancer, Dashwood[342] wrote: "In the meantime, the best approach to reducing the risk of colorectal cancer would be to increase the dietary intake of fruits, vegetables and cereals, while reducing the overall intake of fat, particularly from animal sources."

Fats, fatty acids and red meat

Foods from animal sources remain major contributors of total fats, saturated fat and cholesterol in North American and some European diets. Although red meats (i.e. beef, pork and lamb) are often rich in these lipids and have been associated with various cancers, especially of the colon and prostrate,[343] all studies have not. For example, Howe and associates[344] examined the effect of dietary fat intake on colorectal cancer risk in a combined analysis of data from 13 case-controlled studies involving 5287 persons with colorectal cancer and 10,470 non-cancer controls. Although positive associations with total energy intake were found for 11 of the 13 studies, there was minimal, if any evidence that total fat was an important risk factor; the quintile odds ratios of total fat intake and colorectal cancer were 1.00, 0.95, 1.01 and 0.92.

A major interpretive problem here is differentiating the effects of dietary fat from total energy intake. There are several mechanisms whereby dietary fat and specific fatty acids may affect the risk of colon cancer in addition to total energy intake. In a population-based study, Slattery *et al.*[345] compared 1993 colon cancer cases with 2410 controls in three areas of the US. They found that the most commonly consumed fatty acid was oleic acid and that one-third of dietary fats consumed were from additions to other foods or from the preparation of other foods. Their results showed that neither total dietary fat nor specific fatty acids was associated with an increased risk of colon cancer after adjusting for total energy intake, level of physical activity, or body size. However, fats from food preparation were associated with an increased risk for colon cancer among older women, although fats from foods themselves were not. Moreover, population subgroups were at "slightly greater risk if they consumed a high-fat diet."

Several reports have also suggested that frequent eating may be a risk factor for colon cancer. To further investigate this possible relationship, Favero and associates[346] reported their case-control study from six areas of Italy involving 1225 incident cancer cases less than 75 years of age and 4154 control subjects. After controlling for the level of physical activity, education, vegetable intake and major energy sources, they found a direct correlation between colon cancer and eating frequency. Interestingly, coffee intake reversed the association. The authors suggested that whereas eating increases the excretion of bile acids, which may be carcinogenic, coffee decreases bile acid excretion.

The intake of red meat has frequently been regarded as a stronger risk factor for colon cancer than total fat. To examine the relative effects of fat, meat, fiber and vegetable intake, 47,949 American male health professionals, aged 40 to 75 years and free of cancer in 1986, were followed until 1992.[347] The results showed that intakes of total fat, saturated fat and animal fat, were not risk factors of colon cancer. However, the relative cancer risk was directly associated with red meat intake (relative risk 1.71). Men who ate pork, beef or lamb as a main serving five or more times per week had a relative risk of 3.57 compared with men who consumed these foods less than once each month. The mechanism whereby red meat increases the risk of colon cancer is probably not mediated through its total fat content. Rather, other factors such as heterocyclic aromatic amines formed from cooking meat and fish most likely have an important role in colon carinogenesis.[348] Indeed, chronic administration of heterocyclic amine mutagens (e.g. 2-amino-1-methyl-6-phenylimidazo [4,5-b]pyridine and 2-amino-3methylimidazo[4,5-f]quinoline) induces tumors in rats at several sites, including colonic adenocarcinomas.[349] Importantly, these heterocyclic animes are products of cooking meat and fish. Moreover, Wu *et al.*[350] found that the incidence of colon cancer was significantly higher in humans whose dietary exposure to these amines was increased. Thus, people who preferred well-cooked red meat and had higher frequencies of frying, barbecuing, broiling, or using meat drippings had significantly higher colon cancer rates compared with those less inclined to these characteristics. Indeed, the risk of colon cancer was increased three-fold among persons who preferred well-done red meat and was increased over two-fold among those who frequently fried, barbequed, or broiled their meats, or used meat drippings.

To further evaluate the association between several foods and nutrients and the development of colon and rectal cancers, Fung *et al.*[351] prospectively assessed dietary information from 76,401 women over a 12-year follow-up period and identified two major dietary patterns: "prudent" (higher intake of fruits, vegetables, legumes, fish, poultry and whole grains) and "Western" (higher intake of red and processed meats, sweets and desserts, french fries and refined grains). After adjusting for potential confounders, the relative risk for colon cancer among those consuming the Western diet was 1.46 (highest versus lowest quintiles). The prudent diet was not associated with a significant relative risk for the highest versus the lowest quintiles. They found no association between dietary patterns and rectal carcinoma.

Folic acid and methionine

In an early clinical study,[352] 47,931 American male professionals aged 40 to 75 years and free of cancer in 1986, were followed for six years. These investigators found that alcohol intake was directly related to the risk of colon cancer. Thus, for persons who consumed two or more daily drinks, the relative risk was 2.07 compared with those whose alcohol intake was less than 0.25 drinks per day. Moreover, combinations of high alcohol and low methionine and folate intakes showed a relative risk of 3.30 for total colon cancer. When they compared high-methyl diets (i.e. folate and methionine) with low-methyl diets in high alcohol users, the relative risk for distal colon cancer was striking — 7.44. Conversely, there was no increased colon cancer risk for individuals with a high intake of methionine and folate and two or more daily alcohol drinks. Importantly, the increased risk of colon cancer associated with alcohol intake and diets deficient in folate and methionine was not confounded by smoking, level of physical activity, BMI, intakes of red meat, fat, fiber, multivitamins, or aspirin.

A subsequent study[353] involved 88,756 women (Nurses Health Study) free of cancer in 1980 and supplemented with a multivitamin from 1980 to 1994. During this time, 442 women developed colon cancer. Folic acid intake greater than 400 ug/day compared with an intake of less than 200 ug/day resulted in a relative risk of 0.69 after controlling for age, family history of colorectal cancer, aspirin use, smoking, BMI, physical activity and intakes of red meat, alcohol, methionine and fiber. In addition, the results were similar when intakes of vitamins A, C, D and E and calcium were controlled for. Importantly, the reduced risk of colon cancer was evident only after four years of supplementation which then continued to decrease with time. Thus, the relative risk was 0.83 for five to nine years, 0.80 for ten to 14 years, but 0.25 for 15 or more years. The authors suggested that the inverse relation between long-term multivitamin use and colon cancer was perhaps related to the folate contained in multivitamins. Two additional recent studies provide further evidence that folate intake is inversely associated with colon cancer risk.[354,355]

The likely mechanism whereby folic acid appears to decrease the risk of colon cancer and other malignancies is because it is essential for regenerating methionine, which can donate a methyl group for DNA methylation and the synthesis of purine and pyrimidine bases which are required for DNA synthesis. As shown by Blount *et al.*,[356] folate deficiency causes an extensive incorporation of uracil into human DNA (four million/cell) and increases the frequency of micronuclei, a measure of chromosome breaks. These events presumably promote carcinogenesis. However, the nuclear changes are reversed by folate administration (see discussion under vitamins and cancer). A proposed mechanism explaining how folate may reduce carcinogenesis was recently published.[457]

Calcium and vitamin D

The global geographic distribution of colon cancer is similar to that of rickets. That is, colon cancer rates are highest in regions where winter ultraviolet radiation is significantly reduced. For example, the incidence of colon cancer is highest in the northeast and north central areas, and lowest in the southern, southwestern and intermountain regions of the US.[358] Based on the geographic epidemiology of death rates from colon cancer, it was first suggested in 1980 that calcium and vitamin D may reduce the risk of this malignant disease.[359] Subsequent epidemiologic studies added support to this hypothesis in that low intakes of both calcium and vitamin D reportedly increased the incidence of colon cancer.[360,361] More specifically, a 19-year prospective study by Garland *et al.*[360] found that a daily intake of 3.75 ug or more of vitamin D resulted in a 50% reduction in the incidence of colorectal cancer; a daily intake of 1200 mg or more of calcium reduced the incidence by 75%. More recently, a five-year case-control study[362] involving 1953 incident colorectal carcinoma cases and 4154 controls showed a mild inverse relationship between both calcium and vitamin D intake (odds ratios 0.85 and 0.93, respectively) and colorectal carcinoma. However, when the combined effects of high calcium, vitamin D and selected antioxidants were considered in both men and women, the odds ratio was 0.46 compared with subjects whose intakes of these nutrients was low. In another recent clinical study,[363] calcium supplementation (1200 mg/day) was associated with a significant, albeit "moderate," reduction in the risk of colorectal adenomas in both men and women. The adjusted ratio of the mean number of recurrent adenomas in the calcium supplemented group, compared with the placebo group, was 0.76. Importantly, the protective effect was noted as early as one year after supplementation began. In a recent review of this topic, Garland and associates[364] suggested that most cases in colorectal cancer can be prevented by a daily intake of 1800 mg of calcium and 800 IU (20 ug) of vitamin D.

The mechanism whereby calcium and vitamin D reduce the incidence of colorectal cancer is unknown. However, as noted earlier, diets rich in red meat and animal fat increase the risk of colon cancer by increasing the production of potentially carcinogenic bile acids. Calcium, however, may inhibit carcinogenesis by binding bile acids and fatty acids in the bowel or possibly by the direct inhibition of colonic epithelial cell proliferation.[365] Studies in laboratory animals support this proposed mechanism since dietary calcium is protective of bile-induced mucosal damage and experimental carcinogenesis.[366]

Green tea

Tea is widely consumed and generally believed to decrease the risk of various diseases including some cancers and CHD, among others. The major reason for this belief is that tea leaves are rich in antioxidant polyphenols (mainly catechins). However, there are several major categories of tea (i.e. white, green, black and oolong) which are produced by different processing (fermentation) methods. Although fresh tea leaves are rich in these compounds, they become oxidized during fermentation resulting in polymerization to form larger and more complex polyphenols. Hence, the availability of the active antioxidants may vary depending on the type of tea.

As noted above, cooking meat and fish results in the formation of carcinogenic heterocyclic amines. In experimental studies with rats, Dashwood and associates have repeatedly shown that both green and black tea catechins have anti-carcinogenic activity in the colon.[349,367,368] It is not surprising, therefore, that a recent literature review found that three of five clinical studies showed an inverse association between colon cancer and green tea consumption.[369]

Anti-inflammatory drugs

An adenomatous polyp, a benign intermediate in the development of colorectal cancer, is reportedly present in about 33% of the general population by age 50 years and in about 50% by age 70.[370] Recent studies suggest that the prevention of adenomatous polyps and their subsequent progression to colorectal cancer is possible by various pharmacologic agents (chemoprevention). In this regard, aspirin and other non-steroidal anti-inflammatory drugs (NSAIDs) have been widely studied. Several mechanisms have been suggested whereby these agents might inhibit prostaglandin synthesis [i.e. cyclooxygenases 1 and 2 (COX-1, COX-2)]. Thus, various clinical studies have shown that COX-2 is elevated in up to 40% of colorectal adenomas and 90% of sporadic colon carcinomas but is not increased in normal colonic epithelial cells.[371,372] Moreover, NSAIDs may also act by other mechanisms including inhibition of the activation of nuclear factor-kappa B (NFkB)[373] or other mechanisms.[374]

A review of a series of case-controlled clinical studies found a 40% to 50% risk reduction for colonic adenomas and carcinomas among patients who regularly took aspirin.[375] The Cancer Prevention Study II,[376] which involved 662,424 participants between 1982 and 1989, reported a relative risk for death due to colon cancer in those with infrequent aspirin use (i.e. less than once each month) of 0.77 for men and 0.73 for women. The risk was reduced further if aspirin was taken more than 16 times per month. The Health Professional Follow-up Study[377] involved 47,900 men who completed a questionnaire twice each year regarding aspirin use. The results showed that the relative risk for colorectal cancer was 0.68 when regular aspirin use (i.e. more than twice/week) was reported on a single questionnaire; the relative risk was 0.35 when regular use was reported on three or more successive questionnaires. Furthermore, a study involving

89,446 women (Nurses' Health Study)[378] found that regular aspirin use (two or more times/week) had a relative risk of 0.62 compared with those who were not regular aspirin users. Although there was little risk reduction during the first nine years, the relative risk was 0.56 after 20 or more years of use.

Summary

The incidence of colorectal cancer has continued to decrease since 1986. The exact role played by diet is complex since the relationship between diet and colon cancer is multifactorial. As a result, studies have been somewhat inconsistent. Nevertheless, the scientific data generally shows that low dietary intake of fruit and vegetable fiber, calcium, folic acid and perhaps other micronutrients, and increased intake of red meat significantly increase the risk of colorectal cancer. Conversely, regular use of aspirin and other non-steroidal anti-inflammatory drugs appear to significantly reduce the risk of colorectal cancer. Thus, when a "healthy diet" is combined with weight control and moderate physical activity, the risk of colorectal cancer can be significantly lowered.

Stomach and esophageal cancers

Prior to 1930, stomach cancer was the leading cause of cancer-related deaths in most countries, including the US. Since then, however, there has been a steady decrease in gastric cancer throughout the world, but the decrease in the West has been especially high. Although the reasons for this dramatic decrease are not fully understood, decreased consumption of salt-preserved food, increased dietary intake of fresh fruits and vegetables, and the availability of refrigeration are most likely important factors. In addition, considerable epidemiological data indicates that the microorganism, *Helicobacter pylori*, is a strong risk factor for gastric cancer. However, the exact carcinogenic mechanisms remain to be elucidated, but could be due to toxic substances produced by the bacterium or it may be secondary to the host inflammatory response to the infection.

Unfortunately, in some countries the incidence of stomach cancer has fallen much more slowly. For example, gastric carcinoma remains the most common type of cancer in both men and women in Japan and accounts for 18% of all cancer-related deaths (52.6 deaths/100,000 men and 27.5/100,000 women compared with 6.3/100,000 men and 4.2/100,000 women in the US).[379] The estimated number of stomach cancer cases in the US in 2002 was 21,600 (men, 13,300; women, 8300) with 12,400 deaths (men, 7200; women, 5200).[321] Esophageal cancer is significantly less frequent but far more lethal than gastric cancer (96% mortality rate). The estimated number of US cases in 2002 was 13,100 (men, 9800; women, 3300) with 12,600 deaths (men, 9600; women, 3000).[321]

Cereal fiber

When taken together, two case-control studies of adenocarcinomas of the esophagus and gastric cardia found that total dietary fiber intake significantly lowered the risk of both cancers.[380,381] Since *in vitro* studies have shown that cereal fiber might act as a scavenger of nitrite, a presumed carcinogen, under similar conditions that exist in the stomach, Terry and coworkers[382] studied the possible association between dietary cereal fiber and risk of esophageal and gastric cardia cancers. In this population-based case-control study, they found a strong dose-dependent inverse association between total dietary fiber and risk of gastric cardia adenocarcinoma, of which cereal fiber was the most important. The odds ratio among those in the highest quartile of cereal fiber intake compared with the lowest quartile was 0.3. Although a high intake of cereal fiber was also significantly associated with a decreased risk of esophageal adenocarcinoma, a linear dose-risk trend was not observed. Moreover, no association was found between dietary fiber and esophageal squamous cell carcinoma.

Vegetables and fruits

Frequent consumption of fruits and vegetables has also been associated with reduced risk for stomach cancer in most case-control studies, although prospective reports have been less consistent. In a recent prospective study that evaluated the role of fruits and vegetables in fatal gastric cancer, McCullough *et al.*[383] reported their findings from a cohort of 1.2 million American men and women over a 14-year follow-up period (Cancer Prevention Study II). After controlling for various confounders, the results showed that a high overall intake of plant foods (sum of vegetables, citrus fruit and whole grains) was associated with a modest risk reduction of stomach cancer in men but not women. Others,[384] however, reported an inverse association between esophageal adenocarcinoma with dietary intakes of vegetables, citrus fruits and juices, dairy products, fish and dark bread. As with colorectal cancer, they found that diets high in meats may increase the risk of distal stomach cancer.

Micronutrients

In contrast with a significant decline in gastric cancer over the past several decades, Mayne and associates[385] indicated that the incidence rates of esophageal and gastric cardia adenocarcinomas have been rising. To further investigate the possible risk factors for this phenomenon, these workers examined the intake of various nutrients as risk factors for several subtypes of esophageal and gastric cancers (gastric cardia, non-cardia gastric, esophageal adenocarcinoma and esophageal squamous cell carcinoma) in a population-based case-control study in three states (Connecticut, New Jersey and western Washington state). Their findings indicated that fiber, beta-carotene, folate and vitamins C and B_6 were all significantly inversely associated with the risk of all four cancer types. They concluded that diets rich in plant-based foods that contain these nutrients were associated with a reduced risk of gastric and esophageal cancers, whereas a higher intake of nutrients found mainly in foods of animal origin was associated with an increased cancer risk.

As noted in a large clinical study, the people of Linxian County, China have very high rates of esophageal and gastric cardia cancer and a persistently low dietary intake of various micronutrients. To determine whether supplementation with micronutrients might lower the mortality from, or incidence of cancer in these people, Blot and associates[386] studied 29,584 adults aged 40 to 69 years and followed them from 1986 to 1991. Their findings showed that those who received daily supplementation with beta-carotene, vitamin E and selenium had significantly lower overall cancer rates, but this was especially true for stomach cancer. In a companion publication,[387] this research group reported that although multiple vitamin/mineral supplementation in this same population lowered the cumulative esophageal/gastric cardia cancer death rate by 8% and total mortality by 7%, the results were not statistically significant. The authors suggested that perhaps a longer follow-up period would be more informative with respect to the effects of multivitamin/mineral supplementation and esophageal cancer. Indeed, in a follow-up study this group of researchers found a highly significant inverse association between serum selenium levels and the incidence of both esophageal and gastric cardia cancers.[388]

Various laboratory experiments and human case-control studies suggest that the consumption of green tea, which is rich in polyphenolic antioxidants, may decrease the risk of gastric cancer. However, the studies have yielded missed results. For example, a recent review[369] of ten studies that examined the association between green tea and stomach cancer, six suggested an inverse association while three reported a positive relation. Although the most comprehensive of these reports support an inverse association between green tea and stomach cancer, a large recent study involving 26,311 men and women in northern Japan found no association between green tea consumption and risk of stomach cancer.[389] Since green tea has been shown to be protective against several different malignant tumors, more carefully controlled studies are needed to clarify its association with stomach cancer.

Helicobacter pylori, a well established etiologic factor for gastritis and peptic ulcers, is now believed to enhance the risk of gastric cancer. Hence, eradification of this microorganism would presumably reduce the incidence of this tumor. In this regard, a recent study showed that sulforaphane, a substance rich in certain varieties of broccoli and broccoli sprouts, was a potent bacteriostatic agent against three reference strains and 45 clinical isolates of *H. pylori*.[390] Further, sulforaphane was bacteriocidal for *H. pylori* in a human epithelial cell line and blocked experimental fore-stomach tumors in mice. Hence, future clinical trials are needed to evaluate the relationship between broccoli and stomach cancer.

Cancer of the lung and bronchus

Worldwide, lung cancer has the highest incidence and mortality rates among all malignancies.[391] In the US, lung/bronchus cancer is the third most common malignancy after breast and prostate, but it is clearly the most common cause of death due to cancer in both men and women. There were 169,000 estimated cases in 2002 (men, 90,200; women 79,200) and 154,900 deaths (men, 89,200; women, 65,700).[321] Smoking is, of course, well recognized as the primary cause of lung cancer. Importantly, every puff on a cigarette results in the formation of more than one billion free radicals.[392] Hence, it is not surprising that numerous studies have shown that various foods, mainly those rich in antioxidants, lower the risk of this malignancy.

Fruits and vegetables

Flavonoids are potent antioxidants and are particularly rich in brightly colored fruits and vegetables. As antioxidants, they are at least in theory, protective against various epithelial malignancies. Indeed, several early studies concluded that diets high in fruits and vegetables are associated with lower risk of lung cancer.[393,394] More specifically, Knekt *et al.*[395] studied 10,000 Finnish men and women over a 20-year follow-up period in which there were 1000 incident cancer cases (151 involved the lung). Although there was a modest inverse association between dietary flavonoids and the incidence of all cancers (0.80 relative risk of highest quartile versus lowest quartile), the association was mainly a result of the decreased incidence of lung cancer (0.54 relative risk between quartiles). Moreover, the protective effect of flavonoids persisted after adjustment for smoking, total energy intake, vitamins C and E and beta-carotene. Additionally, the association was strongest in persons under 50 years of age and in non-smokers (relative risks, 0.33 and 0.13 respectively). Interestingly, apple consumption was an effective independent factor in decreasing the risk of lung cancer. However, the association between dietary fruits and vegetables and lung cancer from another recent study involving 77,283 women (Nurses' Health Study) and 47,778 men (Health Professional Follow-up Study) showed mixed results.[396] In the entire study group, total dietary fruit and vegetable intake was associated with a modestly lower risk of lung cancer among women but not men (relative risk 0.79 for highest versus lowest quartile of intake). Among both men and women who never smoked, increased fruit and vegetable intake was associated with a significantly lower lung cancer risk.

Micronutrients

As with other population dietary studies, the association between micronutrients and lung cancer has been mixed. In 1994, Mayne *et al.*[397] reported that dietary beta-carotene-rich raw fruits and vegetables, as well as vitamin E supplements, significantly reduced the risk of lung cancer in non-smoking men and women. However, another study published during the same year indicated that supplementation with vitamin E and beta-carotene did not decrease the risk for lung cancer in male smokers.[398] A subsequent report[399] found that beta-carotene produced neither benefit nor harm with respect to lung cancer while others suggested that supplementation with both beta-carotene and vitamin A may increase the risk for lung cancer in smokers and workers exposed to asbestos.[400] In agreement with latter report, the Alpha-Tocopherol, Beta-Carotene Cancer Prevention (ATBC) Study group recently reported that supplemented beta-carotene increased the risk of lung cancer in men, especially among smokers.[401] However, increased serum vitamin E levels were shown to be associated with a lower risk for lung cancer.[402] The decreased risk was even stronger in younger people and among those with a shorter time exposure to cigarette smoke. Increased vitamin E levels were especially protective if present during the critical early stages of tumorigenesis.

Green tea

As with brightly colored fruits and vegetables, green tea is rich in polyphenols (mainly epicatechins and flavonols). A growing body of evidence from studies with laboratory animals indicate that green tea is protective against a variety of cancers. For example, Chung[403] recently reported that both green and black tea and caffeine were protective against lung cancer in both mice and rats. Early clinical studies evaluating the association between tea intake and lung cancer have been mixed, possibly in part due to inadequate statistical adjustment for active smoking. In a population-based case-control study, Zhong et al.[404] reported that among non-smoking women, consumption of green tea was associated with significant reduced risk of lung cancer (odds ratio, 0.65); the risk decreased with increasing tea consumption. However, there was minimal association between green tea consumption and lung cancer in women who smoked. Moreover, in a recent study involving several organ cancers (i.e. stomach, colon, liver and pancreas), including the lung, women who drank 10 cups of green tea/day developed cancer 8.7 years later and men 3.0 years later than women and men who drank <3 cups/day.[405] Similarly, a prospective cohort study of 8552 Japanese men and women was followed for 11 years.[406] During this time, 285 men and 203 women developed cancer. The cohort was divided into three groups depending on their consumption of green tea: <3 cups/day, 4–9 cups/day, and ≥10 cups/day. Those who consumed ≥10 cups/day showed a highly significant reduced risk for lung, colon and liver cancers.

Breast cancer

Breast cancer is the second most common worldwide malignancy among women; it is the most common cancer in developed countries. In 2002, an estimated 205,000 cases were diagnosed in the

Table 4.12: Major Risk Factors of Breast Cancer

Family history
Increasing age
Hormones (exogenous/endogenous)
Lifestyle (physical inactivity, smoking, alcohol)
Obesity
Diet

US and all except 1500 were women.[321] However, compared with lung and other major cancers, early diagnosis and treatment have greatly improved the prognosis (40,000 death/year; 19.5% of total breast cancers). There are numerous risk factors for breast cancer, including increasing age, positive family history, increased exogenous and endogenous hormones, lifestyle, obesity and diet among others (Table 4.12).[407] The association between obesity and physical inactivity and breast cancer are discussed in Chapters 2 and 3, respectively. In the following sections, the role of nutrition in breast cancer prevention is presented.

Fruits, vegetables and micronutrients

Rates of breast cancer are well known to vary greatly among countries suggesting that there are potentially modifiable determinants such as the micronutrients found in fruits and vegetables. Indeed, various experimental studies have supported a role for some micronutrients in reducing the risk of breast cancer. As implied in several previous discussions, oxidative free radical damage to DNA is an important contributor to cancer development in several organs. In this regard, vitamins C and E have been suggested to play a role in breast cancer prevention due to their antioxidative properties. A recent experimental study[408] indicated that alpha-tocopherol (vitamin E), but not vitamin C, inhibits the proliferation of breast epithelial cells and may, therefore, decrease the risk of breast cancer. Nevertheless, a role for vitamin E in breast cancer prevention in both animal experiments and human epidemiologic studies have been mixed.[409] Additionally, other tocopherols and tocotrienols may be more effective than alpha-tocopherol in breast cancer prevention. Schwenke[410] noted that alpha-, gamma- and delta-tocotrienols have potent anti-proliferative and proapoptotic effects on breast cancer cells. Hence, they might be expected to reduce the risk of breast cancer.

Clinical studies, however, have been considerably less consistent; some reported that diets rich in various micronutrients decreased the risk of breast cancer while others found no correlation, indicating that is still much to learn about this complex multifactorial relationship. Several examples will be presented to demonstrate this confusing problem. In 1993, Hunter *et al.*[411] reported their eight-year prospective study of 89,484 women aged 34 to 69 years who were free of cancer at baseline. After evaluating the intakes of dietary vitamins C, E and A from foods and supplements, they concluded that high intakes of these vitamins did not protect women from breast cancer. Similarly, a recent analysis of eight prospective studies that included 7377 incident breast cancer cases indicated that fruit and vegetable consumption did not significantly reduce the risk of this malignancy.[412] Others,[413] however, reported that premenopausal women who ate five or more daily servings of fruits and vegetables had a modestly lower risk of breast cancer compared with women who consumed less than two daily servings (relative risk, 0.77). This inverse association was considerably stronger among premenopausal women who had a positive family history of breast cancer (relative risk, 0.29), as well as in women who consumed 15 g or more of alcohol each day (relative risk, 0.53).

As with colorectal cancer, folic acid deficiency appears to be an important risk factor for breast cancer, at least in some women. For example, the Nurses' Health Study[414] involving 88,818 women with a 16-year follow-up period indicated that folic acid was not associated with an overall risk of breast cancer. However, a significant increase in breast cancer was associated with women who consumed 15 g or more of alcohol daily and had an inadequate dietary intake of folic acid. The authors suggested that women who regularly consume alcohol may reduce their risk of breast cancer by increasing their daily folate intake. Similar findings were recently reported in Canadian women.[415] Here, there was no association between dietary folate intake and breast cancer risk either in postmenopausal women alone or in women overall. However, there were "marked reductions in risk association with folate intake among those consuming more than 14 g of alcohol/day ..."

Other epidemiologic studies, however, have reported a positive effect of folic acid on breast cancer risk in non-alcohol consumers. For example, data from a recent population-based case-control study of breast cancer conducted in Shanghai during 1996–1998 and involving 1321 cases and 1382 controls aged 25 to 64 years who never drank alcohol regularly or used vitamin supplements, showed that folate intake was inversely associated with breast cancer.[416] Moreover, this inverse association was significantly higher among women who also consumed high levels of folate cofactors (i.e. methionine and vitamins B_{12} and B_6). Importantly, these cofactors were not independently related to the risk of breast cancer. Similarly, a study involving 32,826 women (Nurses' Health Study) found that "higher serum levels of folate and possibly vitamin B_6 may reduce the risk of developing breast cancer.[417] A recent literature review summarizing the evidence for the association between folate status and breast cancer risk has been published.[418]

Dietary fat

Early studies in laboratory animals and humans reported a strong correlation between dietary fat intake and breast cancer risk. Subsequent studies, however, have yielded mixed results. For example, an early large case-control study[419] (2024 cancer cases) found no significant difference in dietary fat intake between women who developed breast cancer and the control group. Conversely, a combined analysis from 12 case-control studies, with a total of 4312 cancer cases, reported a significant positive association between total and saturated fat intake and the risk of breast cancer.[420] A similar study[421] evaluated the data from seven prospective studies in four countries. Dietary information from 4980 breast cancer patients and 337,819 women without cancer was available for analysis. When women in the highest quintile of energy-adjusted total fat intake were compared with those in the lowest quintile, the multivariate pooled risk for breast cancer was not significantly increased. Moreover, increased dietary consumption of saturated, monounsaturated and poly-unsaturated fatty acids did not increase the relative risk for breast cancer. Similarly, Velie *et al.*[422] evaluated a dietary questionnaire from 40,022 postmenopausal women and followed them for an average of 5.3 years. A positive association between the percentage of energy from total fat was noted only in women with no prior history of benign breast disease (relative risk, 2.20). Interestingly, the increased risk was mainly attributed to higher intakes of unsaturated fat and oleic acid. Conversely, others[423] reported that high intakes of polyunsaturated fatty acids and some unsaturated fatty acids (i.e. oleic acid) were associated with a decreased risk of breast cancer (odds ratio for highest versus lowest quintile was 0.70 and 0.74, respectively). The intakes of saturated fatty acids, protein and fiber were not associated with an increased risk.

The association between breast cancer and dietary intake of fat and fatty acids was reported from the Nurses' Health Study (88,795 women free of breast cancer followed up for 14 years).[424] The authors "… found no evidence that lower intake of total fat or specific major types of fat was associated with a decreased risk of breast cancer." Of some interest here, Newmark[425] noted that this latter study was not representative of the American female population as a whole. The participants were better educated, more health conscious and their regular intake of multivitamins was higher than the average female population. More recently, data from 88,691 women in the Nurses' Health Study was evaluated to determine whether high intakes of dairy products, calcium, or vitamin D were associated with breast cancer risk.[426] Although no association between consumption of dairy products and breast cancer was found in postmenopausal women, there was a significant reduction in the risk of developing breast cancer in premenopausal women with a high intake of low-fat dairy foods, especially skim/low-fat milk. There was also a similar inverse association between breast cancer risk and dairy food components (i.e. calcium and vitamin D), "but their independent associations with breast cancer are difficult to distinguish."

It should also be noted that there is extensive evidence that estrogens are important in breast cancer development. To further increase the understanding of the possible relationship between dietary fat and breast cancer, Wu and associates[427] recently reviewed the "nature of the evidence" in various prospective studies of fat intake and risk of breast cancer. They found statistically significant reductions in serum estradiol levels in both premenopausal and postmenopausal women (-7.4% and -23.0%, respectively). The greatest reductions were present in two studies in which dietary fat was reduced to 10–20% of total calories compared with 18–25% in the other studies. They concluded that dietary modifications that significantly decrease estrogen levels may reduce the incidence of breast cancer. Thus, although the association between breast cancer risk and fat intake is complex, there does appear to be a direct correlation, albeit not a clear one. As such, more studies are needed to clarify this important matter.

Cooked meat

Epidemiologic and large cohort studies[428,429] found that high meat consumption was associated with an increased risk of breast cancer. Although the exact mechanism for this association is not fully understood, considerable evidence suggests that heterocyclic amines, which are mutagenic agents, have been identified in well-cooked meats and fish.[430,431] In addition, various animal studies and *in vitro* experiments suggest that well-done meats may be associated with human breast cancer. To study this possible relationship, Zheng and coworkers[432] conducted a case-control study among 41,836 women (Iowa Women's Health Study). Their results showed a dose-response association between "doneness" levels of meat consumed and breast cancer risk. Thus, the adjusted odd ratios for very well-done meat versus rare or medium-done meat were 1.54 for hamburger, 2.21 for beef steak and 1.64 for bacon. For women who consistently ate these three meats very well done, the risk was 4.62 times higher than for women who consumed rare or medium-done meats. As discussed previously under colon cancer (i.e. "Fats, Fatty Acids and Red Meat"), the production of carcinogenic heterocyclic amines by cooking meat may be the mechanism whereby the consumption of red meat increases the risk of breast cancer.

Prostate cancer

Prostate cancer is the second most common cancer in the US after breast cancer. In 2002, there were an estimated 189,000 new cases and 30,200 deaths.[321] As with breast cancer, there is a remarkable variation in prostate cancer incidence and mortality across ethnic and geographic groups suggesting that lifestyle differences are probably important.

Fruits and vegetables

Evidence from laboratory, epidemiologic and clinical studies is accumulating that supports the concept that various dietary antioxidants may be effective in reducing the risk for this common malignancy. The carotenoids comprise a very large group of natural pigments that, along with the flavonoids, provide considerable color to our environment (fall leaves, colored vegetables, flowers, etc.). Some dietary carotenoids, such as beta-carotene, serve as an important source of vitamin A, although most, including lycopene, are devoid of provitamin A activity. Interest in the carotenoids, and especially lycopene, a potent antioxidant that is rich in tomatoes, has increased considerably due to its potential role in decreasing the risk of various malignancies including prostate cancer.

An early study of Adventist men suggest that high tomato consumption was associated with a decreased risk for prostate cancer.[433] The following year, it was found that men with lycopene serum levels in the highest quartile had a 50% lower risk for prostate cancer than men in the lowest quartile.[434] Although this study was quite small, and the findings could have been related to chance, a subsequent large nested case-control study of healthy men (Physicians' Health Study) reported similar results.[435] The odds ratios for all prostate cancers declined slightly with increasing quintile of plasma lycopene levels (odds ratio for highest quintile, 0.75). However, the odds ratio for this quintile was 0.56 for aggressive prostate cancer. In addition, a recent study from Greece found that both cooked and raw tomatoes were inversely associated with prostate cancer.[436] Raw tomatoes were found to be less effective than cooked tomatoes because the latter have a higher concentration of lycopene. Review articles on the role of tomatoes and lycopene in cancer prevention have been recently published.[437,438] Moreover, a more recent Health Professionals Follow-up Study among 47,365 men over a 12-year period confirmed the inverse association between prostate cancer and frequent tomato or lycopene intake (relative risk, 0.84 for high versus low quintiles).[439] Interestingly, the dietary intake of tomato sauce, the major source of bioavailable lycopene, was associated with a greater decrease in prostate cancer risk (relative risk for ≥ 2 servings/week versus <1 serving/week was 0.77).

Micronutrients

Vitamin E has also been inversely associated with prostate cancer. The Alpha-Tocopherol, Beta-Carotene Cancer Prevention (ATBC) Study[440] of Finnish male smokers reported that men randomly assigned to 50 mg of alpha-tocopherol had a statistically significant 32% reduction in the incidence of prostate cancer and a 41% reduction in death from prostate cancer compared to men who were not supplemented. In a recent post-intervention follow-up assessment, the ATBC Study Group again reported that participants receiving alpha-tocopherol supplements had a reduced risk of prostate cancer, although they indicated that confirmation requires more studies.[401] Others[402] also evaluated the association of alpha-tocopherol and gamma-tocopherol with prostate cancer in a nested case-control study. Here, the risk of prostate cancer decreased with increasing serum and toenail concentrations of alpha-tocopherol (odds ratio of highest versus lowest quintile, 0.65). The inverse correlation between gamma-tocopherol and prostate cancer was even stronger. Men in the highest quintile had a five-fold reduction in prostate cancer risk compared with those in the lowest quintile.

Selenium is an essential trace metal; it is a cofactor to glutathione peroxidase, an important antioxidant enzyme that may protect DNA from oxidative damage. Although it is toxic at high doses, moderate supplementation has been shown to significantly decrease the frequency of various chemically-induced cancers in laboratory animals. Decreased dietary intake has also been associated with various human cancers, including prostatic carcinoma. For example, an early study by Willett *et al.*[442] reported a significant inverse association between serum selenium levels and gastrointestinal and prostate cancers. In a later placebo-controlled, double-blind cancer trial,[443] the administration of 200 ug of selenium/day was inversely associated with the incidence of prostate, lung and colorectal cancers. More recently, the Health Professionals Follow-up Study also reported that higher selenium intakes significantly reduced the risk of prostate cancer.[444]

Dietary fat, total energy consumption and body weight

Early epidemiologic studies suggested that dietary fat was an important risk factor for prostate cancer. However, as epidemiologic evidence has increased, the support for this association has declined somewhat, although not eliminated. For example, Whittemore *et al.*[445] conducted a population-based case-control study of prostate cancer among blacks (very high risk), white (high risk) and Asian-Americans (low risk) who resided in various cities in the US and Canada. They concluded that there was a causal role for saturated fat in prostate cancer, but only a weak association was found with monounsaturated fat and no association with polyunsaturated fat or total food energy. The authors suggested, however, that other factors are primarily responsible for the risk differences in various ethnic groups.

A recent experimental study also supports a role for fat and energy intake in prostate cancer.[446] These investigators transplanted androgen-responsive prostate cancers from donor rats to recipient rats and then fed the recipients either fat- or carbohydrate-restricted diets. They also injected human prostate cancer cells into severe combined immunodeficient mice to create tumors and then fed the latter different diets. Energy was restricted in one of three ways: (1) reducing fat energy while keeping all other nutrients essentially equal to animals fed *ad libitum*; (2) reducing energy from carbohydrates and keeping other nutrients constant; and (3) reducing total energy from all sources but keeping other nutrients constant. The results showed that energy restriction reduced proliferation of both rat and human prostate cancer cells. Moreover, the reduction in tumor growth was similar in all three types of energy-restricted animals. Thus, as long as total energy was restricted, tumor growth was independent of the amount of dietary fat.

A prior clinical study also reported a significant positive trend for prostate cancer risk with total energy consumption.[447] Here, the odds ratio was 2.22 for men whose total food consumption was "somewhat more" and 3.89 for those whose consumption was "much more" than men in general. These investigators also found an increased trend for body weight. The odds ratios were 1.44 and 1.80 for those whose BMI was 26–29 kg/m^2 (i.e. overweight) and >29 kg/m^2 (i.e. obese), respectively. Total food consumption and BMI remained independent risk factors in a multivariate analysis that included various food items, as well as alcohol and tobacco use.

Non-steroidal anti-inflammatory drugs

Experimental studies have shown that non-steroidal anti-inflammatory drugs (NSAIDs) inhibit the proliferation of prostate cancer cells and reduce prostatic cancer metastasis. To evaluate the possibility that aspirin might reduce the incidence of prostate cancer in men, 47,882 participants in the Health Professionals Follow-up Study were evaluated from 1986 to 1996.[448] Although no association between aspirin intake and total prostate cancer was detected, there was a suggestive decrease in risk among men reporting greater use of aspirin and metastatic prostate cancer (relative risk among men using aspirin ≥22 days/month was 0.73). The results of this cohort study

suggest that other NSAIDs should probably be examined to determine if they might reduce the risk for this common malignancy.

Miscellaneous malignancies

Although several dietary patterns have been associated with various
other malignant disorders, the number of studies is relatively scarce.
However, a few examples will be presented.

Non-Hodgkin's lymphoma

In 2002, there were an estimated 53,900 cases of non-Hodgkin's lymphoma in the US (28,200 men; 25,700 women) with 24,400 deaths
(12,700 men; 11,700 women).[321] Although there has been a steady
increase in the incidence of this malignancy in recent years, the reasons
are not well understood. However, non-Hodgkin's lymphoma is known
to be increased in immunocompromised patients. Several experimental
studies have identified dietary fat and, in particular n-6 polyunsaturated
fatty acids, as suppressors of the immune system.[449] In addition, fat
intake not exceeding 25% of total energy, mainly due to reduced saturated fat, was shown to improve the immune status in women.[450] In a
relatively early large cohort study of postmenopausal women, the risk of
non-Hodgkin's lymphoma was increased with higher intakes of total animal fat, saturated and monounsaturated fat, but not polyunsaturated fat.[451]
To further evaluate the relation between dietary fat and non-Hodgkin's
lymphoma, Zhang *et al.*[452] studied 88,410 women (Nurses' Health Study)
over a 14-year period during which they identified 199 incident cases.
They found that saturated fat was associated with an increased relative
risk of 1.4 for the highest versus the lowest quintile of fat intake. Moreover, the intake of beef, pork, or lamb as a main dish was associated with
a relative risk of 2.2 if the consumption of one of these meats occurred at
least once daily compared with less than once per week. In addition, a
higher intake of trans fatty acids (e.g. margarine) was statistically significantly associated with an increased risk.

These latter authors also studied the relation between non-Hodgkin's
lymphoma and dietary intake of fruits and vegetables in the same

cohort.[453] They reported that a higher intake of these foods was associated with a lower risk for non-Hodgkin's lymphoma; the multivariate relative risk was 0.62 for women who consumed six or more daily servings compared with those who consumed less than three servings/day. Additionally, when examined separately, vegetable consumption was most clearly associated with a reduced risk; cruciferous vegetables were particularly effective in reducing the risk of this form of lymphoma.

Urinary bladder

Cancer of the urinary bladder is a very common malignancy, especially in men where it is the fourth leading type of cancer. In 2002, there were an estimated 56,500 cases (41,500 men; 15,000 women) and 12,600 deaths (8600 men; 4000 women) in the US.[321] The causes of bladder cancer are not well understood, but appear to be related at least in part to direct contact of the bladder lining cells with urinary carcinogens.[454]

Studies with laboratory animals have shown that urination frequency lowers the level of potential carcinogens. Hence, an increase in fluid intake in humans may also dilute urinary toxic waste products and reduce the risk of bladder cancer. To evaluate this possible relationship, Michaud and associates[455] studied 47,909 men in the Health Professional Follow-up Study over a period of ten years. Indeed, their findings revealed that total daily fluid intake was inversely associated with the risk of bladder cancer. Those who drank 2531 ml or more per day had a relative risk of 0.51 compared with those whose daily fluid intake was 1290 ml or less. Moreover, the consumption of water was more effective than drinking other fluids (relative risk 0.49 versus 0.63).

Kidney

Renal cell cancer accounts for an estimated 2% of all cancers worldwide. The incidence of this malignancy has been increasing over the past few decades in North America, western Europe and the

Scandinavian countries, but apparently not in other areas of the world. There were an estimated 31,800 cases of kidney and renal pelvis cancers in the US in 2002 (19,100 men; 12,700 women) with 11,600 deaths (7200 men; 4400 women).[321] The increase in renal cell cancer in America has been about 3% per year with the highest rate among African Americans.[456] Various possible etiologic factors include cigarette smoking, occupational hazards (e.g. asbestos, aromatic hydrocarbons and organic solvents), high intake of fried meats and poultry, hypertension and obesity, the latter especially in women.[457] However, several studies have suggested that increased consumption of fruits and vegetables may reduce the incidence of renal cancer, although the evidence is not as strong as for other cancers. In addition, although tea consumption was recently found to modestly decrease the risk of bladder cancer, it had no apparent effect on renal cancer.[458]

Pancreas

In 2002, there were an estimated 30,300 cases of pancreatic cancer in the US (14,700 men; 15,600 women), 98% of which resulted in 29,700 deaths (14,500 men; 15,200 women).[321] As noted by McCarty,[459] the marked increase in age-adjusted mortality in Japan and among African Americans during the past 100 years suggests that pancreatic cancer is preventable to a significant degree.

A cohort study of the association between dietary folate and pancreatic cancer in 27,101 healthy male smokers aged 50 to 69 years (Alpha-Tocopherol, Beta-Carotene Cancer Prevention Study) was recently published.[460] During the 13-year follow-up period, 157 developed pancreatic cancer. The adjusted hazards ratio comparing the highest with the lowest quintile of dietary folate was 0.52. No significant associations were noted between dietary methionine, vitamins B_6 and B_{12}, or alcohol intake and pancreatic cancer risk. Of the several possible risk factors, cigarette smoking has been repeatedly linked to this lethal malignancy. Indeed, as with earlier studies, this latter report[460] also showed that cigarette smoking significantly increased the risk for pancreatic cancer (hazards ratio 1.82 for highest versus lowest quintile of cigarettes smoked per day).

Of three studies regarding green tea consumption and pancreatic cancer, two found an inverse association.[369] The largest of these studies found that the risk of cancer was particularly decreased in women with regular green tea intake; among both men and women, there was an inverse association with an increased amount and duration of green tea consumption.

Ovary

There were an estimated 23,300 new cases of ovarian cancer in the US in 2002, of which 13,900 died.[321] Although the etiology of ovarian cancer is unknown, several of the risk factors generally believed to be important include increasing age, genetics, physical inactivity, obesity and oral contraception therapy. Numerous studies also suggest that nutrition is an important risk factor for this malignancy.

An early study by Cramer *et al.*[461] indicated that women with a high dietary intake of animal fat and a low intake of vegetable fat had a significantly increased incidence of ovarian cancer. However, coffee, alcohol and tobacco use were not associated with an increased risk. In agreement with this, a meta-analysis of eight observational studies showed that diets rich in total fat, saturated fat and animal fat were all independently and significantly associated with an increased incidence of epithelial ovarian cancer (relative risks 1.24, 1.20 and 1.70, respectively).[462] Conversely, epidemiologic data from the Nurses' Health Study found "no evidence of a positive association between intake of any type of fat and ovarian cancer risk, even after adjustment of fat subtypes for one another."[463] Thus, more studies are clearly needed to clarify the relation between dietary fat intake and ovarian cancer.

Several studies have also suggested that high levels of antioxidant micronutrients (i.e. vitamins C, E and beta-carotene) decrease the risk for ovarian cancer. For example, a multivariate analysis showed that the highest supplemented intake levels of vitamins C and E were protective of ovarian cancer (odds ratios 0.4 and 0.33 respectively compared with non-supplemented controls).[464] The authors noted that the protective effects of vitamins C and E required intakes "well above the current US Recommended Dietary Allowances." Others also showed inverse associations between ovarian cancer and vitamin E (odds ratio, 0.6), and calcium (odds ratio, 0.7) intakes for the highest compared with the lowest quintiles.[465] When vitamin E and calcium intakes were combined, the odds ratio was 0.4 for subjects in the highest versus the lowest tertile of both nutrients. Other recent studies reported that diets rich in green tea,[466] fish[467] and vegetables[467] are inversely associated with ovarian cancer. This latter group also found a direct association between red meat consumption and ovarian cancer (see under colon cancer section for possible explanation of this association).

Micronutrients and cancer

(1) Vitamin C

Vitamin C (ascorbic acid) is a potent water-soluble antioxidant. As such, it is not surprising that it has been studied for a possible role in cancer prevention. Indeed, studies have shown that vitamin C inhibits carcinogenesis induced by radiation and various carcinogens present in smoke.[468] Human studies have shown that vitamin C is rapidly depleted in smokers because of the tremendous number of free radicals present in each puff. The loss of this protective antioxidant results in reducing body defenses, increasing the burden of oxidative stress, and thereby increasing the risk for smoke-related cancers.

Prior to 1991, about 90 epidemiologic studies examined the role of vitamin C or vitamin C-rich foods in cancer prevention.[469] The great majority of these studies reported that vitamin C had statistically significant protective effects, especially in cancers of the oral cavity, esophagus, stomach and pancreas. Several studies have also indicated that vitamin C may decrease the risk of cancers of the rectum, breast, and uterine cervix. Nevertheless, these findings have not been consistent. For example, 19,496 men and women aged 45 to 79 years were prospectively examined over a four-year period to evaluate the relation between plasma ascorbic acid levels and mortality due to all causes, heart disease and cancer.[470] The findings showed that plasma ascorbic acid levels were inversely related to all-cause mortality and heart disease in both men and women. Interestingly, the vitamin C levels were inversely related to cancer mortality in men but not in women. Recent follow-up studies on populations at high risk for stomach cancer, however, suggest that vitamin C protects against this malignancy where infection with *H. pylori* is a significant risk factor.[471]

(2) Vitamin E

Vitamin E (alpha-tocopherol, other tocopherols and tocotrienols) a lipid-soluble vitamin, is also a potent antioxidant. As such, it is especially efficient in neutralizing the peroxyl and alkoxyl radicals generated in the bilipid cell membranes (i.e. lipid peroxidation); it also effectively neutralizes the hydroxyl radical and singlet oxygen. Vitamin E also inhibits the cyclooxygenase pathway and thereby reduces the concentration of prostaglandins which are, at least experimentally, important in carcinogenesis. Both animal and human studies have generally supported a role for vitamin E in cancer prevention. However, Schwenke[472] recently questioned a role for alpha-tocopherol (usual form of vitamin E) in breast cancer prevention. He noted that studies in experimental animals indicate that alpha-tocopheral alone has little effect on breast tumors. Conversely, alpha-, gamma- and delta-tocotrienols have potent anti-proliferative and proapoptotic effects that reduce the risk of breast cancer. He suggested that any protection from breast cancer by dietary vitamin E may be primarily due to the effects of other tocotrienols and tocopherols present in the diet. On the other hand, an Italian case-control study recently showed the dietary vitamin E significantly reduced the risk of ovarian cancer (odds ratio 0.6 for the highest versus lowest tertile of vitamin E intake).[473] Vitamin E was also recently shown to inhibit malignant melanoma in mice.[474]

Ultraviolet (UV) radiation is a major cause of skin cancer, solar erythema and premature skin aging,[475,476] a phenomenon presumably due to the generation of reactive oxygen species (e.g. singlet oxygen, hydroxyl free radicals and hydrogen peroxide).[477,478] Severe depletion of skin antioxidants during prolonged exposure to UV radiation results in insufficient protection and leads to cellular damage. Thus, an intake of anti-oxidants is a promising method to counteract UV radiation-induced oxidative damage. Indeed, vitamin E has been shown to minimize UV radiation-induced skin erythema,[479] tumori-genesis[480] and epidermal lipid peroxidation.[481]

Recent studies also suggest that tea consumption may be beneficial in preventing sun-induced skin cancers. In an animal study, Conney *et al.*[482] reported that oral administration of tea or caffeine to hairless mice increased the apoptotic cells in the epidermis. A similar effect was observed when caffeine was topically applied immediately after UV radiation. Moreover, oral administration of green or black tea to UV-pretreated high risk mice inhibited tumorigenesis. Interestingly, the administration of decaffeinated teas had little or no effect, although adding caffeine to the decaffeinated teas restored their inhibitory effects. These researchers also reported that topical treat-ment with either caffeine or (-) epigallocatechin gallate, a polyphe-nolic component of green tea, five days per week for 18 weeks, resulted in significantly fewer benign and malignant tumors in mice (44% and 72%, respectively).[483]

(3) Beta-carotene, lycopene and lutein

Beta-carotene and the other carotenoids (e.g. lutein, lycopene, etc.) have been extensively studied with respect to their possible role in cancer prevention. These compounds deactivate various reactive oxygen species (e.g. singlet oxygen, free radicals and triplet photo-chemical sensitizers) and may, therefore, be expected to prevent some cancers. Thus, a recent experimental study found that beta-carotene strongly inhibited the growth of cultured human colon cancer cells by apoptosis.[484]

An early literature review of the epidemiologic evidence indicated that low consumption of fruits and vegetables that are rich in carotenoids consistently showed an inverse relation to various cancers.[485] The reviewer emphasized, however, the need for both prospective and retrospective clinical trials to further evaluate the role of carotenoids in cancer prevention. Unfortunately, more recent studies have shown mixed results. In a study involving 30,000 Chinese, Blot and associates[486] reported that supplementation with vitamin E, beta-carotene and selenium decreased the risk of both esophageal and stomach cancers by 13%. Others[487] studied the effect of beta-carotene supplementation and the incidence of all cancers in women (Women's Health Study). This large randomized, double-blind, placebo-controlled trial showed no significant protective effect in the supplemented group versus those not supplemented. Nevertheless, as noted in the earlier section on prostate cancer, recent studies indicate that increased lycopene consumption significantly decreases the risk of prostate cancer. Moreover, increased dietary lutein was recently shown to be inversely associated with colon cancer in both men and women.[488] Here, the greatest inverse association was noted among those in whom colon cancer developed in younger subjects and among those with tumors located in the proximal colon segment. Other carotenoids, however, were not effective in reducing the risk of colon cancer.

(4) Vitamin D

Recent experimental studies suggest that vitamin D and calcium may protect against cancer by reducing cell proliferation and inducing cell differentiation.[489] In addition, several recent studies provide evidence that dietary vitamin D and calcium impede the development of colorectal and possibly other human cancers.[490,491]

(5) Other vitamins

Other vitamins have also been inversely associated with various human malignancies. For example, several cancers previously discussed in this chapter were noted to be inversely associated with increased levels of folic acid. Indeed, a very recent report further supports a protective role for folate in colorectal cancer.[492] In addition, Slattery *et al.*[493] recently reported that dietary vitamin B$_6$, thiamin and niacin were all inversely associated with colon cancer in women (men were not included in this study).

Olshan *et al.*[494] recently reported their findings on the association between childhood neuroblastoma and maternal vitamin and mineral use. Their results showed that daily maternal intake of vitamins and minerals in the month before pregnancy and in each trimester resulted in a 30–40% reduction in the risk of neuroblastoma in early childhood. However, no specific vitamins or minerals responsible for the decreased tumor risk were identified.

(6) Selenium

In addition to the references noted above, numerous other studies have shown an apparent protective role for most antioxidants against cancer. For example, over 50 published reports have demonstrated a reduced incidence of experimental cancer in laboratory animals supplemented with selenium at dietary levels above the usual nutritional range. Early human epidemiologic studies in Finland[495] and the US[496] also support the hypothesis that selenium deficiency results in decreased intracellular levels of glutathione peroxidase, a critical antioxidant enzyme, which presumably results in increased free radical formation and increased cancer risk. These studies showed that decreased serum selenium levels were associated with an increased incidence of prostate, breast or colon cancers. More recently, selenium deficiency has been associated with an increased risk for colon,[497] liver[498] and prostate[499] cancers. These latter authors also reported significant reductions in the incidence of total, lung and colorectal cancers as well as total cancer mortality. However, this study and a previous one [443] found that selenium intake did not reduce the incidence of either basal or squamous cell carcinoma of the skin.

(7) Summary

Numerous epidemiological and clinical studies have clearly shown that populations whose diets are high in fruits and vegetables and low in animal fat, meat and calories have a significantly reduced risk of the most common types of cancer. Thus, the American Cancer Society recommends the following broad dietary guidelines to reduce the risk of several common malignancies.[500]

(1) Eat a variety of healthful foods with an emphasis on plant sources (i.e. fruits, vegetables, 100% fruit/vegetable juices, and limit French fries, snack chips, etc.).
(2) Choose whole grains in preference to processed (refined) grains and sugars.
(3) Limit consumption of red meats, especially those high in fat and processed. Choose fish, poultry or beans in preference to pork, beef and lamb.
(4) Choose foods that help maintain a healthful weight (i.e. low in fat, sugar and calories and avoid large portions).

Nutrition and the Immune System

It is widely recognized that there is a loss of immune function with advancing age. As a result, the immune theory of aging was proposed. Indeed, there is considerable evidence that a degenerating immune system is a significant contributor to the aging process. Thus, older people are more prone to various infectious diseases, autoimmune phenomena, primary amyloidosis, myelomatosis, chronic lymphoproliferative disorders, and various forms of cancer. It has also been suggested that aging is the most common immunodeficiency syndrome. However, the immune system is as vigorous in many elderly people as it was when they were young.[501] In addition, a major problem with the immune theory of aging is in determining which changes are primary (i.e. due to aging *per se*) and which are secondary (i.e. poor nutrition, physical inactivity, etc.). For example, Mazari and Lesourd[502] compared the immune response of healthy elderly persons (mean age 80 years) with different nutritional status to young healthy adults (mean age 25 years). They concluded that "the influences of aging and undernutrition in humans are cumulative and suggest that some changes in the immune response that have been attributed to aging may, in fact, be related to nutrition and not aging."

It is now widely recognized that nutrition is an important determinant of immune responses. Numerous epidemiologic and clinical studies suggest that poor nutrition alters immunocompetence and increases the risk of infections in both children and adults in the industrialized nations as well as the underdeveloped countries. As discussed earlier in this chapter, undernutrition is very common in aged populations in Europe and North America. More specifically, undernutrition induces lower immune responses, particularly, but not exclusively, in cell-mediated immunity (i.e. T-lymphocyte functions). However, a decreased capacity to synthesize antibodies is also often present in the elderly (i.e. decreased antibody reponse to various vaccines). To determine the frequency of micronutrient deficiency in the elderly, Ravaglia *et al.*[503] studied 62 healthy free living and well nourished Italian men and women aged 90 years and above. They found that 50% of both sexes were selenium deficient, 52% of men and 41% of women were zinc deficient, 40% of men and 59% of women were vitamin B_6 deficient, and 16% of men and 27% of women were vitamin A deficient. These deficiencies were significantly associated with decreased numbers and function of natural killer cells, which are important in natural immunity against cancer and infectious diseases.

Caloric restriction

Since the initial publication reporting that caloric restriction in young rats significantly increases their longevity,[504] numerous studies in a wide range of laboratory animals have demonstrated that lifespan can be significantly prolonged by decreasing total food intake but assuring that essential micronutrients are adequate. Thus, the lifespan of various laboratory animals can be increased 30–50% by reducing their caloric intake to 60% of the amount normally consumed by those given food *ad libitum.*[505] Current observations over a decade or more at the University of Wisconsin-Madison and the National Institute on Aging suggest that the same holds for non-human primates.[506] As such, there is little reason not to believe this is also true for humans. Furthermore, caloric restriction reportedly increases stress resistance from numerous sources including oxidative stress, protection of mitochondrial membranes, resistance to various carcinogens and irradiation, and exercise-induced stress.[507]

Although the mechanisms whereby caloric restriction increases longevity, as well as improving the immune system are unknown, early animal studies are adding considerable information that presumably applies to humans. Thus, interleukin (IL)-6, an inflammatory cytokine, has hematologic, immune, hepatic, endocrine and metabolic functions. More specifically, it stimulates the hypothalamic-pituitary-adrenal axis and is under the tonic negative control glucocorticoids. The administration of IL-6 reportedly results in fever, anorexia and fatigue and is important in the pathogenesis of osteoporosis.[508] Conversely, IL-2, which stimulates the production of T-lymphocytes, decreases with increasing age. A recent report indicates that this cytokine dysregulation is health-related and begins in "healthy" adults at age 60 to 70 years for IL-2 and between 36 and 59 years for IL-6.[509]

The serum concentration of IL-6 is very low in young adults but increases with age. However, Kim *et al.*[510] reported that caloric restriction in mice attenuates this age-associated increase; it also attenuates the oxidative stress-induced IL-6 increase in circulating leukocytes in monkeys. Others have also demonstrated that caloric restriction lowers serum levels of both IL-6 and tumor necrosis factor-alpha in old mice to levels comparable to those of young mice.[511]

Protein-energy malnutrition

In protein-energy malnutrition, which is very common in older people, most host defense mechanisms are impaired. There is atrophy of lymphoid tissues and decreased numbers of circulating lymphocytes (total lymphocyte count less than 2000/uL). These individuals become anergic to skin tests and are more susceptible to various microorganisms (e.g. Mycobacterium, Salmonella, Listeria, etc.).[512] In addition, protein undernutrition is associated with both reduced and increased cytokine release (e.g. IL-2 and -6 respectively) and lower antibody response to vaccines.[513] These individuals are often hypoalbuminemic and some may be mildly anemic. Protein undernutrition also impairs several complement system components, mucosal secretory IgA antibodies, antibody affinity, and the ability of phagocytes to kill ingested bacteria and fungi.[514]

Micronutrients

Cell membrane-dependent functions are affected by physical state and fluidity, both of which are determined by the fatty acid profile of the bilipid membrane. These unsaturated fatty acids are readily modified by reactive oxygen species (ROS), a process known as lipid peroxidation. An increase in ROS, which occurs with aging and various diseases, is presumed to negatively affect membrane functions including cell-mediated immune reactions. However, various micronutrients, including those with antioxidant properties, have been shown to improve and/or prevent the loss of immune function that is often associated with the aging process.

Micronutrient combinations

Penn and associates[515] supplemented a group of healthy elderly people with vitamins A, C and E and compared the results with an age-matched placebo group. The supplemented group showed the following improved responses: (1) increased total number of circulating T-cells; (2) increased number of helper cells (CD4+); (3) increased helper cell to cytotoxic cell ratio (i.e. CD4+ to CD8+); and (4) increased lymphocyte response to phytohemagglutinins. Similarly, Chandra[516] randomly assigned a group of healthy elderly individuals to receive placebo or a multivitamin/trace-element supplement. Their nutrient status and several immunologic variables were assessed at baseline and after six and 12 months. Compared with the placebo group, those receiving the supplement showed the following: (1) increased number of T-cell subsets; (2) increased number of natural killer cells; (3) increased killer cell activity; (4) increased serum IL-2 levels; and (5) improved antibody response to an antigenic stimulus. In addition, the supplemented group had significantly fewer infectious sick days during the year.

More recently, the results of a randomized, double-blind, placebo-controlled trial of two groups of community-dwelling adults, one with type 2 diabetes and one without diabetes, in which the participants received either placebo or a multivitamin and mineral supplement were published.[517] After one year follow-up, those receiving placebo had significantly more infectious illnesses than those receiving multivitamin and mineral supplements (73% versus 43%). Infection-related absenteeism was also higher in the placebo group (57% versus 21%). Among the diabetic participants receiving placebo, 93% had an infection during the study period compared with 17% of those receiving supplements. Others[518] compared delayed-type hypersensitivity skin test (DHST) responses in elderly subjects who received a placebo to those who received a micronutrient supplement. DHST and circulating concentrations of nine micronutrients were measured at baseline and after six and 12 months. After 12 months, the micronutrient-supplemented group showed a significant increase in DHST responses to a panel of seven recall antigens; there were no changes in the placebo group.

Single micronutrients

(1) Vitamin E
Vitamin E is an efficient lipid soluble antioxidant that functions as a "chain breaker" in lipid peroxidation of cell membranes and various lipid particles (e.g. LDL). As with other critical micronutrients, vitamin E is a common deficiency, especially in the elderly. As a result, low vitamin E levels lead to unstable immune cell membranes which lead to enhanced production of immunosuppressors (e.g. prostaglandins); however, supplementation readily corrects the problem.[519]

In a double-blind, placebo-controlled study of healthy people 60 years and older, Meydani *et al.*[520] reported that vitamin E supplementation resulted in the following improvements compared to the placebo group: (1) increased plasma and mononuclear cell vitamin E levels; (2) increased positive antigen response to delayed-type hypersensitivity skin tests; (3) increased IL-2 production; (4) increased mitogenic response to concanavalin A; (5) decreased synthesis of prostaglandin (PGE-2); and (6) decreased plasma lipoperoxy levels. In a follow-up randomized, double-blind, placebo-controlled intervention study of free-living healthy subjects 65 years and older, these latter researchers assigned subjects to a placebo group or to groups consuming 30, 200 or 800 mg/day of vitamin E and followed them for 235 days.[521] Compared with the placebo group, those receiving 200 mg/day had a 65% increase in delayed-type hypersensitivity skin response (DTH) and a six-fold increase in antibody titer to hepatitis B, as well as a significant increase in antibody response to tetanus vaccine. The 60 mg/day group had a 41% increase in DTH and a three-fold increase in hepatitis B antibody titer, while those receiving 800 mg/day increased their DTH by 49% and antibody titer by 2.5-fold. Thus, 200 mg/day of vitamin E, which is well above the current minimum recommended intake, significantly enhanced *in vivo* indexes of T cell-mediated functions. In addition, optimal vitamin E supplementation has been shown to significantly improve blood clearance of *E. coli* in cases of bacteremia.[522] Conversely, a recent study involving non-institutionalized well-nourished individual 60 years and older found that neither a daily multivitamin-mineral supplement nor 200 mg of vitamin E had a favorable effect on the incidence or severity of acute respiratory tract infections.[523] Thus, as is often the case with clinical studies, some confusion remains.

(2) Vitamin C
Vitamin C (ascorbic acid) is a water-soluble antioxidant; it also regenerates vitamin E in cell membranes and maintains LDL particle integrity.[524,525] Vitamin C is also important in neutrophil functions, which perhaps explains its normally high concentration in circulating leukocytes.

In an *in vitro* study, Anderson and Lukey[526] showed that extracellularly-released reactive oxygen species are mutagenic, immunosuppressive and autotoxic to phagocytes. Here, ascorbate efficiently neutralized phagocyte-derived extracellular oxidants while the intracellular antimicrobial oxidants remained unchanged. They noted that ascorbate causes a dose-related inhibition of lucigenin-enhanced chemiluminescense of neutrophils activated by various leuko-attractants as well as by a cell free superoxide (O_2^-·) radical generating system. Others showed that vitamin C alleviates the glu-cocorticoid suppressive effect on neutrophil function in cattle,[527] and Gross and associates[528] found that ascorbate supplementation in chicks with *E. coli* pericarditis significantly reduced mortality compared to non-supplemented controls.

(3) Vitamin A and carotenoids

Beta-carotene, lycopene, lutein and other structurally-related caro-tenoids are important antioxidants. Lycopene and beta-carotene effectively neutralize singlet oxygen while the latter also quenches peroxyl radicals.[529] Numerous experimental animal studies have dem-onstrated that carotenoids modulate host defense systems. For example, Chew[530] observed that beta-carotene supplementation increased the (1) total number of circulating mononuclear cells; (2) number of helper T-cells; (3) natural killer cell cytotoxicity; and (4) tumor necrosis factor-alpha and IL-1. In humans, Alexander *et al.*[531] reported that beta-carotene supplementation increases both total lymphocytes and percent of T-helper cells without affecting the percentage of T-cell subsets. More recently, others[532] studied the effects of beta-carotene on photosuppression of the immune response induced by ultraviolet light. The group supplemented with beta-carotene showed no significant change in delayed-type hypersensi-tivity (DTH) response to ultraviolet light, while the placebo group experienced a significant decrease in DTH response.

Until relatively recently, vitamin A research was focused mainly on the prevention of xerophthalmia and blindness in children in under-developed countries, as well as on the development of synthetic retinoids with lower toxicity than vitamin A for the treatment of skin disorders. More recently, there has been an increased focus on child-hood mortality from infectious diseases that accompany xerophthalmia since vitamin A treatment of this visual disorder has also been somewhat effective against the accompanying infectious diseases. This raised the possibility that vitamin A has some influence on the immune system. Indeed, Semba *et al.*[533] conducted a randomized double-blind placebo-controlled clinical trial among 55 Indonesian children aged three to six years. Thirty of the children had xerophthalmia and 25 did not. The researchers found that children with xerophthalmia had lower CD4/CD8 ratios, lower proportions of CD4 naive T-cells, and higher levels of CD8 and CD45RO cells than those without xerophthalmia. However, five weeks of vitamin A supplementation resulted in higher CD4/CD8 ratios, higher levels of CD4 naive T cells, and lower proportions of CD8 and CD45RO T-cells compared with the placebo group.

(4) Zinc

Zinc (Zn) is an essential trace element, being a cofactor for about 200 enzymes, including the cytoplasmic antioxidant copper-zinc superoxide dysmutase (Cu-ZnSOD). Thus, zinc is closely involved with and has a diversity of roles in the fundamental processes of cellular growth and differentiation. More specifically, Zinc (1) competes directly with copper, iron and other transition metal cations and thereby decreases production of the potent hydroxyl and other radicals; (2) protects protein sulfhydryl groups from oxidation; and (3) stimulates the immune system. Moreover, Zn deficiency is associated with lymphoid atrophy, decreased thymic hormone activity, decreased dermal delayed-hypersensitivity response and delayed homograft rejection.[534]

Plasma Cu-ZnSOD activity correlates inversely with age,[535] and plasma Zn levels are commonly decreased in elderly humans. For example, 49% of a group of 260 institutionalized patients ages 60 to 101 were found to have zinc intakes below two-thirds of the recommended dietary allowance (RDA).[536] In another study, 67% of men and 81% of women ages 60 to 89 years had zinc intakes that were less than two-thirds of the RDA.[537]

Zn supplementation reportedly stimulates both B- and T-cell activity. For example, Duchateau and associates[538] supplemented an elderly group aged 70 years and over with daily oral $ZnSO_4$. Compared with the non-supplemented control group, those receiving Zn daily showed significant improvement in the following areas: (1) increased number of circulating T-cells; (2) improved delayed-hypersensitivity response; (3) increased antibody response to tetanus vaccine; and (4) improved lymphocyte mitogen responsiveness. Moreover, Fortes *et al.*[539] reported that with Zn supplementation, a healthy group of elderly people showed significantly increased levels of both CD4+DR+ and cytotoxic T-cells. The topic of zinc and immune function has been recently reviewed.[540]

Zinc deficiency is very common in children of developing countries. Because of zinc's fundamental roles in cell growth and differentiation, young growing children are very vulnerable to the adverse effects of zinc deficiency. Thus, cells with a rapid turnover rate, especially those of the immune and gastrointestinal systems, are most vulnerable to zinc deficiency. As a result, it contributes significantly to diarrheal illnesses, which in turn contribute to growth retardation and early death.[541] However, Zn supplementation of infants and young children with acute diarrhea reportedly reduces the severity and duration of the diarrhea, as well as pneumonia.[540–543] Others[544] found that Zn supplementation improved T cell-mediated responses, which are critical for host protection against parasitic infections.

Numerous studies have recently been reported on the use of zinc salts lozenges in humans with the common cold. These early studies have generally showed mixed results. The authors of a meta-analysis of eight clinical trials before 1997 concluded that "the evidence for effectiveness of zinc salts lozenges in reducing the duration of common colds is still lacking."[545] In two more recent reports, one indicated that zinc gluconate lozenges were not effective in treating cold symptoms in children or adolescents,[546] whereas the other concluded that zinc lozenges were "associated with reduced duration and severity of cold symptoms, especially cough."[547]

(5) Selenium
Selenium (Se) is an essential trace element, being a cofactor for several enzymes, including glutathione peroxidase (GPx), an antioxidant enzyme. Se levels and GPx activity are both commonly

decreased in the serum of elderly individuals.[548] Beck[549] studied a mouse model of coxsackie virus B3 (CVB3)-induced myocarditis and showed that Se-deficient mice were more susceptible to the virus than Se-supplemented mice. He also found that a normal benign strain of CVB became virulent in Se-deficient mice, suggesting that oxidative stress may be an important factor. Others[550] reported depressed natural killer cell activity and depressed T cell-mediated cytotoxicity by either Se or vitamin E deficiency, or their combination. Se deficiency in mice has also been shown to produce a decreased lymphocyte response to concanavalin A.[551] The importance of selenium for a healthy immune response in humans, as well as other critical health roles for this essential element (e.g. cancer, CHD, etc.), was recently reviewed.[552]

(6) Glutamine

Glutamine is generally considered to be a non-essential amino acid. Nevertheless, glutamine is a very important antioxidant since it is the precursor of glutathione (GSH), which is necessary to remove hydrogen peroxide (H_2O_2) by converting it to water in the presence of the selenoenzyme, glutathione peroxidase (GPx); this prevents the formation of the potent hydroxyl free radical.

$$H_2O_2 + 2GSH - GPx \rightarrow 2H_2O + GSSG$$

In an experimental study, the effects of glutamine-rich total parenteral nutrition (TPN) was compared with standard TPN in rats who were challenged with intraperitoneally introduced bacteria (*E. coli*).[553] The results showed that the number of *E. coli* in systemic blood at two hours after intraperitoneal challenge was significantly lower in the glutamine-TPN than those receiving standard TPN. In addition, the glutamine-TPN group had higher tumor necrosis factor levels in the peritoneal lavage fluid and liver, higher splenic interferon-gamma levels, and lower plasma IL-8 levels compared with those receiving standard-TPN.

Severely ill surgical patients undergo glutamine depletion which reportedly results in immune dysfunction. To investigate this further,

O'Riordain *et al.*[554] carried out a random clinical trial of surgical patients on total parenteral nutrition who underwent colorectal resection. They found that glutamine supplementation resulted in a significant T-cell mitogenic response compared with those not supplemented. Moreover, glutamine supplementation increased T-cell production in patients with severe acute pancreatitis compared with a non-supplemented group. A review of the evidence supporting the positive effects of glutamine on the immune system, as well as in human trauma cases, has been recently published.[555]

Cataract and Macular Degeneration

Cataract

A cataract is an opacification of the lens that results in decreased visual acuity and may lead to blindness. Cataracts increase with increasing age and are an important cause of disability among the elderly. Moreover, cataract extractions are the most common surgical procedure performed in the US, and perhaps the most costly item on the Medicare budget since well over one million cataract extractions are performed annually in the US.[556] The identification of factors that might delay or prevent cataract formation would, therefore, be highly important for increasing the well-being of older people and reducing the associated medical costs.

The fact that oxidative damage of lens proteins is a major factor in the pathogenesis of the cataract development has led to speculation that various dietary factors, especially micronutrients with antioxidant capabilities, may slow or even prevent cataract development.[557] Indeed, most recent studies support this supposition. In a case-control study, 207 Italians with cataracts were compared with 706 cataract-free control subjects.[558] After controlling for alcohol, coffee, tea and cola, along with age, sex, education level, smoking status, weight and diabetes, there was a significant inverse risk trend of cataracts for intakes of meat, cheese, cruciferous vegetables, spinach, tomatoes, citrus fruits, peppers and melon. Conversely, a significant increase in risk was found for those consuming increased quantities of butter, total fat and salt. Others[559] conducted a case-control study to investigate the association of various antioxidants and the risk of cataract in a Mediterranean population. Here, blood samples were analyzed for vitamin C in 343 individuals with cataracts and 334 age-sex-matched controls without cataracts. After correction for potential confounders (i.e. smoking, alcohol intake and education level), they found that blood vitamin C levels of 49 umol/L and higher were associated with a 64% reduced risk for cataract.

An early Canadian study suggested that the risk of cataract may be reduced by 50% with dietary supplements of vitamins C and E.[560] Similarly, the Beaver Dam Eye Study evaluated the association between cataracts and multivitamins in a population-based cohort aged 43 to 86 years.[561] They found that, compared with vitamin non-users, the five-year risk of cataract was 60% lower among those who reported the use of multivitamins or any supplement containing vitamin C or E for more than ten years. However, use of vitamin supplements for a shorter time period was not associated with a reduced cataract risk. Jacques *et al.*[562] also reported that multivitamin supplements reduced the prevalence of nuclear cataract (odds ratio 0.60). For both nuclear and cortical cataract, a longer duration of multivitamin use was associated with reduced prevalence of both cataract types.

Prospective cohort studies of carotenoid intake and risk of cataract extraction involving 36,684 male professionals[563] (Health Professionals' Follow-up Study) aged 45 to 75 years and 77,466 female nurses[564] (Nurses' Health Study) aged 45 to 71 years were recently published. The results showed that men in the highest quintile of lutein and zeaxanthin (carotenoids) intake had a 19% lower risk of cataract extraction relative to men in the lowest quintile; the corresponding decreased risk for women in the highest quintile compared with the lowest was 22%. Nevertheless, all studies do not support a protective role for antioxidants against age-related cataracts. For example, the Age-Related Eye Disease Study (AREDS) recently published their findings in a randomized, placebo-controlled clinical trial of high-dose antioxidant supplementation and age-related cataract.[565] This study group concluded that the use of high doses of vitamins C and E and beta-carotene "in a relatively well-nourished older adult cohort had no apparent effect" on the development or progression of age-related cataract. They noted, however, that the AREDS participants were relatively well nourished compared with the general population. Hence, the study participants may have already been relatively well protected against cataract formation. Similarly, a randomized, double-blind, placebo-controlled trial involving current non-smoking American male physicians found no significant difference in cataract formation in the beta-carotene-supplemented group compared with those receiving placebo.[566] Among current smokers, however, beta-carotene decreased the cataract risk (relative risk, 0.74).

In an interesting study involving 60,657 women aged 43 to 63 years, Hu and associates[567] hypothesized that cataract development might be a marker for CHD since oxidative damage to proteins is important in cataract formation and to lipids in arteriosclerosis. After a ten-year follow-up period, they found that cataract extraction was significantly associated with an increased risk for CHD (relative risk, 1.88). This association was even greater among women with a history of diabetes (relative risk, 2.80). Thus, there appears to be related risk factors for these disorders.

Macular degeneration

Age-related macular degeneration (AMD), a chronic progressive loss of central vision due to damage to the retinal cells, is the leading cause of blindness in the US and other developed countries. Over 25% of people 75 years of age and older have some signs of age-related maculopathy and 6% to 8% have advanced stages of AMD that are associated with visual loss.[568] Although the causes of AMD are not known, there are many risk factors including smoking, hypertension, carotid and lower extremity arterial diseases, increased serum cholesterol, increased saturated fat and trans-fatty acid consumption, and BMI; importantly, all of these are risk factors for CHD. Moreover, as emphasized earlier in this chapter, oxidative reactions have been proposed as a causative factor in aging and numerous diseases, including CHD and AMD. In addition, there is increasing evidence that the accumulation of lipofuscin, a product of lipid perioxidation, in the retinal pigment epithelium is involved in the development of AMD.[569] This suggests that dietary antioxidants may reduce lipofuscin production and AMD. Indeed, these latter investigators reported a significant reduction in lipofuscin with the addition of lutein, zeaxanthin, lycopene, or alpha-tocopherol to rabbit and calf retinal epithelial cells exposed to increased oxidative stress.

In an early multicenter Eye Disease Case-Control Study[570] of subjects 55 to 80 years of age, individuals in the highest quintile of carotenoid intake had a 43% lower risk for AMD compared with those in the lowest quintile (odds ratio, 0.57). This decreased incidence was especially significant for those with a high dietary consumption of lutein and zeaxanthin (rich in dark green leafy vegetables). However, the intake of neither preformed vitamin A (retinol) nor vitamin E was statistically associated with decreased AMD risk, while a higher intake of vitamin C only suggested a possible lowered risk for AMD. More recently, a larger double-masked clinical trial was carried out involving persons aged 55 to 80 years over a 6.3-year period.[571] The participants were randomly assigned to one of four groups to receive daily oral tablets containing: (1) antioxidants (vitamin C, 500 mg; vitamin E, 400 IU; beta-carotene, 15 mg); (2) zinc (80 mg as zinc oxide) and copper, (2 mg as cupric oxide); (3) antioxidants plus zinc; and (4) placebo. The findings showed a reduction in AMD in those who received antioxidants plus zinc (odds ratio, 0.72), zinc alone (odds ratio, 0.75), or antioxidants alone (odds ratio, 0.80). The demonstrated benefit of the combination of antioxidants plus zinc in protecting against progression to advanced AMD was 25% to 30%. Thus, although increased dietary intake of various antioxidants may slow the progression of AMD, they cannot prevent the disease. As noted in a recent editorial,[572] "further advances will require a better understanding of the pathogenesis of the condition and the development of new interventions."

With respect to the pathogenesis of AMD, recent studies have evaluated a possible role for dietary fat and fatty acids. Smith and associates[573] carried out a cross-sectional, urban population-based study with 3654 participants aged 49 years and older. The results showed that a higher frequency intake of fish was associated with a decrease in AMD (odds ratio 0.5 for frequency of fish intake of more than once per week versus less than once per month). In addition, those with a high consumption of cholesterol were significantly more likely to develop late age-related maculopathy (odds ratio 2.7 for the highest quintile compared with the lowest quintile). Others also reported that diets high in omega-3 fatty acids and fish were inversely associated with the risk for AMD, but only when the intake of linoleic acid was low.[574] However, a higher intake of specific types of fat, including monounsaturated and polyunsaturated fat and linoleic acid were all associated with a higher risk for AMD.

In addition to dietary fat intake, increased body weight has been associated with AMD. In a recent Physicians' Health Study, the authors found after adjusting for age, randomized aspirin and beta-carotene intake and cigarette smoking, the incidence for visually significant dry age-related maculopathy was lowest in men with a "normal" BMI (22.0–29.9 kg/m^2).[575] Compared with the target BMI, the relative risks for maculopathy were 1.24 for overweight men (BMI 25.0–29.9 kg/m^2) and 2.15 for the obese (BMI $\geq$30 kg/m^2). Interestingly, the study produced a J-shaped curve, indicating that very lean men (BMI <22 kg/m^2) are also at increased risk for AMD (relative risk 1.43).

Type 2 Diabetes Mellitus

Type 2 diabetes (non-insulin-dependent diabetes mellitus; NIDDM) is increasing throughout the world at a striking rate. According to the World Health Organization (WHO), the number of diabetics is estimated to double from 143 million to almost 300 million between 1997 and 2025.[576] There are an estimated 17 million cases in the US, but only about half have been diagnosed. Although type 2 diabetes is reportedly the sixth leading cause of death in the US, it is probably higher since it is an important risk factor for CHD, cerebrovascular disease, hypertension and renal failure.

A recent highly significant study from the Nurses' Health Study involving 84,941 women over a 16-year period found that 91% of the cases were lifestyle-related and therefore preventable.[577] The major risk factor was overweight/obesity although physical inactivity, poor diet and current smoking were also independent risk factors even after adjustment for body weight. Indeed, a recent review of diet and risk of type 2 diabetes reported that the most important lifestyle risk factors were excess adiposity, especially centrally distributed, high intake of saturated and trans fatty acids and physical inactivity.[578] Here, Mann concluded that reduced saturated fatty acids and lifestyle intervention "aimed at lowering rates of obesity are the changes most likely to reduce the epidemic" of type 2 diabetes. Similarly, van Dam *et al.*[579] reported that total and saturated fat intake increased the risk of type 2 diabetes in men (Health Professionals Follow-up Study). As probably expected, however, these associations were not independent of BMI. The authors also reported that "frequent consumption of processed meats may increase the risk of type 2 diabetes." Interestingly, a recent report from the Nurses' Health Study suggested potential benefits of "high nut and peanut butter consumption in lowering risk of type 2 diabetes in women."[580] Nuts are rich in unsaturated fat and other nutrients, but high in caloric content. The authors, therefore, recommended regular nut consumption as a replacement for intake of refined grain products or red and processed meats in order to avoid excess caloric intake.

Diabetes is characterized by a decrease in the effect of insulin on peripheral tissues (insulin resistance) and by the inability of the pancreatic islets to compensate for this resistance. In addition to a positive family history and the diabetic risk factors noted above, there is some evidence that various dietary factors may increase insulin resistance and, over the long term, influence the risk of type 2 diabetes. An example is a six-year study that involved 65,173 women 40 to 65 years of age who were free of all major diseases at baseline.[581] After adjustments for age, BMI, smoking, physical activity, positive family history, alcohol and cereal fiber and total energy intake, the dietary glycemic index (the area under the blood glucose response curve for each food expressed as a percentage of the area after taking the same amount of carbohydrate as glucose), was positively associated with diabetes (relative risk 1.37 comparing the highest with the lowest quintiles. The glycemic load, an indicator of global dietary insulin demand, was also positively associated with diabetes (relative risk, 1.47). Conversely, some dietary substances appeared to decrease insulin resistance and lower the risk for type 2 diabetes. Thus, cereal fiber intake was inversely associated with diabetes risk (relative risk 0.72 for highest versus lowest quintile). Moreover, the combination of a high glycemic load and a low consumption of cereal fiber significantly increased the risk for diabetes when compared with a low glycemic load and high cereal fiber intake (relative risk, 2.50).

More recently, these latter investigators prospectively compared the relation between whole and refined grains and risk of type 2 diabetes in a cohort of 75,521 women aged 38 to 63 years.[582] After a ten-year follow-up, the age and energy-adjusted relative risks were 0.53 for whole grain, 1.31 for refined grain, and 1.57 for the ratio of refined to whole grain intake. Others[583] evaluated the possibility that isocaloric replacement of refined rice with whole grains and other plant products might reduce insulin demand and lipid peroxidation in patients with coronary artery disease. After 16 weeks, serum levels of glucose and insulin decreased by 24% and 14% respectively in the whole-grain group. In addition, whole grains and legume powder consumption in coronary artery disease patients without diabetes significantly decreased their fasting glucose and insulin levels. There was also a significant reduction in plasma homocysteine levels.

Studies have consistently indicated that low magnesium intake is also associated with diabetes mellitus. Indeed, the incidence of hypomagnesemia in type 2 diabetes reportedly varies from 25% to 39%.[584,585] In a recent study involving a large group of white individuals, low serum magnesium levels were found to be a "strong independent predictor of incident type 2 diabetes."[586] Moreover, Humphries *et al.*[587]

studied magnesium intake and insulin resistance in a sample of young non-diabetic African American adults and found that dietary magnesium intake is inversely associated with insulin resistance.

Early studies indicated that increased blood glucose levels in both diabetic humans and animals were associated with increased oxidative stress. As such, it has been suggested that a free radical process involving lipid peroxidation in cell membranes may be involved in the altered glucose transport and microangiopathic disease associated with diabetes.[588] Indeed, Paolisso *et al.*[589] studied the effects of a pharmacologic dose of vitamin E on the action of insulin in healthy subjects and in patients with type 2 diabetes. They concluded that the administration of vitamin E (900 mg/day) "is a useful tool to reduce oxidative stress and improve insulin action." In a separate publication,[590] these authors reported that vitamin E supplementation for three months reduced plasma levels of glucose, free fatty acids, triglycerides, total cholesterol, low-density lipoproteins and apolipoprotein B; plasma glycosylated hemoglobin levels (HbA1C) were also significantly reduced. In addition, pharmacological doses of vitamins C (1250 mg/day) and E (680 IU/day) taken four weeks reportedly lowered the urinary albumin excretion rate in type 2 diabetics by 19%.[591]

Alpha-lipoic acid is also an excellent antioxidant in both aqueous and lipid phases; as such, it regenerates vitamins C and E that had previously neutralized various reactive oxygen species. A recent report[592] found that alpha-lipoic acid (600 mg/day) significantly improved the imbalance between increased oxidative stress and depleted antioxidant defense even in diabetic patients with albuminuria and poor glycemic control. Moreover, the increased oxidative stress noted in early diabetic rat kidney cortex can be prevented by alpha-lipoic acid.[593] On the other hand, beta-carotene supplementation for12 years had no effect on the risk of type 2 diabetes in a large randomized double-blind, placebo-controlled trial (Physician's Health Study).[594]

Hypertension

Increased blood pressure is a very common disorder in the US and other developed countries. A 1995 survey indicated that 24% of

American adults (about 43 million) were hypertensive while only 47% had an optimal blood pressure (i.e. systolic pressure ≤ 120 mm Hg; diastolic pressure ≤ 80 mm Hg).[595] Furthermore, among American adults aged 50 years and older, a significantly higher proportion were hypertensive and a much lower proportion had an optimal blood pressure. Current guidelines to prevent hypertension include weight control, increased physical activity, reduced salt intake and alcohol consumption, and possibly increased dietary potassium. Clinical studies have also indicated that other dietary patterns may be important in reducing the risk of hypertension.

Sodium

Observational epidemiologic studies have repeatedly identified dietary sodium intake as an important risk factor for hypertension. Randomized controlled clinical trials have also demonstrated that reduced sodium intake results in blood pressure lowering in both hypertensive and normotensive individuals. In a meta-analysis of 56 clinical trials in which urinary sodium excretion was monitored as a measure of sodium intake, the mean decrease in systolic and diastolic blood pressure for a 100 mmol/day reduction in sodium excretion was 3.7 mm Hg and 0.9 mm Hg, respectively.[596] However, blood pressure reduction was significantly greater in studies of older hypertensive people.

In the Dietary Approaches to Stop Hypertension (DASH) study,[597] 459 adults with systolic blood pressures less than 160 mm Hg and diastolic blood pressures of 80 to 95 mm Hg were fed a three-week control diet that was low in fruits, vegetables and dairy products with a fat content typical of an average American diet. The subjects were randomly assigned to receive either the control diet, a diet rich in fruits and vegetables, or a "combination" diet rich in fruits, vegetables and low-fat dairy products with decreased saturated and total fat (DASH diet). Sodium intake and body weight were kept as constant levels. The data showed that the "combination" diet substantially lowered both systolic and diastolic blood pressures (11.4 mm Hg and 5.5 mm Hg, respectively). More recently, Sacks and coworkers[598] randomly assigned a group of

412 persons with and without hypertension to a typical American diet (control diet) or the DASH diet. As in the previous study,[597] the DASH diet substantially lowered the systolic and diastolic blood pressures. In addition, compared with the control diet with high sodium level (3.5 g/day), the DASH diet with a low sodium level (1.2 g/day) led to a mean systolic blood pressure of 7.1 mm Hg lower in persons without hypertension and 11.5 mm Hg lower in those with hypertension. The negative effects of sodium were also noted in African Americans, other racial/ethnic groups, and in both men and women.

Since an elevated blood pressure is a strong risk factor for CHD and stroke, a high dietary sodium intake might also increase the risk of cardiovascular disease. To evaluate this hypothesis, 14,407 overweight and non-overweight persons aged 25 to 74 years were studied over a 19-year period.[599] The results indicated that a high sodium diet is strongly and independently associated with an increased risk of CHD, as well as all-cause mortality in overweight individuals.

Potassium

The first clinical trial of potassium supplementation in hypertensive individuals was probably reported in 1928.[600] Since then, numerous reports of blood pressure lowering by potassium supplementation have been reported. However, as noted by Whelton and associates,[601] only about half were randomized controlled trials and most were too small for definitive results. As such, this group carried out a meta-analysis of 33 randomized controlled trials involving 2609 individuals. They concluded that the results "support the premise that low potassium intake may play an important role in the genesis of high blood pressure." More recently, it was shown that a daily potassium intake of less than 2.4 g significantly increased the risk of stroke (relative risk, 1.5).[602] Among diuretic users, the relative risk was 2.5 in those with a serum potassium level less than 4.1 mEq/L. Unfortunately, the authors did not evaluate the blood pressure with the potassium intake or blood levels.

Calcium

Over the past two decades, several epidemiologic studies, as well as studies with laboratory animals, have supported the theory of an inverse association between dietary calcium intake and blood pressure. However, in a meta-analysis of 56 published reports on this topic, the pooled analysis showed a systolic pressure reduction of only 1.27 mm Hg and a reduction of diastolic blood pressure of 0.24 mm Hg.[603] The authors concluded that calcium supplementation may lead to a "small reduction in systolic but not diastolic blood pressure." They emphasized, however, that the results do not exclude the possibility that calcium supplementation may be effective in lowering the blood pressure in some subpopulations.

Antioxidants

It has been hypothesized that oxidative stress increases blood pressure and leads to various medical complications. Hence, antioxidants such as vitamin C and E might improve redox-sensitive vascular changes associated with hypertension. Indeed, two recent reports involving spontaneously hypertensive rats indicated that these two antioxidants improve vascular function and structure and prevent the progression of hypertension.[604,605] These positive findings apparently also apply to hypertension in humans. In a randomized double-blind, placebo-controlled study, Duffy and associates[606] reported that vitamin C supplementation (500 mg/day) for 30 days reduced the systolic blood pressure of hypertensive patients by 9% (mean reduction, 13 mm Hg).

More recently, Kurl *et al.*[607] conducted a 10.4-year prospective population-based cohort study of 2419 randomly selected men aged 42 to 60 years with no history of stroke at baseline. The results showed that men with the lowest plasma vitamin C levels (<28.4 umol/L) had a 2.4-fold risk of any stroke (i.e. ischemic or hemorrhagic) compared with those with the highest levels (>64.96 umol/L). Hypertensive and overweight men with the lowest plasma vitamin C levels

(<28.4 umol/L) had 2.6- and 2.7-fold risks for any stroke after adjustment for age and other known risk factors. The possible role of antioxidants in the treatment and prevention of hypertension was recently reviewed.[608]

Osteoporosis

Osteoporosis is a major health threat. An estimated ten million Americans are currently affected by osteoporosis and another 18 million have low bone mass.[609] Osteoporotic fractures are an important cause of both disability and death. For example, hip fracture is reportedly associated with a 20% excess mortality in the year following the fracture.[610] Moreover, the direct medical costs of managing fractures in 1995 was US$13.8 billion[611]; in 2001, the direct costs were US$17 billion.[612] Once believed to be part of the natural aging process, especially in women, osteoporosis is no longer considered to be age- and sex-dependent. Importantly, it is now recognized that this metabolic disorder is largely preventable by optimization of bone health throughout life in both men and women.

Osteoporosis is most prevalent in white postmenopausal women. To determine the rate of bone loss in white women, Hansen *et al.*[613] studied 178 early menopausal women over a 12-year period. The average reduction in bone mineralization during this time was 20%, although some women ("fast losers") lost 10% more than others ("slow losers"). The mean loss for the "fast losers" was 26.6% compared with 16.6% for the "slow losers." Thus, there is a 40% chance that a 50-year-old white woman will have an osteoporosis-associated fracture during her lifetime. Nevertheless, osteoporsis is common in all populations and has significant physical, psychosocial and financial consequences. As a result, many experts recommend that prevention should begin in early life, even in childhood. Certainly, it is important to recognize that osteoporosis is more easily prevented than treated.

One of the major risk factors for osteoporosis is lack of adequate physical activity, especially resistance and high-impact activities

Table 4.13: Risk Factors for Osteoporosis

Age	Increasing age, menopause
Genetic	Family history, Caucasian race, Asian ethnicity, female sex, low BMI, increased height
Endocrine	Estrogen and testosterone deficiency, excess intake of glucocorticoids, corticosteroids and thyroid hormone
Nutrition	Inadequate dietary calcium and vitamin D, high fat intake, excessive caffeine
Lifestyle	Physically inactive, cigarette and alcohol abuse
Drugs/Medications	Thiazide diuretics, antiepileptics (i.e. phenobarbital, phenytoin, etc.), aluminum antacids, anticonvulsants, heparin

(Chapter 3). Sex hormones are also important determinants of peak and lifetime bone mass in women, men and children. Other risk factors include cigarette smoking and alcohol abuse, various medications, lack of sex hormones, and excess glucocorticoid and thyroid hormones. In addition, an adequate intake of vitamin D and calcium is critical. The major osteoporotic risk factors are presented in Table 4.13.[614,615]

General

Numerous studies have demonstrated that obesity, short stature and African American ethnicity are all associated with a significantly decreased incidence of osteoporosis. A recent prospective study[616] of 6250 postmenopausal women with an average follow-up period of 7.6 years found a decreased fracture risk among obese and African American women and an increased risk with advancing age, body height and total fat intake. The relative risk among African Americans was 0.45 compared with non-African Americans; women taller that 170 cm (about 5'7") had a 64% increase in risk compared with women less than 155 cm (about 5'1"). The risk for BMI decreased from 1.00 for BMI $\leq$22 kg/m^2 to 0.80 for BMI = 28 kg/m^2 (overweight). The fracture risk increased from 1.00 for a total daily fat intake of <57.2 g to 1.24 for an intake of $\geq$75.0 g.

Calcium

Nutritional factors, primarily an inadequate intake of calcium and vitamin D, contribute significantly to bone loss. Conversely, numerous studies have shown that supplemental calcium reduces bone loss in middle-aged, postmenopausal women and lowers the rate of vertebral fractures in women. A review and analysis of the medical literature found that calcium supplementation reduces the rate of bone loss in premenopausal women by about 0.8% per year.[617] This represents a 40% decrease when compared with untreated women. The authors also compared results of the administration of oral estrogen in conjunction with additional calcium intake either through diet or supplements with those of estrogen alone. Their findings showed a 1.3% increase in bone mass of the lumbar spine with estrogen alone, but 3.3% per year when estrogen was given in conjunction with calcium (1183 mg/day). The mean increase in bone mass of the femoral neck was 0.9% per year with estrogen alone compared with 2.4% per year with estrogen plus calcium.

The current recommended guidelines of calcium intake for older adults are listed in Table 4.14.[618] The major dietary sources of calcium include dairy products, grains, bony fish and some green leafy

Table 4.14: Recommended Daily Calcium Intake

Age/Sex Group (Years)	Daily Calcium Intake (mg)
Birth 1	400–600
Children 1–10	800–1200
Both sexes 11–24	1200–1500
Men 25–65	1000
Men >65	1500
Women 25–50	1000
Women 50–65	
On estrogens	1000
Not on estrogens	1500
Women >65	1500
Pregnant/Nursing	1200–1500

vegetables. However, the fraction of calcium absorbed from the intestinal tract is inversely related to the daily intake — about 33.7% of a 400 mg/day intake and 22.5% with an intake of 1000 mg/day.[619] Furthermore, calcium supplements contain a variety of salts (carbonate, citrate, lactate, gluconate and phosphate) that vary in the percentage of elemental calcium they contain by weight. That is, calcium carbonate contains 40% elemental calcium whereas tribasic calcium phosphate contains 39%, calcium citrate contains 21%, calcium lactate contains 13%, and calcium gluconate contains 9%. In addition, absorption of the various salts vary depending on a variety of factors [i.e. age, salt solubility, tablet type (chewable, effervescent and regular), achlorhydria versus normal gastric acid, degree of salt ionization, etc.]. In addition, Weaver and associates[620] reported that an adequate calcium intake by vegetarians is impractical for most people unless they add fortified foods or calcium supplements to their diet. The authors also noted that dietary constitutents that decrease calcium retention (i.e. salt, protein and caffeine) can also be high in the vegetarian diet.

Vitamin D

The vitamin D endocrine system, consisting of cholecalciferol (vitamin D_3) and its metabolites, is critical in calcium homeostasis. There is also increasing evidence that calcitriol, the active vitamin D metabolite, functions as a steroidal hormone with other important functions. Inadequate intake of vitamin D leads to reduced calcium absorption, increased serum parathyroid hormone levels and bone loss. Multiple studies have estimated the prevalence of hypovitaminosis D in various groups at increased risk for deficiency (i.e. nursing home residents, sunlight-deprived people and individuals 65 years and older) to be between 25% and 54%.[621] Several studies on vitamin D deficiency in older adults have recently been reported. This vitamin deficiency is a particular problem for those who are homebound, institutionalized, and where the opportunity to spend time outdoors and exposure to sunlight is minimal, as in the winter.[622-624] British investigators found that older community dwelling people also benefit by vitamin D supplementation.[625] In this randomized, double-blind study of men and women aged 65 to 85 years, the relative risk for incident fractures for those supplemented with oral doses of 100,000 IU of vitamin D_3 every four months was 0.78 after a five-year follow-up compared with the placebo group. The risk was 0.67 for first-time fractures in osteoporotic sites (i.e. hip, wrist, forearm and vertebral). Moreover, the relative risk for total mortality in the vitamin D group compared with the placebo group was 0.88. The findings were "consistent in men and women and in doctors and the general practice population." There were no adverse effects.

Occult vitamin D deficiency is also common in women not in the high-risk category. LeBoff and associates[626] studied 68 postmenopausal community-dwelling women with no secondary causes of bone loss admitted for elective hip replacement. Of these, 17 had osteoporosis and 51 did not. An additional 30 patients admitted for elective hip replacement had acute hip fractures. The women with fractures had significantly lower 25-hydroxyvitamin D blood levels than those admitted with and without osteoporosis. Moreover, parathyroid hormone levels were higher in women with a fracture compared with the other two groups. Thus, 50% of women with hip fractures had deficient serum vitamin D levels and 36.7% had increased parathyroid hormone levels. The authors suggested that vitamin D supplementation with suppression of parathyroid hormone at the time of fracture may reduce the risk of future fractures and accelerate fracture repair.

As noted above, vitamin D is necessary to promote calcium absorption and presumably to prevent, or at least delay osteoporosis. In a three-year study, 176 men and 213 women 65 years and older were daily supplemented with 500 mg of calcium and 700 IU of vitamin D (cholecalciferol)[627]; supplementation resulted in moderately reduced bone loss in the femoral neck, spine and total body. In addition, the incidence of non-vertebral fractures was reduced. These findings are in agreement with earlier reports regarding the incidence of hip fractures in elderly women in which supplements of vitamin D and calcium reduced the fracture rate by 30% to 70% over a two- to four-year period.[628,629]

The minimum recommended daily allowance of vitamin D is 400 IU (10 mg) for those aged 51 to 70 years and 600 IU (15 mg) for those aged 71 years and over. However, considerable evidence suggests that these levels are inadequate, and that especially for those at high risk, the recommended daily intake should be 800 IU (20 mg).[630]

Vitamin A

Increased vitamin A intake has been shown to increase the occurrence of spontaneous fracture in laboratory animals.[631] In addition, a high dietary intake of vitamin A during pregnancy reportedly increases the risk of skeletal deformities in human fetuses,[632] as well as hip fractures in postmenopausal women.[633,634] More recently, the risk of fracture was shown to be increased in men with elevated serum levels of retinol.[635] In this study, the risk of fracture in men with retinol levels in the highest 99th percentile was seven times greater than for men in the lowest quintile.

Potassium bicarbonate and bisphosphonate

In normal people, a low level of metabolic acidosis and positive acid balance exists. Sebastian *et al.*[636] postulated that over a lifetime this could lead to a significant decrease in bone mass. To test this possibility, they administered potassium bicarbonate (60–120 mmol/day) for 18 days to a group of postmenopausal women. Their results showed that the oral administration of potassium bicarbonate improved calcium and phosphorus balance, reduced bone resorption and increased the rate of bone formation.

In an initial study, bisphosphonate (alendronate) was shown to decrease the risk of vertebral, hip and wrist fractures by about 50% and all clinical fractures by 28% among women with vertebral fractures.[637] More recently, these investigators reported that bisphosphonate increased bone mineral density (BMD) in postmenopausal women with low BMD but without vertebral fractures; it also decreased the risk of a first vertebral deformity.[638]

Miscellaneous minerals

Zinc deficits have been associated with the development of osteoporosis.[639] Thus, both decreased serum zinc levels[640] and excessive urinary zinc loss[641] have been reported in osteoporotic people. In addition, the hypothesis that zinc deficiency may cause osteopenia in athletes has been recently supported.[642] These researchers studied the effects of zinc deficiency on vertebral and femoral bone mass in rats who exercised strenuously. Their results confirmed the negative effect of strenuous exercise on bone tissue, as well as the effectiveness of zinc supplementation in preventing osteopenia.

It has long been recognized that sodium fluoride stimulates bone formation. Furthermore, when administered to osteoporotic patients in low doses, bone mass reportedly increases and the risk for vertebral fractures decreases. In a recent study, Rubin and associates[643] reported that sustained-release sodium fluoride significantly reduced the risk for vertebral fractures and increased spinal bone mass without decreasing bone mass in the femoral neck and hip bones. Fluoride is also very important in the prevention of tooth decay. Dental caries is a multifactorial transmissible disease that affects 50% of American children aged five to nine years and 67% of adolescents aged 12 to 17 years.[644] In addition, 94% of adults are affected.[645] However, over the past 50 years there has been a major decline in the prevalence of dental caries due to water fluoridation.[646] Unfortunately, many American communities still do not fluoridate their drinking water.

Copper may also be important in bone formation. Early observations indicated that spontaneous fractures were frequent in cattle and sheep grazing on copper-deficient pastures. It was subsequently noted that copper deficiency resulted in skeletal abnormalities and spontaneous fractures in children.[647] In a subsequent study involving elderly patients, Conlan *et al.*[648] reported that serum copper levels were inversely associated with risk for femoral-neck fractures.

Neurologic Disorders

Oxidative stress and reactive oxygen species are widely accepted as major contributors to the aging process and numerous diseases, including several neurodegenerative disorders.[649] Studies with experimental animals have repeatedly shown that antioxidant-rich diets not only improve, but may reverse, various age-related declines including neuronal signal transduction and cognitive, behavioral and motor learning deficits.[650]

Cognitive function and aging

Unsaturated fatty acids

Cognitive function commonly decreases with age. Since polyunsaturated fatty acids and antioxidants have important effects on atherosclerosis and thrombosis, Kalmijn *et al.*[651] investigated the possible association of dietary fatty acids and antioxidants and cognitive function in a cohort of men aged 69 to 89 years (Zutphen Elderly Study). Their findings showed, after adjustment for various confounders, that a high intake of linoleic acid (an n-6 fatty acid) was associated with increased cognitive impairment (odds ratio 1.76 for highest versus lowest tertile). However, an increased intake of n-3 polyunsaturated fatty acids was not associated with cognitive impairment. Indeed, a high fish diet, which is rich in n-3 fatty acids, was inversely associated with cognitive impairment (odds ratios = 0.63) and cognitive decline (odds ratio = 0.45). However, intakes of beta-carotene, vitamins C and E, and flavonoids were not associated with cognitive changes. Others hypothesized that n-3 fatty acids may inhibit neuronal signal transduction pathways and exhibit mood-stabilizing properties in bipolar disorder.[652] Thus, in a four-month, double-blind, placebo-controlled study they found that patients supplemented with n-3 fatty acids had a significantly longer period of remission than the placebo group given olive oil.

Antioxidants

The brain is especially vulnerable to free radical damage because of its high rate of oxygen consumption. Thus long-term oxidative stress is widely believed to be a major factor in cognitive decline in older people.[653] To further evaluate this relationship, Ortega and associates[654] studied a group of men and women aged 65 to 91 years who were free of significant cognitive impairment. The cognitive capacity of each individual was tested using the Pfeiffer's Mental Status Questionnaire (PMSQ). The results showed that subjects with vitamin E intakes lower than 50% of the recommended intake demonstrated a greater number of errors in comparison to those with higher vitamin E intakes. Moreover, subjects who made no errors in the PMSQ test had significantly higher alpha-tocopherol serum levels compared to those who made errors. Thus, the authors concluded that a direct relationship exists between vitamin E intake and cognitive function. A recent longitudinal population-based study adds further support that vitamin E intake slows cognitive decline in older persons.[655] These researchers followed 2889 community-dwelling men and women aged 65 to 102 years over a seven-year period. Cognitive change was measured by the East Boston Memory Test, Mini-Mental State Examination and the Symbol Digit Modalities Test. The test results showed that vitamin E intake, either from foods or supplements, lessened age-associated cognitive decline.

Current studies have also demonstrated that the age-related decline in cognitive and motor-behavioral deficits in rats can be reversed by the consumption of flavonoid-rich spinach, blueberries and strawberries.[656] Others[657] demonstrated that these phenolic antioxidants attenuate neuronal cell death due to oxidative stress and may, therefore, reduce neurodegeneration associated with chronic free radical-associated diseases.

Tardive dyskinesia

Tardive dyskinesia is a late-onset disorder in which there is impairment of the power of voluntary movement resulting in fragmentary movements. It has been theorized that this disorder may in part result from neurotoxic damage due to excess free radical formation. Although several early studies of individuals with this disorder who were supplemented vitamin E were carried out, the results were mixed. To more fully evaluate the possible beneficial effects of vitamin E on tardive dyskinesia, Adler and associates[658] carried out a placebo-controlled, parallel-design study. Their results showed that those with the disorder who were supplemented with vitamin E had a mean 32.5% improvement in the Abnormal Involuntary Movement Scale while the placebo group showed no improvement.

Alzheimer's disease

Alzheimer's disease (AD) is the most common age-associated neurodegenerative disorder. It affects about 15 million people world-wide and the incidence increases from about 0.5% per year at age 65 years to 8% per year at age 85 years.[659,660] If mild cases are included, the prevalence may be as high as 10.3% in non-institutionalized white persons over age 65 years,[661] a figure that may be even higher for black and Hispanic persons.[662] In the US, the estimated average annual cost of care per person is US$35,287; the total annual cost to the US economy is more than US$141 billion (1997 dollars).[663]

AD is characterized by loss of memory, language and other cognitive abilities. These functions are also accompanied by concomitant behavioral, emotional, interpersonal and social deterioration. Moreover, AD may coexist with ischemic dementia,[664] the second most common cause of age-related dementia. AD appears to have a long stage of neuropathological change and cognitive decline before it is diagnosed, at which time there is a significant loss of cholinergic, dopaminergic and noradrenergic neurons. In addition to aging, other risk factors for AD include Down's syndrome, history of head injury, cigarette smoking, diabetes mellitus and the APOE e4 allele.

Oxidative stress and AD

Although the exact cause of AD is not well understood, there is considerable evidence that oxidative stress plays an important role

Table 4.15: Oxidative Stress Markers in AD

Lipid Peroxidation
  Lipid hydroperoxides (e.g. malondialdehyde)
  4-Hydoxynonenal
  Isoprostanes
Protein Oxidation
  Protein carbonyls
  Nitrotyrosine
DNA Oxidation
  DNA strand breaks
  8-Hydroxy-deoxyguanosine (8-OHDG)

in its pathogenesis. Support for increased oxidative stress in AD is because the brain (1) has high energy requirements; (2) has a high oxygen consumption rate; (3) is rich is peroxidizable fatty acids; (4) is rich in transition metals which may catalyze the formation of the potent hydroxyl radical; and (5) has a relative deficit in antioxidative defenses compared with other organs. Moreover, numerous quantitative markers of oxidative stress are increased in AD (i.e. markers of lipid peroxidation, DNA oxidation and protein oxidation (Table 4.15).

Several studies have shown that the onset of AD is usually preceded by an interim phase of mild cognitive impairment (MCI). Moreover, a specific marker of *in vivo* lipid peroxidation (i.e. isoprostane 8 and 12-iso-iPF$_{2-alpha}$ VI) is increased in AD. To further understand this early phase, Pratico *et al.*[665] investigated the urine, plasma and cerebrospinal fluid levels of this marker and found significantly higher levels in subjects with MCI compared with cognitively normal elderly subjects. Further support for an oxidative role in AD pathogenesis comes from a recent caloric intake study of elderly persons free of dementia at baseline who were followed for a mean of four years.[666] Here, compared with individuals in the lowest quartile of caloric intake, those in the highest quartile had an increased risk of AD (hazard ratio, 1.5). For persons with the apolipoprotein E e4 allele, the hazard ratios of AD for the highest quartile of caloric and fat intake were 2.3 and 2.3, respectively compared with the lowest quartiles.

Dietary antioxidants and AD

An early case-controlled study reported that serum levels of vitamin E and beta-carotene were significantly reduced in both Alzheimer's disease and multi-infarct dementia compared with a control group.[667] Vitamin A levels were significantly reduced only in Alzheimer's patients. Since then, numerous studies have shown that increased dietary intake of various antioxidants appear to delay the onset of AD. For example, in a double-blind, placebo-controlled, randomized multicenter trial in patients with Alzheimer's disease of moderate severity, 341 patients received a monoamine oxidase inhibitor (selegiline), vitamin E, both selegiline and vitamin E, or placebo over a two-year period.[668] Using the Mini-Mental State Examination as a covariate, both selegiline and vitamin E significantly slowed the progression of the disease. More recently, Engelhart *et al.*[669] reported that high dietary intake of vitamins C and E was associated with a lower risk of AD, while others[670] reported the "vitamin E from food, but not other antioxidants, may be associated with a reduced risk of AD." However, this latter association was observed only among individuals without the APOE e4 allele.

Perry and associates[671] stressed that "the study of single markers of oxidative damage outside the context of oxidative balance is probably not sufficient to determine oxidative status." In agreement with this concept is a recent report regarding vitamins C and E in Alzheimer's patients.[672] Prior studies indicated that patients with AD have very low cerebrospinal fluid (CSF) levels of vitamins C and E. These investigators set out to determine whether oral supplementation might elevate both plasma and CSF levels and thereby decrease the susceptibility of lipoprotein oxidation. Two AD groups were supplemented daily with either vitamin E (400 IU) and vitamin C (1000 mg) or with vitamin E (400 IU) alone. Supplementation of both vitamins significantly increased their concentrations in plasma and CSF while susceptibility of plasma and CSF lipoproteins was significantly decreased. Although vitamin E supplementation significantly increased its concentration in both plasma and CSF, it did not decrease lipoprotein oxidizability. Hence, supplementation with both vitamins was superior to vitamin E alone. The American Academy of Neurology now recommends 1000 IU of vitamin E twice daily for the treatment of patients with AD.[673]

Flavonoids, a family of antioxidants rich in brightly colored fruits and vegetables, were described in an earlier section of this chapter. However, it should be mentioned here that recent *in vitro* studies have shown that these polyphenolic substances are effective in protecting neuronal cells from oxidative stress[674] and attenuate neuronal cell death following uptake of oxidized LDL.[675]

Folic acid, homocysteine and AD

As discussed earlier in this chapter, an increased plasma homocysteine level is an important risk factor for arteriosclerosis. As such, increased levels are associated with CHD, ischemic stroke and peripheral vascular disease. Moreover, cross-sectional studies indicate that elevated plasma homocysteine levels have been associated with poor cognition and dementia. To study the possible association of plasma homocysteine concentrations and AD, 1092 subjects (425 men; 667 women), mean age 76 years, were followed over an eight-year period (Framingham Study).[676] Their results indicated that individuals whose plasma homocysteine levels were 14 umol/L or greater had nearly twice the risk of AD compared to those with levels below 14 umol/L. However, as noted previously in this chapter, elevated plasma homocysteine levels can usually be significantly reduced by increasing the dietary intake of folic acid.

Dietary fats and AD

Data from an early epidemiologic study suggested that a high intake of total fat, saturated fat and dietary cholesterol may increase the risk of dementia.[677] To better understand this possible association, Morris *et al.*[678] studied 815 community residents aged 65 years and older, who were unaffected by AD at baseline, and followed them for a mean of 3.9 years. Their findings indicated that intakes of saturated fat and trans-unsaturated fat were positively associated with an increased risk of AD whereas intakes of n-6 polyunsaturated fat and monounsaturated fat were inversely associated with AD. In their multivariate analysis adjusted for age, sex, race, education and apolipoprotein E status (i.e. APOE e4 allele), persons in the upper quintile of saturated fat intake are 2.2 times more at risk of incident AD compared to those in the lowest quintile. The AD risk also increased with increased trans-unsaturated fat. Although there was an inverse association between AD and vegetable fat intake, consumption of total fat, animal fat and cholesterol were not associated with AD.

These investigators also evaluated the association of fish and n-3 polyunsaturated fatty acid consumption and risk of AD.[679] In this prospective study, conducted from 1993 through 2000, participants who consumed fish at least once per week had a 60% less risk of AD compared with those who rarely or never ate fish (relative risk, 0.4). Total intake of n-3 polyunsaturated fatty acids was also associated with a reduced risk.

Anti-inflammatory drugs and AD

Numerous epidemiologic studies have demonstrated an inverse association between the use of non-steroidal anti-inflammatory drugs (NSAIDs) and AD.[680] In addition, recent clinical studies have shown that NSAIDs slow the decline in cognitive function in patients with AD.[681,682] More recently, Broe and associates[683] examined the association between NSAIDs dosage with AD progression. Their results confirmed the inverse association between NSAIDs, including aspirin and AD. This inverse association, however, was not present in vascular dementia. Furthermore, high doses of NSAIDs were no more effective than lower doses in slowing AD progression. Similarly, a recent prospective, population-based cohort of 6989 people aged 55 years and older who were free of dementia at baseline was followed for an average of 6.8 years.[684] The relative risk of AD was 0.95 in subjects with short-term NSAIDs use, 0.83 in those with intermediate use, and 0.20 in those with long-term use. As with previous studies, the use of NSAIDs was not associated with a reduction in the risk of vasular dementia. Others,[685] however, recently reported that neither rofecoxib or naproxen, both of which are NSAIDs, slowed cognitive decline in patients with mild-to-moderate AD.

Caffeine and AD

Caffeine is the most widely consumed behaviorly active stimulant in the industrialized nations. Various experimental models have shown that chronically administered low doses of caffeine have neuroprotective effects. To test the possibility that caffeine may be effective in slowing the progression of AD, Maia and De Mendonca[686] carried out a case-control study of 54 patients with AD and compared them with 54 cognitively normal persons matched for age and sex. Their results showed that long-term caffeine intake was significantly inversely associated with AD (odds ratio, 0.40).

Parkinson's disease

Parkinson's disease (PD) is also a chronic neurodegenerative disorder of unknown etiology affecting older persons. As with Alzheimer's disease, considerable evidence suggests that excessive free radical production may be an important factor. Indeed, a recent experimental study showed that repeated intramuscular administrations of vitamin E in a PD rat model resulted in a protective effect on the nigrostriatal dopaminergic neurons.[687] In addition, numerous studies have demonstrated an excess of transition metals, which may increase the production of hydroxyl radicals, in the substantia nigra of individuals with PD. For example, Lin[688] recently showed that zinc and iron, both of which are increased in the substantia nigra of PD patients, result in oxidative injuries to the neurons in this brain area of rats.

However, epidemiologic studies on the effectiveness of dietary antioxidants in preventing or delaying PD progression have been inconsistent. For example, the Rotterdam Study reported that a high intake of vitamin E may protect against PD,[689] as did an earlier report in an American population by Golbe *et al.*[690] Conversely, others found no association between vitamins C and E and PD.[691] More recently, researchers at ten US medical centers randomly assigned 80 patients with early PD to one of four treatment groups: placebo, 300, 600 and 1200 mg/day of coenzyme Q_{10} (a very effective antioxidant).[692] The participants were followed for up to 16 months. The results showed that all groups receiving coenzyme Q_{10} deteriorated more slowly than the placebo group although "the benefit was greatest in subjects receiving the highest dosage." Importantly, there were no adverse side effects.

Several studies have shown an inverse association between coffee intake and PD, although there have been some inconsistencies. For example, a longitudinal study from the Honolulu Heart Program found that coffee intake appeared to reduce the risk of PD, but after adjustment for smoking, there was no protective action.[693] To further evaluate the association of coffee and caffeine intake with PD risk, Ross *et al.*[694] analyzed data from 30 years of follow-up in 8004 Japanese-American men aged 48 to 68 years. Their findings, independent of smoking, "indicate that higher coffee and caffeine intake is associated with a significantly lower incidence of PD."

Folic acid deficiency may also increase the risk for PD. In a recent experimental study, mice fed a folate-deficient diet developed severe Parkinson-like symptoms which were traced to elevated levels of homocysteine in the brain.[695] They postulated that this amino acid, which has also been established as a risk factor for cardiovascular, cerebrovascular and peripheral vascular diseases, damages DNA in the substantia nigra, which is rich in dopamine neurons. Interestingly, they noted that the administration of uric acid, an established antioxidant, also ameliorated the adverse effects of homocysteine.

Nutrition and Miscellaneous Medical Disorders

Hypercalciuria

Idiopathic hypercalciuria is a common risk factor for the formation of kidney stones. Although thiazides can reduce urinary calcium excretion, dietary modification should be the initial step since stone formation is dependent on calcium intake. In addition, most people with hypercalciuria have intestinal hyperabsorption of calcium.[696] As such, a low calcium diet is generally recommended. However, the long-term effect of a low calcium diet in these patients is unknown. To further study this disorder, Borghi *et al.*[697] conducted a five-year randomized trial comparing two diets in 120 men with hypercalciuria and recurrent stone formation. One group (60 men) was assigned a diet containing a normal amount of calcium (30 mmol/day) but reduced amounts of animal protein (52 g/day) and salt (50 mmol of sodium chloride/day). The other group was assigned the traditional low-calcium diet (10 mmol of calcium/day). Interestingly, dietary restriction of animal protein and salt combined with a normal calcium intake provided significantly greater protection against recurring stones and hypercalciuria than the traditional low-calcium diet.

Gallbladder disease

Vitamin C is important in the catabolism of cholesterol to bile acids. Experimental studies have shown that vitamin C-deficient guinea pigs are prone to develop gallstones.[698] To investigate the relationship between vitamin C intake in humans and gallbladder disease (gallstone formation or history of cholecystectomy), data from a large group of men and women enrolled in the Third National Health and Nutrition Examination Survey were analyzed.[699] The results showed that serum ascorbic acid levels were inversely associated with the prevalence of clinical asymptomatic gallbladder disease among women but not among men.

Pre-eclampsia and eclampsia

Pre-eclampsia is an important cause of maternal morbidity and mortality and accounts for over 40% of iatrogenic premature deliveries. Until recently, there has been no effective medical management of these complex cases except elective delivery. However, several empirical therapeutic methods have recently been shown to prevent or delay this traumatic and costly disorder. Although the pathogenesis of pre-eclampsia is unknown, the toxemia hypothesis, which suggests that the compromised placenta produces substances that lead to pre-eclampsia, is a widely accepted theory.

Recent studies suggest the possibility that free radicals may be important in the pathophysiology of this disorder. Indeed, several reports have demonstrated that various serum markers of oxidative stress are increased in patients with both pre-eclampsia and eclampsia relative to normal pregnancies. Moreover, the levels of these markers directly correlate with increased systolic and diastolic blood pressures.[700,701] To clinically evaluate this theory, Chappell *et al.*[702] studied 283 women at increased risk for pre-eclampsia. The women were randomly assigned vitamin C (1000 mg/day) and vitamin E (400 IU/day) or placebo at 16 to 22 weeks' gestation. For those participants who completed the study, there was a significant decrease in pre-eclampsia risk in those supplemented with vitamins C and E compared with the non-supplemented group (odds ratio = 0.24).

Magnesium has also been shown to be an effective first-line treatment in patients with pre-eclampsia since it reduces cerebral vasoconstriction ischemia.[703,704] In a recent study, magnesium sulfate ($MgSO_4$) was compared with nimodipine, a calcium-channel blocker with specific cerebral vasodilator activity.[705] This unblinded, multicenter trial included 1650 women with severe pre-eclampsia. The participants were randomly assigned to receive either nimodipine (60 mg every four hours) or intravenous $MgSO_4$ from enrollment until 24 hours postpartum. The authors concluded the $MgSO_4$ "is more effective than nimodipine for prophylaxis against seizures in women with severe pre-eclampsia.

Birth defects and spontaneous abortion

Over the past two decades, numerous studies have evaluated the association between various birth defects and maternal nutrition. The most commonly noted problems include neural tube defects, spontaneous abortion, and various organ and skeletal abnormalities.

Folic acid and birth defects

A neural tube defect (NTD) is one that involves any malformation of the embryonic brain and/or spinal cord. The neural tube is formed 20 to 28 days after fertilization. The various forms of NTD range in severity from anencephaly (absence of the cerebrum) to incomplete formation of the spinal cord, cranial bones, vertebral arches, meninges and overlying skin. NTD is among the most common of the severe birth defects, the rate of occurrence with the first pregnancy being about one in 1000 live births. In mothers with a previous NTD pregnancy, however, the rate is ten to 20 times higher. Each year, there are an estimated 4000 affected pregnancies in the US and 300,000 to 400,000 worldwide. In 1991, the annual medical expenses of this serious disorder in the US were estimated at US$200 million.[706]

In 1980, Smithells *et al.*[707] published their results of a non-randomized trial suggesting that multivitamin supplementation during the preconceptional period reduced the incidence of NTD. Since then numerous studies have demonstrated a reduced risk among women who took multivitamin supplements containing folic acid.[708,709] As a result of these studies, folic acid deficiency is now widely accepted as a major risk factor for NTD. Indeed, in 1992 the US Public Health Service recommended that women of childbearing age (i.e. aged 15 to 44 years) who might become pregnant should consume 400 ug of folic acid daily to reduce the number of NTDs.[710] In 1998, the Food and Drug Administration required the fortification of enriched cereal grain products with folic acid.[711]

To evaluate the impact of these public health policies on the prevalence of NTDs, Williams *et al.*[712] identified 5630 cases of spina bifida from 24 population-based surveillance systems from 1995 to 1999. Their findings indicated a 31% decrease in the prevalence of spina bifida from the pre- to post-mandatory fortification period; the prevalence of anencephaly decreased by 16%. Unfortunately, many women do not regularly consume cereal grain products. If they did, the prevalence of NTDs would be decreased significantly more. In fact, the incidence of spina bifida and anencephaly could be reduced about 50% by the daily consumption of 400 ug of folic acid before conception and during the early days of pregnancy.[713]

Multivitamins and birth defects

In their review of the relation between multivitamin supplementation and risk of various birth defects, Werler and associates[714] referenced several recent reports that suggested various other birth defects that might be reduced by regular multivitamin intake. These include defects of the lip and palate, heart, limbs, urinary tract, brain and pylorus muscle. Indeed, renewed interest in vitamin K over the past decade has occurred because of concerns that deficiencies may significantly increase the risk of neonatal death in the first six months of life from brain damage.[715] In addition, vitamin K deficiency has been linked to bone metabolism[716] and questions have been raised regarding the possibility that vitamin K deficiency may be important in osteoporosis. Moreover, Lipsky stressed that there is an incorrect theory that diet-induced vitamin K deficiency is non-existent and that the "unsubstantiated" theory that vitamin K deficiency can occur with antibiotic killing of intestinal bacteria.[717] He concluded that "the insistent belief that intestinal bacteria are an important source of vitamin K has led to erroneous conclusions about the source of vitamin K for human nutrition."

Folic acid and spontaneous abortion

Some, albeit not all, early studies found that folic acid deficiency was a significant risk factor for spontaneous abortion. George and associates[718] recently suggested that these "conflicting results could be due to small sample size, highly selected populations, or lack of control for potential confounders such as age, smoking and alcohol consumption." To clarify the risk of spontaneous abortion with folic acid deficiency, these researchers carried out a population-based, matched, case-control study of 468 women with spontaneous abortion and compared them with 921 controls from 1996 through 1998. Their results showed that compared to women with plasma folate levels between 2.20 and 3.95 ng/mL, women with folate levels of 2.19 ng/mL or less were at increased risk of spontaneous abortion (odds ratio 1.47). Moreover, women with plasma folate levels of 3.96 to 6.16 ng/mL or higher showed no increased risk of early spontaneous abortion.

As a final note, acute viral myocarditis was recently shown to be associated with increased oxidative stress and lipid peroxidation.[719] Moreover, these patients had a significant decrease in plasma and erythrocyte antioxidant vitamins C, E and beta-carotene as well as the antioxidant enzymes superoxide dismutase, catalase and glutathione peroxidase. The study results led the authors to recommend that patients with acute viral myocarditis be supplemented with these vitamins and other antioxidants "to alleviate potential oxidative and lipoperoxidative damages in their bodies."

Nutrition and All-Cause Mortality

Life experience is dependent on numerous factors including genetics, diet, BMI, level of physical activity, environmental toxins, and personal habits such as smoking, alcohol and drug abuse, among others. This chapter has focused, to a significant extent, on the role of single nutrients, foods, or food groups on specific diseases. In this section, several examples of the effects of nutrient intake and diet on all-cause mortality will be presented.

Vitamin C is a critical micronturient and has an important role in many biological processes including free radical scavenging, hemostasis, collagen and hormone synthesis, and protection of cellular lipid membranes which presumably affects the risk for various chronic diseases. In an early study, the relation between vitamin C intake and mortality was examined in a cohort of 11,348 non-institutionalized adults aged 25 to 74 years and followed for an average of ten years.[720] The findings showed a strong inverse relation between all causes of death and increasing vitamin C intake in males, but only a weak inverse relation for women. Among men, the standard mortality ratio (SFR) for those with the highest vitamin C intake was 0.65 for all causes, 0.78 for all cancers and 0.58 for cardiovascular diseases. The SFRs for women were 0.90 for all causes, 0.86 for all cancers and 0.75 for cardiovascular disease. More recently, others prospectively studied the relation between plasma vitamin C levels and subsequent all-cause mortality, cardiovascular disease, ischemic heart disease and cancer in 19,496 men and women aged 45 to 79 years.[721] Their results showed a significant inverse relation between plasma vitamin C levels and all-cause mortality, cardiovascular disease and ischemic heart disease in both men and women. However, vitamin C levels were inversely related to cancer mortality only in men.

Noting that relatively few studies have addressed the health effects of dietary patterns comprising interdependent dietary factors, Kant *et al.*[722] prospectively studied a cohort of 42,254 women, mean age 61.1 years, with a median follow-up of 5.6 years. Compared with those in the lowest quartile of the Recommended Food Score (i.e. sum of the number of foods recommended by current guidelines including fruits, vegetables, whole grains, low-fat dairy, lean meats and poultry), subjects in the upper quartiles for all-cause mortality was 0.82 for quartile 2, 0.71 for quartile 3 and 0.69 for quartile 4, after adjusting for the usual confounders (i.e. age, ethnicity, education level, body weight, smoking status, alcohol use, physical activity level, menopausal hormone use and disease history). Thus, the current dietary guidelines, as discussed in the early sections of this chapter, are associated with a decreased risk for various diseases and overall mortality.

To further evaluate the association between diet and cancer, ischemic heart disease and all-cause mortality, Fraser[723] recently summarized the results of a cohort study of 34,192 Seventh-day Adventists, most of whom did not smoke cigarettes or drink alcoholic beverages. About 50% of those studied ate meat products less than once a week or not at all and the vegetarians consumed more legumes, nuts, tomatoes and fruit. The multivariate analysis showed the following: (1) a significant association was present between beef consumption and fatal ischemic heart disease in men who ate beef three or more times a week; (2) a significant protective association existed between nut consumption and fatal and non-fatal ischemic heart disease in both sexes; (3) a reduced risk of ischemic heart disease in those preferring whole grain to white bread; (4) colon and prostate cancers were significantly more common in non-vegetarians; (5) frequent beef consumers had a higher risk for bladder cancer; (6) legume intake was inversely associated with risk for colon and pancreatic cancers; and (7) higher consumption of all fruit and dried fruit was associated with lower risks of lung, prostate and pancreatic cancers. The data also suggested that vegetarian Seventh-day Adventists have lower risks for diabetes mellitus, hypertension and arthritis compared with non-vegetarians.

Aging is associated with an increased frequency of diseases and disorders involving virtually all organ systems which results in increased mortality rates. A recent study examined the relationship between biochemical markers and all-cause mortality in a group of nonagenarians aged 90 to 100 years.[724] Blood and urine were initially analyzed for 50 basic biochemical, hematologic and biologic markers; these analyses were then repeated in six- to 12-month intervals during the four- to 45-month study period. Of the 50 markers, only increased serum vitamin E and calcium levels and significantly lower serum alanine aminotransferase and urinary neopterin levels were associated with the survivors compared to those who died during the study period.

Chapter Summary

Good nutrition is critical for a long, productive and healthy life. Poor dietary habits result in significantly increased risks for numerous diseases and clinical disorders. Protein-energy malnutrition, a common problem in the elderly and lower socioeconomic groups, results in several clinical problems and significantly increases medical costs. In addition, dietary deficiencies of one or more of the 40 important micronutrients are very common. However, all of these nutrients are readily supplied by following the dietary guidelines discussed in the first section of this chapter. These diet and nutrition guidelines serve two important purposes; they guide policy makers and educate consumers. Moreover, dietary supplements may be important, especially in the elderly where diet is often poor due to various reasons. Other important dietary problems include excessive intakes of total fat, saturated fats and trans-fatty acids. Conversely, there is need for increased intake of the omega-3 (n-3) fatty acids, which are rich in fish and some vegetable oils.

In order to improve peoples' diets, as with excess body weight and physical inactivity, it is critical that more national effort be expended in educating the public and medical profession as to the importance of nutrition. Moreover, this education must begin in early childhood if we are to be successful. The exploding elder population puts increasing demands on a health care system already burdened by the elderly and the poor. Nevertheless, these personal and societal costs can be markedly reduced by lifestyle changes, including more nutritious diets. The government publications, *Healthy People 2000* and *Healthy People 2010*, are important steps in this direction.[725] However, this information must be more vigorously and widely distributed if there is to be further improvement in the nation's health and in reducing the escalating medical costs.

References

1. Jelliffe DB. *The Assessment of the Nutritional Status of the Community*. WHO Monograph No. 53, World Health Organization, Geneva, 1966.
2. *Dietary Guidelines for Americans*, 3rd Ed. US Department of Agriculture and Department of Health and Human Services, Home and Garden Bulletin No. 232. Superintendant of Documents, Washington, DC, 1990.
3. Truswell AS. Practical and realistic approaches to healthier diet modifications. *Am J Clin Nutr* 1998;67(Suppl):583S–590S.
4. Russell RM, Rasmussen H, Lictenstein AH. Modified food guide pyramid for people over 70 years of age. *J Nutr* 1999;129:751–753.
5. Willett WC, Stampfer MJ. Rebuilding the food pyramid. *Sci Am*, January 2003, pp. 64–71.
6. Krauss RM, Eckel RH, Howard B, *et al.* AHA guidelines Revision 2000: a statement for health care professionals from the Nutrition

Committee of the American Heart Association. *Circulation* 2000; 102:2284–2299.

7. MRC Vitamin Study Research Group. Prevention of neural tube-defects: results of the Medical Research Council Vitamin Study. *Lancet* 1991;338:131–137.

8. Czeizel AE, Dudas I. Prevention of the first occurrence of neural tube defects by periconceptional vitamin supplementation. *N Engl J Med* 1992;327:1832–1835.

9. Trumbo P, Yates AA, Schlicker S, Poos M. Dietary reference intakes. *J Am Diet Assoc* 2001;101:294–301.

10. Lowenstein FW. Nutritional status of the elderly in the United States of America 1971–1974. *J Am Coll Nutr* 1982;1:165–177.

11. Weir DR. Nutritional deficiency in aging due to protein-calorie semi-starvation. In: *Aging: Its Chemistry*. AA Dietz, (ed.) American Association of Clinical Chemistry, Washington, DC, 1980, pp. 417–424.

12. Posner BM, Jette AM, Smith KW, Miller DR. Nutrition and health risks in the elderly: the nutrition screening initiative. *Am J Public Health* 1993;83:972–978.

13. Nelson K, Brown ME, Lurie N. Hunger in an adult patient population. *JAMA* 1998;279:1211–1214.

14. Wendland BE, Greenwood CE, Weinberg I, Young KW. Malnutrition in institutionalized seniors: the iatrogenic component. *J Am Geriatr Soc* 2003;51:85–90.

15. Krombout D, De Lezenne Coulander C, Oberman-de Boer GL, *et al.* Changes in food and nutrient intake in middle-aged men from 1960–1985 (the Zutphen Study). *Am J Clin Nutr* 1990;51:123–129.

16. Morley JE, Miller DK. Malnutrition in the elderly. *Hospital Pract* 1992;27(No. 7):95–116.

17. Mojon P, Budtz-Jorgensen E, Rapin C-H. Relationship between oral health and nutrition in very old people. *Age Ageing* 1999;28:463–468.

18. Saletti A, Lingren EY, Johansson L, Cederholm T. Nutritional status according to mini nutritional assessment in an institutionalized elderly population in Sweden. *Gerontology* 2000;46:139–145.

19. McWhirter JP, Pennington CR. Incidence and recognition of malnutrition in hospital. *BMJ* 1994;308:945–948.

20. Giner M, Laviano A, Megurd MM, Gleason JR. In 1955 a correlation between malnutrition and poor outcome in critically ill patients still exists. *Nutrition* 1996;12:23–29.

21. Alarcon T, Barcena A, Gonzalez M, *et al.* Factors predictive of outcome on admission to an acute geriatric ward. *Age Ageing* 1999;28:429–432.

22. Goodwin JS. Social, psychological and physical factors affecting the nutritional status of elderly subjects separating cause and effect. *Am J Clin Nutr* 1989;50:1201–1209.

23. Murphy SP, Davis MA, Neuhaus Jm, Lein D. Factors influencing the dietary adequacy and energy intake of older Americans. *J Nutr Edu* 1990;22:224–291.

24. De Graaf C, Polet P, van Staveren WA. Sensory perception and pleasantness of foods flavors in elderly subjects. *J Gerontol* 1994;49:93–99.

25. Krall E, Hayes C, Garcia R. How dentition status and masticatory function affect nutrient intake. *JADA* 1998;129:1261–1269.

26. Bernstein LH, Shaw-Stiffel TA, Schorow M, Brouillette R. Financial implications of malnutrition. *Clin Lab Med* 1993;13:491–507.

27. Garrow JS, James WPT (eds.). *Human Nutrition and Dietetics*, 9th Ed. Churchill Livingstone, Edinburgh, 1993, p. 786.

28. Biena R, Ratcliff S, Barbour GL, Kummer M. Malnutrition in the hospitalized geriatric patients. *J Am Geriatr Soc* 1982;30:433–436.

29. Constans T, Bacq Y, Brechot JF, *et al.* Protein-energy malnutrition in elderly medical patients. *J Am Geriatr Soc* 1992;40:263–268.

30. Volkert D, Kruse W, Oster P, Schlierf G. Malnutrition in geriatric patients. *Ann Nutr Metab* 1992;36:97–112.

31. Potter J, Klipstein K, Reilly JJ, Roberts M. The nutritional status and clinical course of acute admissions to a geriatric unit. *Age Ageing* 1995;24:131–136.

32. Sullivan DH, Sun S, Walls RC. Protein-energy undernutrition among elderly hospitalized patients: a prospective study. *JAMA* 1999; 281:2013–2019.

33. Mowe M, Bohmer T. The prevalence of undiagnosed protein-calorie undernutrition in a population of hospitalized elderly patients. *J Am Geriatri Soc* 1991;39:1089–1092.

34. Sullivan DH, Walls RC, Bopp MM. Protein-energy undernutrition and the risk of mortality within one year of hospital discharge: a follow-up study. *J Am Geriatr Soc* 1995;43:507–512.

35. Rudman D, Feller AG. Protein-calorie undernutrition in the nursing home. *J Am Geriatr Soc* 1989;37:173–183.

36. Friedman PJ, Campbell AJ, Caradoc-Davies TH. Prospective trial of a new diagnostic criterion for severe wasting malnutrition in the elderly. *Age Ageing* 1985;14:149–154.

37. Danesh J, Collins R, Appleby P, Peto R. Association of fibrinogen, C-reactive protein, albumin or leukocyte count with coronary heart disease. *JAMA* 1998;279:1477–1482.

38. Phillips A, Shaper AG, Whincup PH. Association between serum albumin and mortality from cardiovascular disease, cancer and other causes. *Lancet* 1989;2:1434–1438.
39. Sahyoun NR, Jacques PF, Dallal G, Russell RM. Use of albumin as a predictor of mortality in community dwelling and institionalized elderly populations. *J Clin Epidemiol* 1996;49:981–988.
40. Hermann FR, Safran C, Levkoff SE, Minaker KL. Serum albumin level on admission as a predictor of death, length of stay, and readmission. *Arch Intern Med* 1992;152:125–130.
41. Sullivan DH, Walls RC. Protein-energy undernutrition and the risk of mortality within six years of hospital discharge. *J Am Coll Nutr* 1998;17:571–578.
42. McMurtry CT, Rosenthal A. Predictors of two-year mortality among older male veterans on a geriatric rehabilitation unit. *J Am Geriatr Soc* 1995;43:1123–1126.
43. Burness R, Horne G, Purdie G. Albumin levels and mortality in patient with hip fractures. *N Z Med J* 1996;109:56–57.
44. Gibbs J, Cull W, Henderson W, *et al.* Preoperative serum albumin level as a predictor of operative mortality and morbidity. *Arch Surg* 1999;134:36–42.
45. Bienia R, Ratcliff S, Barbour GL, Kummer M. Malnutrition in the hospitalized geriatric patient. *J Am Geriatr Soc* 1982;30:433–436.
46. Grant JP, Custer PB, Thurlow J. Current techniques of nutritional assessment. *Surg Clin North Am* 1981;61:437–463.
47. Oster P, Muchowski H, Heuck CC, Schlierf G. The prognostic significance of hypo-cholesterolemia in hospitalized patients. *Klin Wochenschr* 1981;59:857–860.
48. Noel MA, Smith TK, Ettinger WH. Characteristics and outcomes of hospitalized older patients who develop hypocholesterolemia. *J Am Geriatr Soc* 1991;39:455–461.
49. Gui D, Spada PL, De Gaetano A, Pacelli F. Hypocholesterolemia and risk of death in the critically ill surgical patient. *Intensive Care Med* 1996;22:790–794.
50. Verdery RB, Goldberg AP. Hypocholesterolemia as a predictor of death: a prospective study of 224 nursing home residents. *J Gerontol* 1991;46:M84–M90.
51. Terpenning MS, Bradley SF. Why aging leads to increased susceptibility to infection. *Geriatrics* 1991;46:77–80.
52. Chandra RK. The relation between immunology, nutrition, and disease in elderly people. *Age Ageing* 1990;19:525–531.

53. Polge A, Bancel E, Bellet H, *et al.* Plasma amino acid concentrations in elderly patients with protein energy malnutrition. *Age Ageing* 1997;26:457–462.
54. Lauque S, Arnaud-Battandier F, Mansourian R, *et al.* Protein-energy oral supplementation in malnourished nursing-home residents. A controlled trial. *Age Ageing* 2000;29:51–56.
55. Bos C, Benamouzig R, Bruhat A, *et al.* Short-term protein and energy supplementation activates nitrogen kinetics and accretion in poorly nourished elderly subjects. *Am J Clin Nutr* 2000;71:1129–1137.
56. Reilly JJ Jr., Hull SF, Albert N, *et al.* Economic impact of malnutrition: a model system for hospitalized patients. *JPEN* 1988;12:371–376.
57. Mullen JL, Buzby GP, Mathews DC, *et al.* Reduction of operative morbidity and mortality by combined preoperative and postoperative nutritional support. *Ann Surg* 1980;192:604–613.
58. Bastow MD, Rawlings J, Allison SP. Benefits of supplementary tube feeding after fractured neck of femur: a randomized controlled trial. *Br Med J* 1983;287:1589–1592.
59. Starker PM, LaSala PA, Askanazi J, *et al.* The influence of preoperative total parenteral nutrition upon morbidity and mortality. *Surg Genecol Obst* 1986;162:569–574.
60. Robinson G, Goldstein M, Levine GM. Impact of nutritional status on DRG length of stay. *JPEN* 1987;11:49–51.
61. Brugler L, DiPrinzio MJ, Berstein L. The five-year evolution of a malnutrition treatment program in a community hospital. *J Qual Imp* 1999;25:191–206.
62. Bernstein LH. Managing nutritional care is essential for managing total care. *Am Clin Lab* 2001;20:8–12.
63. Crawford D, Baghurst K. Nutrition information in Australia — the public's views. *Aust J Nutr Diet* 1991;48:40–44.
64. Harris L. *Health Maintenance.* Pacific Mutual Life Insurance Company, 1978.
65. Wechsler H, Levin S, Idelson RK, *et al.* The physician's role in health promotion — a survery of primary care practitioners. *N Engl J Med* 1983;308:97–100.
66. Wechsler H, Levine SD, Idelson RK, *et al.* The physician's role in health promotion revisited — a survey of primary care practitioners. *N Engl J Med* 1996;334:996–998.
67. Hiddink GJ, Hautvast JGAJ, van Woerkum CMJ, *et al.* Nutrition guidance by primary-care physicians: perceived barriers and low involvement. *Eur J Clin Nutr* 1995;49:842–851.

68. Wallace PG, Brennan PJ, Haines AP. Are practitioners doing enough to promote healthy lifestyle? Findings of the Medical Research Council's general practive research framework study on lifestyle and health. *BMJ* 1987;294:940–942.

69. Kreuter MW, Scharff DP, Brennan LK, Lukwago SN. Physician recommendations for diet and physical activity: which patients get advised to change? *Prev Med* 1997;26:825–833.

70. Galuska DA, Will JC, Serdula MK, Ford ES. Are health care professionals advising obese patients to lose weight? *JAMA* 1999;282:1576–1578.

71. Steptoe A, Perkins-Porras L, McKay C, *et al.* Behavioral counseling to increase consumption of fruit and vegetables in low income adults: randomized trial. *BMJ* 2003;326:855–858.

72. Knight JA. *Free Radicals, Anitoxidants, Aging and Disease.* AACC Press, Washington, DC, 1999.

73. Floyd RA, Watson JJ, Harris J, *et al.* Formation of 8-hydroxy-deoxyguanosine, hydroxyl free radical adduct of DNA in granulocytes exposed to tumor promoter, tetradecanoyl phorbolacetate. *Biochem Biophys Res Commun* 1986;137:841–846.

74. Feig DI, Reid TM, Loeb LA. Reactive oxygen species in tumorigenesis. *Cancer Res* 1994;54 (Suppl):1890S–1894S.

75. Ames BN, Gold LS, Willett WC. The causes and prevention of cancer. *Proc Natl Acad Sci USA* 1995;92:5258–5265.

76. Ames BN, Shigenago MK, Hagan TM. Oxidants, antioxidants, and the degenerative diseases of aging. *Proc Natl Acad Sci USA* 1993;90:7915–7922.

77. Harman D. Aging: a theory based on free radical and radiation chemistry. *J Gerontol* 1956;11:298–300.

78. Harman D. The aging process. *Proc Natl Acad Sci USA* 1981;78:7124–7128.

79. Beckman KB, Ames BN. The free radical theory of aging matures. *Physiol Rev* 1998;78:547–581.

80. McKay CM, Crowell MF, Maynard LA. The effect of retarded growth upon the length of life span and upon the ultimate body size. *J Nutr* 1935;10:63–79.

81. Masoro E. Physiology of ageing: nutritional aspects. *Age Ageing* 1990;19:S5–S9.

82. Weindruch R, Walford RL. Dietary restriction in mice beginning at 1 year of age. Effect on life-span and spontaneous cancer incidence. *Science* 1982;215:1415–1418.

83. Yu BP, Masoro EJ, McMahan CA. Nutritional influences on aging of Fischer 344 rats. I. Physical, metabolic and longevity characteristics. *J Gerontol* 1985;40:657–670.

84. Masoro EJ. The role of animal models in meeting the gerontologic challenge of the 21st century. *Gerontologist* 1992;32:627–633.
85. Chung MH, Kasai H, Nishimura S, *et al.* Protection of DNA damage by dietary restriction. *Free Radic Biol Med* 1992;12:523–525.
86. Turturro A, Blank K, Murasko D, Hart R. Mechanisms of caloric restriction affecting aging and disease. *Ann NY Acad Sci* 1994;719:159–170.
87. Koizumi A, Weindruch R, Walford RL. Influences of dietary restriction and age on liver enzyme activities and lipid peroxidation in mice. *J Nutr* 1987;117:361–367.
88. Suzuki K, Oberley TD, Pugh TD, *et al.* Caloric restriction diminishes the age-associated loss of immunoreactive catalase in rat prostate. *Prostate* 1997;33:256–263.
89. Weindruch R. Caloric restriction and aging. *Sci Am* January 1996, pp. 46–52.
90. Lane MA, Baer DJ, Rumpler WV, *et al.* Caloric restriction lowers body temperature in rhesus monkeys, consistent with a postulated anti-aging mechanism in rodents. *Proc Natl Acad Sci USA* 1996;93: 4159–4163.
91. Weed JL, Lane MA, Roth GS, *et al.* Activity measures in rhesus monkeys on long-term calorie restriction. *Physiol Behav* 1997;62:97–103.
92. Lane MA, Ingram DK, Ball SS, Roth GS. Dehydroepiandrosterone sulfate: a bio-marker of primate aging slowed by calorie restriction. *J Clin Endocrinol Metab* 1997;82:2093–2096.
93. Luan X, Zhao W, Chendrasekar B, Fernandes G. Caloric restriction modulates lymphocyte subset phenotype and increases apoptosis in MRL/lpr mice. *Immunol Lett* 1995;47:181–186.
94. Mezzetti A, Lapenna D, Romano F, *et al.* Systemic oxidative stress and its relationship with age and illness. *J Am Geriatr Soc* 1996;44: 823–827.
95. Mecocci P, Polidori MC, Troiano L, *et al.* Plasma antioxidants and longevity: a study on healthy centenarians. *Free Radic Biol Med* 2000;28:1243–1248.
96. Takahashi R, Goto S. Effect of dietary restriction beyond middle age: accumulation of altered proteins and protein degradation. *Microsc Res Tech* 2002;59:278–281.
97. Goto S, Takahashi R, Araki S, Nakamoto H. Dietary restriction initiated in late adulthood can reverse age-related alterations of protein and protein metabolism. *Ann N Y Acad Sci* 2002;959:50–56.
98. Nagai M, Takahashi R, Goto S. Dietary restriction initiated late in life can reduce mitochondrial protein carbonyls in rat livers: western blot studies. *Biogerontology* 2000;1:321, 328.

99. Sohal RS, Weindruch R. Oxidative stress, caloric restriction, and aging. *Science* 1996;273:59–63.

100. Weindruch R, Sohal RS. Caloric intake and aging. *N Engl J Med* 1997;337:986–994.

101. Olshansky SJ, Hayflick L, Carnes BA. No truth to the fountain of youth. *Sci Am*, June 2002, pp. 92–95.

102. Packer L, Witt EH, Tritschler HJ. Alpha-lipoic acid as a biological antioxidant. *Free Radic Biol Med* 1995;19:227–250.

103. Arora A, Nair MG, Strasburg GM. Structure activity relationship for antioxidant activities of a series of flavonoids in a liposomal system. *Free Radic Biol Med* 1998;24:1355–1363.

104. Bray TM, Bettger WJ. The physiologic role of zinc as an antioxidant. *Free Radic Biol Med* 1990;8:281–291.

105. Coassin M, Ursini F, Bindoli A. Antioxidant effect of manganese. *Arch Biochem Biophys* 1992;299:330–333.

106. Richard M-J, Rousell A-M. Micronutrients and ageing: intakes and requirements. *Proc Nutr Soc* 1999;58:573–578.

107. de Groot CPGM, van den Broek T, van Staveren W. Energy intake and micronutrient intake in elderly Europeans: seeking the minimum requirement in the SENECA study. *Age Ageing* 1999;28:469–471.

108. Joosten E, van den Berg A, Riezler R, *et al.* Metabolic evidence that deficiencies of vitamin B-12 (cobalamin), folate, and vitamin B-6 occur commonly in elderly people. *Am J Clin Nutr* 1993;58: 468–476.

109. Naurath HJ, Joosten E, Riezler R, *et al.* Effects of vitamin B12, folate, and vitamin B6 supplements in elderly people with normal serum vitamin concentrations. *Lancet* 1995;346:85–89.

110. Daly LE, Kirke PN, Molloy A, *et al.* Folate levels and neural tube defects. *JAMA* 1995;274:1698–1702.

111. Food and Drug Administration. Food standards: amendments of standards of identity for enriched grain products to require additional of folic acid. *Fed Regist* 1996;61(44):878–897.

112. Baik HW, Russell RM. Vitamin B12 deficiency in the elderly. *Ann Rev Nutr* 1999;19:357–377.

113. Pennypacker LC, Allen RH, Kelly JP, *et al.* High prevalence of cobalamin deficiency in elderly outpatients. *J Am Geriatr Soc* 1992; 40:1197–1204.

114. Metz J, Bell AH, App Sc B, *et al.* The significance of subnormal serum vitamin B12 concentration in older people: a case control study. *J Am Geriatr Soc* 1996;44:1355–1361.

115. Stabler SP. Screening of the older population for cobalamin (vitamin B12) deficiency. *J Am Geriatr Soc* 1995;43:1290–1297.

116. Eggersten R, Nilsson T, Lindstedt G, Lundberg P-A. Prevalence and diagnosis of cobalamin deficiency in older people. *J Am Geriatr Soc* 1996;44:1273–1274.

117. Fata FT, Herzlich BC, Schiffman G, Ast AL. Impaired antibody responses to pneumococcal polysaccharide in elderly patients with low serum vitamin B12 levels. *Ann Intern Med* 1996;124:199–204.

118. Mahmoud MY, Lugon M, Anderon CC. Unexplained macrocytosis in elderly patients. *Age Ageing* 1996;25:310–312.

119. Crystal HA, Ortof E, Frishman WH, *et al.* Serum vitamin B12 levels and incidence of dementia in healthy elderly population: a report from the Bronx Longitudinal Aging Study. *J Am Geriatr Soc* 1994;42:933–936.

120. O'Neill D, Barber RD. Reversible dementia caused by vitamin B12 deficiency. *J Am Geriatr Soc* 1993;41:192–194.

121. Penninx BWJH, Guralnick JM, Ferrucci L, *et al.* Vitamin B12 deficiency and depression in physically disabled older women: epidemiologic evidence from the Women's Health and Aging Study. *Am J Psychiatry* 2000;157:715–721.

122. Chandra RK. Effect of vitamin and trace-element supplementation on cognitive function in elderly subjects. *Nutrition* 2001;17:709–712.

123. Dallman PR. Biochemical basis for the manifestations of iron deficiency. *Annu Rev Nutr* 1986;6:13–40.

124. CDC. Iron deficiency — United States, 1999–2000. *MMWR* 2002;51:897–899.

125. Looker AC, Dallman PR, Carroll MD, *et al.* Prevalence of iron deficiency in the United States. *JAMA* 1997;277:973–976.

126. MacKenzie R, Rafferty T, Beckett G. Selenium: an essential element for immune function. *Immunol Today* 1998;19:342–345.

127. Lloyd-Jones DM, Larson MG, Beiser A, Levy D. Lifetime risk of developing coronary heart disease. *Lancet* 1999;353:89–92.

128. Knight JA. Wellness assessment: a role for laboratory medicine. *Ann Clin Lab Sci* 2000;30:23–32.

129. Fang J, Alderman MH. Serum uric acid and cardiovascular mortality. *JAMA* 2000;283:2404–2410.

130. Straus SE, Majumdar SR, McAlister FA. New evidence for stroke prevention. *JAMA* 2002;288:1389–1395.

131. Goldstein JL, Ho YK, Basu SK, Brown MS. Binding site on macrophages that mediate uptake and degradation of acetylated low

density lipoprotein producing massive cholesterol deposition. *Proc Natl Acad Sci USA* 1979;76:333–337.

132. Berliner JA, Navab M, Fogelman AM, *et al.* Atherosclerosis: basic mechanisms, oxidation, inflammation and genetics. *Circulation* 1995;91:2488–2496.

133. Quinn MT, Parthasarathy S, Steinberg D. Endothelial cell-derived chemotactic activity for mouse peritoneal macrophages and the effect of modified forms of low density lipoprotein. *Proc Natl Acad Sci USA* 1985;82:5949–5953.

134. Quinn MT, Parthasarathy S, Fong LG, Steinberg D. Oxidatively modified low density lipoprotein: a potential role in recruitment and retention of monocytes/macrophages during atherosclerosis. *Proc Natl Acad Sci USA* 1987;84:2995–2998.

135. Steinberg D, Parthasarathy SK, Carew TE, *et al.* Beyond cholesterol: modifications of low-density lipoprotein that increase its atherogenicity. *N Engl J Med* 1989;320:915–924.

136. Ehara S, Ueda M, Naruko T, *et al.* Elevated levels of oxidized low density lipoprotein show a positive relationship with the severity of acute coronary syndromes. *Circulation* 2001;103:1955–1960.

137. Devaraj S, Li D, Jialal I. The effects of alpha-tocopherol supplementation on monocyte function. *J Clin Invest* 1996;98:756–763.

138. Esterbauer H, Puhl H, Dieber-Rutheneder M, *et al.* Effect of antioxidants on oxidative modification of LDL. *Ann Med* 1991;23: 573–581.

139. Jialal I, Fuller CJ, Huel B. The effect of alpha-tocopherol supplementation on LDL oxidation. *Atheroscler Thromb Vasc Biol* 1995; 15:190–198.

140. Belcher JD, Balla J, Balla G, *et al.* Vitamin E, LDL and endothelium: brief oral vitamin supplementation prevents oxidized LDL-mediated vascular injury *in vitro*. *Atheroscler Thromb Vasc Biol* 1993;13: 1779–1789.

141. Yoshida H, Ishikawa T, Nakamura H. Vitamin E/lipid peroxide ratio and susceptibility of LDL to oxidative modification in non-insulin-dependent diabetes mellitus. *Atheroscler Thromb Vasc Biol* 1997; 17:1438–1446.

142. Cominacini L, Young MM, Capriati A, *et al.* Troglitazone increases the resistance of low density lipoprotein to oxidation in healthy volunteers. *Diabetologia* 1997;40:1211–1218.

143. Prasad K, Kalra J. Oxygen free radicals and hypercholesterolemic atherosclerosis: effects of vitamin E. *Am Heart J* 1993;125:958–973.

144. Sun J, Giraud DW, Moxley RA, Driskell JA. Beta-carotene and alpha-tocopherol inhibit the development of atherosclerotic lesions in hypercholesterolemic rabbits. *Int J Vitam Nutr Res* 1997;67:155–163.

145. Verlangieri AJ, Bush MJ. Effects of D-alpha-tocopherol supplementation on experimentally induced primate atherosclerosis. *J Am Coll Nutr* 1992;11:131–138.

146. van Jaarsveld H, Pool GF, Barnard HC. Dietary iron concentration alters LDL oxidatively, the effect of antioxidants. *Res Commun Mol Pathol Pharmacol* 1998;99:69–80.

147. Azen SP, Qian D, Mack WJ, *et al*. Effect of supplementary antioxidant vitamin intake on carotid arterial wall intima-media thickness in a controlled clinical trial of cholesterol lowering. *Circulation* 1996;94:2369–2372.

148. Mezzetti A, LaPenna D, Pierdomenico SD, *et al*. Vitamins E, C and lipid peroxidation in plasma and arterial tissue of smokers and non-smokers. *Atherosclerosis* 1995;112:91–99.

149. Frei B, Stocker R, Ames BN. Antioxidant defenses and lipid peroxidation in human blood plasma. *Proc Natl Acad Sci USA* 1988;85:9748–9752.

150. Retsky KL, Freeman MW, Frei B. Ascorbic acid oxidation product(s) protect human low density lipoprotein against atherogenic modification. *J Biol Chem* 1993;268:1304–1309.

151. Frei B, England L, Ames BN. Ascorbate is an outstanding antioxidant in human blood plasma. *Proc Natl Acad Sci USA* 1989;86:6377–6381.

152. Jialal I, Grundy SM. Preservation of the endogenous antioxidants in low density lipoprotein by ascorbate but not probucol during oxidative modification. *J Clin Invest* 1991;87:597–601.

153. Rifici VA, Khachadurian AK. Dietary supplementation with vitamins C and E inhibits *in vitro* oxidation of lipoproteins. *J Am Coll Nutr* 1993;12:631–637.

154. Heitzer T, Just H, Munzel T. Antioxidant vitamin C improves endothelial dysfunction in chronic smokers. *Circulation* 1996; 94:6–9.

155. Ting HH, Timimi FK, Haley EA, *et al*. Vitamin C improves endothelium-dependent vasodilation in forearm resistance vessels of humans with hypercholesterolemia. *Circulation* 1997;95:2617–2622.

156. Gokee N, Keaney JF Jr., Frei B, *et al*. Long-term ascorbic acid administration reverses endothelial vasomotor dysfunction in patients with coronary artery disease. *Circulation* 1999;99:3234–3240.

157. Heitzer T, Schlinzig T, Krohn K, *et al.* Endothelial dysfunction, oxidative stress, and risk of cardiovascular events in patients with coronary artery disease. *Circulation* 2001;104:2673–2678.

158. May JM. How does ascorbic acid prevent endothelial dysfunction? *Free Radic Biol Med* 2000;28:1421–1429.

159. Burton GW, Ingold KU. Beta-carotene: an unusual type of antioxidant. *Science* 1984;224:569–573.

160. Lynch SM, Morrow JD, Roberts LJ II, Frei B. Formation of non-cyclooxygenase derived prostanoids (F_2-isoprostanes) in plasma and low density lipoprotein exposed to oxidative stress *in vitro*. *J Clin Invest* 1994;93:998–1004.

161. Frei B. Reactive oxygen species and antioxidant vitamins: mechanisms of action. *Am J Med* 1994;97(Suppl):5S–13S.

162. Parthasarathy S, Young SG, Witztum JL, *et al.* Probucol inhibits oxidative modification of low density lipoprotein. *J Clin Invest* 1986;77:641–644.

163. Kita T, Nagano Y, Yokode M, *et al.* Probucol prevents the progression of atherosclerosis in Watanabe heritable hyperlipidemic rabbit, an animal model for familial hypercholesterolemia. *Proc Natl Acad Sci USA* 1987;84:5928–5931.

164. Carew TE, Schwenke DC, Steinberg D. Antiatherogenic effect of probucol unrelated to its hypocholesterolemic effect: evidence that antioxidants *in vivo* can selectively inhibit low density lipoprotein degradation in macrophage-rich fatty streaks slowing the progression of athersclerosis in the WHHL rabbit. *Proc Natl Acad Sci USA* 1987;84:7725–7729.

165. Hertog MGI, Feskins EJM, Hollman PC, *et al.* Dietary antioxidant flavonoids and risk of coronary artery disease: the Zutphen Elderly Study. *Lancet* 1993;342:1007–1011.

166. Luiz da Silva E, Tsushida T, Terao J. Inhibition of mammalian 15-lipoxygenase-dependent lipid peroxidation in low-density lipoprotein by quercetin and quercetin monoglucosides. *Arch Biochem Biophys* 1998;349:313–320.

167. Frankel EN, Kanner JH, German JB, *et al.* Inhibition of oxidation of low-density lipoprotein by phenolic substances in red wine. *Lancet* 1993;341:454–457.

168. Frankel EN, Waterhouse AL, Kinsella JE. Inhibition of human LDL oxidation by resveratrol. *Lancet* 1993;341:1103–1104.

169. Visioli F, Galli C. Oleuropein protects low density lipoprotein from oxidation. *Life Sci* 1994;55:1965–1971.

170. Kagan VE, Shvedova A, Serbinova E, *et al.* Dihydroplipoic acid — a universal antioxidant both in the membrane and in the aqueous phase. *Biochem Pharmacol* 1992;44:1637–1649.

171. Heitzer T, Finckh B, Albers S, *et al.* Beneficial effects of alpha-lipoic acid and ascorbic acid on endothelium-dependent, nitric oxide-mediated vasodilation in diabetic patients: relation to parameters of oxidative stress. *Free Radic Biol Med* 2001;31:53–61.

172. Arivazhagan P, Shila S, Narchonai E, Panneerselvam C. Alpha-lipoic acid enhances reduced glutathione, ascorbic acid and alpha-tocopherol in aged rats. *J Anti-Aging Med* 2002;5:265–269.

173. Fung TT, Willett WC, Stampfer MJ, *et al.* Dietary patterns and the risk of coronary heart disease in women. *Arch Intern Med* 2001; 161:1857–1862.

174. Hu FB, Willett WC. Optimal diets for prevention of coronary heart disease. *JAMA* 2002;288:2569–2578.

175. Rimm EB, Willett WC, Hu FB, *et al.* Folate and vitamin B6 from diet and supplements in relation to risk of coronary heart disease among women. *JAMA* 1998;279:359–364.

176. Simopoulos AP. The Mediterranean diets: what is so special about the diet of Greece? The scientific evidence. *J Nutr* 2001;131:3065S–3073S.

177. Keys A, Menotti A Aravanis C, *et al.* The seven countries study: 2289 deaths in 15 years. *J Prev Med* 1984;13:141–154.

178. Gjonca A, Bobak M. Albania paradox: another example of protective effect of Mediterranean lifestyle? *Lancet* 1997;350:1815–1817.

179. Renaud S, de Lorgeril M, Delaye J, *et al.* Cretan Mediterranean diet for prevention of coronary heart disease. *Am J Clin Nutr* 1995;61(Suppl):1360S–1367S.

180. de Lorgeril M, Renaud S. Mamelle N, *et al.* Mediterranean alpha-linolenic acid-rich diet in secondary prevention of coronary heart disease. *Lancet* 1994;343:1454–1459.

181. de Lorgeril M, Salen P, Martin J-L, *et al.* Mediterranean dietary pattern in a randomized trial: prolonged survival and possible reduced cancer rate. *Arch Intern Med* 1998;158:1181–1187.

182. Joshipura KJ, Hu FB, Manson JE, *et al.* The effect of fruit and vegetable intake on risk for coronary heart disease. *Ann Intern Med* 2001;134:1106–1114.

183. Trichopoulou A, Costacou T, Barnia C, Trichopoulos D. Adherence to a Mediterranean diet and survival in a Greek population. *N Engl J Med* 2003;348:2599–2608.

184. DeBoer SW, Thomas RJ, Brekke MJ, *et al.* Dietary intake of fruits, vegetables, and fat in Olmsted County, Minnesota. *Mayo Clin Proc* 2003;78:161–166.

185. Gey KF, Puyska P, Jordan P, Moser UK. Inverse correlation between plasma vitamin E and mortality from ischemic heart disease in cross-cultural epidemiology. *Am J Clin Nutr* 1991; 53:326S–334S.

186. Stampfer MJ, Hennekins CH, Manson JE, *et al.* Vitamin E consumption and the risk of coronary disease in women. *N Engl J Med* 1993;328:1444–1449.

187. Rimm EB, Stampfer MJ, Ascherio A, *et al.* Vitamin E consumption and the risk of coronary heart disease in men. *N Engl J Med* 1993;328:1450–1456.

188. Loxonczy KG, Harris TB, Havlik RJ. Vitamin E and vitamin C supplement use and risk of all-cause and coronary heart disease mortality in older persons. The established populations for epidemiologic studies of the Elderly. *Am J Clin Nutr* 1996;64:190–196.

189. Knekt P, Reunanen A, Jarvinen R, *et al.* Antioxidant vitamin intake and coronary mortality in a longitudinal population study. *Am J Epidemiol* 1994;139:1180–1189.

190. Stephens NG, Parsons A, Schofield PM, *et al.* Randomized controlled trial of vitamin E in patients with coronary disease: Cambridge Heart Antioxidant Study (CHAOS). *Lancet* 1996;347:781–786.

191. Miwa K, Miyagi Y, Igawa A, *et al.* Vitamin E deficiency in variant angina. *Circulation* 1996;94:14–18.

192. Riemersma RA, Wood DA, MacIntyre CCA, *et al.* Risk of angina pectoris and plasma concentrations of vitamins A, C, and E and carotene. *Lancet* 1991;337:1–5.

193. Regnstrom J, Nilsson J, Moldeus P, *et al.* Inverse relation between the concentration of low-density lipoprotein vitamin E and severity of coronary artery disease. *Am J Clin Nutr* 1996;63:77–85.

194. Kushi LH, Folsom AR, Prineas RJ, *et al.* Dietary antioxidant vitamins and death from coronary heart disease in postmenopausal women. *N Engl J Med* 1996;334:1156–1162.

195. Kuno T, Hozumi M, Morinobu T, *et al.* Anitoxidant vitamin levels in plasma and low density lipoprotein of obese girls, *Free Radic Res* 1998;28:81–86.

196. Mezzetti A, Zuliani G, Romano F, *et al.* Vitamin E and lipid peroxide plasma levels predict the risk of cardiovascular events in a group of healthy very old people. *J Am Geriatr Soc* 2001;49:533–537.

197. Cherubini A, Zuliani G, Constantini F, *et al.* High vitamin E plasma levels and low low-density lipoprotein oxidation are associated with the absence of atherosclerosis in octogenarians. *J Am Geriatr Soc* 201; 49:651–654.

198. The Heart Outcomes Prevention Evaluation Study Investigators. Vitamin E supplementation and cardiovascular events in high-risk patients. *N Engl J Med* 2000;342:154–160.

199. Evans RW, Shaten BJ, Day BW, Kuller LH. Prospective association between lipid soluble antioxidants and coronary heart disease in men. The Multiple Risk Factor Intervention Trial. *Am J Epidemiol* 1998;147:180–186.

200. Pryor WA. Vitamin E and heart disease: basic science to clinical intervention trials. *Free Radical Biol Med* 2000;28:141–164.

201. Salonen JT, Nyyssonen K, Salonen R, *et al.* Anitoxidant supplementation in atherosclerosis prevention (ASAP) study: a randomized trial of the effect of vitamins E and C on three-year progression of carotid atherosclerosis. *J Intern Med* 2000;248:177–186.

202. American Dietetic Association. Position of the American Dietetic Association: food fortification and dietary supplements. *J Am Diet Assoc* 2001;101:115–125.

203. Willet WC, Stampfer MJ. What vitamins should I be taking, doctor? *N Engl J Med* 2001;345:1819–1824.

204. Gey KF. Prospects for the prevention of free radical disease, regarding cancer and cardiovascular disease. *Br Med Bull* 1993;49:679–699.

205. Trout DL. Vitamin C and cardiovascular risk factors. *Am J Clin Nutr* 1991;53:322S–325S.

206. Borek C. Antioxidants and cancer. *Sci Med*, November/December 1997, pp. 52–61.

207. Enstrom JE, Kanim LE, Klein MA. Vitamin C intake and mortality among a sample of the United States population. *Epidemiology* 1992;3:192–202.

208. Harats D, Chevion S, Nahir M, *et al.* Citrus fruit supplementation reduces lipoprotein oxidation in young men ingesting a diet high in saturated fat: presumptive evidence for an interaction between vitamins C and E *in vivo. Am J Clin Nutr* 1998;67:240–245.

209. Nyyssonen K, Parvianen MT, Salonen R, *et al.* Vitamin C deficiency and risk of myocardial infarction: prospective population study of men from eastern Finland. *BMJ* 1997;314:634–638.

210. Vita JA, Keaney JR Jr., Raby KE, *et al.* Low plasma ascorbic acid independently predicts the presence of an unstable coronary syndrome. *J Am Coll Cardiol* 1998;31:980–986.

211. Kritchevsky SB, Shimakawa T, Tell GS, *et al.* Dietary antioxidants and carotid artery wall thickness: the ARIC Study. *Circulation* 1995;92:2142–2150.

212. Hodis HN, Mack WJ, LaBree L, *et al.* Serial coronary angiographic evidence that antioxidant vitamin intake reduces progression of coronary artery atherosclerosis. *JAMA* 1995;273:1849–1854.

213. Jayachandran M, Arivazhagan P, Panneerselvam C. Age-associated plasma lipids, lipid peroxidation, and antioxidant systems in relation to vitamin C supplementation in humans. *J Anti-Aging Med* 2000;3:437–445.

214. Gaziano JM, Manson JE, Buring JE, Hennekins CH. Dietary antioxidants and cardiovascular disease. *Ann N Y Acad Sci* 1992;669:249–259.

215. Olson JA. Vitamin A. In: *Handbook of Vitamins.* IJ Machin (ed.) Marcel Dekker, New York, 1984, pp. 1–43.

216. Diplock AT. Antioxidant nutrients and disease prevention: an overview. *Am J Clin Nutr* 1991;53:189S–193S.

217. Thompson JN, Duval S, Verdier P. Studies on plasma carotenoids in man and animals. *J Micronutr Anal* 1985;1:81–91.

218. DiMascio P, Kaiser S, Sies H. Lycopene is the most efficient biological carotenoid single oxygen quencher. *Arch Biochim Biophys* 1989;274:1–7.

219. Jialal I, Norkus EP, Cristol L, Grundy SM. Beta-carotene inhibits the oxidative modification of low density lipoprotein. *Biochim Biophys Acta* 1991;1086:134–138.

220. Lavy A, Amotz AB, Aviram M. Preferential inhibition of low density lipoprotein oxidation by the all-trans isomer of beta-carotene in comparison with 9-cis beta-carotene. *Eur J Clin Chem Clin Biochem* 1993;31:83–90.

221. Gaziano JM, Hatla A, Flynn M, *et al.* Supplementation with beta-carotene *in vivo* and *in vitro* does not inhibit low density lipoprotein oxidation. *Atherosclerosis* 1995;112:187–195.

222. Reaven PD, Khouw A, Beltz WF, *et al.* Effect of dietary antioxidant combinations in humans: protection of low density lipoprotein by vitamin E but not beta-carotene. *Atheroscler Thromb* 1993;13:590–600.

223. Hennekens CH, Buring JE, Manson JE, *et al.* Lack of effect of long-term supplementation with beta-carotene on the incidence of malignant neoplasms and cardiovascular disease. *N Engl J Med* 1996;334:1145–1149.

224. The Alpha-Tocopherol, Beta-Carotene Cancer Prevention Study Group. The effect of vitamin E and beta-carotene on the incidence of

lung cancer and other cancers in male smokers. *N Engl J Med* 1994;330:1029–1035.

225. Omenn GS, Goodman GE, Thomquist ME, *et al.* Effects of a combination of beta-carotene and vitamin A on lung cancer and cardiovascular disease. *N Engl J Med* 1996;334:1150–1155.

226. Frankel EN, Kanner J, German JB, *et al.* Inhibition of oxidation of human low-density lipoprotein by phenolic substances in red wine. *Lancet* 1993;341:454–457.

227. Geleijnse JM, Launer LJ, Hofman A, *et al.* Tea flavonoids may protect against atherosclerosis: the Rotterdam Study. *Arch Intern Med* 1999;159:2170–2174.

228. Hertog MGL, Faskens EJM, Dromhout D. Antioxidant flavonols and coronary heart disease risk. *Lancet* 1997;349:699.

229. Knekt P, Jarvinen R, Reunanen A, Maatela J. Flavonoid intake and coronary mortality in Finland: a cohort study. *BMJ* 1996; 312:478–481.

230. Rimm EB, Katan MB, Ahscerio A, *et al.* Relation between intake of flavonoids and risk for coronary heart disease in male health professionals. *Ann Intern Med* 1996;125:384–389.

231. Nigdikar SV, Williams NR, Griffin BD, Howard NA. Consumption of red wine polyphenols reduces the susceptibility of low-density lipoproteins to oxidation *in vivo*. *Am J Clin Nutr* 1998; 68:258–265.

232. Stein JH, Keevil JG, Weibe DA, *et al.* Purple grape juice improves endothelial function and reduces the susceptibility of LDL cholesterol to oxidation in patients with coronary artery disease. *Circulation* 1999;100:1050–1055.

233. Castelnuovo DA, Rotondo S, Iacoviello L, *et al.* Meta-analysis of wine and beer consumption in relation to vascular risk. *Circulation* 2002;105:2836–2844.

234. Fuhrman B, Lavy A, Aviram M. Consumption of red wine with meals reduces the susceptibility of human plasma and low-density lipoprotein to lipid peroxidation. *Am J Clin Nutr* 1995;61:549–554.

235. Folts JD. Potential health benefits from the flavonoids in grape products on vascular disease. *Adv Exp Med Biol* 2002;505:95–111.

236. Osman HE, Maalej N, Shanmuganayagam D, Folts JD. Grape juice but not orange or grapefruit juice inhibits platelet activity in dogs and monkeys. *J Nutr* 1998;128:2307–2312.

237. Keevil JG, Osman HE, Reed JD, Folts JD. Grape juice, but not orange juice or grapefruit juice, inhibits human platelet aggregation. *J Nutr* 2000;130:53–56.

238. Freedman JE, Parker C 3rd, Li L, *et al.* Select flavonoids and whole juice from purple grapes inhibit platelet function and enhances nitric oxide release. *Circulation* 2001;103:2792–2798.

239. Castelli WP, Anderson K. A population at risk: prevalence of high cholesterol levels in hypertensive patients in the Framingham Study. *Am J Med* 1986;80 (Suppl 2A):23–32.

240. Tanne D, Yaari S, Goldbourt U. High-density lipoprotein cholesterol and risk of ischemic stroke mortality. *Stroke* 1997;28:83–87.

241. Knopp RH, Walden CE, Retzlaff BM, *et al.* Long-term cholesterol-lowering effect of four fat-restricted diets in hypercholesterolemic and combined hyperlipidemic men. *JAMA* 1997;278:1509–1515.

242. Hu FB, Stampfer MJ, Manson JE, *et al.* Dietary fat intake and the risk of coronary heart disease in women. *N Engl J Med* 1997;337:1491–1499.

243. Oomen CM, Ocke MC, Feskens EJM, *et al.* Association between trans fatty acid intake and 10-year risk of coronary heart disease in the Zutphen Elderly Study: a prospective population-based study. *Lancet* 2001;357:746–751.

244. Hunninghake DB, Stein EA, Dujovne CA, *et al.* The efficacy of intensive dietary therapy alone or combined with lovastatin in outpatients with hypercholesterolemia. *N Engl J Med* 1993;328:1213–1219.

245. Blankenhorn DH, Azen SP, Kramsch DM, *et al.* Coronary angiographic changes with lovastatin therapy. *Ann Intern Med* 1993; 119: 969–976.

246. Hebert PR, Gaziano JM, Chan KS, Hennekens CH. Cholesterol lowering with statin drugs, risk of stroke and total mortality. *JAMA* 1997;278:313–321.

247. Ansell BJ, Watson KE, Fogelman AM. An evidence-based assessment of the NCEP adult treatment panel II guidelines. *JAMA* 1999;282:2051–2057.

248. Ramsey LE, Yeo WW, Jackson PR. Dietary reduction of serum cholesterol concentration: time to think again. *BMJ* 1991;303:953–957.

249. Jenkins DJA, Kendall CWC, Marchie A, *et al.* Effects of a dietary portfolio of cholesterol-lowering foods versus lovastatin on serum lipids and C-reactive protein. *JAMA* 2003;290:502–510.

250. Davidson MH, Dugan LD, Burns JH, *et al.* The hypocholesterolemic effects of beta-glucan in oatmeal and oatbran. *JAMA* 1991; 265:1833–1839.

251. Rimm EB, Ascherio A, Giovannucci E, *et al.* Vegetable, fruit, and cereal fiber intake and risk of coronary heart disease among men. *JAMA* 1996;275:447–451.

252. Pietinen P, Rimm EB, Korhonen P, *et al.* Intake of dietary fiber and risk of coronary heart disease in a cohort of Finnish men. *Circulation* 1996;94:2720–2727.

253. Wolk A, Manson JE, Stampfer MJ, *et al.* Long-term intake of dietary fiber and decreased risk of coronary heart disease among women. *JAMA* 1999;281:1998–2004.

254. Liu S, Stampfer MJ, Hu FB, *et al.* Whole-grain consumption and risk of coronary heart disease: results from the Nurses' Health Study. *Am J Clin Nutr* 1999;70:412–419.

255. Mozaffarian D, Kumanyika SK, Lemaitre RN, *et al.* Cereal, fruit, and vegetable fiber intake and the risk of cardiovascular disease in elderly individuals. *JAMA* 2003;289:1659–1666.

256. Gillman MW, Cupples LA, Gagnon D, *et al.* Protective effect of fruits and vegetables on development of stroke in men. *JAMA* 1996;273:1113–1117.

257. Joshipura KJ, Ascherio A, Manson JE, *et al.* Fruit and vegetable intake in relation to risk of ischemic stroke. *JAMA* 1999;282:1233–1239.

258. Liu S, Manson JE, Stampfer MJ, *et al.* Whole grain consumption and risk of ischemic stroke in women. *JAMA* 2000:284;1534–1540.

259. Bang HO, Dyerberg J, Hjorne N. The composition of food consumed by Greenland Eskimos. *Acta Med Scand* 1976;200:69–73.

260. Simopoulos AP. Omega-3 fatty acids in health and disease and growth and development. *Am J Clin Nutr* 1991;54:438–473.

261. Simopoulos AP. w-3 fatty acids in the prevention-management of cardiovascular disease. *Can J Physiol Pharmacol* 1997;75:234–239.

262. Kromhout D, Bosschieter EB, Coulander CL. The inverse relation between fish consumption and 20-year mortality from coronary heart disease. *N Engl J Med* 1985;312:1205–1209.

263. Burr ML, Fehily AM, Gilbert JF, *et al.* Effects of changes in fat, fish, and fibre intakes in death and myocardial reinfarction: diet and reinfarction trial (DART). *Lancet* 1989;ii:757–761.

264. Daviglus ML, Stamlet J, Orencia AJ, *et al.* Fish consumption and the 30-year risk of fatal myocardial infarction. *N Engl J Med* 1997;336:1046–1053.

265. de Lorgeril M, Renaud S, Mamelle N, *et al.* Mediterranean alpha-linolenic acid-rich diet in secondary prevention of coronary heart disease. *Lancet* 1994;343:1454–1459.

266. Siscovick DS, Raghunathan TE, King I, *et al.* Dietary intake and cell membrane levels of long-chain n-3 polyunsaturated fatty acids and the risk of primary cardiac arrest. *JAMA* 1995;274:1363–1367.

267. GISSI-Prevenzione Investigators. Dietary supplementation with n-3 polyunsaturated fatty acids and vitamin E after myocardial infarction: results of the GISSI-Prevenzione Trial. *Lancet* 1999; 354:447–455.

268. Hu FB, Bronner L, Willett WC, *et al.* Fish and omega-3 fatty acid intake and risk of coronary heart disease in women. *JAMA* 2002; 287:1815–1821.

269. Albert CM, Campos H, Stampfer MJ, *et al.* Blood levels of long-chain n-3 fatty acids and the risk of sudden death. *N Engl J Med* 2002;346:1113–1118.

270. He K, Rimm EB, Merchant A, *et al.* Fish consumption and risk of stroke in men. *JAMA* 2002;288:3130–3136.

271. Rexrode IH, Stampfer MJ, Manson JE, *et al.* Intake of fish and omega-3 fatty acids and risk of stroke in women. *JAMA* 2001;285:304–312.

272. Goodnight SH. The fish oil puzzle. *Sci Med*, September/October 1996, pp. 42–51.

273. McLennan PL, Abeywardena MY, Charnock JS. Dietary fish oil prevents ventricular fibrillation following coronary artery occlusion and reperfusion. *Am Heart J* 1988;116:709–717.

274. Billman GE, Hallaq H, Leaf A. Prevention of ischemia-induced ventricular fibrillation by w-3 fatty acids. *Proc Natl Acad Sci USA* 1994;91:4427–4430.

275. Sellmayer A, Witzgall H, Lorenz RL, Weber PC. Effects of dietary fish oil on ventricular premature complexes. *Am J Cardiol* 1995; 76:974–977.

276. Thies F, Garry JMC, Yaqoob P, *et al.* Association of n-3 polyunsaturated fatty acids with stability of atherosclerotic plaques: a randomized controlled trial. *Lancet* 2003;361:477–485.

277. Winnicki M, Somers VK, Accurso V, *et al.* Fish-rich diet, leptin and body mass. *Circulation* 2002;106:289–291.

278. McCully KS. Vascular pathology of homocysteinemia: implications for pathogenesis of atherosclerosis. *Am J Pathol* 1969;56:111–128.

279. McCully KS. Chemical pathology of homocysteine: I. Atherogenesis. *Ann Clin Lab Sci* 1993;23:477–493.

280. Genest JJ, McNamara JR, Salem DN, *et al.* Plasma homocyst(e)ine levels in men with premature coronary artery disease. *J Am Coll Cardiol* 1990;16:1114–1119.

281. Stampfer MJ, Malinow MR, Willett WC, *et al.* A prospective study of plasma homocyst(e)ine and risk of myocardial infarction in US physicians. *JAMA* 1992;268:877–881.

282. Selhub J, Jacques PF, Wilson PNF, *et al.* Vitamin status and intake of primary determinants of hyperhomocyteinemia in an elderly population. *JAMA* 1993;270:2693–2698.

283. Nygard O, Nordrehaug, JE, Refsum HM, *et al.* Plasma homocysteine levels and mortality in patients with coronary heart disease. *N Engl J Med* 1997;337:230–236.

284. Montalescot G, Ankri A, Chadefaux-Vekemans B, *et al.* Plasma homocysteine and the extent of atherosclerosis in patients with coronary artery disease. *Int J Cardiol* 1997;60:295–300.

285. Bots ML, Launer LJ, Lindemans J, *et al.* Homocysteine, atherosclerosis and prevalent cardiovascular disease in the elderly: the Rotterdam Study. *J Intern Med* 1997;242:339–347.

286. Wald NJ, Watt HC, Law MR, *et al.* Homocysteine and ischemic heart disease. *Arch Intern Med* 1998;158:862–867.

287. Rimm EB, Willett WC, Hu FB, *et al.* Folate and vitamin B6 from diet and supplements in relation to risk of coronary heart disease among women. *JAMA* 1998;279:359–364.

288. Giles WH, Croft JB, Greenlund KJ, *et al.* Total homocyst(e)ine concentration and the likelihood of nonfatal stroke. *Stroke* 1998; 29:2473–2477.

289. Yoo J-H, Chung C-S, Kang S-S. Relation of plasma homocyst(e)ine to cerebral infarction and cerebral atherosclerosis. *Stroke* 1998;29:2478–2483.

290. Botts ML, Launer LJ, Lindemans J, *et al.* Homocysteine and short-term risk of myocardial infarction and stroke in the elderly: the Rotterdam Study. *Arch Intern Med* 1999;159:38–44.

291. Voutilainen S, Alfthan G, Nyyssonen K, *et al.* Association between elevated plasma total homocysteine and increased common carotid artery wall thickness. *Ann Med* 1998;30:300–306.

292. Rassoul F, Richter V, Janke C, *et al.* Plasma homocysteine and lipoprotein profile in patients with peripheral arterial occlusive disease. *Angiology* 2000;51:189–196.

293. Bazzano LA, Jiang H, Ogden LG, *et al.* Dietary intake of folate and risk of stroke in US men and women. NHANES I Epidemiologic Follow-up Study. *Stroke* 2002;33:1183–1189.

294. Morrison HI, Schaubel D, Desmeules M, Wigle DT. Serum folate and risk of fatal coronary heart disease. *JAMA* 1996;275:1893–1896.

295. Schnyder G, Roffi M, Flammer Y, *et al.* Effect of homocysteine-lowering therapy with folic acid, vitamin B12 and vitamin B6 on

clinical outcome after percutaneous coronary intervention. *JAMA* 2002;288:973–979.

296. Boushey CJ, Beresford SAA, Omenn GS, Motulsky AG. A quantitative assessment of plasma homocysteine as a risk factor for vascular disease: probable benefits of increasing folic acid intakes. *JAMA* 1995;274:1049–1057.

297. Robinson K, Arheart K, Refsum H, *et al.* Low circulating folate and vitamin B6 concentrations: risk factors for stroke, peripheral vascular disease and coronary artery disease. *Circulation* 1998;97:437–443.

298. Homocysteine Lowering Trialists' Collaboration. Lowering blood homocysteine with folic acid based supplements: meta-analysis of randomized trials. *BMJ* 1998;316:894–898.

299. Jacobsen DW. Homocysteine and vitamins in cardiovascular disease. *Clin Chem* 1998;44:1833–1843.

300. Peterson JC, Spence JD. Vitamins and progression of atherosclerosis in hyper-homocyst(e)inaemia. *Lancet* 1998;351:263.

301. Brattstrom L, Wilcken DE. Homocysteine and cardiovascular disease: cause or effect? *Am J Clin Nutr* 2000;72:315–323.

302. Klerk M, Verhoef P, Clarke R, *et al.* MTHFR 677C — T polymorphism and risk of coronary heart disease. *JAMA* 2002;288:2023–2031.

303. Altura BM. Introduction: importance of magnesium in physiology and medicine and the need for ion selective electrodes. *Scand J Clin Lab Invest* 1994;54(Suppl 217):5–9.

304. Singh RB, Rastogi SS, Ghosh S, Niaz MA. Dietary and serum magnesium levels in patients with acute myocardial infarction, coronary artery disease and non-cardiac diagnoses. *J Am Coll Nutr* 1994;13:139–143.

305. Touitou Y, Godard J-P, Ferment O, *et al.* Prevalence of magnesium and potassium deficiencies in the elderly. *Clin Chem* 1987;33:518–523.

306. Reinhart RH, Desbiens NA. Hypomagnesemia in patients entering the ICU. *Crit Care Med* 1985;13:506–507.

307. DeCarli C, Sprouse G, LaRosa JC. Serum magnesium levels in symptomatic atrial fibrillation and their relation to rhythm control by intravenous digoxin. *Am J Cardiol* 1986;57:956–959.

308. England MR, Gordon G, Salem M, Chernow B. Magnesium administration and dysrhythmias after cardiac surgery. *JAMA* 1992;268:2395–2402.

309. Turapaty PDMV, Altura BM. Magnesium deficiency produces spasms of coronary arteries. Relationship to etiology of sudden death ischemic heart disease. *Science* 1980;208:198–200.

310. Hanline M Jr. Hypomagnesemia causes coronary artery spasm. *JAMA* 1985;253:342.
311. Woods KL, Fletcher S. Long-term outcome after intravenous magnesium sulfate in suspected acute myocardial infarction. The second Leicester Intravenous Magnesium Intervention Trial (LIMT). *Lancet* 1994;343:815–819.
312. Altura BM, Altura BT. Magnesium in cardiovascular biology. *Sci Am Sci Med*, May/June 1995, pp. 28–37.
313. Singh RB, Gupta UC, Mittal N, *et al*. Epidemiologic study of trace elements and magnesium on risk of coronary heart disease in rural and urban Indian populations. *J Am Coll Nutr* 1997;16:62–67.
314. Kris-Etherton PM, Zhao G, Binkoski AE, *et al*. The effects of nuts on coronary heart disease. *Nutr Rev* 2001;59:103–111.
315. Albert CM, Gaziano JM, Willett WC, Manson JE. Nut consumption and decreased risk of sudden cardiac death in the Physicians' Health Study. *Arch Intern Med* 2002;162:1382–1387.
316. Almario RU, Vonhavaravat V, Wong R, Kasim-Karakas SE. Effects of walnut consumption on plasma fatty acids and lipoproteins in combined hyperlipidemia. *Am J Clin Nutr* 2001;74:72–79.
317. Morgan WA, Clayshulte BJ. Pecans lower low-density lipoprotein cholesterol in people with normal lipid levels. *J Am Diet Assoc* 2000;100:312–318.
318. Feldman EB. The scientific evidence for a beneficial health relationship between walnuts and coronary heart disease. *J Nutr* 2002; 132:1065S–1101S.
319. Jiang H, Ogden LG, Bazzano LA, *et al*. Dietary sodium intake and incidence of congestive heart failure in overweight US men and women: First National Health and Nutrition Examination Survey Epidemiologic Follow-up Study. *Arch Intern Med* 2002;162:1619–1624.
320. Fletcher RH, Fairfield KM. Vitamins for chronic disease prevention in adults: clinical applications. *JAMA* 2002;287:3127–3129.
321. Jemal A, Thomas A, Murray T, Thun M. Cancer statistics, 2002. *CA Cancer J Clin* 2002;52:23–47.
322. Mitka M. Disparity in cancer statistics changing. *JAMA* 2002; 287:703–704.
323. Howe HL, Wingo PA, Thun MJ, *et al*. Annual report to the nation on the status of cancer (1973 through 1998), featuring cancers with recent increasing trends. *J Natl Cancer Inst* 2001;93:824–842.
324. Sporn MB. The war on cancer. *Lancet* 1996;347:1377–1381.
325. Bal DG. Cancer statistics, 2001: quo vadis or whither goest thou? *CA Cancer J Clin* 2001;51:11–14.

326. Khaw K-T, Bingham S, Welch A, *et al*. Relation between plasma ascorbic acid and mortality in men and women in EPIC-Norfolk prospective study: a prospective population study. *Lancet* 2001;357:657–663.

327. Ames BN. Dietary carcinogens and anticarcinogens, oxygen radicals and damage in healthy humans. *Science* 1983;221:1256–1264.

328. Chen L, Bowen PE, Berzy D, *et al*. Diet modification affects DNA oxidative damage in healthy humans. *Free Radic Biol Med* 1999;26:695–703.

329. Platz EA, Willett WC, Colditz GA, *et al*. Proportion of colon cancer risk that might be preventable in a cohort of middle-aged men. *Cancer Causes Control* 2000;11:579–588.

330. Burkitt DP. Epidemiology of cancer of the colon and rectum. *Cancer* 1971;29:3–13.

331. Potter JD. Nutrition and colorectal cancer. *Cancer Causes Control* 1996;7:127–146.

332. Howe GR, Benito E, Castelleto R, *et al*. Dietary intake of fiber and decreased risk of cancers of the colon and rectum: evidence from the combined analysis of 13 case-control studies. *J Natl Cancer Inst* 1992;84:1887–1896.

333. Meyer F, White E. Alcohol and nutrients in relation to colon cancer in middle-aged adults. *Am J Epidemiol* 1993;138:225–236.

334. Negri E, Franceschi S, Parpinel M, La Vecchia C. Fiber intake and risk of colorectal cancer. *Cancer Epidemiol Biomarkers Prev* 1998;7:667–671.

335. Fuchs CS, Giovannucci EL, Colditz GA, *et al*. Dietary fiber and the risk of colorectal cancer and ademoma in women. *N Engl J Med* 1999;340:169–176.

336. Michels KB, Giovannucci E, Joshipura KJ, *et al*. Prospective study of fruits and vegetables consumption and incidence of colon and rectal cancers. *J Natl Cancer Inst* 2000;92:1740–1752.

337. Schatzkin A, Lanza E, Corle D, *et al*. Lack of effect of a low-fat, high-fiber diet on the recurrence of colorectal adenomas. *N Engl J Med* 2000;342:1149–1155.

338. Alberts DS, Martinez ME, Roe DJ, *et al*. Lack of effect of a high-fiber cereal supplement on the recurrence of colorectal adenomas. *N Engl J Med* 2000;342:1156–1162.

339. Terry P, Giovannucci E, Michels KB, *et al*. Fruit, vegetables, dietary fiber, and risk of colorectal cancer. *J Natl Cancer Inst* 2001;93:525–533.

340. Steinmetz KA, Potter JD. Vegetables, fruits, and cancer prevention: a review. *J Am Diet Assoc* 1996;96:1027–1039.

341. Frentzel BR, Chang CJ. Vegetarian diets and colon cancer: the German experience. *Am J Clin Nutr* 1994;59(Suppl):1143S–1152S.

342. Dashwood RH. Early detection and prevention of colorectal cancer (review). *Oncol Rep* 1999;6:277–281.

343. Kushi LH, Lenart EB, Willett WC. Health implications of Mediterranean diets in light of contemporary knowledge. 2. meat, wine, fats, and oil. *Am J Clin Nutr* 1995;61:1465–1527.

344. Howe GR, Aronson KJ, Benito E, *et al.* The relationship between dietary fat intake and risk of colorectal cancer: evidence from the combined analysis of 13 case-control studies. *Cancer Causes Control* 1997;8:215–228.

345. Slattery ML, Potter JD, Duncan DM, Berry TD. Dietary fats and colon cancer: assessment of risk associated with specific fatty acids. *Int J Cancer* 1997;73:670–677.

346. Favero A, Franceschi S, La Vecchia C, *et al.* Meal frequency and coffee intake in colon cancer. *Nutr Cancer* 1998;30:182–185.

347. Giovannucci E, Rimm EB, Stampfer MJ, *et al.* Intake of fat, meat, and fiber in relation to risk of colon cancer in men. *Cancer Res* 1994;54:2390–2397.

348. Giovannucci E, Goldin B. The role of fat, fatty acids, and total energy intake in the etiology of human colon cancer. *Am J Clin Nutr* 1997;66(Suppl):1564S–1571S.

349. Xu M, Dashwood RH. Chemoprevention studies of heterocyclic amine-induced colon carcinogenesis. *Cancer Lett* 1999;143:179–183.

350. Wu AH, Shibata D, Yu MC, *et al.* Dietary heterocyclic amines and microsatellite instability in colon adenocarcinomas. *Carcinogenesis* 2001;22:1681–1684.

351. Fung T, Hu FB, Fuchs C, *et al.* Major dietary patterns and the risk of colorectal cancer in women. *Arch Intern Med* 2003;163:309–314.

352. Giovannucci E, Rimm EB, Ascherio A, *et al.* Alcohol, low-methionine—low-folate diets, and risk of colon cancer in men. *J Natl Cancer Inst* 1995;87:265–273.

353. Giovannucci E, Stampfer MJ, Colditz GA, *et al.* Multivitamin use, folate, and colon cancer in women in the Nurses' Health Study. *Ann Intern Med* 1998;129:512–524.

354. Su LJ, Arab L. Nutritional status of folate and colon cancer risk: evidence from NHANES I epidemiologic follow-up study. *Ann Epidemiol* 2001;11:65–72.

355. Fuchs CS, Willett WC, Colditz GA, *et al.* The influence of folate and multivitamin use on the familial risk of colon cancer in women. *Cancer Epidemiol Biomarkers Prev* 2002;11:227–234.

356. Blount BC, Mack MM, Wehr CM, *et al.* Folate deficiency causes uracil misincorporation into human DNA and chromosome breakage: implications for cancer and neuronal damage. *Proc Natl Acad Sci USA* 1997;94:3290–3295.

357. Choi S-W, Manson JB. Folate and carcinogenesis: an integrated scheme. *J Nutr* 2000;130:129–132.

358. Pickle L, Mason T, Howard N, *et al. Atlas of US Cancer Mortality Among Whites: 1950–1980.* DHHS Publication No. (NIH) 87-2900:52–56, National Cancer Institute, Bethesda, MD, 1987.

359. Garland CF, Garland FC. Do sunlight and vitamin D reduce the risk of colon cancer? *Int J Epidemiol* 1980;9:227–231.

360. Garland CF, Shekelle RB, Barrett-Cannor E, *et al.* Dietary calcium and vitamin D and risk of colorectal cancer: a 19-year prospective study in men. *Lancet* 1985;1:307–309.

361. Slattery ML, Sorenson AW, Ford MH. Dietary calcium intake as a mitigating factor in colon cancer. *Am J Epidemiol* 1988;128:504–514.

362. La Vecchia C, Braga C, Negri E, *et al.* Intake of selected micronutrients and risk of colorectal cancer. *Int J Cancer* 1997;73:525–530.

363. Baron JA, Beach M, Mandel JS, *et al.* Calcium supplements for the prevention of colorectal adenomas. *N Engl J Med* 1999;340:101–107.

364. Garland CF, Garland FC, Gorham ED. Calcium and vitamin D: their potential roles in colon and breast cancer prevention. *Ann N Y Acad Sci* 1999;889:107–119.

365. Lipkin M, Newmark H. Effect of added dietary calcium on colonic epithelial-cell proliferation in subjects at high risk for familial colonic cancer. *N Engl J Med* 1985;313:1381–1384.

366. Pence RC. Role of calcium in colon cancer prevention: experimental and clinical studies. *Mutat Res* 1993;290:87–95.

367. Xu M, Bailey AC, Hernaez JF, *et al.* Protection by green tea, black tea, and indole-3-carbinol against 2-amino-3-methylimidazo[4,5-f] quinoline-induced DNA adducts and colonic aberrant crypts in the F344 rat. *Carcinogenesis* 1996;17:1429–1434.

368. Dashwood RH, Xu M, Hernaez JF, *et al.* Cancer chemopreventive mechanisms of tea against heterocyclic amine mutagens from cooked meat. *Proc Soc Exp Biol Med* 1999;220:239–243.

369. Bushman JL. Green tea and cancer in humans. A review of the literature. *Nutr Cancer* 1998;31:151–159.

370. Williams AR, Balasooriya BA, Day DW. Polyps and cancer of the large bowel: a necropsy study in Liverpool. *Gut* 1982;23:835–842.

371. Eberhart CE, Coffey RJ, Radhika A, *et al.* Up-regulation of cyclooxygenase-2 gene expression in human colorectal adenomas and adenocarcinomas. *Gastroenterology* 1994;107:1183–1188.

372. Fujita T, Matsui M, Takaku K, *et al.* Size- and invasion-dependent increase in cyclooxygenase-2 levels in human colorectal carcinomas. *Cancer Res* 1998;58:4823–4826.

373. Yamamoto Y, Yin M-J, Kin K-M, Gaynor RB. Sulindac inhibits activation of the NF-kappa B pathway. *J Biol Chem* 1999;274:27307–27314.

374. He T-C, Chan TA, Vogelstein B, Kinzler KW. PPARdelta is an APC-regulated target of non-steroidal anti-inflammatory drugs. *Cell* 1999;99:335–345.

375. DuBois RN, Giardiello FM, Smalley WE. Non-steroidal anti-inflammatory drugs, eicosanoids and colorectal cancer prevention. *Gastroenterol Clin North Am* 1996;25:773–791.

376. Thun MJ, Namboodiri MM, Heath CW Jr. Aspirin use and reduced risk of fatal colon cancer. *N Engl J Med* 1991;325:1593–1596.

377. Giovannucci E, Rimm EB, Stampfer MJ, *et al.* Aspirin use and the risk for colorectal cancer and adenoma in health professionals. *Ann Intern Med* 1994;121:241–246.

378. Giovannucci E, Egan KM, Hunter DJ, *et al.* Aspirin and the risk of colorectal cancer in women. *N Engl J Med* 1995;333:609–614.

379. Sano T, Sasako M. Green tea and gastric cancer. *N Engl J Med* 2001;344:675–676 (Editorial).

380. Brown LM, Swanson CA, Gridley G, *et al.* Adenocarcinoma of the esophagus: role of obesity and diet. *J Natl Cancer Inst* 1995;87:104–109.

381. Zhang ZF, Kurtz RC, Yu GP, *et al.* Adenocarcinoma of the esophagus and gastric cardia: the role of diet. *Nutr Cancer* 1997;27:298–309.

382. Terry P, Lagergren J, Ye W, *et al.* Inverse association between intake of cereal fiber and risk of gastric cardia cancer. *Gastroenterology* 2001;120:387–391.

383. McCullough ML, Robertson AS, Jacobs EJ, *et al.* A prospective study of diet and stomach cancer mortality in United States men and women. *Cancer Epidemiol Biomarkers Prev* 2001;10:1201–1205.

384. Chen H, Ward MH, Graubard BI, *et al.* Dietary patterns and adenocarcinoma of the esophagus and distal stomach. *Am J Clin Nutr* 2002;75:137–144.

385. Mayne ST, Risch HA, Dubrow R, *et al.* Nutrient intake and risk of subtypes of esophageal and gastric cancer. *Cancer Epidemiol Biomarkers Prev* 2001;10:1055–1062.

386. Blot WJ, Li J-Y, Taylor PR, *et al.* Nutrition intervention trials in Linxian, China: supplementation with specific vitamin/mineral combinations, cancer incidence, and disease-specific mortality in the general population. *J Natl Cancer Inst* 1993;85:1483–1492.

387. Li J-Y, Taylor PR, Bing L, *et al.* Nutrition intervention trials in Linxian, China: multiple vitamin/mineral supplementation, cancer incidence, and disease-specific mortality among adults with esophageal dysplasia. *J Natl Cancer Inst* 1993;85:1492–1498.

388. Mark SD, Qiao Y-L, Dawsey SM, *et al.* Prospective study of serum selenium levels and incident esophageal and gastric cancers. *J Natl Cancer Inst* 2000;92:1753–1763.

389. Tsubono Y, Nishino Y, Komatsu S, *et al.* Green tea and risk of gastric cancer in Japan. *N Engl J Med* 2001;344:632–636.

390. Fahey JW, Haristoy X, Dolan PM, *et al.* Sulforaphane inhibits extracellular, intracellular, and antibiotic-resistant strains of *Helicobacter pylori* and prevents benzo[a]pyrene-induced stomach tumors. *Proc Natl Acad Sci* 2002;99:7610–7615.

391. World Cancer Research Fund. *Food, Nutrition and the Prevention of Cancer: A Global Perspective.* World Cancer Research Fund/ American Institute of Cancer Research, Washington, DC, 1997.

392. Borek C. Antioxidants and cancer. *Sci Med;* November/December 1997, pp. 52–61.

393. Steinmetz KA, Potter JD. Vegetables, fruit and cancer. I. Epidenmiology. Cancer causes and other malignant neoplasms. *Am J Epidemiol* 1997;146:223–230. *Control* 1991;2:325–357.

394. Ziegler RG, Mayne ST, Swanson CA. Nutrition and lung cancer. *Cancer Causes Control* 1996;7:157–177.

395. Knekt P, Jarvinen R, Seppanen R, *et al.* Dietary flavonoids and the risk of lung cancer and other malignant neoplasms. *Am J Epidemiol* 1997;146:223–230.

396. Feskanich D, Ziegler RG, Michaud DS, *et al.* Prospective study of fruit and vegetable consumption and risk of lung cancer among men and women. *J Natl Cancer Inst* 2000;92:1812–1823.

397. Mayne ST, Janerich DT, Greenwald P, *et al.* Dietary beta carotene and lung cancer risk in US non-smokers. *J Natl Cancer Inst* 1994;86:33–38.

398. The Alpha-Tocopherol Beta Carotene Cancer Prevention Study Group. The effect vitamin E and beta carotene on the incidence of lung

cancer and other cancers in male smokers. *N Engl J Med* 1994;330:1029–1035.

399. Hennekens CH, Buring JE, Manson JE, *et al.* Lack of effect of long-term supplementation with beta carotene on the incidence of malignant neoplasms and cardiovascular disease. *N Engl J Med* 1996;334:1145–1149.

400. Omenn GS, Goodman GE, Thornquist MD, *et al.* Effects of a combination of beta carotene and vitamin A on lung cancer and cardiovascular disease. *N Engl J Med* 1996;334:1150–1155.

401. The ATBC Study Group. Incidence of cancer and mortality following alpha-tocopherol and beta-carotene supplementation: a post-intervention follow-up. *JAMA* 2003;290:476–485.

402. Woodson K, Tangrea JA, Barrett MJ, *et al.* Serum alpha-tocopherol and subsequent risk of lung cancer among male smokers. *J Natl Cancer Inst* 1999;91:1738–1743.

403. Chung FL. The prevention of lung cancer induced by a tobacco-specific carcinogen in rodents by green and black tea. *Proc Soc Exp Biol Med* 1999;220:244–248.

404. Zhong L, Goldberg MS, Gao YT, *et al.* A population-based case-control study of lung cancer and green tea consumption among women living in Shanghai, China. *Epidemiology* 2001;12:695–700.

405. Fujiki H, Suganuma M, Okabe S, *et al.* Cancer inhibition by green tea. *Mutat Res* 1998;402:307–310.

406. Imai K, Suga K, Nakachi K. Cancer-prevention effects of drinking green tea among a Japanese population. *Prev Med* 1997;26:769–775.

407. Hulka BS, Stark AT. Breast cancer: cause and prevention. *Lancet* 1995;346:883–887.

408. Dabrosin C, Ollinger K. Protection by alpha-tocopherol but not ascorbic acid from hydrogen peroxide induced cell death in normal human breast epithelial cells in culture. *Free Radic Res* 1998;29:227–234.

409. Kimmick G, Bell R, Bostick R. Vitamin E and breast cancer: a review. *Nutr Cancer* 1997;27:109–117.

410. Schwenke DC. Does lack of tocopherols and tocotrienols put women at increased risk of breast cancer? *J Nutr Biochem* 2002;13:2–20.

411. Hunter DJ, Manson JE, Colditz GA, *et al.* Prospective study of the intake of vitamins C, E and A and the risk of breast cancer. *N Engl J Med* 1993;329:234–240.

412. Smith-Warner SA, Spiegelman D, Yaun S-S, *et al.* Intake of fruits and vegetables and risk of breast cancer: a pooled analysis of cohort studies. *N Engl J Med* 2001;285:269–276.

413. Zhang S, Hunter DJ, Forman MR, *et al.* Dietary carotenoids and vitamins A, C and E and risk of breast cancer. *J Natl Cancer Inst* 1999;91:547–556.

414. Zhang S, Hunter DJ, Hankinson SE, *et al.* A prospective study of folate intake and the risk of breast cancer. *JAMA* 1999;281:1632–1637.

415. Rohan TE, Jain MG, Howe GR, Miller AB. Dietary folate consumption and breast cancer risk. *J Natl Cancer Inst* 2000;92:266–269.

416. Shrubsole MJ, Jin F, Dai Q, *et al.* Dietary folate intake and breast cancer risk: results from the Shanghai Breast Cancer Study. *Cancer Res* 2001;61:7136–7141.

417. Zhang SM, Willett WC, Selhub J, *et al.* Plasma folate, vitamin B6, vitamin B12, homocysteine, and risk of breast cancer. *J Natl Cancer Inst* 2003;95:373–380.

418. Prinz-Langenohl R, Fohr I, Pietrzik K. Beneficial role for folate in the prevention of colorectal and breast cancer. *Eur J Nutr* 2001;40:98–105.

419. Graham S, Marshall J, Mettlin C, *et al.* Diet in the epidemiology of breast cancer. *Am J Epidemiol* 1982;116:68–75.

420. Howe GR, Hirohata T, Hislop TG, *et al.* Dietary factors and risk of breast cancer: combined analysis of 12 case-control studies. *J Natl Cancer Inst* 1990;82:561–569.

421. Hunter DJ, Spiegelman D, Hans-Olov A, *et al.* Cohort studies of fat intake and the risk of breast cancer — a pooled analysis. *N Engl J Med* 1996;334:356–361.

422. Velie E, Kulldorff M, Schairer C, *et al.* Dietary fat, fat subtypes, and breast cancer in postmenopausal women: a prospective cohort study. *J Natl Cancer Inst* 2000;92:833–839.

423. Franceschi S, Favero A, Decarli A, *et al.* Intake of micronutrients and risk of breast cancer. *Lancet* 1996;347:1351–1356.

424. Holmes MD, Hunter DJ, Colditz GA, *et al.* Association of dietary intake of fat and fatty acids with risk of breast cancer. *JAMA* 1999;281:914–920.

425. Newmark H. Dietary fat and risk of breast cancer. *JAMA* 1999;282:1223 (Letter).

426. Shin MH, Holmes MD, Hankinson SE, *et al.* Intake of dairy products, calcium, and vitamin D and risk of breast cancer. *J Natl Cancer Inst* 2002;94:1301–1311.

427. Wu AH, Pike MC, Stram DO. Meta-analysis: dietary fat intake, serum estrogen levels, and the risk of breast cancer. *J Natl Inst* 1999;91:529–534.

428. Vatten LJ, Solvoll K, Loken EB. Frequency of meat and fish intake and risk of breast cancer in a prospective study of 14,500 Norwegian women. *Int J Cancer* 1990;46:12–15.

429. Toniolo P, Riboli E, Shore RE, Pasternack BS. Consumption of meat, animal products, protein, and fat and risk of breast cancer: a prospective cohort study in New York. *Epidemiology* 1994;5:391–397.

430. Layton DW, Bogen KT, Knize MG, *et al.* Cancer risk of heterocyclic amines in cooked foods: an analysis and implications for research. *Carcinogenesis* 1995;16:39–52.

431. Steineck G, Gerhardsson de Verdier M, Overvik B. The epidemiological evidence concerning intake of mutagenic activity from the fried surface and the risk of cancer cannot justify preventive measures. *Eur J Cancer Prev* 1993;2:293–300.

432. Zheng W, Gustafson DR, Sinha R, *et al.* Well-done meat intake and the risk of breast cancer. *J Natl Cancer Inst* 1998;90:1724–1729.

433. Mills PK, Beeson WL, Phillips RL, Fraser GE. Cohort study of diet, lifestyle and prostate cancer in Adventist men. *Cancer (Phila.)* 1989;64:598–604.

434. Hsing AW, Comstock GW, Abbey H, Polk BF. Serologic precursors of cancer: retinal, carotenoids and tocopherol and risk of prostate cancer. *J Natl Cancer Inst* 1990;82:941–946.

435. Gann PH, Ma J, Giovannucci E, *et al.* Lower prostate cancer risk in men with elevated plasma lycopene levels: results of a prospective analysis. *Cancer Res* 1999;59:1225–1230.

436. Tzonou A, Signorello LP Lagiou P, *et al.* Diet and cancer of the prostate: a case-control study in Greece. *Int J Cancer* 1999;80:704–708.

437. Clinton SK. Lycopene: chemistry, biology, and implications for human health and disease. *Nutr Rev* 1998;56:35–51.

438. Giovannucci E. Tomatoes, tomato-based products, lycopene, and cancer: review of the epidemiologic literature. *J Natl Cancer Inst* 1998;91:317–331.

439. Giovannucci E, Rimm EB, Liu Y, *et al.* A prospective study of tomato products, lycopene, and prostate cancer risk. *J Natl Cancer Inst* 2002;94:391–398.

440. Heinonen OP, Albanes D, Virtamo J, *et al.* Prostate cancer and supplementation with alpha-tocopherol and beta-carotene: incidence and mortality in a controlled trial. *J Natl Cancer Inst* 1998;90:440–446.

441. Helzlsouer KJ, Huang H-Y, Alberg AJ, *et al.* Association between alpha-tocopherol, gamma-tocopherol, selenium, and subsequent prostate cancer. *J Natl Cancer Inst* 2000;92:2018–2023.

442. Willett WC, Polk BF, Morris JS, *et al.* Prediagnostic serum selenium and risk of cancer. *Lancet* 1983;2:130–134.

443. Clark LC, Combs GF Jr, Turnbull BW, *et al.* Effects of selenium supplementation for cancer prevention in patients with carcinoma of the skin. A randomized controlled trial. Nutritional Prevention of Cancer Study Group. *JAMA* 1996;276:1957–1963.

444. Yoshizawa K, Willet WC, Morris SJ, *et al.* Study of prediagnostic selenium level in toenails and the risk of advanced prostate cancer. *J Natl Cancer Inst* 1998;90:1219–1224.

445. Whittemore AS, Kolonel LN, Wu AH, *et al.* Prostate cancer in relation to diet, physical activity, and body size in blacks, whites and Asians in the United States and Canada. *J Natl Cancer Inst* 1995;87:652–661.

446. Mukherjee P, Sotnikov AV, Mangian HJ, *et al.* Energy intake and prostate tumor growth, angiogenesis, and vascular endothelial growth factor expression. *J Natl Cancer Inst* 1999;91:512–523.

447. Gronberg H, Damber L, Damber J-E. Total food consumption and body mass index in relation to prostate cancer risk; a case-control study in Sweden with prospectively collected exposure data. *J Urol* 1996;155:969–974.

448. Leitzmann MF, Stampfer MJ, Ma J, *et al.* Aspirin use in relation to risk of prostate cancer. *Cancer Epidemiol Biomarkers Prev* 2002;11:1108–1111.

449. Kelley DS, Bendich A. Essential nutrients and immunologic functions. *Am J Clin Nutr* 1996;63:994S–996S.

450. Kelley DS, Dougherty RM, Branch LB, *et al.* Concentration of dietary N-6 polyunsaturated fatty acids and the human immune status. *Clin Immunol Immunopathol* 1992;62:240–244.

451. Chu BC-H, Cerhan JR, Folsom AR, *et al.* Diet and risk of non-Hodgkin lymphoma in older women. *JAMA* 1996;275:1315–1321.

452. Zhang S, Hunter DJ, Rosner BA, *et al.* Dietary fat and protein in relation to risk of non-Hodgkin's lymphoma among women. *J Natl Cancer Inst* 1999;91:1751–1758.

453. Zhang SM, Hunter DJ, Rosner BA, *et al.* Intakes of fruits, vegetables, and related nutrients and the risk of non-Hodgkin's lymphoma among women. *Cancer Epidemiol Biomarkers Prev* 2000;9:477–485.

454. Silverman DT, Hartge P, Morrison AS, Devesa SS. Epidemiology of bladder cancer. *Hematol Oncol Clin North Am* 1992;6:1–30.

455. Michaud DS, Spiegelman D, Clinton SK, *et al.* Fluid intake and the risk of bladder cancer in men. *N Engl J Med* 1999;340:1390–1397.

456. McLaughlin JK, Lipworth L. Epidemiologic aspects of renal cell cancer. *Semin Oncol* 2000;27:115–123.

457. D'Amico A, Piacentini I, Righetti R, *et al.* Exogenous risk factors for parenchymal carcinoma of the kidney. *Arch Ital Urol Androl* 2001;73:49–55.

458. Bianchi GD, Cerhan JR, Parker AS, *et al.* Tea consumption and risk of bladder and kidney cancers in a population-based case-control study. *Am J Epidemiol* 2000;15:377–383.

459. McCarty MF. Insulin secretion as a determinant of pancreatic cancer risk. *Med Hypotheses* 2001;57:146–150.

460. Stolzenberg-Solomon RZ, Pietinen P, Barrett MJ, *et al.* Dietary and other methyl-group availability factors and pancreatic cancer risk in a cohort of male smokers. *Am J Epidemiol* 2001;153: 680–687.

461. Cramer DW, Welch WR, Hutchison GB, *et al.* Dietary animal fat in relation to ovarian cancer risk. *Obstet Gynecol* 1984;63:833–838.

462. Huncharek M, Kupelnick B. Dietary fat intake and risk of epithelial ovarian cancer: a meta-analysis of 6689 subjects from eight observational studies. *Nutr Cancer* 2001;40:87–91.

463. Bertone ER, Rosner BA, Hunter DJ, *et al.* Dietary fat intake and ovarian cancer in a cohort of US women. *Am J Epidemiol* 2002; 156:22–31.

464. Fleischauer AT, Olson SH, Mignone L, *et al.* Dietary antioxidants, supplements and risk of epithelial ovarian cancer. *Nutr Cancer* 2001;40:92–98.

465. Bidoli E, Lavecchia C, Talamini R, *et al.* Micronutrients and ovarian cancer: a case control study in Italy. *Ann Oncol* 2001;12:1589–1593.

466. Zhang M, Binns CW, Lee AH. Tea consumption and ovarian cancer risk: a case-control study in China. *Cancer Epidemiol Biomarkers Prev* 2002;11:713–718.

467. Bosetti C, Negri E, Franceschi S, *et al.* Diet and ovarian cancer risk: a case-control study in Italy. *Int J Cancer* 2001;93:911–915.

468. Borek C. Antioxidants and cancer. *Sci Med*, November/December 1997, pp. 52, 61.

469. Block G. Epidemiologic evidence regarding vitamin C and cancer. *Am J Clin Nutr* 1991;54:1310S–1314S.

470. Khaw K-T, Bingham S, Welch A, *et al.* Relation between plasma ascorbic acid and mortality in men and women in EPIC-Norfolk prospective study: a prospective population study. *Lancet* 2001;357: 657–663.

471. Feiz HR, Mobarhan S. Does vitamin C intake slow the progression of gastric cancer in *Helicobacter pylori*-infected populations? *Nutr Rev* 2002;60:34–36.

472. Schwenke DC. Does lack of tocopherols and tocotrienols put women at increased risk of breast cancer? *J Nutr Biochem* 2002;13:2–20.

473. Bidoli E, Lavecchia C, Talamini R, *et al.* Micronutrients and ovarian cancer: a case-control study in Italy. *Ann Oncol* 2001;12:1589–1593.

474. Malafa MP, Fokum FD, Mowlavi A, *et al.* Vitamin E inhibits melanoma growth in mice. *Surgery* 2002;131:85–91.

475. Matsui MS, DeLeo VA. Longwave ultraviolet radiation and promotion of skin cancer. *Cancer Cells* 1991;3:8–12.

476. Fisher GJ, Wang ZQ, Datta SC, *et al.* Pathophysiology of premature skin aging induced by ultraviolet light. *N Engl J Med* 1997;337:1419–1428.

477. Peus D, Vasa RA, Meves A, *et al.* H_2O_2 is an important mediator of UVB-induced EGF-receptor phosphorylation in cultured keratinocytes. *J Invest Dermatol* 1998;110:966–971.

478. Darr D, Fridovich I. Free radicals in cutaneous biology. *J Invest Dermatol* 1994;102:671–675.

479. Fryer MJ. Evidence for the photoprotective effects of vitamin E. *Photochem Photobiol* 1993;58:304–312.

480. Gensler HL, Magdaleno M. Topical vitamin E inhibition of immunosuppression and tumorigenesis induced by ultraviolet irradiation. *Nutr Cancer* 1991;15:97–106.

481. Bissett DL, Chatterjee R, Hannon DP. Photoprotective effect of superoxide-scavenging antioxidants against ultraviolet radiation-induced chronic skin damage in the hairless mouse. *Photodermatol Photoimmunol Photomed* 1990;7:56–62.

482. Conney AH, Lu YP, Lou YR, Huang MT. Inhibitory effects of tea and caffeine on UV-induced carcinogenesis: relationship to enhanced apoptosis and decreased tissue fat. *Eur J Cancer Prev* 2002; 11(Suppl 2):S28–S36.

483. Lu YP, Lou YR, Xie JG, *et al.* Topical applications of caffeine or (-) epigallocatechin gallate (EGCG) inhibit carcinogenesis and selectively increase apoptosis in UVB-induced skin tumors in mice. *Proc Natl Acad Sci USA* 2002;99:12455–12460.

484. Briviba K, Schnabele K, Schwertle E, *et al.* Beta-carotene inhibits growth of human carcinoma cells *in vitro* by induction of apoptosis. *Biol Chem* 2001;382:1663–1668.

485. Ziegler RG. A review of the epidemiologic evidence that carotenoids reduce the risk of cancer. *J Nutr* 1989;119:116–122.

486. Blot WJ, Li JY, Taylor PR, *et al.* Nutrition intervention trials in Linxian China: supplementation with specific vitamin/mineral combination, cancer incidence, and disease-specific mortality in the general population. *J Natl Cancer Inst* 1993;85:1483–1492.

487. Lee I-M, Cook NR, Manson JE, *et al.* Beta-carotene supplementation and incidence of cancer and cardiovascular disease: the Women's Health Study. *J Natl Cancer Inst* 1999;91:2102–2106.

488. Slattery ML, Benson J, Curtin K, *et al.* Carotenoids and colon cancer. *Am J Clin Nutr* 2000;71:575–582.

489. Holt PR, Arber N, Halmos B, *et al.* Colonic epithelial cell proliferation decreases with increasing levels of serum 25-hydroxy vitamin D. *Cancer Epidemiol Biomarkers Prev* 2002;11:113–119.

490. Peters U, McGlynn KA, Chatterjee N, *et al.* Vitamin D, calcium, and vitamin D receptor polymorphism in colorectal adenomas. *Cancer Epidemiol Biomarkers Prev* 2001;10:1267–1274.

491. Lamprecht SA, Lipkin M. Cellular mechanisms of calcium and vitamin D in the inhibition of colorectal carcinogenesis. *Ann NY Acad Sci* 2001;952:73–87.

492. Terry P, Jain M, Miller AB, *et al.* Dietary intake of folic acid and colorectal cancer risk in a cohort of women. *Int J Cancer* 2002;97:864–867.

493. Slattery ML, Potter JD, Coates A, *et al.* Plant foods and colon cancer: an assessment of specific foods and their related nutrients (United States). *Cancer Causes Control* 1997;8:575–590.

494. Olshan AF, Smith JC, Bondy ML, *et al.* Maternal vitamin use and reduced risk of neuroblastoma. *Epidemiology* 2002;13:575–580.

495. Salonen JT, Alfthen G, Huttunen JK, Puska P. Association between serum selenium and the risk of cancer. *Am J Epidemiol* 1984;120:343–349.

496. Willett WC, Polk BJ, Morris JS, *et al.* Prediagnostic serum selenium and risk of cancer. *Lancet* 1983;2:130–134.

497. Finley JW, Davis CD, Feng Y. Selenium from high selenium broccoli protects rats from colon cancer. *J Nutr* 2000;130:2384–2389.

498. Li W, Zhu Y, Yan X, *et al.* The prevention of primary liver cancer by selenium in high risk populations. *Zhonghua Yu Fang Yi Xue Za Zhi* 2000;34:336–338. (Chinese Journal).

499. Clark LC, Dalkin B, Krongrad A, *et al.* Decreased incidence of prostate cancer with selenium supplementation: results of a double-blind cancer prevention trial. *Br J Urol* 1998;81:730–734.

500. Byers T, Nestle M, McTiernen A, *et al.* American Cancer Society guidelines on nutrition and physical activity for cancer prevention: reducing the risk of cancer with healthy food choices and physical activity. *CA Cancer J Clin* 2002;52:92–119.

501. Chandra RK. Nutritional regulation of immunity and risk of infection in old age. *Immunology* 1989;67:141–147.

502. Mazari L, Lesourd BM. Nutritional influences on immune response in healthy aged persons. *Mech Ageing Dev* 1998;104:25–40.

503. Ravaglia G, Forti P, Maioli F, *et al.* Effect of micronutrient status on natural killer cell function in healthy free living subjects ≥ 90 years. *Am J Clin Nutr* 2000;71:590–598.

504. McCay CM, Crowell MF, Maynard LA. The effect of retarded growth upon the length of life span and upon the ultimate body size. *J Nutr* 1935;10:63–79.

505. Masoro EJ. Physiology of ageing: nutritional aspects. *Age Ageing* 1990;19:55–59.

506. Lane MA, Black A, Handy A, *et al.* Caloric restriction in primates. *Ann NY Acad Sci* 2001;928:287–295.

507. Yu B, Chung HY. Stress resistance by caloric restriction of longevity. *Ann N Y Acad Sci* 2001;928:39–47.

508. Mysliwska J, Bryl E, Foerster J, Mysliwski A. Increase of interleukin-6 and decrease in interleukin-2 production during the ageing process are influenced by the health status. *Mech Ageing Dev* 1998;100:313–328.

509. Papanicolaou DA, Wilder RL, Manolagas SC, Chrousos GP. The pathophysiologic roles of interleukin-6 in human disease. *Ann Intern Med* 1998;128:127–137.

510. Kim MJ, Aiken JM, Havighurst T, *et al.* Adult-onset energy restriction of rhesus monkeys attenuates oxidative stress-induced cytokine expression by peripheral blood mononuclear cells. *J Nutr* 1997;127:2293–2301.

511. Spaulding CC, Walford RL, Effros RB. Calorie restriction inhibits the age-related dysregulation of the cytokines TNF-alpha and IL-6 in C3B1ORF1 mice. *Mech Ageing Dev* 1997;93:87–94.

512. Terpenning MS, Bradley SF. Why ageing leads to increased susceptibility to infection. *Geriatrics* 1991;46:77–80.

513. Lesourd BM. Nutrition and immunity in the elderly: modification of immune responses with nutritional treatments. *Am J Clin Nutr* 1997;66:478S–484S.

514. Chandra RK. The relation between immunology, nutrition and disease in elderly people. *Age Ageing* 1990;19:525–531.

515. Penn ND, Purkins I, Kelleher J, *et al.* The effect of dietary supplementation with vitamins A, C and E on cell-mediated immune function in elderly long-stay patients: a randomized controlled study. *Age Ageing* 1991;20:169–174.

516. Chandra RK. Effect of vitamin and trace-element supplementation on immune responses and infection in elderly patients. *Lancet* 1992;340:1124–1127.

517. Barringer TA, Kirk JK, Santaniello AC, *et al.* Effect of a multivitamin and mineral supplement on infection and quality of life: a randomized, double-blind, placebo-controlled trial. *Ann Intern Med* 2003;138:365–371.

518. Bogden JD, Bendich A, Kempt FW, *et al.* Daily micronutrient supplements enhance delayed-hypersensitivity skin test responses in older people. *Am J Clin Nutr* 1994;60:437–447.

519. Meydani SN, Haytek M. Vitamin E and the immune response. In: *International Conference on Nutrition, Immunity and Illness in the Elderly.* RK Changra (ed.) ARTS Biomedical Publications, St. Johns, Newfoundland, 1992, pp. 105–128.

520. Meydani SN, Barklund MP, Liu S, *et al.* Vitamin E supplementation enhances cell-mediated immunity in healthy subjects. *Am J Clin Nutr* 1990;52:557–563.

521. Meydani SN, Meydani M, Blumberg JB, *et al.* Vitamin E supplementation and *in vivo* immune response in healthy elderly subjects: a randomized controlled trial. *JAMA* 1997;277:1380–1386.

522. Schmidt K. Antioxidant vitamins and beta-carotene: effects on immunocompetence. *Am J Clin Nutr* 1991;53:383S–385S.

523. Graat JM, Schouten EG, Kok FJ. Effect of daily vitamin E and multivitamin-mineral supplementation on acute respiratory tract infections in older persons. *JAMA* 2002;288:715–721.

524. Niki E. Interaction of ascorbate and alpha-tocopherol. *Ann NY Acad Sci* 1987;498:186–199.

525. Harats D, Chevion S, Nahir M, *et al.* Citrus fruit supplementation reduces lipoprotein oxidation in young men ingesting a diet high in saturated fat: presumptive evidence for an interaction between vitamins C and E *in vivo. Am J Clin Nutr* 1998;67:240–245.

526. Anderson R, Lukey PT. A biological role for ascorbate in the selective neutralization in extracellular phagocyte-derived oxidants. *Ann N Y Acad Sci* 1987;498:229–233.

527. Roth JA, Kaeberle ML. *In vivo* effect of ascorbic acid on neutrophil function in healthy and dexamethasone-treated cattle. *Am J Vet Res* 1985;46:2434–2436.

528. Gross WB, Jones D, Cherry J. Effect of ascorbic acid on the disease caused by *Escherichia coli* challenge infections. *Avian Dis* 1988;32:407–409.

529. Palozza P, Krinsky NI. Antioxidant effects of carotenoids *in vivo* and *in vitro:* an overview. In: *Methods in Enzymology, Carotenoids.* L Packer (ed.) Academic Press, San Diego, 1992, pp. 403–439.

530. Chew BP. Role of carotenoids in the immune response. *J Dairy Sci* 1993;76:2804–2811.

531. Alexander M, Newmark H, Miller RG. Oral beta-carotene can increase the number of OKT4+ cells in human blood. *Immunol Lett* 1985;9:221–224.

532. Fuller CJ, Faulkner H, Bendich A, *et al.* Effect of beta-carotene supplementation on photosuppression of delayed-type hypersensitivity in normal young men. *Am J Clin Nutr* 1992;56:684–690.

533. Semba RD, Ward MBJ, Griffin DE, *et al.* Abnormal T-cell subset proportions in vitamin-A-deficient children. *Lancet* 1993;341:5–8.

534. Chandra RK. Nutrition and the immune system: an introduction. *Am J Clin Nutr* 1997;66:460S–463S.

535. Ceballos-Picot I, Trivier J-M, Nicole A, *et al.* Age-correlated modifications of copper-zinc superoxide dismutase and glutathione-related enzyme activities in human erythrocytes. *Clin Chem* 1992;38:66–70.

536. Sahyoun NR, Otradovec CL, Hartz SC, *et al.* Dietary intakes and biochemical indicators of nutritional status in an elderly, institutionalized population. *Am J Clin Nutr* 1988;47:524–533.

537. Bogden JD, Oleske JM, Lavenhar MA, *et al.* Effects of one year of supplementation with zinc and other micronutrients on cellular immunity in the elderly. *J Am Coll Nutr* 1990;9:214–225.

538. Duchateau J, Delepesse G, Vrijens R, Collet H. Beneficial effects of oral zinc supplementation on the immune response of old people. *Am J Med* 1981;70:1001–1004.

539. Fortes C, Forastiere F, Agabiti N, *et al.* The effect of zinc and vitamin A supplementation on immune response in an older population. *J Am Geriatr Soc* 1998;46:19–26.

540. Sazawal S, Black RE, Bhan MK, *et al.* Zinc supplementation in young children with acute diarrhea in India. *N Engl J Med* 1995;333:839–844.

541. Hambidge M, Krebs N. Zinc, diarrhea and pneumonia. *J Pediatr* 1999;135:661–664.

542. Shankar AH, Prasad AS. Zinc and immune function: the biological basis of altered resistance to infection. *Am J Clin Nutr* 1998;68(Suppl):447S–463S.

543. Bhutta ZA, Black RE, Brown KH, *et al.* Prevention of diarrhea and pneumonia by zinc supplementation in children in developing countries: pooled analysis of randomized controlled trials. *J Pediatr* 1999;135:689–697.

544. Mitchell GF. T cell dependent effects in parasite infection and disease. *Prog Immunol* 1980;4:794–808.

545. Jackson JL, Peterson C, Lesho E. A meta-analysis of zinc salts lozenges and the common cold. *Arch Intern Med* 1997;157:2373–2376.

546. Macknin ML, Piedmonte M, Calendine C, *et al.* Zinc gluconate lozenges for treating the common cold in children: a randomized controlled trial. *JAMA* 1998;279:1962–1967.

547. Prasad AS, Fitzgerald JF, Bao B, *et al.* Duration of symptoms and plasma cytokine levels in patients with the common cold treated with zinc acetate. *Ann Intern Med* 2000;133:245–252.

548. Berr C, Nicole A, Godin J, *et al.* Selenium and oxygen-metabolizing enzymes in elderly community residents: a pilot epidemiological study. *J Am Geriatr Soc* 1993;41:143–148.

549. Beck MA. Rapid genomic evolution of a non-virulent coxsackievirus B3 in selenium-deficient mice. *Biomed Environ Sci* 1997;10:307–315.

550. Meeker HC, Eskew ML, Scheuchenzuber W, *et al.* Antioxidant effect on cell-mediated immunity. *J Leuk Biol* 1985;38:451–458.

551. Sun E, Xu H, Liu Q, *et al.* The mechanisms for the effect of selenium supplementation on immunity. *Biol Trace Elem Res* 1995;48:231–238.

552. Brown KM, Arthur JR. Selenium, selenoproteins and human health: a review. *Public Health Nutr* 2001;4:593–599.

553. Lin MT, Saito H, Furakawa S, *et al.* Alanyl-glutamine enriched total parenteral nutrition improves local, systemic, and remote organ responses to intraperitoneal bacterial challenge. *J Parenter Enteral Nutr* 2001;25:346–351.

554. O'Riordain MG, DeBeaux A, Fearon KC. Effect of glutamine on immune function in the surgical patient. *Nutrition* 1996; 12(Suppl):582–584.

555. Newsholme P. Why is L-glutamine metabolism important to cells of the immune system in healthy, post injury, surgery, or infections? *J Nutr* 2001;131(Suppl):2515S–2522S.

556. West SK. Who develops cataracts? *Arch Opthalmol* 1991;109:196–197.
557. Christen WG, Glynn RJ, Hennekins CH. Anitoxidants and age-related eye disease: current and future perspectives (review). *Ann Epidemiol* 1996;6:60–66.
558. Tavani A, Negri E, LaVecchia C. Food and nutrient intake and risk of cataract. *Ann Epidemiol* 1996;6:41–46.
559. Valero MP, Fletcher AE, Stavola BL, *et al.* Vitamin C is associated with reduced risk of cataract in a Mediterranean population. *J Nutr* 2002;132:1299–1306.
560. Robertson JM, Donner AP, Trevithick JR. A possible role for vitamins C and E in cataract prevention. *Am J Clin Nutr* 1991;53:346S–351S.
561. Mares-Perlman JA, Lyle BJ, Klein R, *et al.* Vitamin supplement use and incident cataracts in a population-based study. *Arch Ophthalmol* 2000;118:1556–1563.
562. Jacques PF, Chylack LT Jr, Hankinson SE, *et al.* Long-term nutrient intake and early age-related nuclear lens opacities. *Arch Ophthalmol* 2001;119:1009–1019.
563. Brown L, Rimm EB, Seddon JM, *et al.* A prospective study of cartenoid intake and risk of cataract extraction in US men. *Am J Clin Nutr* 1999;70:517–524.
564. Chasan-Taber L, Willett WC, Seddon JM, *et al.* A prospective study of carotenoid and vitamin A intakes and risk of cataract extract in US women. *Am J Clin Nutr* 1999;70:509–516.
565. Age-Related Eye Disease Study Research Group. A randomized, placebo-controlled clinical trial of high-dose supplementation with vitamins C and E and beta-carotene for age-related cataract and vision loss. *Arch Ophthalmol* 2001;119:1439–1452.
566. Christen WG, Manson JE, Glynn RJ, *et al.* A randomized trial of beta carotene and age-related cataract in US physicians. *Arch Ophthalmol* 2003;121:372–378.
567. Hu FB, Hankinson JE, Stampfer MJ, *et al.* Prospective study of cataract extraction and risk of coronary heart disease in women. *Am J Epidemiol* 2001;153:875–881.
568. Klein R, Klein BEK, Linton KLP. Prevalence of age-related maculopathy. *Ophthalmology* 1992;99:933–943.
569. Sundelin SP, Nilsson EG. Lipofuscin-formation in retinal pigment epithelial cells is reduced by antioxidants. *Free Radic Biol Med* 2001;31:217–225.
570. Seddon JM, Ajani UA, Sperduto RD, *et al.* Dietary carotenoids, vitamins A, C and E, and advanced age-related macular degeneration. *JAMA* 1994;272:1413–1420.

571. Age-Related Eye Disease Study Research Group. A randomized, placebo-controlled, clinical trial of high-dose supplementation with vitamins C and E, beta carotene and zinc for age-related macular degeneration and vision loss. *Arch Ophthalmol* 2001;119:1417–1436.

572. Jampol LM. Antioxidants, zinc and age-related macular degeneration. *Arch Ophthalmol* 2001;119:1533–1534 (Editorial).

573. Smith W, Mitchell P, Leeder SR. Dietary fat and fish intake and age-related maculopathy. *Arch Ophthalmol* 2000;118:401–404.

574. Seddon JM, Rosner B, Sperduto RD, *et al.* Dietary fat and risk for advanced age-related macular degeneration. *Arch Ophthalmol* 2001;119:1191–1199.

575. Schaumberg DA, Christen WG, Hankinson SE, Glynn RJ. Body mass index and the incidence of visually significant age-related maculopathy in men. *Arch Ophthalmol* 2001;119:1254–1265.

576. Ruhe RC, McDonald RB. Use of antioxidant nutrients in the prevention and treatment of type 2 diabetes. *J Am Coll Nutr* 2001;20 (Suppl 5):363S–369S.

577. Hu FB, Manson JE, Stampfer MJ, *et al.* Diet, lifestyle, and the risk of type 2 diabetes mellitus in women. *N Engl J Med* 2001;345:790–797.

578. Mann JI. Diet and risk of coronary heart disease and type 2 diabetes. *Lancet* 2002;360:783–789.

579. van Dam RM, Stampfer MJ, Willett WC, *et al.* Dietary fat and meat intake in relation to risk of type 2 diabetes in men. *Diabetes Care* 2002;25:417–424.

580. Jiang R, Manson JE, Stampfer MJ, *et al.* Nut and peanut butter consumption and risk of type 2 diabetes in women. *JAMA* 2002;288:2554–2560.

581. Salmeron J, Manson JE, Stampfer MJ, *et al.* Dietary fiber, glycemic load, and risk of non-insulin-dependent diabetes mellitus in women. *JAMA* 1997;277:472–477.

582. Liu S, Manson JE, Stampfer MJ, *et al.* A prospective study of whole-grain intake and risk of type 2 diabetes mellitus in US women. *Am J Public Health* 2000;90:1409–1415.

583. Jang Y, Lee JH, Kim OY, *et al.* Consumption of whole grain and legume powder reduces insulin demand, lipid peroxidation, and plasma homocysteine concentrations in patients with coronary artery disease: randomized controlled clinical trial. *Atheroscler Thromb Vasc Biol* 2001;21:2065–2071.

584. Rude RK. Magnesium metabolism and deficiency. *Endocrinol Metab Clin N Am* 1993;22:277–394.

585. Nadler JL, Rude RK. Disorders of magnesium metabolism. *Endocrinol Metab Clin N Am* 1995;24:623–637.

586. Kao WHL, Folsom AR, Nieto FJ, *et al.* Serum and dietary magnesium and the risk for type 2 diabetes mellitus. *Arch Intern Med* 1999;159:2151–2159.
587. Humphries S, Kushner H, Falkner B. Low dietary magnesium is associated with insulin resistance in a sample of young non-diabetic black Americans. *Am J Hypertens* 1999;12:747–756.
588. Cabalero B. Vitamin E improves the action of insulin. *Nutr Rev* 1993;51:339–340.
589. Paolisso G, D'Amore A, Giugliano D, *et al.* Pharmacologic doses of vitamin E improves insulin action in healthy subjects and non-insulin-dependent diabetic patients. *Am J Clin Nutr* 1993;57:650–656.
590. Paolisso G, Giugliano D, D'Amore A, *et al.* Daily vitamin E supplements improve metabolic control but not insulin secretion in elderly type II diabetic patients. *Diabetes Care* 1993;16:1433–1437; Effect of combined treatment with vitamin C and E on albuminuria in type 2 diabetic patients. *Diabet Med* 2001;18:756–760.
591. Goede P, Poulsen HE, Parving HH, Pedersen O. Double-blind, randomised study of the effect of combined treatment with vitamin C and E on albuminuria in type 2 diabetic patients. *Diabet Med* 2001;18:756–760.
592 Borcea V, Nourooz-Zadeh J, Wolff SP, *et al.* Alpha-lipoic acid decreases oxidative stress even in diabetic patients with poor glycemic control and albuminuria. *Free Radic Biol Med* 1999;22:1495–1500.
593. Obrosova IG, Fathallah L, Liu E, Nourooz-Zaheh J. Early oxidative stress in the diabetic kidney: effect of DL-alpha-lipoic acid. *Free Radic Biol Med* 2003;34:186–195.
594. Liu S, Ajani U, Chae C, *et al.* Long-term beta-carotene supplementation and risk of type 2 diabetes mellitus. *JAMA* 1999;282:1073–1075.
595. Burr VL, Whelton P, Roccella EJ, *et al.* Prevalence of hypertension in US adult population: results from the Third National Health and Nutrition Examination Survey, 1988–1991. *Hypertension* 1995;25:305–313.
596. Midgley JP, Mathew AG, Greenwood CMT, Logan AG. Effect of reduced dietary sodium on blood pressure: a meta-analysis of randomized controlled trials. *JAMA* 1996;275:1590–1597.
597. Appel LJ, Moore TJ, Obarzanck E, *et al.* A clinical trial of the effects of dietary patterns on blood pressure. *N Engl J Med* 1997;336:1117–1124.
598. Sacks FM, Svetkey LP, Vollmer WM, *et al.* Effects on blood pressure of reduced dietary sodium and the dietary approaches to stop hypertension (DASH) diet. *N Engl J Med* 2001;344:3–10.

599. He J, Ogden LG, Vupputuri S, *et al.* Dietary sodium intake and subsequent risk of cardiovascular disease in overweight adults. *JAMA* 1999;282:2027–2034.

600. Addison WLT. The use of sodium chloride, potassium chloride, sodium bromide and potassium bromide in cases of arterial hypertension which are amendable to potassium chloride. *Can Med Assoc J* 1928;18:281–285.

601. Whelton PK, Jiang H, Cutler JA, *et al.* Effects of oral potassium on blood pressure: meta-analysis of randomized controlled clinical trials. *JAMA* 1997;277:1624–1632.

602. Green DM, Ropper AH, Kronmal RA, *et al.* Serum potassium level and dietary potassium intake as risk factors for stroke. *Neurology* 2002;59:314–320.

603. Bucher HC, Cook RJ, Guyatt GH, *et al.* Effects of dietary calcium supplementation on blood pressure: a meta-analysis of randomized controlled trials. *JAMA* 1996;275:1016–1022.

604. Vasdev S, Ford CA, Parai S, *et al.* Dietary vitamin C supplementation lowers blood pressure in spontaneously hypertensive rats. *Mol Cell Biochem* 2001;218:97–103.

605. Chen X, Touyz RM, Park JB, Schiffrin EL. Antioxidant effects vitamins C and E are associated with altered activation of vascular NADPH oxidase and superoxide dismutase in stroke-prone SHR. *Hypertension* 2001;38:606–611.

606. Duffy SJ, Gokce N, Holbrook M, *et al.* Treatment of hypertension with ascorbic acid. *Lancet* 1999;354:2048–2049.

607. Kurl S, Tumainen TP, Laukkanen JA, *et al.* Plasma vitamin C modifies the association between hypertension and risk of stroke. *Stroke* 2002;33:1568–1573.

608. Digiesi V, Lenuzza M, Digiesi G. Prospects for the use of antioxidant therapy in hypertension. *Ann Ital Med Int* 2001; 16:93–100.

609. NIH Consensus Development Panel on Osteoporosis Prevention, Diagnosis and Therapy. Osteoporosis prevention, diagnosis and therapy. *JAMA* 2001;285:785–795.

610. National Osteoporosis Foundation. Osteoporosis: review of the evidence for prevention, diagnosis and treatment and cost-effectiveness analysis. *Osteoporosis Int* 1998;8(Suppl 4):S1–S88.

611. Ray NF, Chan JK, Thamer M, Melton U. Medical expenditures for the treatment of osteoporotic fractures in the United States in 1995: report from the National Osteoporosis Foundation. *J Bone Miner Res* 1997;12:24–35.

612. Miller SM. *Vitamin D: Bones and Beyond.* Advance/Laboratory, November 2002, pp. 37, 39.

613. Hansen MA, Overgaard K, Riis BJ, Christiansen C. Role of peak bone mass and bone loss in postmenopausal osteoporosis: 12-year study. *BMJ* 1991;303:961–964.

614. Rowe JW, Kahn RL. Human aging: usual and successful. *Science* 1997;237:143–149.

615. Knight JA. *Laboratory Medicine and the Aging Process.* ASCP Press, Chicago, 1996, pp. 227–230.

616. Kato I, Toniolo P, Zeleniuch-Jacquotte A, *et al.* Diet, smoking and anthropometric indices and postmenopausal bone fractures: a prospective study. *Int J Epidemiol* 2000;29:85–92.

617. Nieves JW, Komar L, Cosman F, Lindsay R. Calcium potentiates the effect of estrogen and calcitonin on bone mass: review and analysis. *Am J Clin Nutr* 1998;67:18–24.

618. NIH Consensus Development Panel on Optimal Calcium Intake. Optimal calcium intake. *JAMA* 1994;272:1942–1948.

619. Barger-Lux MJ, Heaney RP, Lanspa SJ, *et al.* An investigation of sources of variation in calcium absorption efficacy. *J Clin Endocrinol Metab* 1995;80:406–411.

620. Weaver CM, Proulx WR, Heaney R. Choices for achieving adequate dietary calcium with a vegetarian diet. *Am J Clin Nutr* 1999; 70(Suppl):543S–548S.

621. Thomas MK, Lloyd-Jones DM, Thadhani RI, *et al.* Hypovitaminosis D in medical inpatients. *N Engl J Med* 1998;338:777–783.

622. Gloth FM, Gundberg CM, Hollis BW, *et al.* Vitamin D deficiency in homebound elderly persons. *JAMA* 1995;274:1683–1686.

623. Liu BA, Gordon M, Labranche JM, *et al.* Seasonal prevalence of vitamin D deficiency in institutionalized older adults. *J Am Geriatr Soc* 1997;45:598–603.

624. van der Wielen RPJ, Lowik MRH, van den Berg H, *et al.* Serum vitamin D concentrations among elderly people in Europe. *Lancet* 1995;346:207–210.

625. Trivedi DP, Doll R, Khaw KT. Effect of four monthly oral vitamin D3 (cholecalciferol) supplementation in fractures and mortality in men and women living in the community: randomised double blind controlled trial. *BMJ* 2003;326:469–472.

626. LeBoff MS, Kohlmeier L, Hurwitz S, *et al.* Occult vitamin D deficiency in post-menopausal US women with acute hip fracture. *JAMA* 1999;281:1505–1511.

627. Dawson-Hughes B, Harris SS, Krall EA, Dallal GE. Effect of calcium and vitamin D supplementation on bone density in men and women 65 years of age and older. *N Engl J Med* 1997;337:670–676.

628. Chapuy MC, Arlot ME, Dubocuf F, *et al.* Vitamin D and calcium to prevent hip fractures in elderly women. *N Engl J Med* 1992;327:1637–1642.

629. Reid JR, Ames RW, Evans MC, *et al.* Long-term effects of calcium supplementation on bone loss and fractures in postmenopausal women: a randomized controlled trial. *Am J Med* 1995;98:331–335.

630. Compston JE. Vitamin D deficiency: time for action. *BMJ* 1998;317:1466–1467.

631. Binkley N, Krueger D. Hypervitaminosis A and bone. *Nutr Rev* 2000;58:138–144.

632. Rothman KJ, Moore LL, Singer MR, *et al.* Teratogenicity of high vitamin A intake. *N Engl J Med* 1995;333:1369–1373.

633. Melhus H, Michaelsson K, Kindmark A, *et al.* Excessive dietary intake of vitamin A is associated with reduced bone mineral density and increased risk for hip fracture. *Ann Intern Med* 1998;129:770–778.

634. Feskanich D, Singh V, Willett WC, Colditz GA. Vitamin A intake and hip fractures among postmenopausal women. *JAMA* 2002;287:47–54.

635. Michaelsson K, Lithell H, Vessby B, Melhus H. Serum retinol levels and the risk of fracture. *N Engl J Med* 2003;348:287–294.

636. Sebastian A, Harris ST, Ottaway JH, *et al.* Improved mineral balance and skeletal metabolism in postmenopausal women treated with potassium bicarbonate. *N Engl J Med* 1994;1776–1781.

637. Black DM, Cummings SR, Karpf DB, *et al.* Randomised trial of effect of alendronate on risk of fracture in women and existing vertebral fractures. *Lancet* 1996;348:1535–1541.

638. Cummings SR, Black DM, Thompson ED, *et al.* Effect of alendronate on risk of fracture in women and low bone density but without vertebral fractures. *JAMA* 1998;280:2077–2082.

639. Rico H. Minerals and osteoporosis. *Osteoporosis Int* 1991;2:20–25.

640. Atik OS. Zinc and senile osteoporosis. *J Am Geriatr Soc* 1983;31:790–791.

641. Herzberg M, Foldes J, Steinberg R, Menczel J. Zinc excretion in osteoporotic women. *J Bone Miner Res* 1990;5:251–257.

642. Seco C, Revilla M, Hernandez ER, *et al.* Effect of zinc supplementation on vertebral and femoral bone mass in rats on strenuous treadmill training excerise. *J Bone Miner Res* 1998;13:508–512.

643. Rubin CD, Pak CYC, Adams-Huet B, *et al.* Sustained-release sodium fluoride in the treatment of the elderly with established osteoporosis. *Arch Intern Med* 2001;161:2325–2333.

644. Kaste LM, Selwitz RH, Oldakowski RJ, *et al.* Coronal caries in the primary and permanent dentition of children and adolescents 1–17 years of age: United States 1988–1991. *J Dent Res* 1996;75: 631–641.

645. Winn DM, Brunelle JH, Selwitz RH, *et al.* Coronal and root caries in the dentition of adults in the United States, 1988–1991. *J Dent Res* 1996;75:642–651.

646. CDC. Achievements in public health, 1990–1999; fluoridation of drinking water to prevent dental caries. *MMWR* 1999;48:933–940.

647. Chapman S. Child abuse or copper deficiency? A radiological review. *BMJ* 1987;294:1370.

648. Conlan D, Korula R, Tallentire D. Serum copper levels in elderly patients with femoral-neck fractures. *Age Ageing* 1990;19:212–214.

649. Joseph JA, Shukitt-Hale B, Denisova NA, *et al.* Reversals of age-related declines in neuronal signal transduction, cognitive and motor behavioral deficits with blueberry, spinach or strawberry dietary supplementation. *J Neurosci* 1999;15:8114–8121.

650. Bickford PC, Gould T, Briederick L, *et al.* Antioxidant-rich diets improve cerebellar physiology and motor learning in aged rats. *Brain Res* 2000;866:211–217.

651. Kalmijn S, Feskens EJM, Launer LJ, Kromhout D. Polyunsaturated fatty acids, antioxidants, and cognitive function in very old men. *Am J Epidemiol* 1997;145:33–41.

652. Stoll AL, Severus E, Freeman MP, *et al.* Omega 3 fatty acids in bipolar disorder: a preliminary double-blind, placebo-controlled trial. *Arch Gen Psychiatry* 1999;56:407–412.

653. Meydani M. Antioxidants and cognitive function. *Nutr Rev* 2001;59: S73–S80.

654. Ortega RM, Requejo AM, Lopez-Sobaler AM, *et al.* Cognitive function in elderly people is influenced by vitamin E status. *J Nutr* 2002;132:2065–2068.

655. Morris MC, Evans, DA, Bienias JL, *et al.* Vitamin E and cognitive decline in older persons. *Arch Neurol* 2002;59:1125–1132.

656. Joseph JA, Shukitt-Hale B, Denisova NA, *et al.* Reversals of age-related decline in neuronal signal tranduction, cognitive and behavioral deficits with blueberry, spinach or strawberry dietary supplementation. *J Neurosci* 1999;19:8114–8121.

657. Schroeter H, Williams RJ, Matin R, *et al.* Phenolic antioxidants attenuate neuronal cell death following uptake of oxidized low-density lipoprotein. *Free Radic Biol Med* 2000;29:1222–1233.

658. Adler LA, Peselow E, Rotrosen J, *et al.* Vitamin E treatment of tardive dyskinesia. *Am J Psychiatry* 1993;150:1405–1407.

659. Geldmacher DS, Whitehouse PJ. Evaluation of dementia. *N Engl J Med* 1996;335:330–336.

660. Mayeux R, Sano M. Treatment of Alzheimer's disease. *N Engl J Med* 1999;341:1670–1679.

661. Evans DA, Funkenstein HH, Albert MS, *et al.* Prevalence of Alzheimer's disease in a community population of older persons. Higher than previously reported. *JAMA* 1989;262:2551–2556.

662. Gurland BJ, Wilder DE, Lantigua R, *et al.* Rates of dementia in three ethnoracial groups. *Int J Geriatr Psychiatry* 1999;14:481–493.

663. Ernst RI, Hay JW, Fenn C, *et al.* Cognitive function and the costs of Alzheimer disease. An exploratory study. *Arch Neurol* 1997;54:687–693.

664. Hofman A, Ott A, Breteler MMB, *et al.* Atherosclerosis, apolipoprotein E and prevalence of dementia, and Alzheimer's disease in the Rotterdam study. *Lancet* 1997;349:151–154.

665. Pratico D, Clark CM, Liun F, *et al.* Increase of brain oxidative stress in mild cognitive impairment: a possible predictor of Alzheimer disease. *Arch Neurol* 2002;59:972–975.

666. Luchsinger JA, Tang M-X, Shea S, Mayeux R. Caloric intake and the risk of Alzheimer disease. *Arch Neurol* 2002;59:1258–1263.

667. Zaman Z, Roche S, Fielden P, *et al.* Plasma concentrations of vitamins A and E and carotenoids in Alzheimer's disease. *Age Ageing* 1992;21:91–94.

668. Sano M, Ernesto C, Thomas RG, *et al.* A controlled trial of selegiline, alpha-tocopherol or both as treatment for Alzheimer's disease. *N Engl J Med* 1997;336:1216–1222.

669. Engelhart MJ, Geerlings MI, Ruitenberg A, *et al.* Dietary intake of antioxidants and risk of Alzheimer disease. *JAMA* 2002;287:3223–3229.

670. Morris MC, Evans DA, Bienias JL, *et al.* Dietary intake of antioxidant nutrients and the risk of incident Alzheimer disease in a biracial community study. *JAMA* 2002;287:3230–3237.

671. Perry G, Raina AK, Nunomura A, *et al.* How important is oxidative damage? Lessons from Alzheimer's disease. *Free Radic Biol Med* 2000;28:831–834.

672. Kontush A, Mann U, Arit S, *et al.* Influence of vitamin E and C supplementation on lipoprotein oxidation in patients with Alzheimer's disease. *Free Radic Biol Med* 2001;31:345–354.

673. Ishige K, Schubert D, Sagara Y. Flavonoids protect neuronal cells from oxidative stress by three distinct mechanisms. *Free Radic Biol Med* 2001;30:433–446.

674. Doody RS, Stevens JC, Beck C, *et al.* Practice parameter: management of dementia (an evidence-based review). Report of the Quality Standards Subcommittee of the American Academy of Neurology. *Neurology* 2001;56:1154–1166.

675. Schroeter H, Williams RJ, Matin R, *et al.* Phenolic antioxidants attenuate neuronal cell death following uptake of oxidized low-density lipoprotein. *Free Radic Biol Med* 2000;29:1222–1233.

676. Seshadri S, Bieser A, Selhub J, *et al.* Plasma homocysteine as a risk factor for dementia and Alzheimer's disease. *N Engl J Med* 2002;346:476–483.

677. Kalmijn S, Feskens EJ, Launer LJ, Kromhout D. Polyunsaturated fatty acids, antioxidants and cognitive function in very old men. *Am J Epidemiol* 1997;145:33–41.

678. Morris MC, Evans DA, Bienias JL, *et al.* Dietary fats and the risk of incident Alzheimer disease. *Arch Neurol* 2003;60:194–200.

679. Morris MC, Evans DA, Bienas JL, *et al.* Consumption of fish and n-3 fatty acids and risk of incident Alzheimer disease. *Arch Neurol* 2003;60:940–946.

680. McGeer PL, Schulzer M, McGeer EG. Arthritis and anti-inflammatory agents as possible protective factors for Alzheimer's disease: a review of 17 epidemiologic studies. *Neurology* 1996;47:425–432.

681. Rich JB, Rasmusson DX, Folstein MF, *et al.* Nonsteroidal anti-inflammatory drugs in Alzheimer's disease. *Neurology* 1995;45:51–55.

682. Stewart WF, Kawas C, Corrada M, Metter EJ. Risk of Alzheimer's disease and duration of NSAID use. *Neurology* 1997;48:626–632.

683. Broe GA, Grayson DA, Creasey HM, *et al.* Anti-inflammatory drugs protect against Alzheimer disease at low doses. *Arch Neurol* 2000;57:1586–1591.

684. Veld BA, Ruitenberg A, Hofman A, *et al.* Non-steroidal anti-inflammatory drugs and the risk of Alzheimer's disease. *N Engl J Med* 2001;345:1515–1521.

685. Aisen PS, Schafer KA, Grundman M, *et al.* Effects of rofecoxib or naproxen versus placebo on Alzheimer disease progression. *JAMA* 2003;289:2819–2826.

686. Maia L, De Mendonca A. Does caffeine intake protect from Alzheimer's disease? *Eur J Neurol* 2002;9:377–382.

687. Roghani M, Behzadi G. Neuroprotective effect of vitamin E on the early model of Parkinson's disease in rats: behavioral and histochemical evidence. *Brain Res* 2001;892:211–217.

688. Lin AMY. Coexistence of zinc and iron augmented oxidative injuries in nigrostriatal dopaminergic system of SD rats. *Free Radic Biol Med* 2001;30:225–231.

689. de Rijk MC, Breteler MMB, den Breeijen JH, *et al.* Dietary antioxidants and Parkinson's disease. *Arch Neurol* 1997;54:762–765.

690. Golbe LI, Farrell TM, Davis PH. Case-control study of early life dietary factors in Parkinson's disease. *Arch Neurol* 1988;45:1350–1353.

691. Logroscino G, Marder, K, Cote L, *et al.* Dietary lipids and antioxidants in Parkinson's disease: a population-based case control study. *Ann Neurol* 1996;39:89–94.

692. Shults CW, Oakes D, Kieburtz K, *et al.* Effects of coenzyme Q_{10} in early Parkinson disease. *Arch Neurol* 2002;59:1541–1550.

693. Grandinetti A, Morens D, Reed D, MacEachem D. Prospective study of cigarette smoking and the risk of developing idiopathic Parkinson's disease. *Am J Epidemiol* 1994;139:1129–1138.

694. Ross GW, Abbott RD, Petrovitch H, *et al.* Association of coffee and caffeine intake with the risk of Parkinson disease. *JAMA* 2000;283:2674–2679.

695. Duan W, Ladenheim B, Cutler RG, *et al.* Dietary folate deficiency and elevated homocysteine levels endanger dopaminergic neurons in models of Parkinson's disease. *J Neurochem* 2002;80:101–110.

696. Broadus AF, Insogna KI, Lang R, *et al.* Evidence for disordered control of 1,25-dihydroxyvitamin D production in absorptive hypercalciuria. *N Engl J Med* 1984;311:73–80.

697. Borghi L, Schianchi T, Meschi T, *et al.* Comparison of two diets for the prevention of recurrent stones in idiopathic hypercalciuria. *N Engl J Med* 2002;346:77–84.

698. Jenkins SA. Biliary lipids, bile acids and gallstone formation in hypovitaminotic C guinea-pigs. *Br J Nutr* 1978;40:317–322.

699. Simon JA, Hudes ES. Serum ascorbic acid and gallbladder disease prevalence among US adults: the Third National Health and Nutrition Examination Survey (NHANES III). *Arch Intern Med* 2000;160:931–936.

700. Yanik FF, Amanvermez R, Yanik A, *et al.* Pre-eclampsia associated with increased lipid peroxidation and decreased serum vitamin E levels. *Int J Gynaecol Obstet* 1999;64:27–33.

701. Sagol S, Ozkinay E, Ozsener S. Impaired antioxidant activity in women with pre-eclampsia. *Int J Gynaecol Obstet* 1999;64:121–127.

702. Chappell LC, Seed PT, Briley AL, *et al.* Effect of antioxidants on the occurrence of pre-eclampsia in women at increased risk: a randomised trial. *Lancet* 1999;354:810–816.

703. Belfort MA, Anthony J, Saade GR, Allen JC Jr. A comparison of magnesium sulfate and nimodipine for the prevention of eclampsia. *N Engl J Med* 2003;348:304–311.

704. Pritchard JA, Cunningham FG, Pritchard SA. The Parkland Memorial Hospital protocol for treatment of eclampsia. Evaluation of 245 cases. *Am J Obstet Gynecol* 1984;148:951–963.

705. Sibai BM. Eclampsia VI: maternal perinatal outcome in 254 consecutive cases. *Am J Obstet Gynecol* 1990;163:1049–1055.

706. Center for Disease Control. Use of folic acid for prevention of spina bifida and other neural tube defects — 1983–1991. *MMWR* 1991;40:513–516.

707. Smithells RW, Sheppard S, Schorah CJ, *et al.* Possible prevention of neural tube defects by periconceptional vitamin supplementation. *Lancet* 1980;1:339–340.

708. Berry RJ, Li Z, Erickson JD, *et al.* Prevention of neural-tube defects with folic acid in China. *N Engl J Med* 1999;341:1485–1490.

709. Botto LD, Moore CA, Khoury MJ, Erickson JD. Neural-tube defects. *N Engl J Med* 1999;341:1509–1519.

710. CDC. Recommendations for the use of folic acid to reduce the number of cases of spina bifida and other neural tube defects. *MMWR* 1992;41(No. RR-14).

711. Food and Drug Administration. Food standards: amendment of standards of identity for enriched grain products to require addition of folic acid. *Fed Register* 1996;61:8781–8797.

712. Williams LJ, Mai CT, Edmonds LD, *et al.* Prevalence of spina bifida and anencephaly during the transition of mandatory folic acid fortification in the United States. *Teratology* 2002;66:33–39.

713. Center for Disease Control. Use of folic acid-containing supplements among women of childbearing age — United States, 1997. *MMWR* 1998;47:131–134.

714. Werler MM, Hayes C, Louik C, *et al.* Multivitamin supplementation and risk of birth defects. *Am J Epidemiol* 1999;150:675–682.

715. Shearer MJ. Vitamin K. *Lancet* 1995;345:229–230.

716. Vermeer C, Jie KSG, Knapen MHJ. Role of vitamin K in bone metabolism. *Ann Rev Nutr* 1995;15:1–22.

717. Lipsky JJ. Nutritional sources of vitamin K. *Mayo Clin Proc* 1994;69:462–466.

718. George L, Mills JL, Johansson ALV, *et al.* Plasma folate levels and risk of spontaneous abortion. *JAMA* 2002;288:1867–1873.

719. Chen P, Zhou J. Abnormal metabolism of nitric oxide, oxidative stress and lipoperoxidative stress in patients with acute viral myocarditis. *Chin Med J* 2001;114:1132–1135.

720. Enstrom JE, Kanim LE, Klein MA. Vitamin C intake and mortality among a sample of the United States population. *Epidemiology* 1992;3:194–202.

721. Khaw K-T, Bingham S, Welch A, *et al.* Relation between plasma ascorbic acid and mortality in men and women in EPIC-Norfolk prospective study: a prospective population study. *Lancet* 2001;357:657–663.

722. Kant AK, Schatzkin A, Graubard BI, Schairer C. A prospective study of diet quality and mortality in women. *JAMA* 2000;283:2109–2115.

723. Fraser GE. Associations between diet and cancer, ischemic heart disease, and all-cause mortality in non-Hispanic white California Seventh-day Adventists. *Am J Clin Nutr* 1999;70(Suppl 3):532S–538S.

724. Solichova D, Melichar B, Blaha V, *et al.* Biochemical profile and survival in nonagenarians. *Clin Biochem* 2001;34:563–569.

725. US Department of Health and Human Services. *Healthy People 2010: Understanding and Improving Health*, 2nd Ed. US Government Printing Office, Washington, DC, November 2000.

5

Substance Abuse, Herbal Medicines and Environmental Factors: Their Effect on Aging, Health and Disease

Introduction

The referenced causes of death generally indicate the major pathological conditions identified at the time of death as opposed to their root causes. However, since most clinical diseases, disorders and injuries are multifactorial in nature, it is often very difficult to sort out the relative contributions of the various factors. For example, in 1990 the ten leading causes of death in the United States were reportedly heart disease (720,000), cancer (505,000), cerebrovascular disease (144,000), accidents (92,000), chronic obstructive pulmonary disease (87,000), pneumonia/influenza (80,000), diabetes mellitus (48,000), suicide (31,000), chronic liver disease/cirrhosis (26,000) and human immunodeficiency virus (25,000).[1] In the same year, McGinnis et al.[2] reported that the major non-genetic factors contributing to mortality in the US were tobacco (400,000), diet and activity patterns (300,000), alcohol (100,000), microbial agents (90,000), toxic agents (60,000), firearms (35,000), sexual behavior (30,000), motor vehicles (25,000) and illicit drug use (20,000). Thus, about 50% of all 1990 deaths were attributable to specific external factors. In addition to these health altering factors, atmospheric pollutants, herbs, ultraviolet radiation, among others may negatively contribute to the aging process and increase the risk of various diseases and disorders as well as decrease life expectancy and the quality of life. Moreover, when the number of non-lethal problems are considered, it becomes readily apparent that in addition to the tremendous personal costs, the financial costs are also extensive. The association between these risk factors and various diseases and disorders is presented in the following sections of this chapter.

Cigarette Smoking

Prevalence, economic costs and mortality

Cigarette smoking is the leading cause of preventable death in the US and results in substantial societal health-related economic costs. According to the Centers for Disease Control (CDC), smoking caused 442,398 premature deaths each year from 1995 to 1999 (264,087 men; 178,311 women).[3] The annual health-related economic losses during this time were estimated at US$157 billion (US$3391/year for each smoker). The annual per capita number of cigarettes smoked in 1900 was 54; this increased to 4345 in 1963 and then decreased to 2261 in 1998.[4] According to recent CDC statistics, the percent of US smoking adults in 1997 was 24.7%, a significant decrease from 1965 when an estimated 42% of US adults smoked.[5] However, since 1990, the prevalence of cigarette smoking has remained about the same (approximately 28.0% for men; 22.5% for women).[6] In 1997, the CDC reported the following smoking prevalence among various groups of Americans:[7]

(1) Age: 18–24 years (28.7%); 25–44 years (28.6%); ≥65 years (12%).
(2) Race/Ethnicity: American Indians/Alaska Natives (34.1%); non-Hispanic blacks (26.7%); non-Hispanic whites (25.3%); Hispanics (20.4%); and Asians/Pacific Islanders (16.9%).
(3) Education level: 9–11 years (35.4%); ≥16 years (11.6%).

(4) Economic status: below poverty line (33.3%); at or above poverty line (24.6%).

The smoking-attributable mortality rate also varies considerably with the state of residence, Utah being the lowest (13.4%) and Nevada the highest (24.0%).[8] The goal of Healthy People 2010, the US Department of Health and Human Services' health promotion and disease prevention initiative, is to reduce the smoking prevalence to 12% by the end of the decade. The major diseases/disorders associated with smoking include various neoplasms, cardiovascular and cerebrovascular diseases, respiratory diseases, cataracts/macular degeneration and pregnancy-associated disorders, among others. Smoking also accelerates the aging process (Table 5.1).

The economic and health problems of smoking are not limited to the US. Indeed, China, with 20% of the world's population, now smokes 30% of the world's cigarettes.[9] Moreover, over the past decade several publications have reported a marked smoking increase in China. An early report found that from 1976 to 1986 half of the global increase in tobacco use occurred in China and in 1984, 61% of Chinese males over age 15 years smoked.[10] The changing smoking patterns suggested that by 2025, two million Chinese men will die each year from smoking. Other smoking studies were limited to specific areas of China. For example, a study from the Minhang District, near Shanghai, found that 67% of men but only 2% of women smoke.[11] The cost of smoking represented 60% of the personal income and 17% of household income. The figures were similar in a 1996 country-wide population-based Chinese study in which 63% of men and 3.8% of women smoked.[12]

A significant increase in mortality attributable to smoking has also been noted. According to a recent World Health Report,[13] the annual number of smoking-related deaths in 1998 were as follows: Europe, 1,273,000; Western Pacific, 1,093,000; the Americas, 772,000; Southeast Asia, 580,000; Eastern Mediterranean, 182,000; and Africa, 125,000. In a 16-year prospective study, about 20% of all Chinese deaths during the 1980s were due to smoking.[14] However, it was predicted

Table 5.1: Major Diseases/Disorders Associated with Smoking

Aging
Cardiovascular Diseases
   Hypertension
   Ischemic heart disease
   Aortic aneurysm
Cerebrovascular Disease
Neoplasms
   Oral cavity, pharynx
   Larynx
   Lung, bronchus, trachea
   Esophagus
   Pancreas
   Urinary bladder
   Kidney
   Leukemia, myelodysplastic syndromes
Lung Diseases
   Chronic obstructive pulmonary disease
   Invasive pneumococcal disease
   Pulmonary embolism
Cataract and Macular Degeneration
Osteoporosis
Menopause
Pregnancy-Associated Disorders
Multiple Sclerosis
Thyroid Dysfunction
Type 2 Diabetes Mellitus
Hemoglobin Level
Physical Function
Psychologic Changes

that about 150 million Chinese smokers will die of smoking-related diseases "if urgent tobacco-control measures are not instituted …"[15] Additionally, the proportion of smoking-attributable male deaths in Hong Kong is significantly higher (33%) than in mainland China.[16] Examples of the percentage of 1990 deaths due to smoking in various other countries are as follows:[17] Italy (26%), Ireland (25%), Belgium (31%), The Netherlands (32%), United Kingdom (28%), United States (26%), Canada (27%), Poland (29%), Russian Federation (30%), Ukraine (28%) and Hungary (29%). Except for Canada, US, UK and

Ireland, the percentage of female deaths was less than 10% of the total and most were less than 5%.

In Japan, the smoking prevalence among the general population is reportedly about 54% for men and 14.5% for women; this is about twice the prevalence of Japanese physicians (males, 27.1%; females, 6.8%).[18] However, the smoking prevalence is higher among Japanese male physicians than for male physicians in several other countries (US, 3–10%; UK, 4–5%; New Zealand, 5%). An important mortality study of British male physicians over a 40-year period found that about 50% of those who smoked died of causes secondary to smoking.[19] A later report indicated that half of the regular smokers in the US also die prematurely of a tobacco-related disease.[20]

The prevalence of cigarette smoking among American high school students increased during the early-mid 1990s,[21] and over 80% of adults that currently smoke began before aged 18 years.[22] According to the National Youth Tobacco Survey, the overall prevalence of tobacco use during this time was 12.8% among middle school students (grades 6–8) and 34.8% among high school students (grades 9–12).[23] However, in 2001 the percent of high school students who smoked had decreased to 28.5% (males, 29.2%; females, 27.7%).[24] Nevertheless, a significant progressive increase with each grade still exists (grades 9–12; 23.9%, 26.9%, 29.8%, 35.2%, respectively).

From 1993 to 1997, there was also a significant increase in cigarette smoking among college students.[25] Over this four-year period, cigarette smoking increased from 22.3% to 28.5% in 99 of 116 college studies; the increased smoking rate rose faster in public schools (from 22% to 29.3%) than in private schools (from 22.9% to 26.8%). The problem is even more serious in other countries. For example, cigarette smoking among secondary school students aged 14 to 18 years in Budapest, Hungary increased from 36% in 1995 to 46% in 1999.[26]

Exposure to environmental tobacco smoke has been associated with acute and chronic diseases among non-smokers; these include an increased incidence of lung cancer, asthma, respiratory infections, coronary heart disease (CHD) and decreased pulmonary function.[27] These workers reported that 43% of American children aged two months to 11 years lived in a home with at least one smoker and 37% of adult non-tobacco users lived in a home with at least one smoker or were exposed to tobacco smoke at work. Lam *et al.*[28] also reported that smoke exposure among Hong Kong police officers who never smoked had a significant increase in serious health disorders associated with smoke exposure at work.

Smoking prevention and treatment

Smoking cessation reduces the risk of tobacco-related diseases, increases life expectancy and the quality of life even when smoking stops after the age of 65 years or after the development of a smoking-related disease.[29] However, smoking has complex physiological and psychological determinants. Hence, stopping smoking requires more than just willpower. As a result, smoking is best regarded as a chronic disease that requires a long-term management strategy. Less than 10% of smokers who attempt to quit on their own are successful over the long term.[29,30] Moreover, although one-third of smokers try to stop smoking each year, only about 20% seek professional help. The major obstacle to quitting is the addictive nature of nicotine, which causes tolerance and physical dependence. Thus, when smoking is stopped, a withdrawal syndrome characterized by irritability, anger, restlessness, impatience, anxiety, difficulty concentrating, insomnia, increased appetite and depression often develops.[31] However, pharmacotherapy and physician counseling are both individually effective in getting people to quit smoking, although a combination of the two is most effective.[32] Nevertheless, addiction treatments "should be regarded as being long term, and a 'cure' is unlikely from a single course of treatment."[33]

In 1980, the American Medical Association Council on Scientific Affairs recommended that physicians routinely assess their patients' smoking habits and encourage them to quit by offering either direct assistance or referring them to community clinics.[34] To evaluate the success of these recommendations, Anda *et al.*[35] analyzed data from two random surveys of Michigan adults. Of the smokers who had seen a physician in the previous year, 44% indicated that they had ever been advised to quit smoking, although only 30% of young male smokers had been so advised. In addition, smokers who were hypertensive, obese, diabetic, sedentary, or users of oral contraceptives were no more likely to be advised to quit smoking than smokers without these CHD risks. The authors concluded that "most smokers do not perceive physicians to be even minimally involved in their efforts to quit." Unfortunately, studies continue to document the failure of physicians and other health care providers to intervene with their patients who smoke. Indeed, only about half of current smokers indicate they were encouraged to stop smoking and significantly fewer received specific counseling.[36]

Since the hazards of smoking are well understood by physicians, why is counseling their patients to stop smoking not more frequent? According to Pearson *et al.*,[37] the four major barriers are as follows: (1) physicians do not believe they are effective; (2) physicians lack behavioral counseling skills; (3) a belief that patients do not want their physicians to intervene; and (4) inadequate time to counsel, especially since reimbursement is not available. In addition, physicians have generally not received adequate intervention training in medical school. Thus, Spangler and associates[38] recently reported that although various education methods have been used in some medical schools to train medical students in smoking intervention, there are significant shortcomings including the following: (1) lack of integration of tobacco dependence information in all four years; (2) lack of intervention training in smokeless tobacco; (3) tobacco intervention that addresses cultural issues; and (4) long-term evaluation to demonstrate that the acquired skills are retained.

Nevertheless, interventions by primary care physicians have consistently yielded cessation rates of 10% to 20%, a three- to five-fold increase over the one-year maintained cessation rate of 4% seen in the general population.[39] Thus, randomized controlled trials have demonstrated that advice from a physician to stop smoking increases the rate of smoking cessation by about 30%. This is especially so when the physician spends a few minutes (three or less) counseling rather than just advising the patient to quit.[40] Moreover, more than half of smokers aged 50 years and over welcome physician advice to quit.[41] Unfortunately, as with obesity and physical inactivity (Chapters 2 and 3), physicians are more likely to advise patients to stop smoking after they have developed a smoking-related disease.

Early studies indicated that pharmacotherapy may be effective in smoking cessation and five products have been approved by the Food and Drug Administration (sustained-release bupropion and four nicotine replacement products).[42] Thus, when both counseling and drug therapy were combined, typical smoking cessation rates were 40% to 60% at the end of drug treatment and 25% to 30% after one year.[40] More recently, however, Pierce and Gilpin[43] examined the trends in smoking cessation, pharmaceutical cessation aid use and cessation success in the general California population in 1992, 1996 and 1999. They concluded that nicotine replacement therapy, since becoming available over-the-counter, "appears no longer effective in increasing long-term successful cessation in California smokers."

The major features of the American Heart Association guidelines for health professionals to assist their patients in ways to quit smoking are as follows:[44]

(1) counsel smoking patients to quit at every office visit;
(2) ask every patient about their tobacco use and record and update this information on a regular basis;
(3) smoking interventions are helpful in as little as three minutes/visit, but more successful with intense intervention;
(4) clinicians should receive training in patient-centered counseling techniques; and
(5) establish links with other health professionals and organizations to provide smoking cessation interventions.

The routine treatment of smokers by American physicians was a national health objective for the year 2000. Unfortunately, these objectives "fell far short of national health objectives and practice guidelines."[45]

More important than quitting smoking is, of course, to never start. Several studies have examined various methods to stimulate children and adolescents not to begin smoking. In a cross-sectional longitudinal cohort study, Sargent and Dalton[46] recently published their findings as to whether parental disapproval of smoking prevents adolescents from becoming chronic smokers. After controlling for various confounding influences, adolescents who perceived strong parental disapproval of their smoking were less than half as likely to become established smokers. Additionally, the study suggested that the peer smoking effect is attenuated when both parents strongly disapprove of smoking "suggesting that parent disapproval makes adolescents more resistant to the influence of peer smoking." Others[47] found that adolescents who lived in smoke-free households were 74% less likely to smoke than those who lived in households with no smoking restrictions. In addition, adolescents who worked in a smoke-free workplace were 68% less likely to smoke as adolescents whose workplace had no smoking restrictions. Unfortunately, the promotion of smoking by the tobacco industry "appears to undermine the capability of authoritative parenting to prevent adolescents from starting to smoke."[48]

Another major factor that influences young people to begin smoking is the incidence and context of tobacco use in popular movies. In a cross-sectional survey of 4919 children aged nine to 15 years, and after adjustment of confounding factors, the prevalence of ever trying smoking increased as the number of smoking occurences seen in movies increased.[49] Thus, 4.9% tried cigarettes in those who saw 0–50, 13.7% for 51–100, 22.1% for 101–150, and 31.3% for >150. In addition, Tickle *et al.*[50] found that if adolescents' favorite movie stars smoke, they are "significantly more likely to have an advanced smoking status and more favorable attitudes toward smoking than adolescents who choose non-smoking stars." Thus, despite increasing societal anti-smoking sentiments, movies "continue to model smoking as a socially acceptable behavior and portray it as both a way to relieve tension and something to do while socializing."[51]

Coordinated programs to prevent and reduce both youth and adult tobacco use have been implemented in several states. To evaluate its success in Florida, Bauer *et al.*[52] assessed changes in youth cigarette smoking following implementation of the Florida Pilot Program in Tobacco Control. The surveys were completed by 22,540, 20,978 and 23,745 students attending 255, 242 and 243 Florida public middle and high schools in 1998, 1999 and 2000, respectively. After two years, current cigarette use decreased from 18.5% to 11.1% among middle school students, and from 27.4% to 22.6% among high school students. Similar positive findings were reported for cigarette never users, experimenters, current smokers and former smokers. The authors concluded that a comprehensive statewide program "can be effective in preventing and reducing youth tobacco use."

Workplace smoking results in significant employer costs such as increased housekeeping and ventilating expenses, life and safety code expenses, and replacement of computers and furniture.[53] As a result, many employers have addressed the problem with workplace smoking bans. To evaluate smoking ban effectiveness, Longo and associates[54] examined the impact of workplace smoking bans on employee smoking behaviors. This cross-sectional randomized study of five years duration compared current or former smokers employed in smoke-free hospitals with current or former smokers employed in non-smoke-free workplaces. Their findings showed that the quit smoking ratio for those sites that were five years postban was 0.506 in smoke-free workplaces compared with 0.377 in workplaces that allowed smoking. The authors recommended that all industries should examine smoking bans as a method to improve employee health, as well as to reduce medical costs and improve safety and employer operating and maintenance expenses. The Johns Hopkins Medical Institutions' experience is an excellent example of the positive effects of a hospital smoking ban.[55] This prospective cohort study measured changes in employee smoking behavior, environmental fires, smoke-related litter and environmental tobacco pollution exposure. Their findings showed the following: (1) 25% decrease in employee smoking prevalence (21.7% to 16.2%); (2) 25% decrease in the daily number of cigarettes smoked by employees who continued to smoke; (3) significant reduction in the level of public smoking and the quantity of smoking remnants; and (4) decreased concentrations of nicotine vapor in all areas except restrooms.

Smoking and oxidative stress

Increased oxidative stress due to various oxygen-derived free radicals has been associated with over 100 diseases/disorders, including the aging process, atherosclerosis, cancer, cataracts, diabetes and immune deficiencies, among many others.[56] Cigarette smoking has also been associated with many of these disorders. Indeed, each puff of a cigarette reportedly contains over one trillion free radicals in both the tar phase ($\sim 10^{14}$) and gas phase ($\sim 10^{15}$).[57] Cigarette smoking also contains increased levels of nitrogen oxides.[58] As a result, smokers have significantly less antioxidant protection against the effects of oxidative stress. However, the exact biochemical mechanisms involved in the contributions of tobacco smoke to the various diseases are not fully understood, although recent studies have significantly increased our understanding of this association. For example, Reddy *et al.*[59] have shown that exposure of tobacco smoke results in rapid depletion of reduced glutathione (GSH), the major cellular thiol and an important antioxidant in respiratory tract lining fluids. Moreover, the activity of oral peroxidase, the "pivotal enzyme" in the salivary antioxidant system, is significantly decreased in persons after smoking a single cigarette.[60]

Smokers may also have worse dietary habits. For example, French male smokers eat less fruit and vegetables than non-smokers leading to decreased levels of essential antioxidants (i.e. vitamins C and E and beta-carotene).[61] These smokers also had lower plasma levels of ascorbic acid and beta-carotene than non-smokers. Moreover, cigarette smoking accelerates the lowering of plasma vitamin E levels.[62] Environmental tobacco smoke is also associated with decreased serum ascorbic acid levels in both adults[63] and children.[64] In this latter study, the authors noted that children exposed to tobacco smoke have an increased risk of respiratory diseases, asthma, sudden infant death syndrome, lower birth weight and adverse lipid profiles. However, supplementation with dietary antioxidants, such as ascorbic acid, has been shown to modulate the negative effects of tobacco smoke.[65]

Tobacco smoke and atherosclerosis

Cardiovascular disease

Tobacco smoke damages vascular endothelium, a primary antecedent to atherosclerosis.[66,67] Smoking also has negative effects on coronary artery vaso-occlusive factors, such as platelet aggregation, vasomotor reactivity and a prothrombotic state.[68] In addition, studies have consistently demonstrated that smokers have increased plasma levels of cholesterol and decreased levels of high-density lipoprotein cholesterol (HDL-C).[69,70] Furthermore, the negative effects of plasma lipid levels are associated with the number of daily cigarettes smoked. A major theory of the pathogenesis of atherosclerosis is oxidative modification of low-density lipoproteins by free radicals.[71,72] The scientific support for this theory has been recently reviewed.[56]

Atherosclerosis, the major cause of CHD, stroke and gangrene of the lower extremities, is responsible for about 40% of all mortality in the US, Europe and Japan. The 2000 US mortality figures indicated there were 709,894 deaths from heart disease (No. 1 cause of death) and 166,028 deaths from cerebrovascular disease (No. 3 cause of death).[73] Together, they accounted for almost as many deaths as the other eight major causes of death together (Chapter 1, Table 1.1). A relation between cigarette smoking and CHD was first reported at the Mayo Clinic in 1940.[74] Since then, clinical studies have consistently shown that cigarette smoking significantly increases the risk for CHD and acute myocardial infarction (AMI), cerebrovascular disease and stroke, peripheral vascular disease and aortic aneurysm.[75] Indeed, in women with type 2 diabetes mellitus there is a dose-response association between current smoking status and risk for CHD.[76] Compared with never smokers, the relative risks for CHD were 1.21

for past smokers, 1.66 for current smokers (one to 14 cigarettes per day) and 2.68 for current smokers of 15 or more cigarettes per day. The study strongly suggests that diabetic women who stop smoking significantly reduce their risk of CHD. Unfortunately, smokers too often deny the personal consequences of continued smoking. As emphasized by Ayanian and Cleary,[77] "most smokers do not view themselves at increased risk of heart disease or cancer."

Although CHD has long been considered a "man's disease," it is now apparent that CHD is also the No. 1 cause of death in women. Indeed, following menopause, the prevalence of CHD parallels that of men. Moreover, women are more likely to die after a myocardial infarction than men.[78] They are also more likely to die following coronary artery bypass surgery and coronary angioplasty, although these latter events may, at least in part, be related to other factors including diagnostic procedures, treatments, allocation of health care funds, and society's perception of the importance of CHD in women.[79] Thus, one in eight or nine American women aged 45 to 64 years reportedly has clinical evidence of CHD and this increases to one in three in those 65 years and older. With the aging of the population, more American women now die of CHD each year than men. Furthermore, white postmenopausal American women are ten times more likely to die of heart disease than from breast cancer.[79]

Atherosclerosis begins in early childhood and progresses from subendothelial macrophages filled with oxidized low density lipoprotein cholesterol ("foam cells") to the grossly visible, slightly raised yellowish lesions (fatty streaks), to progressively larger raised and later calcified lesions that progressively narrow the arterial lumen (atherosclerotic plaque). In a forensic autopsy study of adolescents and young adults aged 15 to 34 years who died of external causes, McGill *et al.*[80] reported the following: (1) fatty streaks in the aorta were more common in women than men; (2) raised aortic lesions were equal in both sexes; (3) women and men had comparable fatty streaks in the right coronary artery, however raised lesions were about half the extent in women as in men; (4) fatty streaks were more common in blacks than in whites, but raised lesions were similar;

and (5) smokers had more extensive fatty streaks and raised lesions than non-smokers.

Cigar smoking, also associated with serious health risks, has increased rapidly in the US since 1993. To evaluate its relationship to death from CHD, Jacobs and associates[81] studied 121,178 men, aged 30 years and older, over a ten-year period. Interestingly, the risk was not increased among current cigar smokers aged 75 years and older. However, for younger male cigar smokers, the rate ratio of early death from CHD was 1.30. The major consensus conclusions from a recent American Cancer Society conference regarding the effects of cigar smoking were as follows:[82] (1) cigar smoking rates are rising among both adolescents and adults; (2) cigar smoking does not reduce the risk of nicotine addiction; (3) cigar smoking-related deaths approach that of cigarette smoking as the number of cigars smoked and the amount of smoke inhaled increases; (4) cigar smoke contains more toxic and carcinogenic compounds than cigarettes; and (5) cigar smoking increases the risk for cancers of the lung and upper aerodigestive tract.

After reviewing the available epidemiological, clinical, physiological and biochemical evidence prior to 1991, Glantz and Parmley concluded that environmental tobacco smoke was a significant risk factor for heart disease in non-smokers.[83] In a subsequent literature review, these authors concluded that "passive smoking reduces the blood's ability to deliver oxygen to the heart and compromises the myocardium's ability to use oxygen to create adenosine triphosphate."[84] As such, these effects result in "an increased risk of both fatal and non-fatal cardiac events." More recent prospective studies have confirmed that passive smoking increases the risk of CHD. For example, a cohort study of 34,046 American non-smoking female nurses, aged 36 to 61 years and followed for ten years, showed that regular exposure to passive smoking at home or work significantly increased the risk of CHD.[85] Others[86] compared the relationship between active and passive smoking with the progression of atherosclerosis over a three-year period. The changes in atherosclerosis from baseline were assessed by ultrasound measurement of the intimal-medial thickness of the carotid artery. Their findings indicated that both active and passive smoking are associated with progression of atherosclerosis. The authors further emphasized that tobacco smoke is of particular concern for people with diabetes and hypertension.

Although numerous studies have shown that passive smoke increases the risk of CHD, the acute effects of passive smoking on coronary artery circulation in non-smokers had not been evaluated until a recent study by Otsuka *et al.*[87] These researchers assessed the coronary flow velocity reserve by non-invasive transthoracic Doppler echocardiography in 30 Japanese men, half of whom were smokers and half were non-smokers. Their findings showed that passive smoking significantly reduced the coronary flow velocity reserve in the healthy non-smokers. The results provide direct evidence that passive smoking may cause acute endothelial dysfunction in non-smokers.

Significant advances have been made in the treatment of CHD, peripheral vascular disease, and congestive heart failure, as well as in the development of preventive strategies for these diseases. Clinical studies continue to support primary prevention through aggressive treatment of well defined risk factors including weight control, increased physical activity, control of blood lipids, and diets low in fat and rich in fruits, vegetables, grains, omega-3 fatty acids, and not smoking. With respect to this latter risk factor, it is very important to recognize that the risk of myocardial infarction in former smokers approaches that of non-smokers after three years.[88] Moreover, smoking cessation in patients with established CHD is associated with a significant reduction in risk of all-cause mortality.[89] Indeed, even after having a myocardial infarction, smoking cessation significantly decreases the risk mortalilty.[90]

Ischemic and hemorrhagic stroke

Although cigarette smoking is an independent risk factor for stroke, studies conflict on the strength of the relationship. As noted by

Robbins *et al.*,[91] estimates of relative risk of stroke among current male smokers have ranged from 0.90 to 4.2. To study the association more closely, this group examined the relationship between cigarette smoking and risk of stroke in 22,071 men (Physicians' Health Study) aged 40 to 84 at entry for an average of 9.7 years. Their results showed the following risks relative to never smokers: former smokers, 1.20; current smokers of <20 cigarettes per day, 2.02; and current smokers of >20 cigarettes per day, 2.52.

Silent cerebral infarctions were first noted as part of the evaluation of patients with transient ischemic attacks (TIA). Over 30 studies have now reported the prevalence of silent cerebral infarctions in the TIA population; however, estimates of the prevalence of these silent infarctions based on CT scans have varied from 10% to 40%.[92] More recently, Howard and associates[93] reported the incidence of silent cerebral infarctions to be 11% in the general population aged 55 to 70 years. Moreover, cigarette smoking had an ordered association with the presence of silent infarctions. The odds ratios compared with non-smokers not exposed to environmental smoke were as follows: non-smokers exposed to environmental smoke, 1.06; past smokers, 1.16; and current smokers, 1.88. The authors also reported an increased prevalence of silent cerebral infarctions among black, older and hypertensive persons. Indeed, in combination with hypertension, cigarette smoking reportedly results in a ten- to 20-fold increase in risk of stroke compared with the risk in normotensive non-smokers.[94,95]

As with CHD, smoking cessation is associated with a significant reduction in the risk of ischemic stroke, particularly in those who smoke less than 20 cigarettes per day.[96] However, a "complete loss of risk was not seen in heavy smokers." Moreover, switching from cigarettes to pipe or cigar smoking conferred little benefit. Although these and other studies have established that smoking is a risk factor for ischemic stroke, the impact of smoking on intracerebral hemorrhage has been less clear. However, Kurth and associates[97] recently published their findings in a prospective cohort study among 22,022 American male physicians (Physicians' Health Study). They categorized smoking into four groups: never, past, current smokers of <20 cigarettes/day, and current smokers of ≥20 cigarettes/day. Never smokers and past smokers had equal rates for both subarachnoid and intracerebral hemorrhage. Current smokers of <20 cigarettes/day had relative risks of 1.65 for total hemorrhagic stroke, 1.60 for intracerebral hemorrhage and 1.75 for subarachnoid hemorrhage. Current smokers of ≥20 cigarettes/day had a relative risk of 2.36 for total hemorrhagic stroke, 2.06 for intracerebral hemorrhage and 3.22 for subarachnoid hemorrhage.

Tobacco smoke and cancer

The annual incidence rates and numbers of new cases of 25 different cancers in 23 countries for the year 1990 were recently reported.[98] The number of new cancer cases was 8.1 million (excluding non-melanoma skin cancer), slightly over 50% of which occurred in developing countries. The most common malignancy was lung cancer, which accounted for 18% of cancers in men worldwide, and 21% in men in developed countries. The authors concluded that tobacco smoking and chewing are the major risk factors of cancer throughout the world. They estimated that in 1990 there were 5.2 million worldwide deaths, excluding non-melanoma skin cancers, from these 25 different cancers, 55% of which occurred in developing countries.[99] Worldwide, lung cancer is the most common malignant disease with over 900,000 deaths each year followed by gastric (600,000), colorectal (400,000) and liver cancers (400,000). Worldwide, 20% of all cancers are due to smoking.

Smoking causes about one-third of the cancer cases in the US, being associated with cancers of the lung, mouth, pharynx, larynx, esophagus, pancreas, uterine cervix, kidney, ureter and urinary bladder.[100,101] As such, smoking is responsible for about 30% of all cancer deaths in the US. In addition, the overall death rate from cancer is about twice as high among smokers compared with non-smokers. Without a doubt, tobacco use is the most important preventable cause of cancer in the world today. Tobacco products reportedly contain more than 50 established or identified carcinogens which can cause gene mutations that disrupt cell cycle regulation or via pathways that affect the immune and endocrine systems.[102]

Respiratory tract and oral cavity cancers

Lung cancer is the most common cancer in the world and accounts for over 900,000 annual deaths.[99] The estimated number of cases of cancer of the lung and bronchus in the US in 2002 was 169,400 (men, 90,200; women, 79,200); the number of deaths was 154,900 (men, 89,200; women, 65,700).[103] Smoking was responsible for about 85% of these cases.[104] Moreover, a case-control study suggests that 17% of lung cancer cases among non-smokers can be attributed to exposure to high levels of tobacco smoke during childhood and adolescence.[105] In 1992, an estimated 300 lung cancer deaths were due to environmental tobacco smoke.[106] In addition, there were 8900 cases of laryngeal cancer in 2002 and 3700 deaths.[103] Of these, about 82% were due to cigarette smoking.[75]

Although lung cancer incidence in African American men has decreased by 1.6% per year since 1984, the rate is still higher than in any other racial or ethnic group.[107] However, lung cancer rates have remained stable since 1990 in African American women. As a result, the lung cancer death rate among African American men has decreased significantly due to decreased smoking prevalence, but the death rate has continued to increase in African American women.

An estimated 28,900 cases of cancer involving the oral cavity (i.e. tongue, mouth, lip, salivary gland and pharynx) occurred in 2002; there were 7400 deaths.[103] About 93% of these tumors in men and 61% in women are associated with smoking.[75] However, the greatest risk for oral cavity tumors occurs in smokers who regularly use alcohol. This combination accounts for about 75% of all oral and pharyngeal malignancies.[108] Smokeless tobacco has also been established as an important cause of oral cancer.[109,110]

Esophageal cancer

In 2002, there were an estimated 13,100 cases of esophageal cancer in the US (men, 9800; women, 3300) resulting in 12,600 deaths (men,

9600; women, 3000).[103] About 80% of these cases are attributed to smoking.[75] As with oral cancers, the combination of smoking and regular alcohol consumption significantly increases the risk of this malignancy.[110]

Colorectal and anal cancers

In 2002, there were an estimated 148,300 cases of colorectal cancer in the US (colon, 107,300; rectum, 41,000; 72,600 men, 75,700 women) and 56,600 deaths (48,100 colon, 8500 rectum; 27,800 men, 28,800 women).[103] Although early epidemiologic reports of the association between tobacco use and colorectal cancer yielded mixed results, more recent studies have consistently shown a direct correlation between cigarette smoking and colorectal and anal cancers and colorectal adenomas. Indeed, 20% of colorectal cancers in men may be attributable to smoking.[111] The following recent studies are important examples supporting the relationship between smoking and colorectal and anal cancers.

Heineman *et al.*[112] prospectively evaluated a cohort of 248,046 American veterans for 26 years. Their results showed that both colon and rectal cancers increased significantly with pack years of smoking, earlier age at first use, and numbers of cigarettes smoked. More specifically, they estimated that tobacco use accounted for 16% of colon cancer and 22% of rectal cancer deaths. In 1997, 12% of colorectal cancers among both men and women in the general American population were reported to be secondary to cigarette smoking.[113] In addition, in a population-based case-controlled study conducted in northern California, Utah and Minnesota, a 50% increase in colon cancer risk from smoking a pack of cigarettes per day among both men and women was reported.[114] The death rates were lowest among people who had never smoked, intermediate among ex-smokers and highest among current smokers. Furthermore, the younger a person was when he or she began smoking, the greater the risk. Moreover, those who stopped smoking remained at increased risk even if they had not smoked for more than ten years. Neither cigar nor pipe smoking was associated with colon cancer risk.

An early study in men found that smoking for less than 20 years had a strong relation to small colorectal adenomas, smoking for at least 20 years was related to larger adenomas, while colorectal cancers correlated with smoking for at least 35 years.[115] As a result, the authors emphasized the need to intensify efforts to prevent smoking among young people in order to decrease the risk of colorectal cancer later in life. Although most studies have shown an association between smoking and both colon and rectal cancers, all have not. For example, a large study of Canadian women found that although smoking for 30 years or more was significantly associated with an increased risk of rectal cancer, there was no association with colon cancer risk "even with smoking of very long duration and high intensity."[116]

In 2002, there were an estimated 3900 cases of anal cancer in the US (1700 men, 2200 women) and 500 deaths (200 men, 300 women).[103] As with colorectal cancers, most case-controlled studies have shown that smoking increases the risk of anal cancer by a factor of two to five, independent of sexual practices.[117,118]

Pancreatic cancer

Pancreatic cancer is extremely lethal; the death rate being about 98%. In 2002, there were an estimated 30,300 cases of pancreatic cancer in the US (14,700 men, 15,600 women) and 29,700 deaths (14,500 men, 15,200 women).[103] Increasing age and cigarette smoking are the most consistent risk factors for pancreatic cancer. In a population-based, case-control study from 1986 to 1989 involving people in Georgia, Michigan and New Jersey, Silverman and associates[119] reported that cigarette smokers had a 70% increased risk of this malignancy compared with non-smokers. There was also a significant positive trend in risk with increasing duration of smoking. However, smokers who stopped for more than ten years had a 30% reduction in risk compared with current smokers. The proportion of pancreatic cancer attributed to smoking was 27% (blacks 29%, whites 26%).

More recent studies have confirmed that cigarette smoking is a significant risk factor for this malignancy. In a nested case-control study of male smokers (Alpha-Tocopherol, Beta-Carotene Cancer Prevention Study), the authors observed a significant increased risk with increased cigarette exposure (e.g. number of packs smoked per day times the number of years smoked);[120] the odds ratio was 2.13 for the highest versus the lowest quartile. Importantly, serum folate and pyridoxal-5'- phosphate levels showed significant inverse dose-response relationships with pancreatic cancer risk. Individuals with the highest serum levels had about half the risk compared to those with the lowest levels. In a later report,[121] these researchers again confirmed that cigarette smoking is an important risk factor for pancreatic cancer and that dietary folate intake is inversely associated with the risk of pancreatic cancer in male smokers. However, no significant associations were found between dietary methionine, vitamin B_6 or vitamin B_{12}.

Similar findings between cigarette smoking and pancreatic cancer were recently reported among the Japanese.[122] In this large prospective cohort study involving 110,792 people (46,465 men, 64,327 women), the relative risks for current smokers compared with non-smokers were 1.6 in men and 1.7 in women. Men who smoked more than 40 cigarettes each day had a relative risk of 3.3. The study also found a significantly decreasing risk with increasing years after smoking cessation among male ex-smokers; the relative risk for those who had quit smoking for ten or more years was 0.85.

Urinary bladder and kidney cancers

There are currently about 56,500 new cases of urinary bladder cancer each year in the US (41,500 men, 15,000 women) and 12,600 related deaths (8600 men, 4000 women).[103] The major established risk factors for bladder cancer are cigarette smoking and occupational exposure to arylamines.[123] Almost 50% of all bladder and kidney cancer deaths have been attributed to smoking.[124] Thus, studies have consistently reported cigarette smokers have a two- to three-fold increased risk for bladder cancer compared with non-smokers.[123,125]

In a recent population-based case-control study, researchers analyzed their data to determine whether the risk of bladder cancer in smokers differed between men and women.[126] Their results showed a 2.5-fold higher risk of bladder cancer in smokers compared with never smokers. Moreover, the risk for this malignancy was significantly higher in women than in men who smoked comparable numbers of cigarettes. Indeed, recent data from the Iowa Women's Health Study indicated that the relative risk of bladder cancer in women who were current smokers was 3.58 compared with those who never smoked.[127]

Worldwide, renal cell carcinoma accounts for about 2% of all malignancies. In Europe and North America, in contrast to other areas of the world, it has been increasing in frequency. The rate of increase in the US is about 3% per year;[128] the increased rate among blacks is greater than among whites. There were an estimated 31,800 American cases of kidney and renal pelvis cancers in 2002 (19,100 men, 12,700 women) with 11,600 deaths (7200 men, 4400 women).[103]

Several major risk factors for renal cell carcinoma have been reported; these include smoking, obesity, hypertension and occupational exposure to various toxic chemicals.[129] Poor nutrition, primarily due to inadequate intake of fruits and vegetables, has also consistently been shown to be inversely related to kidney cancer. The association between cigarette smoking and kidney cancer has been observed in numerous early studies.[130] More recently, Chiu *et al.*[125] carried out a population-based case-control study in Iowa. Here, cigarette smoking was associated with an increased cancer risk in men (odds ratio 1.8) and in women, but to a lesser degree (odds ratio 1.2). In an interesting retrospective study, Oh and associates[131] reported that smoking and alcohol use were present in 70% and 62% of patients with clear cell renal carcinoma, respectively. In those with Stage MO (i.e. localized disease), the survival rate was significantly worse among smokers than non-smokers. There was also a trend toward a worse survival rate among regular alcohol users compared with those who were not frequent consumers.

Uterine cervix cancer

An estimated 13,000 cases of uterine cervical cancer occurred in the US in 2002; about 4100 of these resulted in death.[103] The major determinants for cervical cancer include sexual factors and transmitted infections.[130] Winkelstein first theorized that cigarette smoking was also related to cervical cancer.[132] Since then, numerous studies have shown an association between cigarette smoking and this malignant disease. For example, after adjusting for age, educational level, church attendance and sexual activity, an early study found that the adjusted risk for a current smoker was 3.42; for having smoked for five or more pack-years, the risk was 2.81.[133] In addition, the adjusted risk estimate associated with passive smoke exposure for three or more hours per day was 2.96. Others suggested that cigarette smoking accounted for about 30% of cervical cancer cases in the early 1990s.[130,134] Overall, the incidence of cervical cancer in smokers appears to be about twice that of non-smokers.[130] Furthermore, smoking cessation significantly decreases the risk for cervical cancer such that former smokers are not at increased risk compared with non-smokers.

Interestingly, smoking results in lower rates of uterine cancer compared with non-smokers.[135] However, an early Nurses' Health Study found no overall relation between breast cancer and smoking.[136] More recently, these latter researchers also reported no relationship between passive smoking and breast cancer. However, they noted that active smoking is "compatible with a small increase in risk of breast cancer when smoking is initiated at young ages."[137]

Myeloid leukemia and other hematologic malignancies

There are about 30,800 annual total cases of leukemia in the US resulting in 21,700 deaths;[103] the number of acute myeloid leukemia cases is estimated at 10,800 with 7400 deaths. Although leukemia has been studied more than many other malignant diseases, its causes still remain largely unknown. However, increasing evidence, particularly over the past two decades, suggests that certain forms of adult leukemia may be associated with smoking. Brownson *et al.*[138] conducted a meta-analysis of available studies from 1970 to 1992, including seven prospective and eight case-control studies. Their findings indicated that approximately 14% of all US leukemia cases may be due to smoking (17% of myeloid and 14% of acute non-lymphocytic leukemias). However, two studies suggested that 20% to 30% of leukemia cases was attributable to smoking in both men and women.[139,140] In their review of the subject, Newcome and Carbone[130] cited several prospective and retrospective studies suggesting that the risk of lymphoid leukemia among cigarette smokers was increased about two-fold and the smoking risk for myeloid leukemia was increased three-fold.

More recent studies suggest that the risk of leukemia among smokers primarily involves myeloid leukemia (odds ratio, 2.0).[141] However, acute myelogenous leukemia (AML) is a heterogeneous disease with distinct subtypes. Pogoda *et al.*[142] examined the association between smoking and adult AML subtype classified by the French-American-British (FAB) criteria. Although they found that the overall risk for AML was mild (odds ratio, 1.2), a significant risk was present for FAB subtype M2 (odds ratio, 2.3). Moreover, a significant dose-response was associated with total years smoked, cigarettes per day and product filter status (i.e. filtered versus non-filtered). In addition, of the morphologic subtypes of AML, Bjork *et al.*[143] reported that the smoking-associated risk for AML was recently found to be restricted to the cytogenetic subgroup t(8;21)(q22,q22).[144]

What is the specific toxin in smoke that might account for the association between cigarette smoking and leukemia? It has been suggested that benzene, an established leukemogen which is present in cigarette smoke, is the responsible agent. Indeed, a typical smoker reportedly inhales about ten times as much benzene as a non-smoker (i.e. 2 mg/day versus 0.2 mg/day).[145] A recent study[146] combined epidemiologic data on the health effects of smoking with a risk assessment technique for low-dose extrapolation, and assessed the proportion of smoking-induced total leukemia and AML attributable to the benzene in cigarette smoke. The conclusion was that benzene is responsible for 10% to 50% of smoking-induced total leukemia mortality and up to 60% of smoking-related AML mortality.

Tobacco smoking may also be a risk factor for myelodysplastic syndromes (i.e. abnormal maturation of red blood cells, platelets and granulocytes) resulting in anemia, thrombocytopenia or pancytopenia. Thus, Bjork et al.[147] reported that smoking was associated with an increased risk for primary myelodysplastic syndromes with chromosome 7 abnormalities (odds ratio, 5.0), refractory anemia (odds ratio, 2.5), and refractory anemia with ringed sideroblasts (odds ratio, 3.2). In addition, smoking for at least one year at some time 20 years or less before diagnosis was associated with an increased risk of myelodysplasia (odds ratio, 1.8).

Recent studies have also suggested that cigarette smoking may be an important risk factor for hematolymphopoietic malignancies. For example, Stagnaro and associates[148] reported only a slightly increased risk for non-Hodgkins lymphoma in smokers (odds ratio, 1.2), but a consistent positive association for follicular non-Hodgkins lymphoma (odds ratio, 1.8). This increased risk for follicular lymphoma was particularly strong for women smokers (odds ratio, 2.3); the risk was only mildly increased for male smokers (odds ratio, 1.3). No clear association was found between smoking and Hodgkins disease or multiple myeloma.

Aging

Life expectancy

Aging is a very complex multifactorial process associated with an increased risk for many diseases (e.g. atherosclerosis, cancer, decreased immune function, macular degeneration, among others).

The major theories of aging are genetic, hormonal, immune and free radical. Of these, the free radical aging theory[56] is of primary importance with regards to smoking (see "Smoking and Oxidative Stress" section and Chapter 1). As noted previously, a single puff on a cigarette results in the formation of an estimated one trillion free radicals.[57] Hence, it is not surprising that smoking accelerates the aging process. Indeed, Taylor and coworkers[149] recently determined the life extension obtained from stopping smoking at various ages among 877,243 respondents to the Cancer Prevention Study II. Their results showed that life expectancy among smokers who quit at age 35 years exceeded those who continued to smoke by 6.9 to 8.5 years for men and 6.1 to 7.7 years for women. Smokers who quit at younger ages experienced even greater life extension. Furthermore, men who stopped smoking at age 65 years gained 1.4 to 2.0 years of life and women gained 2.7 to 3.7 additional years. The association between cigarette smoking and lifespan was also studied in English male physicians.[150] The results showed that the age at which half of the cigarette smokers had died was eight years less than the age for non-smokers; for heavy smokers, it was ten years less.

The effect of smoking and physical activity on active and disabled life expectancy was estimated in the Established Populations for Epidemiologic Studies of the Elderly (EPESE).[151] Here, population-based samples of 8604 persons aged 65 years and older without disability were assessed at baseline and followed for mortality and disability over six annual follow-ups. Compared with smokers, men and women who never smoked survived 1.6 to 3.9 and 1.6 to 3.6 years longer respectively, depending on the level of physical activity. Physical activity from low to moderate to high was associated with an increased life expectancy in both smokers (9.5, 10.5, 12.0 years in men and 11.1, 12.6, 15.3 years in women at age 65) and non-smokers (110, 14.4, 16.2 years in men and 12.7, 16.2, 18.4 years in women at age 65). In agreement with the examples cited in Chapter 3, this study also found that higher physical activity in both smokers and non-smokers was associated with fewer years of disability prior to death.

Skin wrinkling

Smokers have long been suspected of having characteristic facial changes similar to those in premature aging.[152] In 1971, Daniell[153] suggested that smoking might be an important risk factor for premature skin wrinkling. Subsequent reports also indicated that cigarette smoking may accelerate skin wrinkling, but they did not take into consideration confounding variables such as age, sex, sun exposure, or the amount of smoking. After elimination of these confounding factors, Kadunce *et al.*[154] found that the prevalence of skin wrinkling was independently associated with pack-years of smoking. Persons who smoked 50 or more pack-years were 4.7 times more likely to be wrinkled than non-smokers. When both excessive sun exposure and cigarette smoking were present, the risk for excessive wrinkling was multiplicative (prevalence ratio of 12.0). A subsequent literature review of this topic, entitled "Does cigarette smoking make you ugly and old?", confirmed the association between smoking and skin aging.[155] These latter authors suggested that this information "may be important evidence to convince young persons not to begin smoking and older smokers to quit." In this regard, how aware is the general public of the relation between skin aging and smoking? A recent study of 678 randomly selected adults found that current smokers were less likely to be aware of this association compared with former and never smokers.[156] About 25% of the current smokers believed that most smokers would seriously consider this information in their decision to quit smoking.

Technological advances now make it possible to evaluate skin damage before it is grossly observable. For example, Koh and associates[157] assessed the risk of smoking on the development of premature facial wrinkling using computerized image analysis of skin replicas. Their results showed that current smokers have a higher degree of facial wrinkling than non-smokers or past smokers. After adjusting for age, the relative risk of moderate to severe wrinkling for current smokers compared with non-smokers was 2.72. Using image analysis of facial skin replicas, the mean values of Ra (arithmetic average roughness), Rz (average roughness) and Rt (distance between the highest and lowest values) of current smokers were significantly higher than those of past smokers or non-smokers in all age groups.

Gray hair and baldness

Graying of hair is a natural phenomena that consistently affects aging men and women; hair loss is very common in aging men. However, observations of persons less than age 50 years who looked older than expected for their age led Mosley and Gibbs to test the hypothesis that premature hair graying and hair loss may be associated with cigarette smoking.[158] Indeed, their observational results of 268 men and 338 women, 152 of each sex who smoked, did support an association between smoking and gray hair in both men and women and between smoking and hair loss in men.

Taste and smell

Oral changes associated with aging may include decreased levels of smell and taste perceptions, often making foods tasteless and resulting in a decline in appetite.[159] To further complicate the problem, smoking diminishes the taste of food and makes flavorful food taste flat and unappetizing.[160] Various dental problems are also associated with smoking, including periodontal disease, halitosis, tooth staining, stomatitis nicotina and gingival bleeding.[161] As discussed in Chapter 4, protein energy malnutrition is a major problem among the elderly. As these and other studies indicate, smoking further aggravates the serious problem of protein energy malnutrition in older adults.

Chronic obstructive pulmonary disease (COPD)

Chronic obstructive pulmonary disease (COPD) includes a group of diseases characterized by airflow obstruction that is usually associated with breathing-related symptoms (e.g. cough, exertional dyspnea, expectoration and wheeze). The major diseases associated with COPD are emphysema and chronic bronchitis, although the symptoms may be silent and unrecognized in the early phases. Currently,

COPD is known to affect about 16 million Americans, the majority of whom have chronic bronchitis.[162] However, the latest National Health and Nutrition Examination Survey (NHANES III) estimated that approximately 24 million American adults have evidence of impaired lung function, suggesting that COPD is significantly underdiagnosed.[163] The estimated direct COPD medical cost in 1993 was US$14.7 billion; the indirect morbidity costs (e.g. loss of work time and productivity) and premature mortality was an additional US$9.2 billion (total, US$23.9 billion).[164] The current costs are undoubtedly significantly higher since the prevalence of COPD in men, women and the elderly has increased significantly over the past several years. COPD is now the fourth most common cause of death in the US, accounting for 123,550 deaths in 2000.[73]

The most important risk factor for COPD is cigarette smoking. As noted by Rennard,[165] smoking activates inflammatory mechanisms which damage lung tissue. Active proteases and oxidants are thought to play a major role. In response to the injury, repair mechanisms are activated but may also be negatively affected by cigarette smoking. The severity and extent of emphysema in heavy smokers (>30 pack-years) with normal chest radiographs was recently reported using high-resolution CT (HRCT).[166] These researchers correlated their HRCT findings with spirometric tests and symptomatology. Their results showed that 58% of the participants (29 of 50) had significant emphysema by HRCT. Eleven out of 15 with normal spirometric tests showed emphysema by HRCT and two with airflow obstruction on spirometric tests showed normal CT scores. Fourteen percent of the asymptomatic subjects had severe emphysema compared with 64% that were symptomatic. Thus, a significant percentage of asymptomatic and undiagnosed smokers have emphysema.

Invasive pneumococcal disease

Invasive pneumococcal disease is defined as an illness in which *Streptococcus pneumoniae* is isolated from a normally sterile site (e.g. blood and cerebrospinal fluid). The incidence of invasive pneumococcal disease is highest among the young and elderly. However, smokers reportedly account for about half of otherwise healthy adult patients with this disease.[167,168] Since early studies of this disease were not adjusted for multiple risk factors,[167,169] Nuorti *et al.*[170] conducted a population-based case-control study to evaluate the importance of smoking and other possible risk factors. They found that invasive pneumococcal disease was associated with both active cigarette smoking (odds ratio, 4.1) and passive smoking among non-smokers (odds ratio, 2.5) after adjustment for various confounders (e.g. age, sex, black race, chronic illness and low education level). There were also dose-response relations for the current number of cigarettes smoked per day, pack-years of smoking and time since quitting.

Cataract and macular degeneration

Numerous studies have shown that cigarette smoking is an important independent risk factor for developing age-related cataract.[171–176] For example, an early Physician's Health Study based on five years of follow-up showed that current smokers of 20 or more cigarettes per day had a two-fold increased risk of cataract compared with never smokers.[174] More recently, this study was extended to more than 13 years of follow-up and focused on smoking cessation and cataract.[177] Compared with current smokers, the relative risks of cataract in post smokers who quit smoking less than ten years, ten to less than 20 years and 20 or more years before the study were 0.79, 0.73 and 0.74. The relative risk for never smokers was 0.64. The authors concluded that "smoking cessation reduces the risk of cataract primarily by limiting total dose-related damage to the lens."

In 1993, age-related macular degeneration (AMD) was responsible for about 1.7 million cases of visual impairment in the US, and was the major cause of new cases of blindness in persons 65 years or older.[178] For more than two decades, researchers have attempted to identify the major risk factors for AMD. Although only tobacco smoking has been consistently demonstrated across various studies, racial, ethnic and environmental factors are other possibilities. In a prospective cohort study of 21,157 American male physicians (Physicians' Health Study) with an average follow-up period of 12.2 years, current smokers of 20 or more cigarettes per day had an increased relative risk of AMD of 2.46 compared with never smokers.[179] For past smokers, the relative risk was reduced to 1.30. Similarly, a prospective cohort study of 31,843 women (Nurses' Health Study) with 12 years follow-up found that women who smoked 25 or more cigarettes per day had a relative risk of AMD of 2.4 compared with women who never smoked.[180] Past smokers of this number of cigarettes also had a two-fold increased risk compared with never smokers. Moreover, there was minimal reduction in risk for women after quitting smoking for 15 or more years. The risk of AMD also increased with increasing numbers of pack-years smoked. The association between smoking and AMD was further demonstrated in the recent Blue Mountains Eye Study.[181] In this cohort, smokers at baseline had a significant increased risk of five-year incident late AMD and retinal pigment abnormalities compared with never smokers. Moreover, current smokers developed AMD at a significantly earlier age than past or never smokers (current smokers, 67 years; past smokers, 73 years; never smokers, 77 years).

Pulmonary embolism

In the absence of established risk factors for pulmonary embolism, such as antecedent cancer, surgery, trauma or immobilization, prospective data on other possible risks are few. This led Goldhaber *et al.*[182] to prospectively investigate other possible risk factors in a group of 112,822 women (Nurses' Health Study) aged 30 to 55 years who were free from diagnosed CHD and cancer at baseline. In a multivariate analysis, cigarette smoking, obesity and hypertension were all independent predictors of pulmonary embolism. The relative risk for obesity was 2.9; the risk for hypertension was 1.9. The relative risk for women who smoked 25 to 34 cigarettes per day was 1.9; the risk for those who smoked 35 or more cigarettes each day was 3.3.

Osteoporosis

Osteoporotic bone fractures are a very important cause of morbidity and mortality among the elderly. The most common sites of osteoporotic fractures are hip, wrist and vertebrae. The incidence of wrist fractures begins in the earliest postmenopausal period when women are in their 50s and are the most common fracture until age 75 years after which hip fractures become the most common.[183] Osteoporotic fractures are significantly decreased in those who are obese, of short stature, and of African American ethnicity.[184] The major risk factors for osteoporotic fractures are increasing age, female sex, increased body height and total dietary fat intake.[184]

Cigarette smoking is also an important risk factor for osteoporotic fractures. In 1997, Law and Hackshaw[185] published a meta-analysis of 29 cross-sectional studies reporting the difference in bone density in smokers and non-smokers according to age and of 19 cohort case-control studies of the risk of hip fractures in smokers and non-smokers. Their results showed the following: (1) bone density in premenopausal women was similar in smokers and non-smokers; (2) postmenopausal bone loss was greater in current smokers than non-smokers by about an additional 2% for every ten-year increase in age, with a difference of 6% at age 80; and (3) after age 50, the risk of hip fracture in current smokers compared with non-smokers was 17% at age 60, 41% at 70, 71% at 80 and 108% at 90. In a more recent population-based case-control study in Sweden, Baron and associates[186] assessed the association of cigarette smoking with hip fracture risk among postmenopausal women. Compared with never smokers, current smokers had an increased risk of hip fracture (odds ratio, 1.66). In addition, smoking duration, especially after menopause, was more important than the amount smoked. Women who stopped smoking had a minimal increased risk of hip fracture compared with never smokers (odds ratio, 1.15).

A cross-sectional study of bone density at the lumbar spine and femoral neck and shaft was carried out in 41 pairs of female twins aged 27 to 73 years of age who were discordant for at least five pack-years of smoking.[187] The results showed that for every ten pack-years of smoking, the bone density of the twin who smoked more heavily was 2.0% lower at the lumbar spine, 0.9% lower at the femoral neck and 1.4% lower at the femoral shaft. For those who were discordant by 20 or more pack-years, the differences in bone density at the three sites were 9.3%, 5.8% and 6.5%, respectively. The authors concluded that women who smoke 20 or more cigarettes per day throughout adulthood will, by the time of menopause, have an average bone density deficit of 5% to 10%.

The mechanism whereby smoking increases the risk for bone fractures is poorly understood. To evaluate this, Krall *et al.*[188] studied the relationship of smoking to rates of bone mineral density (BMD) change at the femoral neck, spine and total body, as well as intestinal calcium absorption, in elderly men and women. After adjusting for various confounders (i.e. BMD, weight, age, gender and calcium intake), the annualized rates of BMD loss were higher in smokers than in non-smokers at the femoral neck and total body. Moreover, the mean calcium absorption was lower in smokers than non-smokers. Thus, their data suggests that smoking accelerates total body and femoral neck bone loss due to decreased intestinal calcium absorption.

Menopause and pregnancy-associated disorders

In addition to menopause-associated osteoporosis, studies have shown that smoking is associated with a wide variety of other disorders such as the time to reach menopause, fertility and fetal disorders, and newborn male to female ratio.

Time of menopause

Smoking has been shown to shorten the time to reach menopause.[189] For example, a population-based random study of white women, aged 45 to 55 years, found that current smokers reached menopause an average of 1.74 years earlier than non-smokers.

Fetal complications

In an early literature review,[190] the author quoted studies showing that women who smoke have higher rates of infertility, fetal growth retardation, neonatal deaths, premature delivery and possible negative effects on lactation. Early human clinical studies and experimental work in rodents suggested that nicotine may alter the hypothalamic-pituitary axis with increased production of growth hormone, cortisol, vasopressin and oxytocin which may inhibit the release of luteinizing hormone and prolactin.

Male to female birth ratio

Studies from numerous developed countries have shown that the newborn male to female ratio has declined significantly over the past several decades. Although the reasons for this phenomenon remains unclear, chronic exposure to various toxic agents that predominantly affect the male reproductive system might explain the lower male : female ratio. Indeed, increased exposure to dioxin[191] and methylmercury[192] both resulted in a reduced male : female ratio. A recent study also found that the male : female ratio was lower when either or both parents smoked more than 20 cigarettes per day compared with parents in which neither smoked.[193] The lowest sex ratio was noted when both parents smoked 20 or more cigarettes per day.

Birth weight

Maternal smoking is a significant risk factor for low-birth-weight infants. This in turn affects infant mortality and the long-term outcome of surviving infants. However, maternal cigarette smoking is the most modifiable risk factor for intrauterine growth restriction in developed countries.[194] However, not all women who smoke cigarettes during pregnancy have low-birth-weight infants. In a recent study,[195] continuous maternal smoking during pregnancy was associated with an average reduction of 377 g in birth weight (odds ratio, 2.1). However, the magnitude of the effect of maternal smoking on birth weight was dependent on their genotype at two genes involved in the metabolism of smoking toxins (CYP1A1 and GSTT 1).

Miscellaneous disorders

Multiple sclerosis

Although environmental factors have long been considered to play a role in the development of multiple sclerosis (MS), few such factors have been positively identified. As noted by Hernan *et al.*,[196] experimental studies have shown that cigarette smoke has both neurotoxic and immunomodulatory effects. In addition, epidemiologic investigations have suggested that cigarette smoking is associated with some autoimmune disorders (e.g. systemic lupus erythematosus and rheumatoid arthritis). Although several studies have supported an association between cigarette smoking and MS, all have not.

Two relatively small prospective studies recently suggested an increased incidence of MS among smokers,[197,198] although neither study attained statistical significance. However, a recent report from both the Nurses' Health Study and Nurses' Health Study II involving 121,700 women aged 30 to 55 years at baseline in 1976 and 116,671 women aged 25 to 42 years at baseline in 1989 reported that cigarette smoking may be an important risk factor.[196] Compared to women who never smoked, the relative rates of MS among current smokers was 1.6; it was 1.2 for past smokers. The relative incidence rate increased with increased smoking. The study was adjusted for age, latitude and family history. The authors concluded that although the biologic basis for the association between smoking and MS is poorly understood, "these results suggest that smoking may increase the risk of developing MS."

Impaired thyroid hormone function

Early studies of the effect of smoking on thyroid function have been controversial, some showing an effect while others did not. To help clarify the problem, 138 normal women, 84 women with subclinical hypothyroidism, and 51 women with overt hypothyroidism were studied to determine the possible effect of cigarette smoking on thyroid function.[199] Among the subclinical hypothyroid group, the smokers had a higher mean serum level of thyrotropin (21.3 ± 16.6 versus 12.7 ± 7.2 mU/L), and a higher ratio of serum triiodothyronine to serum free thyroxine (by 30%) than the non-smokers. Among those with overt hypothyroidism, the serum concentrations of thyrotropin, free thyroxine and triiodothyronine were similar in the smokers and non-smokers. Compared with the non-smokers, however, the smokers had a clinical score indicating a greater degree of hypothyroidism (i.e. higher serum levels of total and low-density lipoprotein cholesterol, longer ankle-reflex time, and higher serum levels of creatine kinase). The authors concluded that "smoking increases the metabolic effects of hypothyroidism in a dose-dependent way." That is, smoking decreases both thyroid secretion and thyroid hormone action.

Type 2 diabetes mellitus

The significance of cigarette smoking with the development of impaired fasting glucose and type 2 diabetes has been unclear. To better understand this association, 1266 Japanese men aged 35 to 59 years without either impaired fasting glucose or type 2 diabetes at baseline were followed for five years (1994–1999)[200] After controlling for possible predictors of diabetes, the relative risks for impaired fasting glucose (fasting serum glucose 110–125 mg/dL) compared with never smokers were as follows: 1.62 for never smokers; 1.14 for those who smoked 1–20 cigarettes per day; 1.33 for those who smoked 21–30 cigarettes per day; and 2.56 for those who smoked ≥31 cigarettes each day. The adjusted relative risks for type 2 diabetes (fasting serum glucose ≥126 mg/dL) compared with never smokers were 1.08, 1.88, 3.02 and 4.09, respectively. The number of pack-years of smoking was also positively related to the development of both impaired fasting glucose and type 2 diabetes.

Hemoglobin level

Cigarette smoking, long known to increase hemoglobin levels, is thought to be due to increased exposure to carbon monoxide (CO). CO binds to hemoglobin to form carboxyhemoglobin, which is inactive and unable to carry oxygen. To adjust for the decreased oxygen delivery capacity, smokers maintain higher hemoglobin levels than non-smokers.[201] To further clarify its clinical importance, a later investigation found that women smokers had a mean hemoglobin level of 13.7 g/dL compared with 13.3 g/dL for never smokers.[202] Among men, the mean hemoglobin levels for smokers and never smokers were 15.6 g/dL and 15.2 g/dL, respectively. This upward shift of the hemoglobin distribution curve reduces the utility of hemoglobin level to detect mild anemia, mainly in women. Thus, the mean prevalence of anemia was 4.8% among women smokers compared with 8.5% among never smokers. The authors suggested that the lower hemoglobin cut-off values should be adjusted for smokers to compensate for "the masking effect of smoking on the detection anemia."

Physical function

Physical function progressively declines with increasing age, thereby limiting their activities and predisposing them to falls and injuries. Some of these lost functions, however, are preventable and include lack of regular physical activity, use of sedatives or tranquilizers, and excessive body weight. In addition, function decline has been associated with cigarette smoking.[203] For example, Nelson *et al.*[204] studied 9704 community-dwelling ambulatory women 65 years and older from four areas of the US. Twelve performance tests of muscle strength, agility and coordination, gait and balance, and self-reported functional status were evaluated. After adjusting for age, history of stroke, body mass index (BMI), physical activity and alcohol use, current smokers had significantly poorer function on all of the performance measures except grip strength compared with never smokers. This functional decrease was 50% to 100% as great as that associated with a five-year age increase. Moreover, most measures worsened with increasing number of pack-years.

Psychological features and cognitive decline

Several early studies linked cigarette smoking with either a negative affect (i.e. tension, anxiety, anger and a depressed mood) or with distinct depressive symptoms. For example, smokers rated higher on symptomatic measures of both anxiety and depression than non-smokers.[205] Moreover, depressive symptoms among 15- and 16-year-old children were associated with their smoking status about a decade later.[206] Others[207] reported that smoking was more common among depressed patients from a psychiatric clinic than in the general population.

Glassman and associates[208] later verified the association of smoking with major depression. They also confirmed their earlier observation that smokers without a psychiatric problem are more successful in cessation efforts than smokers with a lifetime diagnosis of depression (31% versus 14%). Similarly, Anda *et al.*[209] reported that after adjusting for age, sex, number of cigarettes smoked and educational level, depressed smokers were 40% less likely to have quit after nine years compared with non-depressed smokers. In a somewhat related study, Gulliver *et al.*[210] noted an important interrelationship between smoking and alcohol dependence. The study demonstrated the following, among others: (1) alcohol dependence predicted an urge to smoke during alcohol treatment; (2) exposure to alcohol cues increased the urge to smoke; and (3) the urge to smoke was positively correlated with an urge to drink.

Cigarette smoking has also been associated with gambling, but little is known about smoking in disordered gamblers. To better understand the association, Petry and Oncken[211] compared psychosocial problems and gambling in smoking gamblers who sought treatment. Their results showed that daily smokers gambled more often and spent more money on gambling than non-smokers. Smokers also craved gambling more and had lower perceived control over their gambling habits. Moreover, daily smokers were taking more psychiatric medications and experienced more frequent anxiety episodes than non-smokers.

Although several population-based studies of the association between smoking and cognitive impairment have generally shown either weak or no association, others have indicated an increased risk of cognitive decline. Perhaps a major explanation in the inconsistency of these reports is that most the earlier studies were conducted among retired older people. However, a more recent cross-sectional study of mainly middle-aged people showed reduced psychomotor speed and cognitive flexibility among current smokers compared with those who had never smoked.[212] Similarly, in a recent multiple regression study, Richards *et al.*[213] found that smoking in men and women aged 43 to 53 years was associated with faster declines in verbal memory and with slower visual search speeds. These negative effects were primarily associated with individuals who smoked 20 or more cigarettes per day. The results were independent of sex, socioeconomic status, adolescent cognitive ability, as well as various health indicators.

Alcohol Consumption

Prevalence and economic costs

Alcohol is the most commonly abused drug throughout the world. Indeed, alcohol abuse is the third leading preventable cause of death in the US. In 1994, alcoholism claimed about 100,000 American lives and cost over US$100 billion.[214] In 2000, the economic cost of alcohol misuse was estimated at US$185 billion.[215] Of this amount, US$22.5 billion was attributed to underage drinking (12–22 years of age) and US$34.4 billion to excessive adult drinking (>2 drinks/day).[216]

Adams and coworkers[217] reported that among persons admitted to general hospitals, 20% to 40% had alcohol-related problems. Among older people, alcohol-related hospitalizations were as frequent as those due to myocardial infarction. Further evidence of the increased medical costs in heavy alcohol consumers was shown by Cryer *et al.*[218] who randomly surveyed 41,000 adults regarding their use of acute and preventive medical services. The study confirmed that heavy alcohol consumers are disproportionate users of acute medical services (i.e. accident and emergency services). Conversely, these individuals are underusers of preventive medicine services.

Alcohol is regularly consumed by about 50% of adults and an estimated 15 to 20 million Americans are alcoholics. The American Medical Association (AMA) guidelines reported that at least three million Americans over age 60 years are alcoholics or have a major drinking problem.[219] Unfortunately, those in this latter "hidden" group are frequently not identified by their physicians. Rather, the signs of alcohol abuse, such as incontinence, dementia, seizures and falls may be mistakenly attributed to aging. A member of the AMA guidelines advisory panel recently stated, "This problem takes a horrendous toll on society. Not only are the financial implications staggering, but more importantly it results in a tragic loss of productive years — a loss felt by families and communities."[220]

The trends in alcohol consumption in the US between 1984 and 1995 differed among whites, blacks and Hispanics.[221] This report noted that heavy drinking decreased significantly among white males (from 20% to 12%), but remained stable among black (15% on both dates) and Hispanic men (17% and 18%). Frequent heavy drinking also decreased among white women (from 5% to 2%), but again remained stable among black (5% on both dates) and Hispanic women (2% and 3%).

Binge drinking, the consumption of five or more alcoholic beverages on one occasion, usually leads to acute impairment and causes a significant fraction of all alcohol-related disabilities and deaths. The adverse health risks associated with binge drinking reportedly include the following:[222] unintentional injuries (e.g. motor vehicle accidents, falls, drowning, hypothermia and burns), suicide, sudden infant death syndrome, hypertension, myocardial infarction, gastritis, pancreatitis, sexually transmitted diseases and poor diabetic control. In addition, increased homicide, assault, domestic violence, rape, child neglect and abuse, and lost productivity further add to the high social and economic costs.

Detection, screening and counseling

Most physicians care for patients with alcohol-related problems. However, physicians often fail to identify alcoholism, especially in its early stage. Moreover, they frequently feel ill-equipped due to their own inadequate training, attitudinal barriers and perceived lack of skill.[223] Even when routine screening of hospital admissions for alcoholism is recommended, the diagnosis is relatively low and treatment varies significantly depending on the department.[224] Thus, detection rates in patients who screened positive were as follows: surgery and obstetrics & gynecology, <25%; neurology, 25%; medicine, 50%; and psychiatry, >50%. In addition, patients with higher incomes, higher education, private insurance, women and those who strongly denied alcohol intake were less likely to be identified. Patients identified as having alcohol dependence or abuse were significantly more likely to be men, non-white, younger and of low socioeconomic status, suggesting there was a stereotyped image of people with alcohol dependence or abuse.

Unfortunately, the alcohol-related recurring problems, including those associated with impending death, often leaves physicians with the impression that these patients rarely respond to counseling. The fact is, however, several studies in Europe and the US have shown that simple interventions can be very successful. For example, a randomized controlled trial conducted in 47 general practitioners' offices in the UK reported significant reductions in alcohol use by the intervention group compared with the control group.[225] Similarly, the World Health Organization Trial, carried out in ten countries, reported similar findings in alcohol consumption between the intervention and control groups.[226] A more recent randomized controlled clinical study of 17,695 patients screened for problem drinking was carried out in 17 community-based primary care practices in Wisconsin.[227] The intervention consisted of two ten- to 15-minute counseling visits that included advice, education and contracting information. Compared with the control group, which received no intervention, the decreases in reported alcohol intake were substantially and statistically significant and were present at both the six-month and 12-month follow-ups. One simple, practical and somewhat reliable tool used in this and other studies to screen for alcohol abuse is the CAGE questionnaire.[228] Here, alcohol abuse is considered to exist if a person answers "yes" to two or more of the following four questions that begin with, "Have you ever …"

(1) tried to Cut down on your drinking?
(2) been Annoyed by anybody criticizing your drinking?
(3) felt Guilty about your drinking?
(4) had an Eye-opener (drink) in the morning?

Older people are more vulnerable to the adverse effects of alcohol than are younger individuals and are more likely to hide their alcohol use.[229] Although the CAGE questionnaire has been recommended for primary care physicians,[230] it is reportedly insufficient when used as the sole screening tool, at least in older patients.[231] In this study, 5065 consecutive persons over 60 years completed a self-administered questionnaire that included beverage-specific questions about the quantity and frequency of regular alcohol consumption over the previous three months, the number of binge drinking episodes (≥ 6 drinks/occasion), and the CAGE questionnaire. The study showed that 15% of men and 12% of women regularly consumed more than the maximum recommended amount (i.e. >7 drinks/week for women; >14 drinks/week for men). The CAGE questionnaire identified only 9% of men and 3% of women that consumed more than the recommended amount. Moreover, the CAGE was relatively ineffective in detecting heavy or binge drinkers.

Researchers from the Mayo Clinic used the Self-administered Alcoholism Screening Test (SAAST) in a study involving 795 adult in-patients at two teaching hospitals.[232] The records of SAAST-positive patients were reviewed to determine the number receiving laboratory screening tests, addiction consultative services, and a discharge diagnosis of alcoholism. Of the SAAST participants, 42 (7.4%) had a positive alcohol-dependent score. Of these, 13 (31%) received addictive or psychiatric consultative services during their hospitalization. However, only 11% of the alcoholics received an alcohol screening test and 7% had a discharge diagnosis of alcoholism. The authors concluded that laboratory screening tests in hospitalized patients are underutilized and that there are persistent problems in physician detection, assessment and diagnosis of alcoholism. Indeed, "...diagnosis of alcohol dependence had not improved from similar observations more than 20 years earlier."

Other alcohol-abuse screening methods include laboratory testing. Indeed, gamma-glutamyltransferase (GGT), aspartate aminotransferase (AST), alanine aminotransferase (ALT), and the mean red cell volume (MCV) are common markers of alcohol abuse.[233] These tests are, however, not highly sensitive and are more often within the reference range unless there is liver damage (i.e. GGT, AST and ALT) or nutrition deficiencies, especially folic acid (i.e. MCV). Several more recent markers, such as carbohydrate deficient transferrin, are more sensitive and specific for alcohol abuse.[234]

Alcohol-related diseases and disorders

The major diseases and disorders related to excess alcohol consumption include all-cause mortality, malnutrition, cardiovascular diseases, stroke, various cancers, liver diseases, injuries, suicide, psychiatric disorders, newborn abnormalities, dementia and cognitive dysfunction among others (Table 5.2).

Mortality

Alcohol consumption has both adverse and beneficial effects on survival. Modest alcohol intake is associated with increased life expectancy, primarily due to decreased CHD and ischemic stroke. However, excess consumption increases mortality from accidents, violence, suicide, poisoning, liver disease and certain cancers. Numerous studies have shown that the relationship between mortality and quantity of alcohol intake follows either a U- or J-shaped curve. For example, in a prospective study of 7234 women and 6051 men aged 30 to 79 years and followed for ten to 12 years, the U-shaped curve nadir occurred in those who consumed "one to six

Table 5.2: Major Alcohol-Related Diseases and Disorders

All-Cause Mortality
Cancer
  Breast
  Colon
  Kidney
  Liver
  Oropharyngeal, esophageal
  Pancreas
Cardiac Diseases
  Cardiomyopathy
  Coronary heart disease
  Hypertension
Gastritis, Pancreatitis
Injuries, Accidents
Liver Diseases
  Alcoholic hepatitis
  Cirrhosis
Malnutrition
Newborn-Associated Disorders
  Fetal alcohol syndrome
  Birth defects
  Neurodevelopmental disorders
Psychiatric Disorders
Stroke
Type 2 Diabetes Mellitus

alcoholic beverages per week (a "beverage" was defined as one bottle of beer, glass of wine, or measure of spirits).[235] Thus, abstainers had a relative risk of 1.37 whereas those drinking more than 70 beverages per week had a relative risk of 2.29. Sex, age and BMI did not significantly change the risk level. Similarly, Doll *et al.*[236] Dementia/ Cognitive Dysfunction prospectively studied a large group of British doctors over a 13-year period. After the data was standardized for age, calendar year and smoking habit, their results showed a U-shaped relation between all-cause mortality and the average amount of alcohol consumed. Those who averaged 1–2 units/day (a unit was defined as one glass of beer, lager, or wine and 1/2 glass of spirits or liqueur) had the lowest risks, mainly due to decreased ischemic heart disease. However, all-cause mortality progressively increased when the amount consumed exceeded 3 units/day.

Additional important data regarding alcohol consumption and mortality came from a very large group of men and women (490,000) aged 30 to 104 years (mean, 56 years).[237] Here, as with other studies, diseases associated with drinking were cirrhosis and alcoholism, various cancers including mouth, esophagus, pharynx, larynx and liver in both men and women, breast in women, and injuries and other external causes in men. However, the rates of death from cardiovascular diseases were 30% to 40% lower among both sexes who consumed at least one drink per day compared with non-drinkers. Moreover, the overall death rates were modestly lower among men and women who consumed about one drink each day. However, all causes-mortality increased with heavier drinking.

In a recent study, Gronbaek *et al.*[238] compared the type of alcohol consumed (i.e. beer, wine and spirits) with mortality among 13,064 men and 11,459 women aged 20 to 98 years. The results showed J-shaped relations between total alcohol consumption and mortality at various levels of wine intake. Compared with non-drinkers, light drinkers who avoided wine had a relative risk for all-cause mortality of 0.90 while those who drank wine had a relative risk of 0.66. Heavy drinkers who avoided wine were at higher risk for all-cause mortality compared with heavy drinkers who included wine with other alcoholic beverages. Moreover, wine drinkers had significantly lower mortality rates from both CHD and cancer than did non-wine drinkers (see "Polyphenols," Chapter 4).

The mortality-related benefits of light-to-moderate alcohol consumption begin to outweigh the risks among men in their 40s[239,240] and women in their 50s.[241] However, the authors of this latter study concluded that the increased survival among women with light-to-moderate alcohol consumption may be largely confined to those at greatest risk for CHD. Moreover, in men and women less than 40 years, alcohol consumption is associated with an increase in all-cause mortality even at low levels of drinking. Although young adults have a very low risk of CHD, their risk of injuries is high. For example, in a 15-year follow-up of 18- to 19-year-old Swedish male military conscripts, CHD risk was lower in drinkers than in non-drinkers.[242] However, this accounted for only 4% of all deaths while violent deaths, mainly from suicide and road traffic accidents, was positively associated with alcohol even in those drinking <12 units/week, and accounted for 75% of all deaths. More recently, Hingson *et al.*[243] studied the magnitude of alcohol-related morbidity and mortality among 18 to 24-year-old college students. They estimated that over 1400 students died in 1998 from alcohol-related unintentional injuries, including motor vehicle accidents. In addition, over 500,000 full-time students were unintentionally injured while under the influence of alcohol and over 600,000 were struck or assaulted by another student who had been drinking.

Malnutrition

About 15% of older outpatients and about 50% of all hospitalized elderly persons are protein-calorie malnourished (Chapter 4).[244] The prevalence is even greater in those who are excessive alcohol consumers. Select vitamin (e.g. D, C, E, etc.) and mineral (e.g. magnesium, potassium, zinc, calcium, phosphorus, etc.) deficiencies are also all very common in older alcoholics. For example, vitamin D deficiency and fat malabsorption impairs vitamin D metabolism. This may result in osteomalacia with increased risk of bone pain and fractures. In addition, the Wernicke-Korsakoff syndrome is due to thiamine deficiency, a common problem in alcoholism. Here, cognitive symptoms may be mistaken for delirium or dementia if alcohol abuse is not recognized. Thus, malnutrition is clearly linked to increased morbidity, prolonged hospital stays, more frequent readmissions, susceptibility to pressure ulcers and increased mortality.

Alcohol is a substantial source of energy with 7.1 kcal per gram, a value that significantly exceeds the energy content of carbohydrates and proteins. As a result, ethanol accounts for about 50% of an alcoholic's daily caloric intake. As such, it displaces critical nutrients including folic acid, thiamine and other essential vitamins such as A, B_1, B_6, B_{12}, C, D, E and various important antioxidants (e.g. beta-carotene, lycopene, lutein and flavonoids). It also results in a deficiency of essential minerals such as magnesium, zinc, selenium, iron and copper among others. Malabsorption due to gastrointestinal complications is also common in alcoholics (e.g. pancreatic insufficiency and impaired liver metabolism of nutrients). Although alcohol is rich in calories, long-term consumption of up to 2000 calories per day in the form of ethanol does not produce the expected gain in body weight.[245] This is due, at least in part, to the poor yield of energy produced from the oxidation of fat in damaged mitochondria and to microsomal pathways that oxidize alcohol without conserving chemical energy.

Alcoholic liver disease

Alcoholic liver disease is one of the most common causes of chronic liver disease in the world. Indeed, alcoholism and alcohol-related diseases affect over ten million Americans and, after heart disease and cancer, represents the third largest health problem in the US.[246] Because of the intrinsic toxicity of alcohol, it can injure the liver even in the absence of dietary deficiencies.[247] The quantity of alcohol consumption required to produce clinically significant liver disease varies with age, sex, race and body size. It may also vary within a given person at different times. Studies vary as to how much alcohol is needed to produce hepatocellular damage. Some reports show an increased risk of cirrhosis with 40–60 g of ethanol/day in males and 20 g/day in females. Other studies suggest that ≥80 g of ethanol/day are required (i.e. eight 12-ounces of beer, one liter of wine, or a half-pint of 80-proof whiskey). Thus, it appears that a limited subpopulation of alcoholics is predisposed, probably by genetics, to develop severe liver disease.

The liver changes associated with chronic excessive alcohol consumption are certainly well established. The first manifestation of alcoholic liver disease, the accumulation of fat within hepatic cells (steatosis), can begin to develop within days of heavy alcohol intake. This is followed by early fibrosis, which in turn may be associated with alcoholic hepatitis, the most common type of hepatitis in the US and other industrialized nations. Continued heavy alcohol intake leads to irreversible damage characterized by severe fibrosis and subsequently to cirrhosis.

The mechanisms whereby ethanol exerts its toxic effects are not fully understood. However, DiLuzio[248] first reported that ethanol-induced fatty liver could be partially prevented by the administration of anti-oxidants and hypothesized that ethanol-induced hepatic injury resulted from lipid peroxidation, a free radical process. Since then, abundant experimental data indicate that free radical mechanisms contribute significantly to ethanol-associated liver damage. Moreover, free radicals have also been implicated in ethanol toxicity on various extrahepatic tissues. An extensive review of the experimental evidence supporting the role of free radicals in alcohol-induced hepatotoxicity has been published.[249]

Cardiovascular diseases

(1) Coronary heart disease

Early studies[250] indicated that light-to-moderate alcohol consumption (1–2 alcoholic drinks/day) is protective against CHD, the number one cause of death in the US among both women and men. Since then, numerous studies have confirmed this protective effect. Furthermore, regular moderate alcohol drinking in the year prior to an acute myocardial infarction is associated with a significant decrease in mortality in both men and women.[251] A recent study also indicated that modest alcohol consumption decreases the risk of peripheral arterial disease in men.[252] The suggested explanation of the protective effect of ethanol on CHD is that it increases the serum level of "good" cholesterol (i.e. HDL-C), which is anti-atherogenic. Moreover, red wine contains polyphenolic antioxidants (i.e. flavonoids) which have also been reported to be protective against CHD (Chapter 4).[253]

Although numerous studies have shown that moderate alcohol consumption decreases the risk of myocardial infarction (MI), the effects of the drinking pattern and type of alcoholic beverage consumed is somewhat unclear. Mukamal *et al.*[254] studied the association of alcohol intake with the risk of MI among 38,077 men (Health Professionals Follow-up Study) who were free of cancer and cardiovascular disease at baseline and were followed from 1986 to 1998. Their findings showed that compared with men who consumed alcohol less than once per week, those who consumed alcohol 3–4 or 5–7 days/week had significantly decreased risks of MI. The risk was similar in those who consumed less than 10 g of alcohol/drinking day and those whose intake was $\geq$30 g/drinking day. Interestingly, no single type of beverage (i.e. beer, red wine, white wine and liquor) conferred additional benefit, nor did drinking with meals. However, these results conflict to some extent with other studies, including the one referred to earlier.[253] For example, a pilot study from Spain showed a significant increase in plasma HDL-C levels and decreased low-density lipoprotein (LDL) oxidation after ingestion of red wine compared with the same amount of alcohol consumed as spirits.[255] Moreover, the relation between blood lipid levels and the consumption of different types of alcoholic beverages among French women and men showed that wine drinkers had higher HDL-C levels than non-wine drinkers.[256]

Type 2 diabetes is an established major risk factor for CHD. However, a recent report suggests that alcohol consumption decreases the risk of CHD in older patients with type 2 diabetes.[257] Here, the mortality rates from CHD in never drinkers, former drinkers, alcohol intake <2 g/day, 2–13 g/day and >14 g/day were 43.9, 38.5, 25.3, 20.8 and 10.0 per 1000 person years, respectively. After controlling for various common risk factors (i.e. age, sex, cigarette smoking, etc.), the relative risks for former drinkers, those who drank <2 g/day, 2–13 g/day and >14 g/day were 0.69, 0.54, 0.44 and 0.21 compared with never drinkers.

Although these and other studies clearly indicate that moderate daily alcohol consumption has a protective effect on CHD, higher intakes result in various other medical and social problems. As noted by Criqui and Golomb,[258] alcohol intake by diabetics may induce, or even mask, hypoglycemia by exaggerating hypoglycemic effects caused by other factors (e.g. insulin, exercise and various medications). Furthermore, about half of regular alcohol consumers will experience some alcohol-associated problem in their lifetime, including cancer, liver disease, depression, injuries, social discord and drug interactions. High levels of alcohol consumption have also been associated with paroxysmal supraventricular arrhythimia. Suggested possible mechanisms for this latter relationship include subclinical alcohol cardiomyopathy, electrolyte abnormalities and increased catecholamine levels.[259]

(2) Cardiomyopathy

Alcohol-related cardiomyopathy was recognized over 100 years ago. For example, Bollinger,[260] in discussing cardiac hypertrophy in habitual beer drinkers, noted in 1884 that "with excessive habitual use of beer, one has to take into account the direct effect of alcohol on the heart." Nevertheless, alcoholic cardiomyopathy is still somewhat difficult to clinically distinguish from other cardiomyopathies. However, since 1960 the circumstantial evidence for an association between chronic alcohol abuse and cardiomyopathy has been very strong and includes autopsy studies showing abnormalities in a high percentage of alcoholics, acute and chronic functional and metabolic abnormalities, and structural changes related to alcohol consumption.[259] Indeed, long-term heavy alcohol consumption is the leading cause of non-ischemic, dilated cardiomyopathy among both sexes in the US.[261] According to this literature review, alcoholics who consume >90 g of alcohol/day (7–8 drinks/day) for five or more years are at risk of developing asymptomatic cardiomyopathy. Those who continue to drink at this level may become symptomatic and develop heart failure. Others have shown an inverse dose-dependent relationship between ethanol consumption and cardiac ejection fractions.[262] In addition, women develop alcoholic cardiomyopathy as frequently as men although they usually consume significantly less alcohol.[263,264] Moreover, women are more sensitive to the toxic effects of alcohol on striated muscle (alcoholic myopathy).[263]

The prognosis of alcoholic cardiomyopathy has generally been thought to be better than idiopathic cardiomyopathy if these individuals abstain from alcohol. Fauchier *et al.*[265] have, however, recently reported that patients with alcoholic cardiomyopathy do not have a better prognosis than those with idiopathic cardiomyopathy. Since alcoholism without abstinence in these patients is strongly related to cardiac death, these researchers stressed the need for "a more aggressive approach to alcohol cessation."

(3) Hypertension

An association between high intakes of alcohol and hypertension was first observed in French servicemen in 1915.[266] However, this relationship received little attention until epidemiologic studies over the past few decades linked increasing alcohol intake, along with obesity and increased salt intake, as an important risk factor for hypertension. The association between high alcohol intake and hypertension has been reported in both prospective and cross-sectional studies. For example, the major independent hypertensive risk factors in a recent large cross-sectional study of 19,961 individuals were overweight, current smoking, physical inactivity and high alcohol consumption.[267] A large prospective study of the level of alcohol intake and risk of hypertension in women aged 25 to 42 years was recently reported (Nurses' Health Study II).[268] The findings showed a J-shaped curve; light drinkers (0.5–1.0 drinks/day) had a modest decrease in risk while more regular heavy drinkers (≥ 1.5 drinks/day) demonstrated an increased risk. A review of the relevant literature associating hypertension with alcohol intake has been published.[269]

Cerebrovascular disease and stroke

Cerebrovascular disease is a major cause of disability and is the third leading cause of death in the US.[73] In addition, stroke is a huge financial burden for patients, their families and the health care system. The cost of stroke in the US in 2002 was estimated to be US\$49.4 billion.[270] The personal costs are also extensive since about 30% of stroke survivors are permanently disabled and 20% require institutionalized care.[270] The epidemiologic study of stroke is, however, difficult because of multiple clinical subsets and variations in diagnostic criteria. In addition, low autopsy rates have resulted in the loss of the exact pathologic diagnosis in innumerable cases. The major risk factors for stroke are hypertension, diabetes mellitus, myocardial infarction and smoking.[271] As with CHD, studies in Europe and North America have reported a U- or J-shaped association between alcohol consumption and stroke.

Two recent studies, both published in 1999, found that moderate alcohol intake significantly decreases the risk of ischemic stroke.[272,273] In a population-based case-control study involving a multi-ethnic population aged 40 years and older, Sacco *et al*.[272] reported that moderate alcohol intake (up to 2 drinks/day) was significantly protective for ischemic stroke. After controlling for cardiac disease, hypertension, diabetes, current smoking, BMI and education level, the odds ratio was 0.51 for those consuming up to 2 drinks/day compared with never drinkers. The protective effect was present in both sexes, younger and older groups, and in whites, blacks and Hispanics. However, the risk of stroke was increased significantly among those who consumed ≥ 7 drinks/day (odds ratio, 2.96). Similarly, a prospective cohort study followed 22,071 men (Physicians' Health Study) aged 40 to 84 years for an average of 12.2 years.[273] After controlling for the common stroke risk factors, the relative risks, compared with those who drank <1 drink/week, were 0.78, 0.75, 0.83 and 0.80, for those who averaged 1 drink/week, 2–4 drinks/week, 5–6 drinks/week and ≥ 1 drink/day, respectively. Interestingly, the benefit was apparent with as little as 1 drink/week and did not improve up to 1 drink/day. There was no statistically significant association between alcohol consumption and hemorrhagic stroke. However, this study did not include the potential negative consequences of excessive alcohol intake and stroke. As noted above,[272] the odds ratio for stroke was 2.96 for persons who consumed ≥ 7 drinks/day compared with non-drinkers. Unfortunately, these authors did not differentiate ischemic from hemorrhagic stroke. However, prior studies of stroke in heavy drinkers suggest that most of these were likely hemorrhagic.[259]

Hypertension is generally considered the major risk factor for intracerebral hemorrhage. The use of non-invasive imaging techniques are very useful since hemorrhagic strokes constitute about 10% of stroke cases. For example, in a case-control study, 73 cases of cerebral hematoma were diagnosed by CT scan.[274] Here, the most important risk factor was chronic alcoholism. Other risk factors were a history of hypertension, presence of liver disease and EKG abnormalities. The authors noted, however, that alcohol abuse is an important risk factor for hypertension. In addition, chronic alcoholics with liver disease often have a bleeding disorder which may be an additional causal factor in spontaneous intracerebral hemorrhage.[275] Furthermore, in an early literature review of moderate alcohol intake and stroke, Camargo[276] concluded that moderate drinking increases the risk of both intracerebral and subarachnoid hemorrhage, although there were population variations (e.g. increased in white populations, decreased among Japanese).

Reynolds and associates[277] recently reported a meta-analysis of 35 cohort and case-control studies published between 1966 and 2002 in which total stroke, ischemic stroke or hemorrhagic stroke was the endpoint. Their findings showed the following: (1) compared with non-drinkers, consumption of >60 g of alcohol/day was associated with increased relative risk of total stroke (1.64), ischemic stroke (1.69) and hemorrhagic stroke (2.18); (2) consumption of <12 g/day was associated with a reduced relative risk of total stroke (0.83) and ischemic stroke (0.80); and (3) consumption of 12–24 g/day was associated with a reduced relative risk of ischemic stroke (0.72).

Cancer

Increased alcohol intake has been associated with several cancers, including breast, liver, upper digestive tract (oropharyngeal and esophageal), colon and pancreas, among others. However, the mechanism(s) whereby alcohol induces cancer is not well understood, although alcohol intake clearly results in the production of reactive oxygen species (e.g. hydroxyethyl radicals) and products of lipid peroxidation,[278] which are probably important in some cases.

(1) Breast cancer

The generally accepted risk factors for breast cancer are age, heredity, estrogen metabolism, tobacco smoke and increased alcohol consumption. Although over 50 epidemiologic studies have examined the association between breast cancer and alcohol intake, the exact relationship has been somewhat controveresial.[279] Nevertheless, most studies have shown that alcohol consumption is associated with an increased risk of breast cancer. Indeed, a recent pooled analysis of six prospective studies conducted in Canada, the Netherlands, Sweden and the US has been published.[280] The results showed that for alcohol intakes <60 g/day, the risk increased linearly with increasing consumption. The pooled relative risk for an increment of 10 g/day (0.75–1.0 drink) was 1.09, whereas the relative risk for intakes of 30 to less than 60 g/day (2–5 drinks) was 1.41. Although an intake of $\geq$60 g/day did not show an increased prevalence, the authors had only limited data. They later wrote that "self-reported alcohol intakes may be less reliable at higher alcohol intakes, which may contribute to the appearance of a plateau at these higher levels."[281]

Several mechanisms whereby alcohol consumption increases the risk of breast cancer have been proposed, including disruption of cell membrane integrity, direct cytotoxic effect, interference with DNA repair, impairment of liver metabolism of carcinogens, altering circulating hormonal levels, dietary deficiencies and oxidative stress. In a large 12-year prospective cohort study of postmenopausal women, Sellers *et al.*[282] reported the relative risks of breast cancer with low dietary folate intake were 1.08 among non-drinkers, 1.33 among those who drank $\leq$4 g/day and 1.59 among drinkers of $\geq$4 g/day. Yu[283] proposed that since insulin-like growth factors (IGFs) are "potent mitogens for a variety of cancer cells including most breast cancer lines," moderate alcohol consumption may increase the production of IGFs, which then may increase the risk of breast cancer. Others[284] noted that the enzymes xanthine oxidoreductase (XOR) and alcohol dehydrogenase (DH) are expressed and regulated in breast tissue, and that aldehyde oxidase (AOX) may also be present. Furthermore, these enzymes have been shown to generate highly reactive and potentially destructive reactive oxygen species (ROS). Thus, their reported data suggests the following: (1) expression of ADH and XOR or AOX in breast tissue generates ROS; (2) alcohol metabolism produces acetaldehyde and NADH, both of which can be substrates for XOR or AOX with resultant ROS formation; and (3) the generated ROS can induce carcinogenic mutations and DNA damage found in breast tissue. A recent review[285] of potential mechanisms based on recent epidemiologic data included increased estrogen levels in alcohol consumers, enhanced mammary gland susceptibility to carcinogenesis, increased DNA damage and greater metastatic potential of breast cancer cells, the magnitude of which likely depends on the amount of alcohol consumed.

Physiologic evidence suggests that increased alcohol consumption may increase the risk of breast cancer through a hormonal mechanism. Thus, Gavaler *et al.*[286] suggested that postmenopausal women who are moderate drinkers have higher basal estradiol levels than postmenopausal women who abstain from alcohol. Moreover, a subsequent study[287] showed that acute alcohol ingestion resulted in a 300% increase in circulating estradiol in postmenopausal women who were using estrogen replacement therapy. However, alcohol consumption did not significantly change the estradiol levels in postmenopausal women who were not on estrogen replacement therapy. More recently, Chen *et al.*[288] reported the results of their prospective cohort study of 44,187 postmenopausal women (Nurses' Health Study) that examined the relation between concurrent alcohol and postmenopausal hormone use and invasive breast cancer. Their findings indicated that "both alcohol consumption and postmenopausal hormone use were associated with an increased incidence of breast cancer." Thus, postmenopausal women taking hormones should seriously consider the added risks of regular alcohol consumption.

(2) Hepatocellular carcinoma

Hepatocellular carcinoma accounts for about 90% of liver cancers, 60% to 80% of which arise in cirrhotic livers. Although relatively uncommon in North America and Western Europe, it may be the most common worldwide malignancy. The risk of hepatocellular carcinoma is particularly high with postnecrotic cirrhosis associated with hepatitis B infections, although other etiologic factors include hepatitis C infection, hemochromatosis, alpha-1-antitrypsin deficiency and alcoholic cirrhosis. In regions of low incidence, men are two to three times as likely to develop liver cancer as women, perhaps due to the increased frequency of hepatitis B infections, chronic liver disease and chronic alcoholism in men.

Age at presentation, ethanol consumption, serologic hepatitis viral markers and fibrosis were recently evaluated in 118 consecutive German patients with hepatocellular carcinoma.[289] The male to female ratio was 4:1 and the mean age at presentation was 61.8 years. Alcohol abuse and chronic hepatitis C were the most frequent important risk factors (49.2% and 17.8%, respectively). The authors concluded that chronic alcohol abuse remains the leading risk factor for hepatocellular carcinoma in Germany and other European populations where the prevalence of hepatitis is low. The same assumption is presumably true for Canada and the US.

(3) Colon cancer

Although numerous studies have focused on the association between various foods and colon cancer, most have evaluated two major nutrient hypotheses: high fat intake increases the risk of colon cancer and dietary fiber decreases the risk. Meyer and White[290] assessed the relation between nutrients and the incidence of colon cancer in a population-based case-control study involving 424 colon cancer cases and 414 controls. They found that alcohol consumption was strongly related to colon cancer in both men and women. For alcohol intakes of 0, <10, 10–29 and ≥30 g of ethanol/day, the odds ratios were 1.0, 1.9, 1.7 and 2.6 for men and 1.0, 1.3, 1.8 and 2.5 for women. For both sexes, a high dietary fiber intake was associated with significantly lower risk for colon cancer.

In an interesting study, Jacobs and associates[291] examined the association between daily multivitamin use and colon cancer among 806,397 men and women who were followed from 1982 to 1998 (Cancer Prevention Study II). After multivariate adjustment, use of a multivitamin containing folic acid slightly decreased the risk for colon cancer mortality (rate ratio 0.89). Consistent with prior studies, however, association was stronger among those who consumed two or more alcoholic drinks per day (rate ratio, 0.71). Others reported similar findings in a Polish population.[292] Here, alcohol consumption was a significant risk factor for colon cancer and the risk increased with increasing alcohol intake. However, the risk was even greater among alcohol consumers with a deficient intake of retinol, carotene and vitamins C and E (odds ratio, 6.79).

(4) Renal cell carcinoma

Renal cell cancer is responsible for a small percentage of total cancer cases and deaths throughout the world. However, in contrast to several other cancers which have decreased or stabilized, kidney cancer has steadily increased over the past decade. The major risk factors associated with renal cell carcinoma include genetics, smoking, obesity and hypertension. Most of the early case-control and cohort studies showed no association between alcohol intake and renal cell cancer. However, a more recent large international, multicenter case-control study showed that alcohol intake at least once per week significantly decreased the risk of renal cell carcinoma in women (odds ratio, 0.60), although there was no association in men.[293] Similarly, in a recent population-based case-control study, Parker *et al.*[294] reported their data regarding alcohol consumption and renal cell carcinoma in 261 men and 145 women with this malignancy and compared them with 1598 men and 837 women controls. The results also showed a significant decrease in risk for women who consumed >3 servings of alcohol/week compared with never drinkers (odds ratio, 0.5). Again, however, there was no association between alcohol intake and renal cell cancer in men.

(5) Esophageal and oropharyngeal cancers

Several epidemiological studies have reported a significant association between cancers of the upper digestive tract and alcohol intake. For example, in a prospective study of 6701 American men of Japanese ancestry living in Hawaii who developed cancers of the upper aero-digestive system (i.e. oropharynx, esophagus and larynx) and other organs, consumed significantly larger amounts of total alcohol, mainly beer, compared with cancer-free controls.[295] Those who developed oropharyngeal and esophageal cancers also consumed larger amounts of wine and spirits. Since these latter tumors are also associated with cigarette smoking, age-adjusted relative risks were calculated based on joint exposure to cigarette smoking and heavy alcohol intake ($\geq$30 ml/day). The relative risk was markedly increased among those who were both heavy alcohol drinkers and smokers (relative risk, 17.3) compared with non-smokers and modest drinkers. The cancer risk was also greatly increased among heavy drinkers who were non-smokers (relative risk, 8.6). Others,[296] in a population-based case-control study of esophageal cancer in Shanghai, reported that the risk of esophageal cancer was increased among tobacco smokers and alcohol consumers. The odds ratios for smoking were 2.1 and 1.6 for men and women respectively, and increased with the number of cigarettes smoked each day, duration of smoking, number of pack-years and decreasing age when smoking began. For current male alcohol consumers, the odds ratio was 1.4 with excess risk mainly among heavy drinkers. Since few women drank alcoholic beverages, no data was available. The combined effect of heavy smoking and alcohol intake was marked; the odds ratio was 12.0 for men who smoked >1 pack/day and drank $\geq$750 g of ethanol/week.

The relationship between different types of alcoholic drinks (beer, wine and spirits) and upper digestive tract cancers was examined in a population-based Danish study involving 15,117 men and 13,063 women.[297] Compared with non-drinkers, the relative risk was 3.0 for persons who drank 7–21 beers or spirits/week but no wine; the relative risk was 5.2 for those who consumed >21 beer or spirits/week, but without wine. However, those who had the same total alcohol intake but with wine exceeding 30% of the total intake, the risks were 0.5 and 1.7, respectively. The authors concluded that (1) increased alcohol consumption is a strong risk factor for upper digestive tract cancers; (2) resveratrol, an antioxidant rich in grapes and wine, inhibits the initiation, promotion and progression of cancer; and (3) wine drinkers may be at lower risk of developing oropharyngeal and esophageal cancers than drinkers who have a similar intake of beer and spirits.

Launoy *et al*,[298] noting that in various geographic areas in France there are major variations in the prevalence of esophageal cancer, studied 208 men with cancer and compared them with 399 male controls. Their results showed that the link between esophageal cancer and alcohol intake varied greatly according to the type of alcoholic beverage; aniseed aperitifs, hot spirits (especially hot Calvados) and beer had the greatest risk. After adjusting for all other alcoholic beverages, hot Calvados accounted for about 50% of esophageal cancer cases in Northwest France (Normandy and Brittany).

(6) Pancreatic cancer

Most epidemiological studies do not support a role for alcohol as a risk factor of pancreatic cancer, although an increased risk among heavy drinkers is less well established. To answer this question, Ye and coworkers[299] retrospectively studied a large cohort of Swedish patients with chronic alcoholism, alcoholic chronic pancreatitis, non-alcoholic chronic pancreatitis, alcoholic liver cirrhosis and non-alcoholic liver cirrhosis. Their results showed that alcoholics had only a modest excess risk of pancreatic cancer compared with the general population. The authors suggested that the excess risk among alcoholics might be attributed to smoking which may be over-represented among alcoholics. A recent Japanese study also found no association between pancreatic cancer and alcohol intake.[300]

Type 2 diabetes

Modest alcohol consumption (1–2 drinks/day) has been associated with a reduced risk for type 2 diabetes, reduced fasting insulin concentration and improved insulin sensitivity.[301–303] Others[304] recently reported that the risk of developing diabetes over a six-year period for those who consumed up to 10 g of alcohol/day was 8.0% compared with 12.9% for non-drinkers. In addition, Davies *et al.*[305] studied the effects of moderate alcohol consumption on fasting insulin and glucose levels and insulin sensitivity in postmenopausal women. Here, the consumption of 30 g of alcohol (2 drinks)/day had beneficial effects on insulin and triglyceride levels and insulin sensitivity in non-diabetic postmenopausal women.

Alcohol and miscellaneous medical disorders

Chronic alcohol abuse is often associated with acute erosive gastritis. However, chronic alcoholic gastritis is most often due to *Helicobacter pylori* infections and generally resolves with antimicrobial therapy.[306] Other negative medical effects of chronic alcohol abuse include protein-calorie malnutrition, male impotence, cardiomyopathy and fibrosis,[307] and diarrhea. This latter disorder reportedly exacerbates lactase deficiency, especially in people of African descent.[308]

Maternal alcohol use and fetal alcohol syndrome

Prenatal alcohol exposure is one of the leading preventable causes of birth defects, mental retardation and neurodevelopmental disorders in the US.[309] From 1991 to 1999, alcohol intake by pregnant women increased substantially while alcohol use by non-pregnant women of child-bearing age increased slightly.[310] Although alcohol use (i.e. at least one drink) during pregnancy declined significantly from 1995 to 1999, 12.8% of women still consumed alcohol during pregnancy.[311] Moreover, the rates of binge drinking (i.e. ≥5 drinks on any single occasion) and frequent drinking (i.e. ≥7 drinks/week or ≥5 drinks on any one occasion) did not decrease during pregnancy and remains higher than the 2010 Healthy People objectives. Moreover, unmarried and older pregnant women had the highest rates of alcohol consumption.

The fetal alcohol syndrome, first described in the scientific literature in 1973,[312] is caused by increased alcohol consumption during pregnancy and is one of the major causes of preventable birth defects and developmental disabilities.[313] This syndrome is characterized by a combination of growth deficiency, central nervous system dysfunction, facial dysmorphology and alcohol use during pregnancy. The prevalence varies from 0.2 to 1.0 per 1000 live births due to different study variations, as well as among racial/ethnic populations. In a recent Centers for Disease Control (CDC) study of four states (Alaska, Arizona, Colorado and New York), the prevalence rates varied from

0.3 to 1.5 per 1000 live births and were highest in black and American Indian/Alaska Native populations.[314] This latter report suggested that the number of infants adversely affected by pregnancy-associated alcohol exposure is probably underestimated for the following reasons: (1) some cases may not be diagnosed because of the "syndromic" nature of the disorder, lack of pathognomonic features and negative perceptions of the diagnosis; (2) lack of documentation in the medical records; (3) some children might not be diagnosed until they reach school age, at which time they are recognized to have central nervous system abnormalities and learning disabilities; and (4) some children with this syndrome may have left the surveillance area before being identified. The recommendations of the Task Force on fetal alcohol syndrome and other alcohol-related prenatal effects were recently published.[315]

Cognitive impairment and dementia

Atherosclerotic vascular disease is presumably an important risk factor for both ischemic and non-ischemic dementia.[316] Since moderate alcohol consumption decreases the risk for CHD, it might be expected to lower the risk of dementia. However, very low blood alcohol levels (0.02%) are well-known to impair automobile driving and, as noted in an earlier section, heavy alcohol drinkers have a significantly higher risk of hemorrhagic stroke. Conversely, light-to-moderate alcohol intake reduces the risk of CHD and ischemic stroke. Until recently, however, few studies have examined the effect of alcohol on cognition and dementia. Ruitenberg *et al.*[317] carried out a prospective population-based examination of 7983 persons aged 55 years and older. After adjustment for various confounders (age, sex, blood pressure, education level, smoking and BMI), light-to-moderate drinking (1–3 drinks/day) was associated with a significantly lower risk of any level of dementia (hazard ratio, 0.29). They also found no relation between dementia and the type of alcoholic beverage. Similarly, Mukamal *et al.*[318] found that, compared with abstention, the odds for dementia among older adults whose average weekly alcohol intake was <1 drink were 0.65; 1–6 drinks, 0.46; 7–13 drinks, 0.69; and

≥14 drinks, 1.22. Thus, compared with abstention "consumption of 1 to 6 drinks weekly is associated with a lower risk of incident dementia among older adults."

An Italian study also reported that the probability of cognitive impairment decreased with moderate alcohol consumption (<40 g/day for women; 80 g for men) compared with abstinence.[319] However, cognitive impairment increased significantly for older individuals who consumed more than one wine-equivalent liter per day among men and 0.5 liter among women. Similarly, a cohort study of Canadians aged 65 years and older found that alcohol abuse was significantly associated with cognitive impairment and independently associated with increased short term mortality.[320] The study also noted that alcohol abuse occurred more often in men than women.

Magnetic resonance imaging (MRI) carried out in alcoholic men have consistently shown that excessive alcohol consumption shrinks male brains, especially the white matter.[321] Moreover, there is a corresponding increase in the cerebrospinal fluid (CSF) volume. Recent studies have also shown brain shrinkage in women. For example, Hommer *et al.*[322] reported that alcoholic women have reduced gray and white matter and have correspondingly greater CSF volumes than healthy women. In addition, their data suggested that alcohol-related brain shrinkage is greater in women than men. Conversely, another study published in the same journal issue suggested that men have the greatest shrinkage, especially in the frontal cortex.[323] These conflicting studies emphasize the complexity of the research techniques and will require further studies to clarify the different effects of chronic alcohol intake on brain shrinkage in men and women.

Alcohol and accident-related injuries/fatalities

It is widely recognized that alcohol abuse is a major cause of automobile accidents and crash fatalities. In 2001, there were 17,448 alcohol-related traffic deaths.[324] Moreover, the relative risk of death in a vehicle accident increases steadily with increasing blood alcohol concentration in every age and gender group. A recent study of 40,000 Norwegian male conscripts, born in 1932–1933 and followed until 1991, found that most common causes of death were cardiovascular diseases, cancer and accidents, respectively.[325] However, the relative risks of death for alcohol abusers from accidents, cardiovascular diseases and malignant tumors were 3.2, 2.4 and 1.8, respectively. In an early study, Zador[326] reported on driver fatalities in single-vehicle crashes. Here, for each 0.02% in blood alcohol concentration (BAC), the risk of a fatal crash doubled. The crash risk increased with increasing BAC among all age and sex groups. For BACs in the 0.05–0.09% range, the likelihood of a crash was about nine-fold higher than with a BAC of 0.00%.

Motor-vehicle crashes are the leading cause of death in the US for persons aged 16 to 24 years and a significant proportion of these crashes are alcohol-related. Indeed, alcohol-impaired driving is highest among persons aged 21 to 24 years[327] and the percentage of alcohol-related fatal crashes is highest for this age group.[328] However, drivers less than 21 years of age are more likely to be involved in fatal crashes than older drivers and their added risk for a fatal crash increases more sharply at all levels of alcohol use.[328] Thus, younger drivers with a BAC of 0.05–0.09% were found to be at a significantly higher risk than older drivers and women had higher relative risks than men. For BACs of 0.15% or greater, the risk of an auto crash was 300 to 600 times the risk at zero BAC.[329] More recently, these researchers confirmed and expanded their earlier findings.[330] Thus, among 16- to 20-year-old male drivers, a BAC increase of 0.02% more than doubled the relative risk of a fatal single-vehicle crash injury. At the midpoint of the 0.08–0.10% blood alcohol level, the relative risk of a fatal single-vehicle accident injury varied between 11.4 (drivers aged ≥35 years) and 51.9 (male drivers aged 16–20 years). However, in contrast to the previous report, women had a lower fatality risk than men of the same age. These studies clearly indicate that drivers with blood alcohol levels less than 0.10% are at a significantly elevated risk to themselves and to others. Importantly, due to several public interventions to reduce alcohol-impaired driving, the rates of alcohol-related deaths decreased significantly during 1982–2001 across all age groups, although the largest decrease was among drivers less than 21 years old.[324]

Serious cycling accidents are also associated with alcohol abuse.[331] In this study, intoxicated cyclists were not only more likely to sustain injuries than sober cyclists, but were more likely to sustain the injuries at night, on the weekends, on their way to and from a party, pub or restaurant, in single accidents, and experience more serious injuries to the face and head. In addition, the intoxicated cyclists cycled less during the year, were more often unfamiliar with the route or bicycle, had bicycles without a hand-brake or gears, and were less likely to wear a helmet.

Other studies have shown that the risk of drowning also increases with increased blood alcohol concentrations. Smith *et al.*[332] studied the association between alcohol consumption and recreational boating fatalities. Compared with a referent blood alcohol concentration of 0, the relative risk of death increased with an alcohol concentration as low as 10 mg/dL (odds ratio, 1.3). The odds ratio was 52.4 for a blood alcohol concentration of 250 mg/dL. Importantly, the risk of death associated with alcohol use was similar for passengers and boat operators. Moreover, the type of boat and whether it was moving or stationary did not alter the results. Others[333] reported on the relation between alcohol consumption and drowning among US Army male soldiers on active duty. They found that drowning victims were disproportionately young, black, single, had less time in service, and no college experience. Alcohol consumption was also involved in at least one-third of the cases. Alcohol intake was associated with a ten-fold increase in reckless behavior and was most common among drowning in Europe.

Alcohol, drugs and chemical interactions

Genetics appears to play a major role in alcohol abuse and dependence. The importance of heredity in alcoholism is supported by several observational basic research studies. For example, the prevalence of this disorder is reportedly three- to four-fold higher in first-degree relatives of alcoholics and increases another two-fold in identical twins of alcoholics.[334] Other support involves key enzymes in alcohol metabolism. Ethanol is initially converted to acetaldehyde by alcohol dehydrogenase (ADH), of which two genetic variants (ADH2 and ADH3) produce a more rapid metabolic rate. Acetaldehyde blood levels are usually very low because of the enzyme aldehyde dehydrogenase (ALDH2). About 10% of Asians (homozygotes) carry a variation of ALDH2 (ALDH2-2), which is biologically inactive and therefore have an intense adverse reaction to even low doses of alcohol.[334] Moreover, the 40% of Asian women and men who are heterozygotes for this enzyme also have a significant negative reaction to ethanol. As a result, less than 10% of Japanese alcoholics are heterozygotes compared with 40% of the Japanese population.[335] Other ethnic groups, including Jewish people, reportedly have a lower alcoholism risk due to the presence of either ADH2 or ADH3 isoenzymes.[336]

Chronic ethanol consumption also induces the microsomal alcohol-oxidizing system.[337] The induction of this oxidizing system contributes to the metabolic tolerance of alcohol in abusers. It also affects the metabolism of other drugs, including pentobarbital, propranolol, meprobamate, tolbutamide, warfarin, diazepam, rifamycin and meprobamate.[338] A major enzyme of the P-450 "mixed function oxidase system" involved in ethanol metabolism is cytochrome P-4502E1 (CYP2E1), which also converts a wide variety of foreign compounds into highly toxic metabolites. These substances include anesthetic agents (e.g. methoxyflurane), industrial solvents (e.g. bromobenzene and vinylidene chloride), common medications (e.g. isoniazid and phenylbutazone), illicit drugs (e.g. cocaine) and analgesics (e.g. acetaminophen).[339]

Acetaminophen (paracetamol), one of the most widely used analgesics and antipyretics in the world, is generally considered to be safe. However, even therapeutic amounts can cause serious hepatocellular injury in chronic alcoholics. Moreover, the negative effects of acetaminophen, ethanol and fasting are synergistic since all three contribute independently to the depletion of reduced glutathione (GSH), a critical antioxidant.[340] Ethanol also inhibits the synthesis of GSH. Furthermore, patients with alcoholic cirrhosis are often deficient in vitamin E (alpha-tocoherol), a potent lipid-soluble antioxidant, which adds to the negative effects of ethanol.[341] The fact that even recommended doses of acetaminophen, with appropriate therapeutic blood levels, can cause severe hepatocellular necrosis in alcoholics often makes it very difficult for physicians to explain the extensive increase in serum liver enzyme activities (AST usually >20 times the upper reference level and AST > ALT). For example, Kumar and Rex[342] described five such cases in which the diagnosis was initially missed due to "inadequate knowledge of the distinct clinical presentation of acetaminophen toxicity in chronic alcoholics."

Recent studies have added additional information on the relation between acetaminophen and alcohol abuse. For example, Schiodt *et al.*[343] reported that although chronic alcohol intake enhances acetaminophen hepatic toxicity, acute alcohol intake does not influence the clinical course. Indeed, others[344] reported that acetaminophen-induced heptotoxicity and mortality in chronic alcoholics could be counteracted by concomitant acute alcohol ingestion. These authors also presented data suggesting that chronic alcoholics with suspected acetaminophen intake should be routinely treated with intravenous N-acetylcysteine. They found the longer the interval between N-acetylcysteine treatment and acetaminophen intake, the greater the mortality risk (<12 hours, 0.42%; 12–24 hours, 6.1%; 24–48 hours, 13%; and >48 hours, 19%).

To further complicate the issue, a recent randomized, double-blind, placebo-controlled trial concluded that "repeated administration of the maximum recommended daily doses of acetaminophen to long-term alcoholic patients was not associated with evidence of liver injury."[345] Thus, more studies are clearly needed to fully understand the relation between acetaminophen intake and liver damage in chronic alcoholics.

Herbal Products

So called "alternative," "complementary," and "unconventional" medical therapies, generally recognized as interventions neither widely taught in medical schools nor available in most American hospitals, are extensively used in the US and other industrialized countries. For example, the use of at least one of 16 alternative therapies increased from 33.8% in 1990 to 42.1% in 1997 and the probability of users visiting a practitioner of alternative medicine increased from 36.3% to 46.3%.[346] Indeed, about 427 million people visited alternative medicine practitioners in 1990 compared with over 629 million in 1997, thereby exceeding the total visits to all American primary care physicians (about 357 million and 385 million, respectively). Furthermore, the total out-of pocket expenditures relating to alternative therapies in 1997 were about US$27 billion, which is comparable with the out-of-pocket expenditures for all American physicians and exceeded the total out-of-pocket expenses for all hospital services. The most popular therapies during this time were herbal medicines, massage, chiropractic, acupuncture, megavitamins, self-help groups, folk remedies, energy healing and homeopathy.

A type of alternative therapy that has become almost mainstream is the use of herbal medicines. Indeed, consumer interest in dietary supplements "has exploded into a US$15 billion a year industry …"[347] In a recent study of adults entering an emergency department, 56% reported they had tried alternative therapies and 87% believed that they were effective.[348] Of these, 24% indicated that they had used herbal products. Importantly, 71% did not inform their physicians that they had tried alternative therapies. The authors strongly recommended that emergency room physicians routinely question their patients regarding the use of alternative therapies, especially herbal products, since they may cause serious adverse problems. Indeed, children entering emergency departments have often been given herbal products.[349] In this report, the mean patient age was 5.3 years (range three weeks to 18 years). Forty-five percent of the caregivers reported giving their child an herbal product. The most common therapies used were aloe plant (44%), echinacea (33%) and sweet oil (25%).

Moreover, 77% either did not believe or were uncertain if herbal products had any possible side effects and only 27% could name a possible side effect. Of those who gave their children an herbal product, 80% of their primary information source was from a friend or relative and only 45% had discussed their use with a primary health care provider.

The herbal products most commonly used today, along with their intended benefits, are listed in Table 5.3. Representatives of the less commonly used herbal products are listed in Table 5.4.

Unfortunately, to many people "natural" means "safe" despite abundant evidence to the contrary. Indeed, overuse or wrongful use of

Table 5.3: Commonly Used Herbal Products and Intended Benefits

Herbal Product	Intended Benefits
Aloe	Wound healing, burns, psoriasis, constipation
Chapparal	Retard aging, acne, prevent various diseases
Echinacea	Treat/prevent colds and respiratory tract infections
Ephedra	Athletic enhancer, asthma, decongestant, stimulant
Garlic	Hypercholserolemia, hypertension, cancer prevention
Ginger	Prevent motion and morning sickness, nausea
Ginkgo	Dementia, memory loss, claudication, circulatory disorders
Ginseng	General health promotion, sexual function, increase energy
Kava	Relieve anxiety and stress, sedative
Saw palmetto	Benign prostatic hypertrophy
Silymarin	Liver diseases/disorders
St. John's wort	Depression, insomnia
Valerian	Insomnia, anxiety

Table 5.4: Miscellaneous Herbal Products

Borage oil	Feverfew
Cat's claw	Goldenseal
Chan su (FDA banned)	Licorice
Comfrey	Pycnogenol
Chamomile	Senna
Danshen	Uzara root
Dong quai	

herbal medicines may result in death. In contrast to pharmaceuticals, herbal medicines are not standardized. As a result, the type and quantities of active ingredients may vary significantly depending on the region the herb is grown, the time in season when it is harvested, and the plant species. Furthermore, herbs contain many substances of uncertain biological activity and no reliable data exists on the safety, drug interactions, or medical efficacy of many herbal products. Herbal products are covered under the Dietary Supplement Health and Education Act of 1994 and categorized as "dietary supplements." As such, they are treated as foods, not drugs. Therefore, they do not undergo the rigorous testing required by the US Food and Drug Administration (FDA) for pharmaceutical drugs. As a result, little is known about their effectiveness, optimal dosage, side effects, or interactions with other medications. The labels on herbal products must indicate that they do not "diagnose, treat, cure, or prevent any disease." Unfortunately, many consumers use these products to do just that. As a result, certain herbal products merit close attention because their use is widespread and includes settings where polypharmacy is common. The major products in this latter area are saw palmetto, St. John's wort, *Ginkgo biloba*, echinacea and ginseng. Examples of important herbal toxic effects are summarized in Table 5.5. Common herb-drug interactions are summarized in Table 5.6.

In addition to possible herb-drug interactions, herbal medicines may negatively affect laboratory test results in the following three

Table 5.5: Possible Adverse Effects of Major Herbal Products

Adverse Effect	Herbal Products
Allergic responses	Aloe, Cat's claw, Echinacea, Garlic
Cardiovascular	Ephedra
Coagulation	Feverfew, Ginger, Garlic, Ginkgo
Dermatologic	Garlic, Kava, St. John's wort
Kidney	Chaparral, Ephedra, Licorice, Cat's claw
Liver	Chaparral, Comprey, Echinacea, Ephedra, Valerian
Neurologic	Ephedra, Ginkgo, Kava, St. John's wort
Psychologic	St. John's wort
Transplant rejection	St. John's wort

Table 5.6: Common Herb-Drug Interactions

Herbal Product	Interacting Drug	Disorder(s)
Feverfew	Warfarin	Bleeding
Garlic	Warfarin	Bleeding
Ginger	Warfarin	Bleeding
Ginkgo biloba	Aspirin, Warfarin	Bleeding
	Thiazide	Hypertension
Ginseng	Warfarin	Decrease warfarin effectiveness
	Phenelzine	Headache, insomnia, irritability
Kava	Alprazolam	Additive effects of depressants, alcohol
St. John's wort	Paxil	Lethargy, incoherency, nausea
	Cyclosporine	Possible transplant rejection
	Theophylline	Decreases efficacy of theophylline

categories:[350] (1) abnormal test results due to direct herbal interference with the assay; (2) unexpected concentration of a therapeutic drug due to drug-herb interaction; and (3) abnormal test results due to toxic effects of the herbal product.

St. John's wort (*Hypericum perforatum*)

Hypericum perforatum, an aromatic perennial herb, produces golden yellow flowers which reportedly are particularly abundant on June 24, the celebrated birthday of John the Baptist; hence, the plant is commonly known as St. John's wort. The plant is native to Europe, but is prevalent in America. Numerous chemicals have been isolated from St. John's wort, including hypericin, pseudohypericin and various flavonoids (e.g. quercetin, isoquercetin and rutin), among others. Melatonin, the human pineal gland hormone, is also present.[351] However, the principle ingredient is hypericin, which inhibits the re-uptake of serotonin, norepinephrine and dopamine. The major product sold in the US is a dried alcoholic plant extract which is widely available in health food and vitamin stores. Wagner *et al.*[352] reported that users of St. John's wort do so for three reasons: treat depression, easy access and a history of exposure to and belief in the safety of herbal medicines.

Clinical uses

St. John's wort has long been used in folk medicine for numerous disorders (e.g. bronchitis, burns, cancer, gastritis, insomnia, kidney disease, etc.). However, its current worldwide use is mainly as an antidepressant.[353] The estimated lifetime prevalence of depression in the US is about 17%.[354] Linde *et al*.[355] reported a meta-analysis of 23 published randomized clinical trials involving 1757 patients with mild to moderate depression who were treated with either placebo or St. John's wort. They concluded that the herbal extract was significantly superior to placebo and similarly effective as standard antidepressants, although they noted that methodological flaws limit the generalizability of the data. Others[356] compared the efficacy and tolerability of St. John's wort with imipramine in patients with mild to moderate depression and concluded that the two medications were therapeutically equivalent. Moreover, St. John's wort was better tolerated.

More recently, Shelton and associates[357] carried out a randomized controlled double-blind trial with 200 adults with major depression and concluded that St. John's wort "was not effective for treatment of major depression." Similarly, the Hypericum Depression Trial Study Group[358] carried out a randomized controlled trial conducted in 12 academic and community psychiatric research clinics. The patients were randomly assigned to receive St. John's wort, placebo, or sertraline for eight weeks. The group also concluded that the study "fails to support the efficacy of *H. perforatum* in moderately severe major depression." Thus, the evidence suggests that St. John's wort is modestly effective in cases of mild depression, but ineffective when depression is moderate to severe.

Safety

When taken alone, St. John's wort generally has a good safety record and is reportedly superior in this regard to conventional antidepressants.[359] However, several adverse clinical effects have been reported along with drug interactions that may arise when it is taken with other medications (Table 5.5). St. John's wort activates the hepatic cytochrome P-450 mixed function oxidase system which can decrease the plasma level of a wide variety of prescribed medications (e.g. anticoagulants, oral contraceptives, antiviral agents, etc.) with possible serious consequences.[360] For example, in a study involving healthy volunteers, St. John's wort reduced the area under the curve of indinavir, an HIV-1 protease inhibitor used to treat patients positive for HIV, by 57% and decreased the eight-hour indinavir trough by 81%.[361] The researchers concluded that this degree of inhibition could lead to drug resistance and treatment failure. Moreover, other protease inhibitors (e.g. amprenevir, nelfinavir, ritonavir and saquinavir) used to treat HIV are also presumably affected. Numerous other drugs are also metabolized through the hepatic P-450 system and are presumably similarly affected. These include medicines to treat heart disease (e.g. digoxin, digitoxin, nifedipine and beta-blockers), seizures (e.g. carbamazepine, phenytoin and phenobarbital), depression (e.g. amitriptylene, imipramine and amoxapine), certain cancers (e.g. cyclophosphamide, tamoxifen, taxol and etoposide), or to prevent pregnancy (e.g. ethinyl estradiol) or transplant rejection (e.g. cyclosporine, rapamycin and tacrolimus).[362]

Several reports indicate that St. John's wort may have negative effects on organ transplant patients taking cyclosporine. Thus, St. John's wort resulted in organ rejection in heart,[363] kidney and pancreas[364] transplant patients. Studies have also linked St. John's wort with psychotic relapse in schizophrenic patients,[365] hypertensive crisis,[366] acute toxicity,[367] acute neuropathy[368] and mania.[369] Other reported less serious effects include headache, allergic reactions, gastrointestinal irritations, tiredness and restlessness.[370]

Ginkgo (*Ginkgo biloba*)

Ginkgo, a leaf extract often referred to as EGb761, is prepared from the ginkgo tree which was introduced into Europe from China. The extract, used in China for about 5000 years, is now sold as a dietary supplement to improve blood circulation in the brain and peripheral tissues. Thus, it is used primarily to treat and/or prevent dementia, especially in Germany where it is officially approved to treat this disorder. It has also been used to treat tinnitus, intermittent claudication, impotence and vertigo.

EGb761 contains numerous flavone glycosides and terpenoides. As such, it has an antioxidant action as a free radical scavenger, a relaxing effect on vascular walls which improves blood flow and stimulates neurotransmitters.[371] Moreover, several experimental studies with laboratory animals have shown that *Ginkgo biloba* inhibits the formation of beta-amyloid, possibly through to its antioxidant properties.[372–374] EGb761 also exerts an anti-inflammatory effect by suppressing the production of active oxygen and nitrogen species by inflammatory cells and prolongs blood coagulation since it inhibits platelet aggregation. The antioxidant properties are considered useful for the treatment of free radical-associated diseases such as CHD, ischemic stroke, chronic inflammation and aging among others.

Clinical uses

The authors of a systematic review of 40 controlled trials of *Ginkgo biloba* for memory impairment suggested that only eight were of acceptable methodologic quality.[375] Of these, seven showed mild improvement in cognitive function with ginkgo compared with placebo. Thus, although encouraging data existed from early studies, the evidence was not compelling. Indeed, a very recent randomized controlled study strongly indicated that ginkgo "provides no measurable benefits in memory or related cognitive function in adults with healthy cognitive function."[376] More specifically, this study showed that ginkgo did not facilitate performance on standard tests of memory, learning, attention and concentration or naming, and verbal fluency in elderly people.

Most early studies suggested that EGb761 is at least modestly effective in treating patients with both Alzheimer's and ischemic dementia.[371] For example, Wettstein[377] reported that EGb761 is effective as the second generation cholinesterase inhibitors (e.g. donepezil, rivastigmine and metrifonate). In an earlier study involving 18 elderly people with mild memory loss, ginkgo extract improved the speed recall of three word lists.[378] In a subsequent 52-week randomized, placebo-controlled, double-blind trial involving 309 mildly to severely demented patients with Alzheimer's disease or multi-infarct dementia, EGb761 stabilized and modestly improved the cognitive performance and social functioning "in a substantial number of cases."[379] Moreover, the herbal treatment was reportedly safe. In addition, Oken *et al.*[380] conducted a meta-analysis of four randomized double-blind, placebo-controlled clinical trials of *Ginkgo biloba* to treat Alzheimer's disease. They concluded that there is "a small but significant effect" of treatment with *Ginkgo biloba* extract on cognitive function in patients with Alzheimer's disease. More recently, however, van Dongen *et al.*[381] randomly allocated EGb761 or placebo to 214 elderly patients and assessed the outcomes after 12 and 24 weeks. The authors concluded the EGb761 "is not effective as a treatment for older people with mild to moderate dementia or age-associated memory impairment." Thus, more careful studies involving large numbers of elderly people suffering from memory loss and mild to moderate dementia are needed to determine if there are truly functional improvements with this extract. As emphasized by Grundman *et al.*[382] the clinical value of *Ginkgo biloba* and other antioxidants for treating persons with Alzheimer's disease "is ambiguous and will remain so until properly designed human trials have been performed."

Since *Ginkgo biloba* has been shown to improve blood flow, several studies have compared its effect with placebo in persons with intermittent claudication. In a meta-analysis of eight randomized, double-blind, placebo-controlled clinical trials, Pittler and Ernst[383] concluded that compared with placebo, *Ginkgo biloba* has a moderate, clinically relevant effect on intermittent claudication. However, they noted that ginkgo was significantly less effective than walking exercise.

Ginkgo biloba has also been used to treat tinnitus. In a meta-analysis of five randomized clinical trials, Ernst and Stevinson[384] concluded that there was a moderate statistically significant positive effect. However, they noted that since few rigorous studies have been carried out, the therapeutic value of ginkgo for tinnitus was still somewhat uncertain. More recently, 60 patients with chronic tinnitus underwent ten days of infusion treatment with 200 mg/day of EGb761 after which they were randomized to double-blind, oral treatment with either 80 mg EGb761 twice daily or placebo for 12 weeks.[385] The researchers concluded that a combination of infusion therapy followed by oral administration of EGb761 "appears to be effective and safe in alleviating the symptoms associated with tinnitus aurium."

Safety

Although EGb761 is generally considered to be safe, adverse effects such as spontaneous bleeding,[386-388] gastric disturbances and convulsions[389] have been reported. In addition, interaction between non-steroidal anti-inflammatory drugs (NSAIDs), including aspirin[390] and various anticoagulants, clearly indicate that they should not be taken concurrently. *Ginkgo biloba* has also been recently associated with bleeding complications after liver transplantation[391] and enhanced cytotoxicity in conjunction with amikacin.[392]

Ginseng

The genus *Panax* consists of several species including Chinese ginseng (*P. ginseng*), American ginseng (*P. quinquefolius*) and Japanese ginseng (*P. japonicus*). Most studies have used Chinese ginseng, so the material presented here primarily refers to that species. The common ginseng preparations are from the ginseng root, which can be purchased as capsules, tablets, dried root or root extract. Saponins (ginsenosides or panaxosides) are the major chemical substances in ginseng and at least 28 ginsenosides have been identified.[393] Ginseng also contains maltol, vanillic acid, various peptides and polysaccharides.

Clinical uses

An extensive literature about ginseng has accumulated over the past several centuries. As such, it has been used for its alleged sedative, hypnotic, aphrodisiac, antidepressant, demulcent and diuretic activities.[394] It has also been used to improve stamina, vigilance, concentration and well-being. Its pharmacologic properties reportedly vary from central nervous system stimulation, modulation of the immune system and anabolic effects.[394] Despite these alleged beneficial effects, Cupp[395] recently wrote that "little scientific evidence shows that ginseng is effective for any purpose." This comment is in agreement with Lewis' earlier statement: "Unfortunately, ginseng remains a medical enigma with no proven efficacy for humans."[396]

Safety

The incidence of serious adverse effects of Chinese ginseng appears to be relatively low although it has reportedly been responsible for several negative conditions including nausea, insomnia, diarrhea, vaginal bleeding, headache and hypotension.[394] Ginseng was also recently implicated in a manic episode in a patient on antidepressant medication.[397] American ginseng reportedly lowers blood glucose levels in both diabetic and non-diabetic people.[398] Hence, American ginseng should be taken with a meal to prevent hypoglycemia in non-diabetic persons. In addition, ginseng interacts with warfarin and thereby lowers the international normalized ratio.[399]

Saw palmetto (*Serenoa repens*)

Saw palmetto, a dwarf palm tree, is present in the Southern United States. It contains, among others, a variety of alcohols[400] and biologically active acylglycerides (e.g. 1-monoalaurin and 1 monomyristin).[401]

Clinical uses

Early native Americans used saw palmetto to treat various genitourinary conditions and in the early part of the 20th century it was used as a mild diuretic in conventional medicine. It has subsequently been used to enhance sperm production, libido, breast size and as a mild diuretic. However, its major use is to treat men with symptomatic benign prostatic hyperplasia (BPH) and chronic prostatitis. Indeed, the ripe berry extract from saw palmetto has been officially approved in Germany to treat BPH. However, "over-the-counter" supplements may result in significantly different results due to the apparent variability in the amount of active ingredients in different products. For example, Feifer and associates[402] found that six saw palmetto samples were within a range of -97% to $+140\%$ of the labeled dosages, and three of these contained less than 20% of the stated dosages. The researchers concluded that "saw palmetto demonstrated tremendous variability. Some samples contained virtually no active ingredients."

In a multicenter study, 1098 men with moderate BPH were randomly assigned to receive saw palmetto or finasteride (a 5-alpha reductase inhibitor) over a six-month period.[403] The authors found no significant difference between the two groups. Wilt *et al.*[404] later carried out a literature review and meta-analysis of saw palmetto extracts in men with symptomatic BPH. They concluded that although the literature on saw palmetto for the treatment of BPH "is limited in terms of the short duration of studies and variability in study design," the extract improves both urologic symptoms and urine flow. Moreover, compared with finasteride, it produced similar improvement in urinary tract symptoms and urine flow and "was associated with fewer adverse treatment events." However, as noted above, the clinical results may vary significantly due to the variability in the amount of active ingredients of different saw palmetto products.

Safety

Serious adverse effects of saw palmetto are apparently very uncommon. However, several modest negative effects include constipation, decreased libido, diarrhea, headache and nausea.[394]

Echinacea

Echinacea, a genus that includes nine different species in the US, is a member of the daisy family. These perennial herbs are present throughout North American prairies, plains and woodlands. Echinacea products vary considerably since different parts of the plants, albeit mainly the roots, are used in the various preparations. In addition, commercially available products are primarily prepared from three different *Echinacea* species (*E. angustifolia, E. pallida and E. purpurea*) and include fresh herb, freeze dried herb and an alcoholic extract. The active ingredients include polysaccharides, glycoproteins, alkylamides, alkaloids and various flavonoids. Although both *E. pallida* and *E. purpurea* have been officially approved by the German Commission, *E. angustifolia* root has not.

Clinical uses

Common uses for echinacea include both topically applied and orally administered preparations for wound healing, abscesses, burns, leg ulcers and eczema.[394] In the US, the major use of echinacea is to stimulate the immune system to increase the resistance to colds and upper respiratory tract infections. However, in a randomized, double-blind, placebo-controlled trial with 302 volunteers from an industrial plant and several military institutions, there was no statistically significant difference to the time of onset of upper respiratory infections between echinacea and placebo.[405] Grimm and Muller[406] also examined the efficacy of echinacea in preventing colds and respiratory tract infections and reported no difference in the incidence, duration or severity between the placebo group and those who were supplemented with a fluid extract of *E. purpurea*. After an extensive literature search that included over 100 published articles, books and book chapters, Barrett *et al.*[407] reported that only nine treatment trials and four prevention trials fit the criteria for evaluating the effectiveness of echinacea extracts in reducing the incidence, severity and duration of upper respiratory tract infections (URIs). They concluded that echinacea "may be beneficial for the early treatment of URIs" although they noted that "the influence of publication bias on those results is unknown." They also concluded that "there is little evidence supporting the prolonged use of echinacea for the prevention of URIs."

Safety

Adverse effects to echinacea preparations are reportedly very uncommon and consist primarily of allergic reactions, some of which may be serious. For example, between July 1996 and September 1997, the Australian Adverse Drug Reactions Advisory committee received 11 reports of adverse reactions associated with echinacea.[408] These reactions were as follows: asthma (three cases), rash (one case), rash with myalgia and nausea (one case), hepatitis (three cases), dizziness with swollen tongue (one case), and anaphylaxis (one case).

Kava (*Piper methysticum*)

Kava is prepared from the dried rhizome of the kava plant and is traditionally used in the South Pacific as a recreational beverage. There are 72 different kava plants which differ in appearance and chemical composition. The neurological effects of kava have been attributed to a group of substituted dihydropyrones (kavapyrones), including yangonin, desmethoxyyangonin, 11-methoxyyangonin, kavain and dihydroxykavain. These compounds are present in the lipid-soluble kava extract or kava resin.[409] The major pharmacologic properties of kava are as an anti-convulsant and a central muscle relaxer.[394] The exact mechanism whereby kava is believed to produce its anxiolytyic effect is unclear due to conflicting reports with regard to kava's effect on gamma-aminobutyric acid receptors.

Clinical uses

In an early double-blind study, kava was found to be similarly efficacious with oxazepam in treating patients with anxiety disorders.[410] Scherer,[411] in an observational study, reported that 42 of 50 patients indicated that kava was effective in relieving their anxiety. More recently, Pittler and Ernst[412] carried out a systematic review and meta-analysis of seven randomized, double-blind, placebo-controlled clinical trials in which kava was compared with placebo. They concluded that kava was superior to placebo and that short-term treatment is effective is reducing anxiety. In addition, the combined use of kava extract and hormone replacement therapy was found to be effective in reducing menopausal anxiety.[413]

Safety

Although most clinical studies suggest that adverse effects of kava are relatively uncommon, reported negative effects include visual disturbances, dizziness, stupor, gastrointestinal and hepatic disturbances. Most of the reported adverse effects have been dermatologic. For example, Jappe *et al.*[414] reported that sun exposure to individuals taking kava resulted in skin itching followed by erythematous plaques and papules on the face, chest and back. In addition, when taken in excessive amounts, kava may cause a reversible yellowish discolorization of the skin, nails and hair ("kava dermopathy").[415] However, since 1999 hepatic toxicity has been associated with excessive amounts of kava intake.[416] Indeed, a total of 11 patients from the US, Germany and Switzerland who used kava products developed liver failure and underwent subsequent liver transplantation.[417] As a result, the US Food and Drug Administration now advises consumers and health care providers about the possible risks associated with the intake of products containing kava.

Valerian (*Valeriana efficinalis*)

Valerian is a perennial herb present in North America, Europe and Western Asia. The dried valerian root and root extract are available in capsules, as an oral solution, or tea. The chemical composition of valerian is complex and consists of over 100 compounds including valeranone, valerenic acid, valepotriates, isovaltrate and didrovaltrate. It is generally thought that the valepotriates are responsible for the sedative activity of valerian.

Clinical uses

Valerian is believed to inhibit the degradation and re-uptake of gamma-aminobutyric acid (GABA) and thereby may reduce stress and anxiety. Hence, it is often used to promote sleep. Indeed, valerian has been approved in Germany as a sleep promoting and calming agent. However, as noted by Mar and Bent,[418] only two small randomized clinical trials comparing valerian with placebo have been reported. Although both studies suggested that valerian root decreased sleep latency and improved sleep quality, the reviewers stated that "these studies were poorly done, however, and definitive conclusions cannot be drawn from them."

Safety

Since valerian binds the same cell receptors as benzodiazepines and causes sedation, it "should not be used in combination with benzodiazepines, barbiturates, or other sedative-hypnotics."[418] Other reported adverse effects include gastrointestinal upset, allergies, restless sleep, headache and mydriasis.[419]

Garlic (*Allium sativum*)

Garlic, a worldwide herb commonly used to flavor food, has been cultivated for several thousand years. It has also been used to treat a variety of clinical disorders. There are several sulfur-containing compounds in garlic including cysteine and others derived from allicin, the substance responsible for the garlic odor. However, odorless garlic tablets, which lack allicin, can also be purchased.

Clinical uses

Historically, the Chinese used garlic to lower blood pressure, the Egyptians to increase physical strength and the Europeans to prevent plague.[418] An extensive literature has accumulated, particularly over the past couple of decades, regarding the association between garlic intake and cancer, atherosclerosis, hypertension and blood lipid levels. Some of the positive effects of garlic are presumably related to the antioxidants present in aged garlic extract (AGE), which contains both water and lipid soluble antioxidants, as well as selenium which is essential for the action of glutathione peroxidase, a critical anti-oxidant enzyme.[420] Thus, AGE inhibits lipid peroxidation and reduces ischemia/reperfusion injury and oxidative modification of low-density lipoproteins.[421] As such, it protects endothelial cells and prevents or slows atheroscloerosis. Moreover, AGE protects DNA from free radical-mediated mutations and the subsequent development of some cancers. Indeed, a recent critical literature review suggests that garlic consumption decreases the risk of stomach and colorectal cancers.[422] With respect to gastric ulcers and cancer, garlic reportedly has an antimicrobial effect on *Helicobacter pylori*.[423]

The effect of garlic on blood lipids is somewhat controversial. Early studies in both animals and humans suggested that garlic was effective in lowering blood cholesterol and triglyceride levels. For example, in 1987 Lau *et al.*[424] reported that garlic extract lowered the blood level of both of these lipids. Moreover, two subsequent meta-analyses of randomized placebo-controlled trials also indicated that garlic intake reduced total cholesterol levels,[425,426] although the latter analysis suggested that the cholesterol-reducing effect was modest. Conversely, Berthold *et al.*[427] performed a double-blind, placebo-controlled study of the effect of garlic oil on blood lipid levels. After 12 weeks of garlic therapy, the authors concluded that "the commercial garlic preparation investigated had no influence on serum lipoproteins, cholesterol absorption, or cholesterol synthesis" and that "garlic therapy for treatment of hypercholesterolemia cannot be recommended ..." In a similar multicenter, randomized, placebo-controlled trial using garlic powder, Issacsohn and associates[428] also concluded that garlic is ineffective in lowering cholesterol levels in hypercholesterolemic patients. A recent review of the effect of garlic on cardiovascular disorders has been published.[429]

Garlic has also been used for its anti-platelet and anti-hypertensive activities. With respect to garlic intake and hypertension, Silagy and Neil[430] published a meta-analysis of eight prospective randomized studies and reported that, compared with placebo, persons taking garlic had a mean systolic blood pressure reduction of 7.7 mmHg and a diastolic reduction of 5.0 mmHg. The authors concluded, however, that since these changes were mild and variable, further studies are needed to determine whether garlic significantly lowers blood pressure in hypertensive individuals as well as an antibacterial, antiviral, and antifungal agent. Although garlic can prevent *in vitro* microbial growth, as well as gastric *Helicobacter pylori*, no studies have shown it is effective in the prevention or treatment of other infectious disorders.

Several epidemiologic and laboratory studies suggest that the active ingredients of garlic have an anticarcinogenic effect. Although the mechanism whereby garlic may be anticarcinogenic is not fully understood, some data suggest that it may prevent the suppression of the immune response that is associated with an increased risk for cancer. Examples of the cancers that may be inhibited by garlic and allium vegetables include prostate,[431] colorectal and stomach [432] and urinary bladder.[433] In their review of the epidemiologic literature of garlic and cancer, Fleischauer and Arab[434] concluded that although there is probably a preventive effect of garlic consumption in stomach and colorectal cancers, "low study power, lack of variability in garlic consumption categorization within studies, and poor adjustment for potential confounders may limit the reliability of any conclusions regarding garlic supplements." In addition, there was an indication of publication bias.

Safety

Garlic is generally very well tolerated although common side effects include halitosis, body odor and topical irritation. However, its use should be avoided in patients taking warfarin due to its possible antiplatelet activity.[418] Allergies, including asthma, have also been reported.

Chaparral (*Larrea tridentata*)

Chaparral is prepared by grinding the leaves of the creosote bush ("greasewood"), an evergreen desert shrub. The leaves, stems and bark can be brewed for tea; capsules and tablets are also commercially available.

Clinical uses

Chaparral has been recommended in non-scientific publications for use as an "antioxidant" or "free radical scavenger." As such, it has been promoted to prevent various diseases, skin conditions (e.g. acne), and to slow the aging process.[435] The active agent is reportedly nordihydroguaiaretic acid, a potent antioxidant which, depending on the dosage, can inhibit the lipoxygenase and cyclooxygenase pathways and thereby decrease the formation of oxidants.[435]

Safety

Several published reports have clearly shown that chaparral can cause severe hepatotoxicity. Gordon and associates[436] reported a case of a 60-year-old woman who took chaparral for ten months and developed severe toxic hepatitis that required orthotopic liver transplantation. Others[437] reported a chaparral-induced case of cholestatic hepatitis. In addition, Sheikh *et al.*[438] reviewed 18 cases of chaparral-associated adverse effects reported to the FDA between 1992 and 1994. Of these, there were 13 cases of hepatoxicity. The predominant pattern was characterized as toxic- or drug-induced cholestatic hepatitis. The authors concluded that "the use of chaparral may be associated with acute to chronic irreversible liver damage with fulminant hepatic failure...."

These and other reported cases, although relatively uncommon, highlight the need to alert the public and health care and other health professionals of the potential hazards associated with the use of this and other herbal supplements. Since up to 50% of patients in some studies of fulminant hepatitis could not be attributed to infection by the various hepatitis viruses (e.g. A, B, B mutants, C, D or E), Koff[439] appropriately raised the question as to whether some of these cases might be due to chaparral or other herbal supplements. Importantly, chaparral has not been approved by the German E Commission.

Ephedra (Ma huang)

Ephedra is commonly present in herbal weight-loss products and is often referred to as "herbal fen-phen." Ephedra is a small perennial shrub, the major species being *Ephedra sinica* and *Ephedra equisentina* (collectively known as Ma huang). Ephedrine, a potent central nervous system stimulant, is the predominant alkaloid of ephedra plants.

Clinical uses

Ephedra-containing products are marketed as decongestants, bronchodilators and stimulants. Other promoted uses include weight loss, body building and athletic enhancement. "Herbal-ecstasy," also an ephedra-containing product, may produce a euphoric state.[440]

In a recent extensive literature review and meta-analysis of the efficacy and safety of ephedra and ephedrine for weight loss and athletic performance, the authors concluded that "ephedrine and ephedra promote modest short-term weight loss (~0.9 kg/month more than placebo) in clinical trials."[441] With respect to athletic performance, they concluded that the "evidence to support use of ephedra for athletic performance is insufficient."

Safety

Ephedra should not be used by patients with heart disease, hypertension, diabetes, thyroid disease, or by those taking monoamine oxidase inhibitors. Moreover, numerous studies have shown that ephedra-containing products may produce a variety of toxic disorders. Holler and Benowitz[442] evaluated 140 reports of probable ephedra-related toxicity and concluded that 31% were definitely related to ephedra; another 31% were probably related. Of these, almost half involved the cardiovascular system and 18% affected the central nervous system. Hypertension was the single most common adverse reaction followed by palpitations, tachycardia, stroke and seizure. There were ten deaths and 13 cases of permanent disability. Similarly, Samenuk *et al.*[443] evaluated the possible toxic effects associated with ephedra in 37 cases referred to the FDA from 1995 to 1997. Ephedra-associated diseases were stroke (16), myocardial infarction (10) and sudden death (11). The authors' conclusions were: (1) use of ephedra is temporally related to stroke, myocardial infarction and sudden death; (2) underlying heart or vascular disease is not a prerequisite for adverse ephedra-associated effects; and (3) the cardiovascular toxic effects of ephedra are not limited to massive doses.

More recently, Bent *et al.*[444] compared the relative safety of ephedra with other herbal products. They reported that products containing ephedra accounted for 64% of all adverse reactions to herbs in the US even though these products represented less than 1% (0.82%) of herbal product sales. In persons using ephedra products, the relative risks for an adverse reaction, compared with other herbs, ranged from 100 for kava to 720 for *Ginkgo biloba*.

Ephedra use has also been associated with psychosis and delirium,[445] hypersensitivity myocarditis[446] and acute hepatitis.[447] Nevertheless, despite continuing evidence of the negative effects of ephedra products, they are still marketed in the US and the FDA has been reluctant to take appropriate action to make them illegal. As a result, Wolfe[448] recently wrote, "We call on the FDA as an agency of the Public Health Service to fulfill their legal responsibility and to stop the occurrence of further preventable deaths and injuries by banning ephedra products." In response to the increased concern regarding this product, the US Justice Department is reportedly conducting a criminal investigation into whether Metabolife, the leading ephedra-containing supplement on the market, lied about the safety of this product (August 2002).[449]

Ginger (*Zingiber officinale*)

The ginger plant, native to Asia, is grown in the tropics. Ginger root has been used in China as a flavoring agent and medicinal herb for about 2500 years. The most pharmacologically active component of ginger are gingerol and its derivatives. It is available as the powdered root, tea, capsules, oral solution and as a spice.

Clinical uses

In the US, ginger is promoted to prevent nausea, vomiting, vertigo, motion sickness and morning sickness during pregnancy. Ginger has been reported to reduce nausea and vomiting in some, but not all clinical studies. Phillips *et al.*[450] studied the effectiveness of ginger in preventing nausea and vomiting in 120 postoperative patients. The incidence of nausea and vomiting was 21% with ginger, 27% with the drug metoclopramide and 42% with placebo. Conversely, two later double-blinded randomized controlled trials found that ginger was not effective in preventing nausea and vomiting after laparoscopic gynecologic surgery.[451,452]

In an early randomized trial of the effect of ginger on seasickness, ginger powder reduced vomiting and sweating significantly better than placebo.[453] In another double-blind cross-over, placebo-controlled study, the volunteers were subjected to artificially-induced vertigo.[454] The results showed that powdered ginger root was significantly more effective than placebo in reducing vertigo. Moreover, an early controlled trial found that ginger was more effective in preventing motion sickness than dimenhydrinate,[455] but was not found to be effective in a later similar study.[456] The inconsistencies of these types of studies are related, at least in part, to the difficulty of measuring nausea and motion sickness since these symptoms are often subtle and difficult to fully evaluate.

Safety

Ginger appears to be quite safe since its use has not been associated with any serious side effects. However, its inhibition of platelet aggregation and synthesis of prostaglandins and leukotrienes has been demonstrated *in vitro*. Hence, when used in conjunction with other anti-platelet substances (e.g. garlic, ginkgo, vitamin E, aspirin and other pharmaceuticals), bleeding problems are possible.

Aloe (*Aloe vulgari, Aloe barbadensis*)

Aloe plants are native to Eastern and Southern Africa. Gel from the leaves' inner central zone and latex from the pericyclic cells are used for medicinal purposes. Medicinal use in Mesopotamia extends back to 1750 BC and Egyptians began using aloe for skin infections in about 550 BC. Use in the US began in about 1820.

Clinical uses

Gel from the aloe leaves are used topically for wound healing, skin irritation, burns, sunburn and psoriasis. The latex, consumed orally, is used for constipation and peptic ulcer. The results of wound healing studies in humans have been somewhat inconsistent. For example, Syed and associates[457] reported that aloe was beneficial for the rapid healing of genital herpes, and aloe extract was found to be effective in the treatment of psoriasis.[458] Moreover, Hayes[459] reported a case in which aloe vera was successful in treating a patient with lichen planus, a disease that involves the skin and mucus membranes. Conversely, aloe was ineffective for the prevention of radiation-induced dermatitis[460] and the topical use of aloe reportedly delayed the healing of surgical abdominal wounds.[461]

In an early study, aloe vera and the "Husk of Isabol" were added to the diet of 5000 patients with angina pectorus.[462] After a follow-up of five years, there was a reduction in the frequency of anginal attacks and the patients' drug dosages (i.e. verapamil, nifedipine, beta-blockers and nitrates) were slowly decreased. The author also reported "a marked reduction in total serum cholesterol, serum triglycerides, fasting and postprandial blood sugar level in diabetic patients, total lipids, and also increase in HDL were noted." The author's suggested mechanism whereby these two substances acted were probably related to "their high fibre contents." Further studies of the effects of these two substances on CHD are certainly warranted.

Safety

Aloe is a relatively safe herbal medicine. However, topical use of the gel may delay wound healing. Moreover, oral consumption of aloe may produce diarrhea and hypokalemia.[418] As such, it should not be used in patients with bowel obstruction or irritable bowel syndrome.

Silymarin (*Silybum marianum, Milk Thistle*)

For more than 2000 years, the seeds of this prickly-leaved, purple-flowered plant have been used to treat chronic liver diseases. More specifically, silymarin is currently used by some to treat chronic viral hepatitis and alcoholic cirrhosis. As a polyphenolic flavonoid antioxidant, silymarin has also been used to protect against various hepatoxic agents and reportedly has anti-inflammatory, cytoprotective and anti-carcinogenic effects.

Clinical uses

Various animal studies have shown that silymarin protects liver cells against hepatotoxic substances including drugs (e.g. acetaminophen and amitriptylene),[463,464] toxins (e.g. carbon tetrachloride and alcohol),[465] viruses and radiation.[466] Recent experimental studies also indicate that silymarin protects dopaminergic neurons against lipopolysaccharide-induced neurotoxicity,[467] prevents ultraviolet light-induced immune suppression in mouse skin,[468] and has anti-proliferative and apoptotic effects in rat prostate cancer cells.[469]

In clinical studies, the effects of silymarin on cirrhosis have been inconsistent. For example, in a randomized controlled trial, Ferenci *et al.*[470] reported a 30% decrease in the four-year mortality rate in cirrhotic patients treated with silymarin. The effects were greatest in those with alcoholic cirrhosis. Conversely, a more recent double-blind randomized multicenter study found no difference in progression or mortality in alcoholic cirrhotics after two years of silymarin treatment.[471] Silymarin therapy was, however, shown to reduce hyperinsulinemia and the daily insulin need in cirrhotic diabetic patients.[472]

Safety

Silymarin appears to have a good safety record. Case reports of gastrointestinal disturbances and allergic skin rashes have been uncommon.

Herbal supplementation summary

The use of herbal remedies is an increasingly common worldwide form of alternative medicine. A 1997 survey estimated that 12.1% of American adults used an herbal supplement in the previous 12 months at a personal cost of US$5.1 billion.[346] In 1990, only 2.5% of US adults used herbal medicines. Most herbal products sold in the US are considered dietary supplements and are not, therefore, regulated as medicines. As such, they are not required to meet the drug standards as specified in the Federal Food, Drug and Cosmetic Act.

Contrary to popular belief, the use of these "natural products" can pose serious health risks. This is not surprising since these substances are complex mixtures of chemicals, many of which are toxic. In addition to possible direct adverse effects and serious drug-herb interactions, there is an indirect risk that herbal medicines may compromise, delay or even replace an effective form of treatment.[473] In 2001, the FDA received about 500 reports of adverse effects related to dietary supplements and the US poison-control centers received 19,468 reports.[474] These numbers, however, probably represent less than 1% of the adverse events caused by dietary supplements, including herbal products. Moreover, only a fraction of these cases are properly investigated. The drawbacks to the surveillance system of adverse events associated with dietary supplements have been recently published.[475]

Although some studies have shown herbal medicines to be beneficial in treating certain disorders, others have been inconsistent and serious questions have been raised regarding the methods used and the reliability of the data. Systematic reviews and meta-analyses of these trials usually show that the reported effects are limited and require confirmation by randomized controlled studies. Indeed, only a small fraction of the thousands of medicinal plants used world-wide have undergone rigorous testing in controlled clinical trials. Nevertheless, these products have great appeal to many people, a fact that cannot be ignored. As such, it is imperative that physicians and other health care providers ask patients whether they are taking herbal products, especially when they present with an unexplained health problem.

Because of the potentially serious medical effects related to herbal medicines, there is a definite need for new regulations regarding these products. Indeed, several countries (e.g. France, Germany, Sweden and Australia) have implemented strategies for licensing herbal medicines. Marcus and Grollman[476] recently emphasized this need in the US because of the increasing number of reports of "adverse effects and deaths associated with botanical health products, the distribution and widespread sale of adulterated products, and the marked increase in misleading promotional claims on the Internet demand prompt action to protect the public health."

Prescription and Illicit Drugs

Substance abuse may cause a wide variety of human illnesses and diseases including ischemic heart disease (angina pectorus and acute myocardial infarction), chemical hepatitis and cirrhosis, acute and chronic renal disease and various mental disorders, among others. Moreover, substance abuse imposes severe personal and societal financial burdens. For example, the 1988 losses to the economy related to alcohol and drug abuse were US$129.3 billion and US$58.3 billion, respectively.[477] In 1995, the economic costs of substance abuse was estimated at US$428.1 billion: US$175.9 billion for alcohol and US$114.2 billion for drugs.[478]

Adverse prescription drug reactions

The marked increase in prescription drug use over the past few decades has caused widespread concern on the grounds of inappropriateness of prescribing, adverse drug reactions which result in significant patient morbidity and mortality, as well as increased medical costs. Early studies indicated that the elderly are primarily involved in increased prescription drug use and may have higher adverse reaction rates.[479,480] At this time, the suggested reasons for a higher risk in the elderly were (1) increasing percent of elderly in the population; (2) increased number of multiple illnesses; (3) multiple stresses such as low income, loneliness and widowhood; (4) decreased capacity to metabolize and excrete some drugs; and (5) increased tissue sensitivity.

An early British multicenter study found that 15.3% of older people admitted to Geriatric Departments who were taking prescribed drugs suffered adverse reactions, and in 84% of these cases adverse reactions were an important factor in their hospital admission.[481] The major adverse drug reactions were due to hypotensives, anti-Parkinsonian drugs, psychotropics and diuretics. In a subsequent review of this subject,[482] the authors stressed that the major factors which influence patient susceptibility to adverse drug reactions were (1) multiple drug therapy which increases exponentially rather than linearly with the number of drugs taken; (2) multiple disorders and disease severity can alter drug disposition by increasing steady state concentration or increasing drug half-life; (3) type of prescribed drug; (4) altered pharmacokinetics in that most adverse drug reactions are dose-related and affected by changes in drug metabolism, renal elimination and distribution; and (5) the effect of age on altered pharmacodynamics, which may be increased or decreased depending on the drug. Importantly, these researchers concluded that "remarkably little data is available to support the commonly held view that the incidence of adverse reactions increases with patient age." Rather, "severe illness, multiple pathology and the associated high level of prescribing is much more important than age itself."

Although most early studies of adverse drug reactions involved hospitalized patients, several recent reports have examined adverse drug events in ambulatory community-dwelling residents. For example, Willcox *et al.*[483] examined the incidence of inappropriate drug prescribing for older community-dwelling Americans. Using explicit criteria developed by 13 US and Canadian geriatrics experts, they reported that 23.5% (i.e. 6.64 million people) received at least one of the 20 contraindicated drugs. Moreover, 20.4% of these individuals received two or more contraindicated drugs. The major adverse effects were cognitive impairment and sedation. Similarly, Zhan and associates[484] reported that 21.3% of community-dwelling elderly Americans received at least one of 33 potentially inappropriate medications. These authors concluded that "overall inappropriate medication use in elderly patients remains a serious problem."

Similarly, in a recent prospective study of 661 outpatients, 162 (25%) had adverse drug events.[485] Of these, 24 (13%) were serious, 51 (28%) were ameliorable and 20 (11%) were preventable. Of the ameliorable events, 32 (63%) were due to physician failure to respond to medication-related symptoms and 19 (37%) to patient failure to inform the physician of the problems. The drug classes most frequently involved were selective serotonin-reuptake inhibitions (10%), beta-blockers (9%), angiotensin-converting enzyme inhibitors (8%) and non-steroidal anti-inflammatory drugs (8%).

Prescription errors are also an important health problem. Indeed, from 1983 to 1998, US fatalities from acknowledged prescription errors increased by 243% (2876 to 9856), which is a greater percentage increase than for most other causes of death.[486] However, serious adverse reactions and death are not uncommon even when drugs are prescribed and administered properly. For example, Lazarou and associates[487] carried out a meta-analysis of 39 prospective studies from US hospitals. The incidence of serious adverse drug reactions was 6.7%; fatal events occurred in 0.32%. The estimated number of serious adverse drug reactions in 1994 was 2,216,000 and the estimated number of deaths was 106,000. Thus, adverse drug reactions was the fifth leading cause of death in the US at that time (although not listed as a major cause of death[488]).

The financial cost of adverse drug reactions is also highly significant. Thus, a recent study of surgical intensive care patients showed that for each adverse drug event, the average length of stay was increased by 2.31 days.[489] In addition, Hohl *et al.*[490] studied polypharmacy, frequency of adverse drug events leading to emergency department presentations and the frequency of potential adverse drug interactions in medication regimens of patients 65 years and older. Their results showed that 90.8% of patients were taking one or more medications (prescribed or over-the-counter), the number consumed varying from 0 to 17 (average 4.2 per patient). The adverse drug events accounted for 10.6% of all emergency department visits. The most frequent medication classes were non-steroidal anti-inflammatory drugs, antibiotics, anticoagulants, diuretics, hypoglycemics, beta-blockers, calcium channel blockers and chemotherapeutic agents. At least one potential adverse drug interaction was identified in 31% of cases.

A significant percentage of adverse drug reactions are, however, preventable. A large elderly cohort (30,397 person years) was studied to evaluate the incidence and preventability of adverse drug events in an ambulatory setting during a 12-month period.[491] Here, 1523 adverse drug events were identified of which 27.6% were considered preventable. Of the adverse reactions, 38% were serious, life-threatening or fatal; 42.2% of these more severe events were preventable compared with 18.7% of the significant adverse drug reactions. Cardiovascular drugs (24.5%), followed by diuretics (22.1%), nonopioid analgesics (15.4%), hypoglycemics (10.9%) and anticoagulants (10.2%) were the most common medication categories associated with preventable adverse reactions. The authors noted that the more serious adverse drug reactions are "more likely to be preventable" and that "prevention strategies should target the prescribing and monitoring stages of pharmaceutical care."

Individual differences in drug response is affected by age, sex, disease and drug interactions. However, genetic factors also influence a drug's efficacy and the likelihood of an adverse reaction (pharmaco-genetics). That is, after being absorbed, the drug is metabolized and then excreted. Each of these processes could be affected by ge-netic variation. To examine this factor, Phillips *et al.*[492] evaluated 18 adverse drug reaction studies and 22 variant allele review articles. Here, 27 frequently cited drugs involved in adverse medical events were identified. Of these, 59% are metabolized by at least one enzyme with a variant allele known to cause poor metabolism. How-ever, only 7% to 22% of randomly selected drugs are known to be metabolized by enzymes with this genetic variability. The results sug-gested that drug therapy based on individuals' genetic makeups "may result in a clinically important reduction in adverse outcomes." Indeed, it is now possible to individualize therapy in the case of a few drugs.[493] Further advances in understanding the genetic variations in the proteins involved in drug uptake, distribution, metabolism and action will allow physicians to select the proper drug at the optimal dose for each patient.

Substance abuse and addiction

The abuse of both prescription and illicit drugs is a widely recog-nized and serious problem in the general population. As such, drug abuse is both a health and social issue. It not only affects the individual's mental and physical health, but the health of the public. Over the past two decades, it has been shown that drug addiction is a chronic, relapsing disorder that results from prolonged drug effects on the brain. Early reports regarding the effects of chronic drug use on cognition and comparisons of various drug users have been inconsistent, perhaps due to methodological flaws. To clarify the effects of chronic drug use on cognition, Block *et al.*[494] studied a group of substance users categorized as stimulant, alcohol or polydrug users. Their performance on academic achievement, verbal memory and abstraction tests was compared with the performance of community-dwelling controls. The groups were matched on demo-graphic and psychiatric characteristics. The results showed signifi-cant impairment on each of the achievement tests, abstraction ability and decreased total recall in all drug users compared with the controls. Moreover, stimulant users performed more poorly on several tests compared with the other drug use groups.

Numerous studies have also demonstrated a significant link between both prescription and illicit drug use and psychopathology. Indeed, drug users have both higher rates and more severe levels of psychological impairment than people who do not use drugs. Since it has been unclear as to whether drug use precedes the development of psychiatric disorders, Brook *et al.*[495] carried out a longitudinal study of subjects at mean ages of 14, 16, 22 and 27 years. Their results showed that tobacco use by adolescents and young adults was associated with a significantly increased risk of alcohol dependence and substance use disorders by age 27 years. Moreover, early use of alcohol, marijuana and other illicit drugs predicted a later major depressive disorder even after statistically controlling for age, sex, parental education level, family income and prior episodes of a major depressive disorder.

Drug abuse is also directly or indirectly an important vector for the transmission of several major infectious diseases, especially acquired immunodeficiency syndrome (AIDS), hepatitis and tuberculosis. The reported risk factors for addiction include substance availability, heritability, family, environment, previous psychopathology, childhood/adolescent behavior and previous substance use.[496]

Prescription drug abuse

Opioid analgesics are generally prescribed for pain control and patients with moderate to severe chronic pain commonly present in those with cancer and chronic, long-lasting back pain. The major prescription drugs for these conditions are the opioid agonists (Table 5.7). Unfortunately, these drugs are moderately to highly addictive. In addition to the analgesic effects, their pharmacologic effects include euphoria and various other classic signs and symptoms. Those associated with intoxication include depressed mental state, bradycardia,

Table 5.7: Major Analgesic Prescription Drugs

Codeine	Meperidine
Dihydrocodeine	Methadone
Fentanyl	Morphine
Hydrocodone	Oxycodone
Hydromorphone	Oxymorphone
Levorphanol	

hypotension, coma, hypothermia, depressed respiration and decreased gastrointestinal motility. Withdrawal effects include agitation, vomiting, diarrhea, diaphoresis, hypertension, tachycardia, tachypnea and muscle cramps.

Prescription drug abuse is a serious and rapidly growing problem resulting in a dramatic increase in hospital admissions and deaths, mainly from drug overdose. Indeed, prescription drug overdoses are responsible for more deaths than illegal drugs such as cocaine and heroin.[497] Oxycodone, hydrocodone and methadone abuse continues to increase. Data from the Florida Medical Examiner's office[497] during the first six months of 2002 reportedly showed that: (1) oxycodone, present in 267 cases, caused 112 deaths; (2) hydrocodone, present in 248 cases, caused 61 deaths; (3) benzodiazepine, present in 734 cases, caused 150 deaths; and (4) methadone, present in 254 cases, caused 133 deaths.

According to the National Household Survey on Drug Abuse, almost three million 12- to 17-year olds and seven million young adults (18–25 years old) reported abusing prescription medications in 2001.[498] Indeed, the annual number of new prescriptions for pain relievers increased from about 400,000 in the mid-1980s to two million in 2000. As a result of their increased availability, emergency department visits increased remarkably between 1994 and 2001 for narcotic prescription drugs. Thus, oxycodone increased 352%, methadone 230%, morphine 210% and hydrocodone 131%.[497] Moreover, many of these people were regularly consuming more than one drug.

In addition to the direct toxic effects of these and other prescription drugs, they may cause serious injuries, including death and significantly increase medical costs. For example, benzodiazepines are used by many elderly people to treat anxiety and insomnia. Adverse effects of these drugs include drowsiness, sedation, confusion and impaired motor function. To determine whether the use of benzodiazepines of either long- or short-elimination half-life increases the risk of motor vehicle injuries, a large cohort of Canadians, aged 67 to 84 years, were studied from 1990 to 1993.[499] Here, the adjusted rate ratio of crash involvement within the first week of long half-life benzodiazepine use was 1.45; the ratio was 1.26 for continuous use of longer duration (i.e. up to one year). However, there was no increased risk with short half-life benzodiazepine use. Moreover, as noted above, oxycodone is a potent narcotic and its overuse often leads to drug dependence. Thus, if regularly used during pregnancy, it may result in withdrawal symptoms in the neonate.[500] Furthermore, controlled-release oxycodone is a very expensive drug and contributes significantly to the marked increase in pharmacy costs.[501] This recent review examined 16 clinical trials to determine whether this agent offered clinical benefits over other drugs that would justify its greater cost. The authors concluded that "for patients requiring a controlled-release opioid treatment, controlled-release morphine and methadone should be considered because they appear to be as effective as oxycodone and cost considerably less."

Although substance abuse is widely recognized in the general population, it is largely under-diagnosed and under-treated in people aged 65 years and older, leading to what some have referred to as "an invisible epidemic." The major behavioral signs/symptoms associated with drug abuse in the elderly include the following:[502] (1) inability to cope with occupation loss, (2) mood swings (irritability and depression), (3) loss of physical mobility, (4) hygienic problems, (5) insomnia and hypersomnia, (6) unexplained accidents, falls and trauma, (7) decreased cognitive function, and (8) chronic pain. Most studies of substance abuse in the elderly outpatients, were found to be prescription drug abusers.[503] The major abused drugs were diazepam, codeine, meprobamate and flurazepam. Moreover, 92% of these patients had abused the drugs for over five years. The major risk factors in this group were female sex, social isolation, chronic illness, polypharmacy, and a history of psychiatric problems and alcohol abuse. More recently, Edgell *et al.*[504] found that 4% of geriatric veteran inpatients had non-alcoholic drug abuse disorders (prescription drugs, 3%; illicit drugs, 1%). It is, perhaps, not surprising that the benzodiazepines were the most commonly misused prescription drugs. The high rate of benzodiazepine dependence suggests that physicians should consider alternative treatments for anxiety and depression in the elderly.

Illicit drug use

Cognitive deficits associated with the chronic abuse of marijuana, opiates and stimulants have important theoretical and clinical significance. These deficits result from changes in the cortical, subcortical and neuromodulatory mechanisms that underpin cognition; they also directly interfere with rehabilitation programs. The most commonly used illicit drugs are listed in Table 5.8.

Cocaine

Cocaine, an alkaloid extracted from the leaf of the *Erythroxylon coca* bush, grows in South America. It is available in two forms: the hydrochloride salt and the "free base." Cocaine hydrochloride, which can be taken orally, intravenously, or intranasally is commonly referred to as "chewing," "mainlining" and "snorting," respectively. The free-base form is heat-stable and melts at 98°C, which allows it to be smoked. This form is commonly referred to as "crack cocaine" because of the popping sound it makes when heated.

Table 5.8: Common Illicit Drugs

Cocaine	Heroin
Cannabis (Marijuana)	Methamphetamine
Ecstasy	Steroids

In 1999, about 25 million Americans had used cocaine at least once, 3.7 million had used it within the previous year and 1.5 million were current users. Moreover, 30% of all drug-related emergency department visits was attributed to cocaine.[505] Although cocaine use reportedly declined in the early to mid-1980s, its use increased 82% between 1994 and 1998 (514,000 to 934,000 users).[506] These authors attributed the increased use to its ease of administration, availability and drug purity, reduced cost and the misperception that its use is safe. Cocaine use is also common in middle and high school students. Indeed, a recent government report found that 9.4% of students aged 18 years and younger had used cocaine in some form during their lifetime.[507] Overall, Hispanic and white male students (14.9% and 9.9%, respectively) were also more likely than black male students (2.1%) to report lifetime cocaine use. Hispanic and white female students (13.1% and 9.2%, respectively) were more likely than black female students to report lifetime use (1.3%). Cocaine use also increased with advancing student age. Thus, students in grade 12 were more likely to report lifetime cocaine use than those in grade 9 (12.1% and 7.2%, respectively).

(1) Cocaine and cardiovascular events

Cocaine-related cardiovascular events include accelerated atherosclerosis, angina pectorus, myocardial infarction, cardiomyopathy, myocarditis, arrhythmias, hypertension, aortic dissection and endocarditis.[508] In 1982, Coleman and associates[509] first reported an association between myocardial ischemia and infarction and cocaine use. Since then, numerous studies have verified cocaine-associated myocardial ischemic events. For example, a retrospective cohort study at 29 US hospital centers from 1987 to 1993 identified 130 patients with cocaine-associated myocardial infarction.[510] These patients were relatively young (average age 38 years), non-white (72%) and tobacco smokers (91%) with a history of cocaine use in the past 24 hours (88%). The major complications were congestive heart failure (nine patients), ventricular tachycardia (23 patients), supraventricular tachycardia (six patients) and bradycardia (23 patients). Ninety percent of the complications occurred within 12 hours of presentation. The acute in-hospital mortality was 0%. This is in contrast to a recent Florida Medical Examiner's report of 579 deaths in which cocaine was present. Of these, 180 deaths (31%) were attributed to cocaine.[497]

The suggested mechanisms whereby cocaine induces myocardial ischemia and infarction are as follows:[506] (1) patients with atherosclerotic plaques have increased myocardial oxygen demand but a limited blood supply resulting in increased heart rate, blood pressure and myocardial contractility; (2) increased alpha-adrenergic stimulation, increased endothelin production and decreased nitric oxide results in coronary artery vasoconstriction; and (3) increased plasminogen-activator inhibitor, increased platelet activation and aggregability, and increased endothelial permeability accelerates atherosclerosis and stimulates thrombosis. A recent study also showed that cocaine induces transient erythrocytosis that "may increase blood viscosity while maintaining tissue oxygenation during vasoconstriction."[511] In addition, cocaine increased von Willebrand factor which, without a compensatory change in endogenous fibrinolysis, "may trigger platelet adhesion, aggregation and intravascular thrombosis."

Most cocaine-related cases of myocardial infarction occur in young, non-white male cigarette smokers without other arteriosclerotic risk factors but who have a history of repeated cocaine use.[506] Nevertheless, "myocardial infarction may develop in first-time users, occasional users and long-term users."[508] Moreover, the risk of acute myocardial infarction is increased by a factor of 24 during the 60 minutes following cocaine use in persons who are otherwise at relatively low risk.[512]

(2) Cocaine use and miscellaneous clinical disorders

Ischemic liver damage is a well-known complication of heart failure, but it may also be caused by hypotension associated with cocaine-induced cardiac events.[513] This negative effect on the liver is presumably due to hepatic ischemia, the result of systemic hypotension induced by coronary and systemic arterial vasospasm which leads to congestive heart failure. In addition to these cocaine-associated ischemic events, decreased cerebrovascular blood flow has also been described. Thus, a recent study showed increased hypoperfusion in cocaine abusers compared with controls, presumably due to vasospasm and potential compensations in cerebral blood flow.[514]

Hsue *et al.*[515] reviewed 38 hospital records of acute aortic dissection that occurred from 1981 to 2001. Of these, 14 (37%) were related to cocaine use (crack cocaine in 13 cases; powder cocaine in one). The mean interval between cocaine use and symptom onset was 12 hours. Those with cocaine-associated aortic dissection were younger, black and had a history of hypertension. Cocaine use has also been associated with heat stroke.[516] In this report, eight patients entered the emergency department during the June 1998 heat wave in New Orleans [heat index reached 112°F (44.5°C)]. All had elevated drug levels, codeine being the most common. Six patients had rhabdomyolysis; three of these also had disseminated intravascular coagulation. There were two deaths (25%).

Cocaine use during pregnancy is also a significant public health problem, particularly in US urban areas and among women of low socio-economic status.[517] These researchers reported that "cocaine exposed children had significant cognitive deficits and a doubling of the rate of developmental delay during the first two years of life." They suggested that these children will continue to have learning difficulties at school age.

Marijuana (cannabis)

More than 60 dibenzpyrene compounds known as cannabinoids have been identified in extracts of the hemp plant, *Cannabis sativa*. Most of these compounds are not psychoactive, and only one form of tetrahydrocannabinol (THC) is both active and present in substantial amounts. As with anesthetic agents, cannabinoids are hydrophobic and depress central neurosystem function and induce analgesia. Two receptors have recently been identified to which THC binds and through which it exerts its effects.

Over seven million Americans reportedly use cannabis weekly or more often.[518] In addition, 42.4% of American high school students in 2001 had used marijuana during their lifetime.[507] Overall, male students were significantly more likely to report the lifetime use of marijuana than female students (46.5% and 38.4%, respectively). This sex difference was found for both Hispanic and white students, as well as in students in grades 9, 10 and 11. Moreover, there was a progressive increase in marijuana use from grades 9 to 12 (32.7%, 41.7%, 47.2%, 51.5%, respectively). In addition, 23.9% of students admitted they had used marijuana one or more times during the 30 days preceding the survey.

What are the most common risk factors for cannabis use and progression in abuse and dependence? A four-year prospective community study of adolescents and young adults designed to answer this question was recently published.[519] The findings confirmed the previously well-established risk factors such as peer pressure, drug availability and low self-esteem. In addition, family history (e.g. parental mental disorders and early parental death) and prior experiences with legal drugs both played a significant role in marijuana use and the subsequent transition to cannabis use disorders.

(1) Marijuana use and cognitive function

Although early studies indicated that gross neurologic impairments to chronic marijuana use did not occur, the evidence was inconclusive with regard to the presence of more specific deficits, such as impaired cognition.[520] Thus, recent studies have clearly demonstrated changes in cognition and brain function associated with frequent or long-term use of cannabis. For example, the results of a multi-site retrospective cross-sectional study of 102 "near-daily" cannabis users was recently reported.[518] The findings showed that long-term cannabis users (mean, 23.9 years of use) performed significantly less well than shorter-term users (mean, 10.2 years of use) and controls on memory and attention tests. The authors concluded that "long-term heavy cannabis users show impairments in memory and attention beyond the period of intoxication and worsen with increasing years of regular cannabis use."

(2) Marijuana use and mental disorders

Roeloffs *et al.*[521] studied the characteristics associated with substance abuse in patients with either depressive symptoms (44%) or depressive disorders (56%) in six primary care clinics. Their findings showed that sedative misuse (14% of all patients) was associated with greater wealth, social phobia and misuse of prescription drugs. However, marijuana use (11% of all patients) was associated with younger age, male gender, single marital status, white ethnicity, less education, recurrent depression, agoraphobia and hazardous alcohol use. In an Australian study,[522] 1601 adolescents (mean age, 14.5 years) were followed for seven years. By age 20, about 60% had used marijuana and 7% were daily users. Although early depression and anxiety did not predict later cannabis use, weekly use predicted a two-fold increase in later depression and anxiety. Moreover, the risk of depression and anxiety was increased five-fold in women who used marijuana daily.

Further follow-up of a previously described Swedish cohort of 50,087 men (aged 18 to 19 years) showed a dose-dependent relation between marijuana use and risk of developing schizophrenia.[523] Among those who had used only marijuana, and had used it 50 or more times, the adjusted odds for developing schizophrenia was 6.7. Another long-term study relating schizophrenia to cannabis use involved 759 children who were 11 years old at baseline.[524] Psychotic symptoms were assessed at baseline and at age 26; drug use was assessed at ages 15 and 18. The results showed that frequent cannabis users (36%) had a significantly greater likelihood of showing schizophrenic symptoms at age 26 than those who rarely or never used cannabis (65%). In an accompanying editorial, Rey and Tennant[525] addressed the following three questions: (1) Is the association between cannabis use and mental health problems dose-related? (2) Do people use cannabis to self-medicate existing mental problems? and (3) Could other drugs cause the observed relation between cannabis and schizophrenia and depression? They concluded that there is a dose-related association between cannabis use and serious mental health problems. However, the answers to questions 2 and 3 were "no." Nevertheless, it is still unknown whether long-term marijuana use is a primary cause of mental disorders or whether it unmasks a preexisting predilection to mental health problems.

To further study the association between long-term marijuana use and schizophrenia, Buhler and associates[526] evaluated the onset and lifetime prevalence of substance abuse in a population-based sample of 232 first schizophrenic episodes. Here, schizophrenics were twice as likely as controls to have a lifetime history of substance abuse at the age of first admission (alcohol, 23.7% versus 12.3%; drug abuse, 14.2% versus 7.0%). Of the drug abusers, 88% used cannabis and 62% began the habit before the onset of schizophrenia. The authors concluded that "a small proportion of schizophrenics might have been precipitated by substance, mainly cannabis, abuse." Others[527] concluded that continuous heavy marijuana use can induce a psychotic disorder similar to, but "distinct from" schizophrenia and that these "two clinical entities share some features but they differ in others."

(3) Marijuana use and cardiovascular events
Although it is well known that smoking marijuana has hemodynamic consequences, including a dose-dependent increase in heart rate, supine hypertension and postural hypotension, a possible association between marijuana use and serious cardiac events was not appreciated until recently. To investigate the possible association between marijuana use and acute myocardial infarction, Mittleman et al.[528] interviewed 3882 men and women who had an acute myocardial infarction. Of these, 124 (3.2%) reported smoking marijuana in the prior year, 37 within 24 hours and nine within an hour of symptoms. Marijuana users were mainly men (94% versus 67%), current cigarette smokers (68% versus 32%) and obese (43% versus 32%). Cannabis users were also less likely to have had prior angina or hypertension. The authors concluded that "smoking marijuana is a rare trigger of acute myocardial infarction." Others[529] reported an association between acute cardiovascular deaths following marijuana use. This report identified six cases in which cannabis was the only drug detected in postmortem blood samples, thereby documenting recent marijuana use. In addition, an

interesting report described the case of acute myocardial infarction in a young man following the combined use of cannabis and Viagra (sildenafil citrate), a widely prescribed vasodilator for male erectile dysfunction.[530] Viagra is mainly metabolized by the hepatic cytochrome P4503A4 microsomal enzyme. As such, its vasodilator effects can be potentiated by an inhibitor of this enzyme. Indeed, cannabis inhibits cytochrome P4503A4 enzyme. Other reports have also associated Viagra use with myocardial infarction in patients with cardiovascular disease. Nevertheless, marijuana's cardiovascular effects are clearly not associated with serious cardiac problems for most healthy young users. However, cannabis use by individuals with cardiovascular disease increases their risk of an adverse cardiac event "because of the consequences of the resulting increased cardiac work, increased catecholamine levels, carboxyhemoglobin and postural hypotension."[531]

(4) Marijuana and immunity

Numerous studies of the effects of marijuana on the immune system suggest that cannabinoid intake is associated with an increased incidence of viral infections and allergic symptoms. In a literature review of the effects of marijuana on the immune system, Klein *et al.*[532] reported that marijuana modulates (1) the function of T and B lymphocytes as well as natural killer (NK) cells and macrophages; (2) the host resistance to various infectious agents (e.g. herpes simplex virus and bacterial agents, such as those of the genera *Staphylococcus*, *Listeria*, *Treponema* and *Legionella*; and (3) the production and function of acute phase and immune cytokines as well as the activity of network cells such as macrophages and T helper cells. Thus, cannabinoids can be immunomodulatory and thereby enhance the disease process. More recently, Friedman and Klein[533] updated their prior literature review on the effects of marijuana on the immune system. In addition to their earlier findings, human studies showed that cannabinoids decrease T-cell rosette formation, increase the CD4$^+$/CD8$^+$ratio, increase IgE levels and decrease IgG levels. In human cell cultures, cannabinoids decrease T-cell production, increase B cell production and decrease macrophage phagocytosis and NK cell cytolysis.

(5) Cannabis and use of other drugs

The title of a recent editorial asked the question, "Does Marijuana Use Cause the Use of Other Drugs?"[534] Here, Kandel noted that there are "regular sequences and stages of progression in which the use of alcohol and cigarettes precedes the use of marijuana and, in turn, the use of marijuana precedes the use of other illicit drugs ..." Thus, very few people who have used cocaine and heroin did not previously use marijuana beforehand, a phenomenon known as the "gateway hypothesis." This hypothesis assumes the following three interrelated propositions:[535] (1) *sequencing*, in which there is a fixed relationship between two substances where one is initiated before the other; (2) *association*, whereby the initiation of one substance increases the initiation likelihood of the second substance; and (3) *causation*, in which the use of the first substance is the cause of the use of the second substance. Whether or not there is a direct causal link between the use of marijuana and other drugs, an association between the two is well established.

A recent study by Lynskey *et al.*[536] further supports this association. They examined whether early marijuana use and subsequent progression to other drug use and abuse/dependence persists after controlling for shared environmental and genetic influences. Their results showed that by age 17 years, the odds of other drug use, alcohol dependence and drug abuse/dependence were 2.1 to 5.2 times greater for marijuana users than those of their co-twins who did not use cannabis before age 17 years. They concluded that the "association between early cannabis use and later drug use and abuse/dependence cannot solely be explained by common predisposing genetic or shared environmental factors."

(6) Medicinal uses of marijuana

The potential of cannabinoids as medical therapeutics has long been known. The ability of this diverse family of compounds to modulate neurotransmission and act as antiinflammatory antioxidative agents led to increased scientific interest in their potential as neuroprotective agents. Thus, recent literature reviews suggest that cannabinoids may be clinically useful in treating patients with Parkinson's disease, multiple sclerosis, increasing appetite in patients with HIV wasting disease, reduction of intraocular pressure in glaucoma, bronchodilation in asthma, and relief of chronic nausea and vomiting. Moreover, experimental studies suggest that various cannabinoids may be effective in rescuing dying neurons in cases of acute neuronal injury as occurs in cerebral ischemia and traumatic brain damage.[537-539] Nevertheless, most researchers agree that considerably more basic research is needed to better understand cannabinoid neurobiology, as well as properly designed clinical trials to assess their usefulness in treating various clinical conditions.

Cannabis has also been widely used as an analgesic to relieve chronic pain. The authors of a recent small selected study of patients who smoked cannabis for chronic pain relief concluded that their study results "must be interpreted with caution."[540] They emphasized that clinical trials are needed to fully evaluate whether cannabis is useful in treating patients with chronic pain. Indeed, in a literature review of randomized controlled trials, Campbell *et al.*[541] concluded that "cannabinoids are no more effective than codeine in controlling pain and have depressant effects on the central nervous system that limit their use." As such, the widespread use of cannabinoids for chronic pain management "is therefore undesirable." They also suggested that cannabinoids should not be used in patients with acute postoperative pain.

(7) Marijuana, cocaine, and cancer

Does chronic use of crack cocaine or marijuana cause cancer? Fliegel *et al.*[542] reported that both hyperplasia and squamous cell metaplasia were found substantially more frequently in the lungs of crack cocaine smokers and marijuana smokers than in the lungs of nonsmokers. Moreover, those individuals who smoked both crack cocaine and tobacco or both marijuana and tobacco had an even higher frequency of histopathologic abnormalities. In a later study, Barsky and associates[543] demonstrated that marijuana and crack cocaine smokers have an increased frequency of molecular abnormalities in bronchial epithelium that are similar to those present in cigarette smokers (i.e. Ki-67, a cell proliferation marker; EGFR, a growth factor receptor; P53, a tumor suppressor protein; and DNA ploidy).

Since it took several decades to prove that cigarette smoking causes cancer, it may also take decades to determine whether smoking marijuana and/or crack cocaine are also important risk factors for lung cancer.

Methamphetamine and amphetamine

Methamphetamine use is an increasingly serious problem in the US. Gibson *et al.*[544] recently published the results of their study of methamphetamine use in California's Central Valley, mainly in Sacramento, which may be the most severely affected American city. Their results showed that, in contrast to Seattle and San Francisco, methamphetamine users in the Central Valley are mainly heterosexual and of mixed racial/ethnic heritage. At least 75% began their drug use while in their teens; more than 25% were 15 years or younger. Indeed, a recent CDC report[507] indicated that 9.8% of American students (grades 9 to 12) had used methamphetamine during their lifetime. Overall, Hispanic and white students (9.1% and 11.4%, respectively) were significantly more likely to use methamphetamine in their lifetime than black students (2.1%). This significant racial/ethnic difference applied to both male and female students. The study also showed a three-fold difference in lifetime methamphetamine use across state surveys (5.3% to 15.6%).

Amphetamine and methamphetamine use is also very common in other countries. For example, in New Zealand the National Drug Surveys of people aged 15 to 45 years were conducted in 1998 and 2001.[545] The findings showed that stimulant use (i.e. amphetamine and methamphetamine) increased from 2.9% in 1998 to 5.0% in 2001; the use of methamphetamine increased from 0.1% to 0.9%. Thus, these stimulants moved from the third most popular illicit drug type in 1998 to the second most popular in 2001. Moreover, 41% thought that these stimulants were easier to obtain in 2001 and 20% said they cost less. The availability and use of methamphetamine has also increased since 1998 in Sydney, Australia. Here, the Illicit Drug Reporting System reported the emergence of at least three different forms of "potent" methamphetamine; methamphetamine powder ("speed"), base methamphetamine ("base") and crystalline methamphetamine ("ice", "shabu" and "crystal meth").[546]

(1) Methamphetamine use and HIV infection

As noted by Gibson and associates,[544] since methamphetamine enhances libido, especially if injected, the users typically have many more sexual partners and are more likely to be HIV-infected. A study of 807 California prison inmates, 32% of whom used methamphetamine prior to incarceration, showed a "dramatically higher" sex-related HIV/AIDS risk than non-methamphetamine substance abusers.[547] Similarly, the risks of prevalent HIV infection associated with incarceration of injecting drug users in Bangkok, Thailand were recently studied.[548] The documented HIV seropositive participants were drug-injecting users formerly incarcerated for six months or more during the previous five years. Compared with controls, the independent risk factors for HIV infection were methamphetamine injection before detention (odds ratio, 3.3), sharing needles in the holding cell (odds ratio, 1.9), being tatooed while in prison (odds ratio, 2.1) and borrowing needles after release (odds ratio, 2.5).

Since there is limited information about high-risk behaviors among heterosexual African American men infected with HIV, Wohl *et al.*[549] carried out a case-control study of HIV-infected and uninfected self-identified heterosexual African American men. However, a significantly higher number of the HIV positive men reported increased sexual risk behaviors (i.e. anal sex without condom use with both men and women). Moreover, a history of drug injection significantly increased the risk of HIV (amphetamine odds ratio, 4.3; methamphetamine odds ratio, 2.9). Others[550] studied HIV risk and drug use behavior and psychosocial status of Filipino Americans in San Francisco. The methamphetamine users were generally males, had low levels of perceived personal control in their lives, and low levels of shame about their drug use. As such, methamphetamine use was a

significant risk factor for HIV infection. The frequent methamphetamine users also tended to engage in drug use before or during sex
and to use condoms infrequently. Thus, since methamphetamine is
typically used in social events, a social approach to HIV prevention
might be successful in reducing the incidence of this disease.

(2) Methamphetamine use and other clinical disorders

Although perhaps not commonly reported, various clinical disorders
have been associated with methamphetamine abuse including subcortical hemorrhage in a 32-year-old woman[551] and intrauterine fetal
growth retardation.[552]

3,4-Methylenedioxymethamphetamine (MDMA; "Ecstasy")

Webster's New World Dictionary defines ecstasy as "a state or
feeling of overpowering joy; rapture." Thus, users say that MDMA
lowers their inhibitions and relaxes them. In addition, it reportedly increases their awareness, feelings of pleasure and increases
their energy. Ecstasy gained national attention when it became
the drug of choice at club parties known as "raves"; it is now the
third most used illicit drug after cannabis and amphetamines.
Nevertheless, this illicit stimulant, which is chemically related to
meperidine, amphetamine and methamphetamine, can damage
nerve cells in the brain. Indeed, ecstasy may produce side effects
such as headaches, chills, eye twitching, blurred vision and nausea. In addition, high doses may cause dehydration, hyperthermia
and seizures.

Data from a recent national survey of over 14,000 college students at
119 American colleges regarding ecstasy use and related behaviors
from 1997 to 1999 was recently published.[553] The prevalence of
ecstasy use increased from 2.8% in 1997 to 4.7% in 1999, an increase of 69%. A smaller sample of ten colleges indicated that the
increase continued in 2000. Those who used ecstasy were more likely
to smoke cigarettes, use marijuana, engage in binge drinking, have
multiple sexual partners, consider arts and parties as important,

religion as less important, spend less time studying, and more time socializing with friends. Interestingly, unlike other illicit drug users, MDMA users were not academic underachievers and their interest in education did not differ from that of non-ecstasy users.

(1) MDMA and CNS damage

MDMA, first synthesized and patented in 1914 by Merck, a German drug company, was originally used as an appetite suppressant. In the 1970s, MDMA was used to help those undergoing psychotherapy to be more open and express their feelings. The clinical use of MDMA was stopped in the mid-1980s when animal studies showed that it caused brain damage. Indeed, MDMA may damage neurons that use dopamine and serotonin.[554] In this study, primates were given three doses of MDMA to simulate the dosage people take during all-night "raves." When they were examined a few weeks later, the researchers observed "profound dopaminergic neurotoxicity, in addition to less pronounced serotonergic neurotoxicity." They concluded that MDMA users may put themselves at risk for developing neuropsychiatric disorders related to dopamine and/or serotonin deficiency.

(2) Ecstasy use and psychological disorders

MDMA has been implicated in the onset of various psychological disorders and has been associated with a number of psychiatric symptoms that have persisted after drug cessation. After reviewing ten years of psychiatric case studies, Soar *et al.*[555] concluded that "recurring symptoms strongly suggest a causal relationship between the drug and neuropsychiatric manifestations."

Various animal and human studies have shown that chronic use of MDMA is associated with significant cognitive impairments, particularly in laboratory and field tests of memory for previously encoded material. To evaluate the effects of MDMA use on aspects of everyday cognitive function, Heffernan and coworkers[556] compared regular ecstasy users with non-users in prospective memory (i.e. remembering to do something at some future point) and found that ecstasy users had more errors in prospective memory. The authors suggested that these prospective memory deficits may be related to previously reported serotonergic and frontal lobe deficits in chronic MDMA users. In a follow-up study,[557] this group of researchers concluded that MDMA users have impaired prospective memory that "cannot be explained by an increased propensity of exaggerated cognitive failures." They also suggested that this may be partly attributable to frontal lobe damage associated with the use of MDMA. Indeed, in a 15-year empirical review of chronic MDMA users it was concluded that damage to the frontal lobes, temporal lobes and hippocampus remain long after the recreational use of ecstasy has stopped and that "the pharmacological damage may be permanent."[558]

(3) Ecstasy use and miscellaneous adverse effects

The risk of adverse reactions to MDMA is now widely recognized, although the patterns of illness vary and serious events are relatively uncommon. However, as noted by Gowing and associates,[559] it is the unpredictability of the mortality and substantial morbidity risks that makes the health consequences of MDMA use significant. In their literature review, hyperthermia and hyponatremia are the most significant acute adverse effects whereas neurotoxicity is potentially the most important long-term effect.

Other serious adverse effects of MDMA have also been reported including subarachnoid hemorrhage,[560] hepatic toxicity[561,562] and death.[562,563] Henry *et al.*[562] reported seven cases of MDMA hepatotoxicity, of which one died, one required a liver transplant, and two experienced slow recovery. Among seven other fatalities, the toxicity pattern included convulsions, disseminated intravascular coagulation, hyperthermia, rhabdomyolysis and acute renal failure. Others identified eight ecstasy-related deaths from 1997 to 2000 in England and Wales.[552] Although most of these individuals took ecstasy along with various other drugs, six of them died after only taking ecstasy. Ecstasy has also been associated with victims of motor vehicle accidents.[562,564] Weinbroum[564] suggested that in this time of widespread ecstasy abuse, blood concentrations should be measured in motor vehicle accident patients admitted to emergency services with an altered state of consciousness.

Heroin (diacetylmorphine)

Heroin (an old trademark) is an opiate with effects similar to those of morphine, from which it is synthesized by the addition of two acetyl groups. Thus, it is a central nervous system analgesic that reduces a person's reaction to pain; produces euphoria, lethargy and sleep; reduces anxiety; and depresses respiration and the cough reflex. However, heroin produces less nausea but more euphoria than morphine. Hence, its use has long been abused and is illegal in the US, although it was recently approved on prescription in the UK.[565] Heroin's toxic effects are the same as those of morphine. It is metabolized to monoacetylmorphine and morphine.

Over the past decade, epidemiologic population-based studies reportedly show a marked increase in heroin use. According to the Office of National Drug Control Policy, the number of American heroin users increased by more than half in less than a decade, from 600,000 in the early 1990s to 980,000 in 2001.[566] Heroin use is also a problem with teenagers. In the 2001 behavior surveillance of American high school students, 3.1% admitted they had used heroin during their lifetime.[507] Male students were significantly more likely than females to report lifetime heroin use (3.98% versus 2.5%, respectively), a sex difference that applied to both white and black students. Moreover, white and Hispanic students (3.3% and 3.1%, respectively) were more likely to report lifetime heroin use than black students (1.7%). The prevalence of heroin use varied three-fold across state surveys (1.4% to 4.3%) and five-fold across local surveys (2.8% to 8.6%).

(1) Heroin overdose

The marked increase in heroin use has led to a dramatic increase in the incidence of fatal and non-fatal heroin overdose in several countries. In 1993, there were 3805 heroin-implicated deaths in the US;[568] in 1999 there were 4820 reported heroin-related deaths, as well as 16,646 non-fatal heroin overdose cases seen in emergency departments.[568] In 1999, heroin overdose was the leading cause of death among men aged 25 to 54 years in Multnomah County,

Oregon.[569] Here, heroin-associated deaths more than doubled from 1993 to 1999 (46 to 111). The Florida medical examiner reported that heroin was present in 141 deaths in the first six months of 2002; heroin was listed as the cause of death in 121.[497]

In 1997 to 1998, the mean estimate of dependent heroin users in Australia was 74,000, a population prevalence of 6.9/1000 persons aged 15 to 54 years.[570] This is the same number as estimated in Britain (7/1000 persons) and in the European Union (3–8/1000 persons aged 15–54 years). Moreover, opium-associated deaths in Australia increased from 1.3 to 71.5 per million population aged 14 to 44 years, a 55-fold increase between 1964 and 1997.[571] Indeed, about 2% of people who inject heroin die each year, which is six to 20 times the rate seen in peer controls who do not use drugs.[572] There were also a significant number of opiate-related fatalities in Sheffield, UK between 1997 and 2000.[573] Thus, there were 94 deaths due to illicit opiate overuse, most of them associated with intravenous injections.

Since heroin overdose is a leading cause of morbidity and mortality among active heroin injectors, Sporer[568] recently suggested the following strategies for preventing heroin overdose: some combination of increasing treatment with opiate substitutes (i.e. methadone and naloxone), education of drug users, formation of family support groups; and supervised injecting facilities.

(2) Heroin, HIV and viral hepatitis

The risk correlates for prevalent HIV, hepatitis B virus (HBV) and hepatitis C virus (HCV) were recently examined over a five-year period in 483 non-injecting heroin users.[574] Their findings showed that among never-injectors, the statistically significant correlates were unprotected sex with men who were involved in sex with other men (HIV and HBV), unprotected sex with non-injecting heroin users (HIV), self-reported syphilis infection (HBV), longer periods of heroin use (HBV and HCV), blood transfusion before 1986 (HIV), and having been tatooed (HCV). Among former injectors, the significant correlates were syringe-sharing (HIV and HBV), frequent lifetime injection (HCV), longer duration of sexual activity (HBV), and having been tatooed (HCV).

Others in Canada compared the sociodemographic, drug and sexual risk characteristics between HCV baseline positive and negative young drug injectors and sought to identify the prospective risk factors for HCV seroconversion among those aged 13 to 24 years.[575] Of the 232 drug injectors, 107 (46%) were HCV positive at baseline and another 37 seroconverted during the study period. Base positivity was associated with Aboriginal ancestry, older age, greater number of drug-injecting years, recent incarceration, sex trade work, more than 100 lifetime sexual partners, a previous sexually transmitted disease, and injection more than once per day of heroin, cocaine and speedball. The major independent factors associated with HIV seroconversion were having a drug-injecting partner, requiring help to inject, and cocaine injection more than once daily.

In a longitudinal 10.5-year follow-up study of a cohort of 135 heroin addicts in Spain, 34 had AIDS (25%); the average annual morbidity rate was 2.7%.[576] Twenty of the addicts were diagnosed with tuberculosis and 15 were infected with both AIDS and tuberculosis. A marked increase in new HIV cases was also recently reported in China, where women were also increasingly at risk.[577] There were 4677 new cases of HIV in 1999, an increase of 41.5% over 1998. Since 1985, 17,316 Chinese HIV carriers had been identified. Over the previous 15 years, HIV was largely confined to needle-sharing heroin addicts and their sexual partners. However, there is a fear of future HIV outbreaks in the general population because of the significant HIV increase in truck drivers and prostitutes in areas with thriving sex trades.

(3) Heroin use and other clinical diseases

In 2000, there was an outbreak of serious illness and death among heroin drug-injectors in England.[578] Twenty-six definite or probable cases were identified, half of whom died. The investigators suggested that since the outbreak duration was short (a period of five months), the problem might have been related to a particular supply of heroin. *Clostridium novyi*, a spore-forming microorganism, was identified in two cases. During this same period (April to August, 2000), a similar outbreak among heroin-injectors occurred in Scotland.[579] Here, 60 cases were identified, of which 23 were definite and 37 probable. The median age was 30 years and about half were female. Of the definite cases, there were 20 deaths; of the 37 probable cases, three died. *Clostridum novyi* type A was identified in 13 cases.

Gacouin *et al.*[580] reported a case of spongioform leucoencephalopathy in a young man after he inhaled the vapor from heated heroin. Successive computed tomography scans and magnetic resonance imaging over seven months showed "evolution from bilateral extensive involvement of the cerebral white matter to almost complete resolution...."

Anabolic-androgenic steroids (AAS)

Since its discovery in 1935, numerous testosterone derivatives have been synthesized with the goals of prolonging its biological *in vivo* activity, producing orally active androgens and developing anabolic-androgenic steroids (AAS) that are more anabolic and less androgenic than testosterone. Medically, these AAS are primarily used to treat androgen deficiency syndrome and, more recently, catabolic states such as AIDS-associated wasting, obstructive pulmonary disease, severe burn injuries and alcoholic hepatitis, as well as bone marrow failure syndromes, constitutional growth retardation in children and hereditary angioedema.[581] However, with respect to the possible beneficial effects of AAS in alcoholic liver disease, a systematic literature review "could not demonstrate any significant beneficial effects of AAS on any clinically important outcomes of patients with alcoholic liver disease."[582]

The use of AAS to enhance physical appearance, as well as physical and psychological capacities, has increased dramatically over the past several decades in age groups from adolescence to adulthood.

(1) Adolescent use of anabolic-androgenic steroids
There has been a significant increase in the number of adolescent males in the US who have used AAS in order to improve their

personal appearance and athletic performance over the past decade. Many of them also used AAS in combination with alcohol and psychotropic drugs. In the US, 5% of high school students reported they had used illegal steroids (i.e. without a physician's prescription) during their lifetime.[506] Male students were significantly more likely to report lifetime steroid use than females (6.0% versus 3.9%). In addition, white students were significantly more likely than black students to have used steroids during their lifetime (5.3% versus 3.2%). The prevalence of lifetime illegal steroid use varied significantly across both state (2.5% to 6.9%) and local surveys (2.3% to 5.7%).

Wichstrom and Pedersen[583] investigated the prevalence of AAS use among 8508 Norwegian adolescents and evaluated three perspectives on AAS use: performance enhancement in sports competition, body image and eating concerns, and AAS-use as belonging to a cluster of problem behaviors. Their data led them to conclude that adolescent AAS use is primarily another type of problem behavior (i.e. marijuana use and aggressive conduct); it is only secondarily associated with disordered eating and participation in power sports. In order to evaluate the risk profile of AAS use in adolescents, Swedish researchers analyzed the importance of social, personality and health factors in 2700 senior high school students in Uppsala, Sweden.[584] Their findings showed that immigrant status, low to average self-esteem, low to average perceived school achievement, and use of prescription tranquilizers/sedatives were significantly associated with AAS use after controlling for various confounders (e.g. strength training, truancy and alcohol consumption). The authors concluded that, in addition to strength training and multiple drug use, AAS user characteristics "include social, personality and health aspects."

(2) Anabolic-androgenic steroids: athletic performance and body building

Megadoses of illicit AAS are commonly used for body building and enhancement of athletic performance. Indeed, studies with laboratory animals show that AAS increases exercise tolerance. For example, Tamaki *et al.*[585] demonstrated that AAS (nandrolone decanoate) not only enhanced the rate of protein synthesis during recovery after weight lifting, but increased the work capacity and fatigue resistance in rats. Others[586] reported that, compared with controls, AAS-treated animals exhibited increased dominant behavior in a competition test. The authors suggested that, in agreement with earlier studies, AAS abuse may constitute a risk factor for disinhibitory behavior, partly by decreasing brain serotonin levels.

To assess the physiological and psychological states accompanying steroid use, Bahrke *et al.*[587] studied male weight lifters regarding their physical training and perceived behavioral and somatic changes. Both current and previous AAS users reported the following changes: (1) increases in enthusiasm, aggression and irritability; (2) changes in muscle size, muscle density and strength; (3) faster recovery from workouts and injuries; and (4) changes in libido. Indeed, experienced weight lifters with an adequate diet and who continue training during AAS use reportedly increase their lean mass and strength compared with that from training alone.[588]

(3) Anabolic steroids and behavioral traits
Large doses of AAS have been associated with a variety of behavioral characteristics, including increased aggression and violence. For example, a recent report indicated that men who began AAS with intentions of gaining muscle mass and strength frequently became involved in various criminal activities, including violent offenses.[589] However, the question as to whether AAS use causes aggression or whether aggressive individuals are more attracted to AAS has been raised.[590] This study reported that 60% of participants who were AAS users indicated that AAS increased their aggressiveness. However, the authors noted that the increased aggression "appeared more related to irritability and bad temper than acts of physical violence."

(4) Anabolic-androgenic steroids and drug dependence
Recent studies suggest that AAS may cause mood disorders and dependence syndromes. Moreover, they may introduce some people to opioid abuse. Although a recent literature review found no evidence that AAS abuse or dependence develops from their therapeutic uses, there were 165 reported instances of AAS dependence

among weight lifters and body builders.[591] For example, 49 weight lifters, all users of AAS, were evaluated to investigate the addictive patterns of use.[592] Here, at least one dependence symptom was reported by 94% of the group; three or more dependence symptoms were reported in 57%. The dependent users were distinguished from non-dependent users by their use of larger doses, more cycles of use, more dissatisfaction with body size and more aggression. Not only did many of these individuals take large AAS doses, but often other drugs of abuse.

To assess the apparent association between chronic AAS use and other drugs of abuse, Kanayama and associates[593] evaluated 223 male substance abusers who were being treated for alcohol, cocaine and opioid dependence. Of these, 29 (13%) reported prior steroid use but only four were documented on physicians' admission evaluations. Among 88 men listing opioids as their drug of choice, 22 (25%) admitted to prior steroid use versus only seven (5%) of the other 135 men. Of the 24 men who were interviewed in detail, 18 (75%) reported that AAS were the first drugs that they had ever self-administered by injection. The authors concluded that among individuals with opioid dependence, prior steroid use appears to be a common but under-recognized occurrence.

(5) Anabolic-androgenic steroids and medical diseases

As noted earlier in this chapter, there is a significant risk of hepatitis B, hepatitis C and HIV among individuals who inject drugs of abuse. To examine the exposure to these infectious diseases in injectors of illicit anabolic steroids, Aitken et al.[594] examined blood samples from 63 Australian steroid injectors. Their findings showed the following: 9.5% were positive for hepatitis C antibody; 12% were positive for hepatitis B core antibody; but none were positive for anti-HIV. Hepatitis C was associated with heroin injection, imprisonment, sharing needles, number of tattoos and hepatitis B exposure. Hepatitis B exposure was associated with hepatitis C exposure, past imprisonment and age of first injection. The authors concluded that "steroid injectors should not be neglected in blood-borne virus prevention efforts."

Although rhabdomyolysis has many causes, it may also occur after vigorous weight lifting in persons taking AAS.[595]

(6) Summary: anabolic-androgenic steroid use

The myotrophic actions of AAS are their cerebral stimulatory effects which have led to their widespread use by athletes and "recreational" drug users, especially teenagers and young adults. Although all AAS are classified as class III controlled substances, they have some medical benefits including androgen deficiency syndromes, catabolic states (e.g. AIDS-associated wasting), obstructive pulmonary disease, severe burn injuries and bone marrow failure syndromes among others. Nevertheless, illicit use of megadoses of AAS for the purpose of body building and enhancement of athletic performance can lead to a wide variety of serious and irreversible disorders. In addition to the various disorders noted above, the "administration of these agents should be avoided in pregnant women, women with breast cancer or hypercalcemia, men with carcinoma of the prostate or breast, and patients with the nephrotic syndrome or significant liver dysfunction."[581]

Environment and Occupation

Toxic environmental agents include a host of chemicals and pollutants in the atmosphere, the workplace, the food and water supply, solar radiation and various infectious microorganisms. These environmental and occupational toxic substances can lead to a wide range of human illnesses and are important causes of disability and death. They include, among many others, skin cancer from excess sun exposure, leukemia in persons exposed to benzene, asthma and chronic bronchitis in persons exposed to organic dusts, pulmonary fibrosis, lung cancer and mesothelioma in persons exposed to asbestos, kidney failure and hypertension in persons chronically exposed to lead, impairment of reproductive function in persons exposed to certain solvents and pesticides, and chronic musculoskeletal disorders in workers who perform repetitive motions.

Although occupational exposures are significant contributors to the morbidity and mortality of several diseases, they continue to be greatly under-recognized. Rough estimates of the number of new cases of occupational disease in the US in the early 1990s ranged from 125,000 to 350,000 per year as well as 5.3 million work-related injuries.[596] The annual economic cost was estimated at over US$60 billion. In a later more extensive analysis, Leigh *et al.*[597] reported that in 1992 there were approximately 6500 job-related injury deaths, 13.2 million non-fatal injuries, 60,300 deaths from disease and 862,200 illnesses in the US. The total direct costs (US$65 billion) plus indirect costs (US$106 billion) were estimated to be US$171 billion. Moreover, the authors noted that "these estimates are likely to be low, because they ignore costs associated with pain and suffering, as well as those of within-home care provided by family members, and because the numbers of occupational injuries and illnesses are likely to be undercounted."

Job-related diseases and injuries include a wide variety of medical disorders including increased risk of myocardial infarction, cancer, carpel tunnel syndrome, osteoarthritis and various pulmonary diseases among others. Moreover, some job-related injuries may result in death. Several specific examples will be presented.

Leigh and associates[598] estimated that in 1992 there were 841 agricultural job-related deaths and 512,539 non-fatal injuries in the US; the total financial cost was estimated at US$4.59 billion (direct costs, US$1.66 billion; indirect costs, US$2.93 billion). On a per person basis, farming costs contribute about 30% more than the national average. This research group[599] also estimated the 1992 occupational costs for injuries and illnesses in California. Their results showed the following: 660 job-related injury deaths, 1645 million non-fatal injuries, 7079 deaths from diseases, and 0.133 million illnesses. The total cost was estimated to be US$20.7 billion (direct costs, US$7.04 billion; indirect costs, US$13.62 billion). Injuries cost US$17.8 billion and illnesses, US$2.9 billion. The authors noted that "these costs are similar with those of all cancers combined and only slightly less than the cost of heart disease and stroke in California." Osteoarthritis, a good example of a single job-related disease, accounted for about 9% (US$8.3 billion in 1994 dollars) of the total costs for all osteoarthritis in the US (about 51% medical costs; 49% lost productivity).[600]

Occupational diseases reportedly account for about 85% of the deaths due to circulatory disorders.[601] Fatal acute myocardial infarction occurred more frequently on Monday than any other day; the highest frequency occurred in those with low-paying occupations. Carpal tunnel syndrome and hearing loss accounted for the most morbidity (number of cases and days lost). Mental disorders, especially related to stress, generated more morbidity than is generally recognized. These stress-related problems were highest in the transportation and public utility industries, finance, insurance and real estate. Manufacturing contributed significantly more cases than any other industry. The highest costs of job-related injuries and diseases occur among heavy duty truck drivers, non-construction and construction laborers, machine operators, janitors, carpenters and assemblers.[602]

Several respiratory diseases have also been associated with various occupations. These include tracheobronchitis, asthma, chronic obstructive pulmonary disease, interstitial lung disease, pulmonary fibrosis and lung cancer, as well as others.[603] For example, occupational asthma has been associated with more than 250 workplace substances including acid anhydrides (adhesives and paints), acrylates (paints and adhesives), isocyanates (polyurethane paint and roofing foam), dusts (wood, flour and grains) and animal proteins (laboratory animals and farming), among others.[603] Other respiratory disorders are associated with coal dust, crystalline silica, cotton dust, toluene diisocyanate and several metals (e.g. copper, arsenic and cadmium). Several examples will be presented.

Fixed obstructive lung disease was recently reported in workers at a microwave popcorn factory.[604] Results from early animal studies suggest severe airway damage occurs after inhalation exposure to high air concentrations of butter flavoring. Others[605] studied 973 non-smoking women aged 20 to 40 years who were employed in three similar modern Chinese cotton textile mills. All of the women had some exposure to cotton dust; the average employment time was 8.7 years. After adjustment for certain confounders (e.g. home exposure to tobacco smoke and coal heating), the odds ratios for prevalence of frequent current symptoms were as follows: frequent cough, 2.23; frequent phlegm, 3.24; shortness of breath, 4.54; and wheeze, 2.96.

Although cigarette smoking is the major cause of chronic obstructive pulmonary disease (COPD), many occupational dusts can cause, or at least contribute to, chronic airflow limitation or emphysema. These agents include coal dust, crystalline silica, cotton dust, cadmium and toluene diisocyanate.[603] Moreover, when COPD is caused by coal and silica dust, the disease may progress for decades even after exposure has ceased.[606]

Twelve or more substances found in the workplace are classified as human lung carcinogens.[607] Indeed, it has been estimated that 5% of lung cancers in the US are due to occupational exposure.[608] Most of these cancers are attributed to asbestos, radon, silica, chromium, cadmium, nickel, arsenic and beryllium.[609]

Environmental and Occupational Risk Factors

Although most occupational diseases are preventable, few physicians are trained to recognize or prevent these work-related illnesses.[610] Other factors include physician difficulty in dealing with the Workers' Compensation system, the reluctance of some patients to connect health problems with their workplace, and the present managed care environment which significantly reduces the time available for a complete occupational history and counseling.[611] The major environmental and occupational risk factors responsible for morbidity and mortality are listed in Table 5.9.

Solar radiation

The skin is commonly exposed to solar radiation, which causes a variety of negative effects including inflammation, pigmentation,

Table 5.9: Environmental and Occupational Risk Factors

Air Pollution	Solar Radiation	Dusts
Ozone	Trace Elements	Animal protein
Industrial particulates	Arsenic	Silica
Automobile emissions	Aluminum	Coal
Asbestos	Cadmium	Cotton
Organic chemicals	Lead	Pesticides
Toluene diisocyanate	Mercury	
Acrylamide		

immunomodulation, photoaging and cancer.[612] Sunburn, the most common problem associated with solar radiation, has been well studied and various reactive oxygen species (ROS) generated from several sources have been identified. Ultraviolet light homolytically dissociates water to produce the potent hydroxyl radical (HO·).[613] In addition, ROS have been shown to be produced by endogenous photosensitizers, released from inflammatory cells, prostaglandin endoperoxides, and the formation of peroxynitrite from nitric oxide and superoxide.

Solar radiation and skin cancer

Skin cancer is the most common form of cancer in the US.[614] Increased sun exposure due to ozone depletion and more time spent outdoors have been implicated as important factors to explain the increase in skin cancer rates.[615] Indeed, the incidence of squamous cell carcinoma in New Hampshire increased by 235% in men and 350% in women from 1979–1980 to 1993–1994; basal cell carcinoma increased by more than 80% in both men and women.[616] Excess exposure to solar radiation greatly increases the risk of these two common forms of skin cancer, both of which are generally curable. Melanoma, however, the third most common type of skin cancer and one of the most common cancers in young adults, is significantly more malignant. In 2001, an estimated 1.3 million new cases of basal cell or squamous cell carcinoma were diagnosed with approximately 2000 deaths from both cancers combined. By contrast, about 53,600 new cases of melanoma were diagnosed; there were an estimated 7400 deaths.[617] Moreover, the annual incidence rate for melanoma more than doubled from 1973 to 1998 (5.3 cases/ 100,000 persons to 14.1 cases/100,000 persons).[618]

In addition to increased sun exposure, the use of artificial tanning devices, such as sunlamps and tanning beds that emit ultraviolet (UV) radiation, has become significantly more common in the US. Importantly, a recent study showed that any use of tanning devices was associated with odds ratios of 2.5 for squamous cell carcinoma and 1.5 for basal cell carcinoma.[619] This is not surprising since the type and amount of UV radiation emitted from some tanning devices is similar to that of noontime summer sun, and in some cases the amount is even higher than the sun would emit.[620] Artificial UV radiation has also been linked to ocular melanoma.[621]

Most skin cancers can be readily prevented if individuals will adhere to the following recommended guidelines:[618]

(1) minimize sun exposure during the peak hours (10am to 4pm);
(2) seek shade when possible from midday sun (10am to 4pm);
(3) wear hats, clothing and sunglasses that protect the skin;
(4) use broad-spectrum sunscreen (UV-A and UV-B protection) with a sun-protection factor $\geq$ 15; and
(5) avoid sunlamps and tanning beds.

Solar radiation and cataract

In 1637, Gallileo became blind after he repeatedly observed the sun's course without eye protection. Centuries later, in 1912, an estimated 3500 Germans suffered visual impairment after watching a solar eclipse without eye protection. Worldwide, cataract is the leading cause of visual loss.[622] In 1991, cataract surgery accounted for 12% of the US Medicare budget, or US$3.4 billion annually.[623] Moreover, cataract surgery rates have increased significantly since then. As the world population ages, loss of vision and cataract surgery will become an even greater problem unless appropriate preventive steps are taken.

Early epidemiologic studies reported an association between sun exposure and cataract. For example, studies of the Australian aborigines showed a dose-response relation between the prevalence of cataract and levels of ultraviolet-B radiation (UV-B; wavelength, 290 to 320 nm).[624,625] Since some of these early reports reportedly suffered "from a lack of precision both in the definition of cataract and in the quantification of exposure to UV-B radiation," Taylor et al.[626] studied 838 watermen (mean age, 53 years) who worked on the Chesapeake Bay. After calculation of the annual ocular exposure from age 16, the risk of cortical cataract increased by 3.30 in those whose exposure was in the highest quartile compared with those in the lowest quartile. More recently, West et al.[627] reported that even though older people have a relatively low exposure to UV-B in sunlight, there is still an increased risk of cortical cataract. Two recent literature reviews are in agreement that long-term ocular exposure to UV-B radiation in the general populations of developed countries confers a significant risk of cortical cataract.[628,629] The authors of this latter review of 22 epidemiologic studies reported that most of them "support an association between UV-B and the development of cortical cataract and perhaps posterior subcapsular cataract."

Solar radiation comprises light in the infrared (IR), visible and ultraviolet-A (UV-A) ranges, as well as UV-B. Although less damaging than UV-B, UV-A (wavelength, 320–400 nm) may also damage the lens after long-term exposure. A recent study of chronic low level UV-A exposure to guinea pigs was potentially harmful to the lens since it resulted in a significant increase in oxidized products in the nuclear region.[630] This and other studies suggest that UV-A radiation may also increase the risk of cataract in humans.[631] Certainly, the current data indicate that more research is needed to evaluate the possible role of UV-A light in cataract formation.

What is the mechanism whereby UV radiation leads to cortical cataract? Numerous in vitro, animal and human studies indicate that oxidative damage is important in cataract formation.[632] Several examples will be given. Since polyphenolic compounds (flavonoids) present in green tea are well established antioxidants, Gupta and associates[633] evaluated the anti-cataract potential of green tea leaf extract in the development of lens opacification. Enucleated rat lenses were randomly divided into normal, control and treated groups. Oxidative stress was induced by sodium selenite in the culture media of the control and treated groups. The medium of the treated group was supplied with tea extract. They also induced *in vivo* cataract in nine-day-old rat pups of both control and treated groups by subcutaneous injection of sodium selenite. The treated pups were injected intraperitoneally with tea extract. The results showed that tea extract significantly reduced oxidative stress (i.e. measured malondialdehyde and glutathione levels) in the cultured lenses, as well as the incidence of *in vivo* cataract in the rat pups. Similarly, in a lens organ culture cataract model, quercetin, a potent polyphenolic antioxidant, effectively inhibited hydrogen peroxide-induced lens opacity.[634] Finally, Li *et al.*[635] examined the influence of exogenously administered melatonin, an efficient antioxidant normally produced by the pineal gland, in cataract formation and lipid peroxidation in newborn rats treated with buthionine sulfoximine (BSO). BSO depleted the rats of glutathione, a natural antioxidant required in the inactivation of hydrogen peroxide by glutathione peroxidase. In this study, 81% of the rats treated with BSO developed cataracts. However, only 7% of the rats treated with BSO plus melatonin developed cataracts.

In a random clinical trial, Seddon *et al.*[636] studied 17,774 participants (Physicians' Health Study), aged 40 to 84 years, over a five-year period. Compared with physicians who did not use any vitamin supplements, those who took only multivitamins had a relative cataract risk of 0.72. Similarly, others[637] reported that deficiencies of both vitamin C and carotenoids, and possibly vitamin E, are risk factors for senile cataract. Garland[638] also emphasized that vitamin C is protective against oxidative lens damage, particularly photo-induced damage resulting in cortical and posterior subcapsular cataracts. Moreover, smoking, which greatly reduces vitamin C blood levels, is a significant risk factor in cataract formation.[639] After an extensive review of laboratory and clinical studies, Spector[640] concluded that "the data suggest that the epithelial cell layer is the initial site of attack by oxidative stress and that involvement of the lens fibers follows, leading to cortical cataract."

Solar radiation and macular degeneration

Age-related macular degeneration (AMD) is the most common cause of blindness in the elderly. The Beaver Dam Eye Study reported a prevalence of 36.8% in patients 75 years and older.[641] The major risk factors, in addition to age, are genetics, smoking, poor nutrition and degenerative factors. In addition, oxidative stress from solar radiation is also a major risk factor. The macula is highly susceptible to oxidative stress because the photoreceptor cells are metabolically very active since they are rich in mitochondria which results in an increased formation of superoxide radicals. Moreover, the cell membranes have the highest concentration of polyunsaturated fatty acids of any known tissue, making them highly susceptible to lipid peroxidation.[642] Other indirect evidence supporting a role of oxidative stress is that the concentration of lipofuscin ("age pigment"), a polymerization product of lipid peroxidation, is very high in AMD.[643]

In an early study, the National Health and Nutrition Examination Survey reported that individuals with a high intake of fruits and vegetables rich in vitamin A had a 50% reduced risk of AMD.[644] A later cross-sectional analysis of blood-based information from 600 participants in the Baltimore Longetudinal Study of Aging showed that those with high serum levels of vitamin E had about a 60% reduced risk of ADM, although they found no significant protective effect from vitamin C or beta-carotene.[645] Conversely, Seddon and associates[646] reported that individuals in the highest quintile of carotenoid intake had a 43% lower risk for AMD compared with those in the lowest quintile of carotenoid intake. Lutein and zeaxanthin, which are rich in dark green leafy vegetables (e.g. spinach and collard greens), were particularly effective in reducing the risk of AMD. These authors concluded that "increasing the consumption of foods rich in certain carotenoids, in particular dark, green leafy vegetables, may decrease the risk of developing advanced or exudative age-related macular degeneration, the most visually disabling form of macular degeneration among older people." Similarly, data from the Eye Disease Case-Control Study[647] support a protective role for various carotenoids including lutein, zeaxanthin, alpha-carotene, beta-carotene and cryptoxanthin.

Numerous other epidemiologic, case-control and animal studies support a role for oxidative stress in AMD, although it should be noted that not all studies have reported a positive association between anti-oxidants and AMD.[632]

Air pollution

In 1952, stagnant weather conditions caused a rapid increase in the concentration of air pollutants in London, UK. Over several days, more than three times as many people died than expected resulting in an estimated excess death toll of over 4000. Concentrations of smoke and sulfur dioxide reached several thousands of micrograms per cubic meter.[648] Similar events due to extreme air pollution occurred in the Meuse Valley, Belgium and Donora, Pennsylvania.[649,650] Interestingly, a recent re-analysis of the 1952 London data that included the long term events, the number of additional deaths was about 12,000.[651] Although effective steps were taken to eliminate most of the air pollution in industrialized nations since the 1950s, air pollution due to other factors has re-emerged over the past ten to 15 years and is again an important environmental health problem. Indeed, exposure to pollutants such as airborne particulate matter and ozone have been associated with increased morbidity and mortality, particularly due to respiratory and cardiovascular diseases. These pollutants may also be a risk factor for decreased life expectancy.

Ozone, greenhouse gases, and particulates

Ultraviolet radiation from the sun is absorbed in the stratosphere (ten–30 miles above the earth) by molecular oxygen (O_2) which is dissociated into ground-state oxygen atoms which, in the presence of air, reacts with molecular oxygen to form ozone (O_3).[652] Ozone in the stratosphere protects against harmful ultraviolet radiation. Unfortunately, man-made chemicals are responsible for depleting this ozone layer such that more ultraviolet rays now reach the earth's surface which increases the prevalence of skin cancer and cataract, and depletes farm crops. Below the stratosphere is the troposphere, which extends from the earth's surface to an altitude of 10 Km to 18 Km. Here, in association with the sun's ultraviolet rays, an excess of ozone is formed by oxygen reacting with air pollutants such as automobile exhausts, organic solvents and industrial emissions that contribute to photochemical air pollution (smog). Ozone, a potent oxidant, is capable of reacting with a variety of biomolecules, especially those containing thiol (i.e. -SH) or amine ($-NH_2$) groups (e.g. proteins and amino acids) and unsaturated carbon-carbon bonds (e.g. polyunsaturated fatty acids and phospholipids).

In addition to ozone, atmospheric concentrations of greenhouse gases, including carbon dioxide, methane and nitrous oxide are also of considerable importance. The continued increases in these gases is largely attributed to human activities (e.g. fossil-fuel combustion, and change in land use and agricultural practices). Unless significant efforts are made to reduce production, their concentrations will continue to increase.

Particulate air pollution is a mixture of solid particles and liquid droplets that vary in size, composition and origin. Since only very small particles can be inhaled deep into the lungs, the national US health standards for ambient air quality are based on the mass concentration of "inhalable particles," which refers to particles with an aerodynamic diameter of <10 um (particulate matter; PM_{10}). Fine-particulate air pollution includes particles with an aerodynamic diameter ≤ 2.5 um ($PM_{2.5}$). These fine particulates generally contain a mixture of particles including acid condensates, sulfate, nitrate particles and soot. These fine particles are generally believed to pose a significant risk to health since they are more likely to be toxic than the larger particles and can be breathed more deeply into the lungs.[653]

Air pollution, morbidity and mortality

Air pollution in cities has been linked to increased rates of morbidity and mortality in developed and developing countries. Indeed, deaths from air pollution have been ranked as one of the top ten causes of disability by the World Health Organization (WHO). In 1995, WHO estimated that 460,000 avoidable deaths occur annually as a result of suspended particulate matter, mainly from outdoor urban exposures.[654] Two years later, WHO and the World Resources Institute and others estimated that almost 700,000 air pollution-related deaths occur annually and about eight million avoidable deaths will occur worldwide by the year 2020.[655]

A series of early studies indicated that low concentrations of ozone and particulate matter result in day to day variations in mortality, respiratory and cardiovascular hospital admissions, exacerbations of asthmatic symptoms, and decreased lung function in school children.[656] Nevertheless, some have questioned the validity of the tightening of air quality standards with respect to public health. To address this, Samet *et al.*[657] assessed the effects of five major air pollutants (i.e. PM_{10} particulates, ozone, carbon monoxide, sulfur dioxide and nitrogen dioxide) on mortality rates in 20 of the largest areas in the US from 1987 to 1994. Their results showed consistent evidence that the level of PM_{10} was associated with the rate of death from all causes and from cardiovascular and respiratory diseases. There was weaker, albeit still significant, evidence that increased ozone levels also increased the relative death rates in the summer, but not during the winter. Levels of the other pollutants were not significantly related to mortality.

The results of these cross-sectional studies have been supported by more recent large prospective cohort studies. Thus, Dockery *et al.*[658] analyzed mortality data from 8111 adults over a 14- to 16-year period in six American cities. After adjusting for age, sex, smoking, BMI, education level, occupational exposure and other possible risk factors, the adjusted mortality-rate ratio for the most polluted cities compared with the least polluted was 1.26. Air pollution was positively associated with death from lung cancer and cardiopulmonary disease, but not with death from other diseases. Similarly, Pope and associates[659] used air pollution data collected from 151 American metropolitan areas to evaluate the effects of air pollution on mortality during eight years of follow-up of 552,138 adults. Using multivariate analysis controlled for smoking, education level and other possible risk factors, the association between air pollution and all-cause lung cancer and cardiopulmonary mortality was examined. The adjusted relative risk ratios for all-cause mortality for the most polluted areas compared with the least polluted was 1.15 and 1.17 when using sulfate and fine particulates, respectively. Moreover, particulate air pollution was associated with cardiopulmonary and lung cancer mortality but not with mortality due to other causes. In their follow-up study of this large population,[660] which doubled the follow-up time to more than 16 years and tripled the number of deaths, expanded the exposure data including gaseous co-pollutant data and new $PM_{2.5}$ data, improved control of occupational exposure, incorporated dietary variables and used recent advances in statistical modeling, they concluded that "long-term exposure to combustion-related air pollution is an important environmental risk factor for cardiopulmonary and lung cancer mortality." Similarly, Hoek and coworkers[661] studied the association between mortality and traffic-related pollution in 5000 people aged 55 to 69 years over an eight-year period in the Netherlands. The relative risk for cardiopulmonary mortality associated with living near a major road was 1.95; the relative risk for total deaths was 1.41. Non-cardiopulmonary and non-lung cancer deaths were not related to air pollution.

The impact of total outdoor and traffic-related air pollution on public health in Austria, France and Switzerland was also recently evaluated.[662] Cases attributed to air pollution were estimated for mortality, cardiopulmonary hospital admissions, incidence of chronic bronchitis (adults), bronchitis in children, restricted activity days and asthma attacks. The findings indicated that 6% of total mortality (over 40,000 cases/year) was caused by air pollution, about half of which were attributed to motorized traffic. Moreover, there were more than 25,000 new cases of chronic bronchitis (adults), 290,000 episodes of bronchitis in children, 0.5 million asthma attacks and 16 million person-days of restricted activities.

The importance of reducing air pollution was further emphasized by a recent study from Ireland.[663] Here, concentrations of air pollution and "directly-standardized non-trauma, respiratory and cardiovascular death rates were compared for 72 months before and after the ban of coal sales in Dublin." This ban resulted in a 70% reduction in particulate air pollution as measured in black smoke. The adjusted death rates for respiratory and cardiovascular deaths decreased by 15.5% and 10.3%, respectively.

Diseases associated with air pollution

As noted in the mortality studies previously discussed, several diseases including lung cancer, acute and chronic bronchitis, asthmatic episodes and cardiovascular disease have been associated with air pollution, particularly due to fine particulates.

(1) Lung cancer
Numerous epidemiologic studies from various countries have shown that increased urban and industrial pollutants significantly increase the risk of lung cancer, even after adjustment for smoking and other variables. Indeed, recent population-based cohort studies have shown an increased lung cancer risk of 30% to 50% in areas with high ambient air pollution levels compared with areas with lower levels.[658–660,664] Nyberg *et al.*[665] conducted a large population-based case-control study of men aged 40 to 75 years which included all cases of lung cancer from 1985 to 1990 in Stockholm. Their results also showed that urban air pollution increases the risk of lung cancer and that "vehicle emissions may be particularly important."

(2) Coronary heart disease
Fine particulate air pollution <2.5 um in diameter ($PM_{2.5}$) and ozone are associated with increased cardiovascular disease.[656,666] Individuals with cardiopulmonary disease are particularly at risk for acute

cardiac events since even transient $PM_{2.5}$ exposure has been shown to trigger myocardial infarction in susceptible people.[667] In a study of non-fatal myocardial infarction among Swedish men and women aged 45 to 70 years, the authors evaluated their exposure to motor exhaust, other combustion products and organic solvents.[668] After adjusting for smoking, alcohol intake, hypertension, diabetes, overweight and leisure-time physical activity, the relative risk of myocardial infarction was 2.11 among those who were "highly exposed" and 1.42 among those who were "intermediately exposed" to combustion products from organic material.

Since diabetes is associated with an increased risk for coronary heart disease, Zanobetti and Schwartz[669] evaluated the susceptibility of diabetics to cardiovascular damage by airborne particles. Their results showed that diabetics had twice the risk of a PM_{10}-associated cardiovascular hospital admission compared with non-diabetics. Moreover, persons 75 years and older also had an increased cardiovascular risk.

What is the mechanism whereby air pollution increases the risk for cardiovascular events? To help answer this important question, Brook and associates[670] investigated the effect of air pollution on vascular function in 25 healthy adults. In this randomized, double-blind study, the vascular response in the brachial artery to the inhalation of ambient fine particles plus ozone was compared with the response to inhalation of filtered air. The findings showed that short-term inhalation of fine particulates and ozone at concentrations similar to that in an urban environment causes acute artery vasoconstriction.

(3) Asthma and other allergic disorders

The prevalence of allergic diseases has continued to rise in industrialized countries over the past 200 years. The prevalence of hay fever in adolescents was recently estimated to be 38.6% in the UK and 33.6% in the US.[671] Yet, hay fever, a readily recognized allergic disorder, was reportedly unknown in Europe and North America 200 years ago.[672] These diseases account for a significant number of hospital visits, lost productivity and increased medical costs, as well as deaths.

Asthma, a common chronic illness affecting both adults and children in the US, increased in prevalence from 1980 to 1995.[673] However, a follow-up report indicated that the proportions of children and adults with asthma who reported activity limitations has stabilized, although the rate of emergency department visits has increased. Although the rates of hospitalization and death have decreased overall, black Americans continue to have higher rates of emergency department visits, hospitalizations and deaths from asthma than do whites.[674] Thus, the annual number of deaths attributed to asthma were 2891, 3880, 4819, 5637, and 5667 in 1980, 1985, 1990, 1995 and 1996, respectively.

Although the cause or causes of the increased number of allergic disorders remain somewhat controversial, numerous experimental, laboratory and epidemiologic studies have linked high levels of air pollutants to various respiratory health problems, especially asthma. Because asthma is a major health problem, the Healthy People 2010 established the following eight objectives:[675] (1) reduce the asthma-associated death rate; (2) reduce hospitalizations; (3) reduce emergency department visits; (4) reduce activity limitations; (5) reduce the number of missed school and work days; (6) increase formal asthma education; (7) increase the proportion of people who receive appropriate care; and (8) establish a surveillance system for tracking asthma deaths, illnesses, disabilities, impact of occupational and environmental factors on asthma, access to medical care, and asthma management in at least 25 states.

Asthma is a leading cause of morbidity among children in the US with an estimated prevalence of 6.9% in those aged 18 years and younger.[676] This and other respiratory disorders are well known to be aggravated by various inhaled agents. For example, environmental tobacco smoke has been shown to be an important risk factor for asthma.[677,678] Moreover, occupational studies indicate that some workplace air pollutants, such as toluene diisocyanate, can cause asthma.[679,680] Although epidemiologic studies involving industrial and automobile exhaust pollutants have been somewhat inconsistent, most studies have shown a direct correlation.

Pope[681] assessed the association between hospital admissions and fine particulate pollution (PM_{10}) during a time period in which the closure and reopening of a local steel mill occurred. During the winter months when the steel mill was open, PM_{10} levels were nearly double the levels during the winter months when the mill was closed. Moreover, children's hospital admissions were two to three times higher during the time the mill was open compared to when it was closed. PM_{10} levels more strongly correlated with admissions for bronchitis and asthma than with admissions for pneumonia and pleurisy. Kim *et al.*[682] also reported that the prevalence of asthma among children living around a heavily industrialized area was significantly higher than those who lived in a less polluted area despite similar atopic sensitization.

During the 1996 Summer Olympic Games in Atlanta, the number of acute asthmatic events decreased 41.6% in Medicaid claims, 44.1% in a health maintenance organization, 11.1% in two pediatric emergency departments, and 19.1% in the Georgia Hospital Discharge Database.[683] The explanation for this remarkable reduction in asthmatic events was because of efforts to decrease air pollution by significantly reducing downtown traffic congestion. Others[684] also recently reported a direct association between automobile traffic air pollution and several respiratory disorders, including asthma in children.

Air pollution has also been associated with respiratory symptoms in adults. Zemp and associates[685] investigated the association between long-term exposure to ambient air pollution and respiratory symptoms in a cross-sectional study in random population samples of adults (aged 18 to 60 years) at eight study sites in Switzerland. After controlling for age, BMI, sex, parental asthma, parental atopy, education level and foreign citizenship, they found positive associations between respiratory symptoms and annual mean concentrations of NO_2, total suspended particulates and particulates less than PM_{10}. Among never smokers, the odds ratio for a 10 ug/m^3 increase in PM_{10} concentration was 1.35 for chronic phlegm production, 1.27 for chronic cough or phlegm production, 1.48 for daytime breathlessness and 1.32 for dyspnea on exertion. Interestingly, others[686] observed a positive association with a sensitization to pollen that was most pronounced among adults with a duration of residence exposed to road traffic for at least ten years. After adjusting for possible confounders, the odds ratios for traffic exposure compared with the lowest quartile (referent category) were 1.99, 2.47 and 2.83. The data suggested to the authors that living on busy roads is associated with a significantly higher risk for pollen sensitization and "could possibly be interpreted as an indication for interactions between pollens and air pollutants."

Pesticides, trace elements, asbestos and other chemical toxicants

Millions of persons worldwide are continually exposed, occupationally and environmentally, to a wide variety of toxic substances such as metals, pesticides, organic solvents and other chemical toxicants.

Pesticides

There were about 400 synthetic chemical pesticides registered for use on food crops in North America in 1997.[687] Indeed, 80% to 90% of American households use pesticides,[688,689] including organophosphates, chlorpyrifos, diazinon, pyrethroids (i.e. cis- and trans-permethrin), some carbamates, [689,690] and various organochlorine chemicals, among others. As such, the most common route of exposure is through the diet and drinking water. In addition, various pesticides are commonly found in house dust and indoor air.

A study at two non-occupational sites (Jacksonville, Florida and Springfield, Massachusetts) found that indoor, personal and outdoor air sample concentrations were highest in the summer, lower in the spring and lowest in winter.[688] Indoor and personal air concentrations were comparable and significantly higher than outdoor air concentrations. In a nine-home study to evaluate potential exposure to children aged six months to five years, 23 of 30 target pesticides were detected.[689] The most frequently detected pesticides were chlordone, chlorpyrifos, dieldrin, hepachlor and pentachlorophenol.

The greatest number of pesticides and the highest concentrations were found in carpet dust. Because of their play close to the ground, hand-to-mouth behavior and unique dietary patterns, it is not surprising that children consume and absorb significantly more pesticides per kg body weight than adults; and some children consume considerably more.[691] Moreover, children are often more vulnerable than adults to the ingested pesticides.

Six million children in America's inner cities live in poverty. Unfortunately, low-income groups bear a disproportionate share of the health risks from pesticides that are commonly used in urban schools, homes and day-care centers to control roaches, rats and other vermin. Studies with laboratory animals suggest that pesticide exposure during pregnancy and early life may impair neurodevelopment in the offspring. Since pesticide concentrations are particularly high in urban areas, and data are limited in minority populations, Whyatt and associates[692] gathered questionnaire data on home pesticide use during pregnancy from 316 African-American and Dominican women residing in minority communities in New York City. Of these, 72 also underwent personal air monitoring for 48 hours during their third trimester. All that were monitored had detectable levels of organophaphates, diazinon and chlorpyrifos. Diazinon exposures for some of these women "may have exceeded health-based levels…" Other pesticides were also present in a significant number of women. Landrigan *et al.*[688] reported that the heaviest use of pesticides in all counties of New York State was in the boroughs of Manhattan and Brooklyn.

Chronic exposure to persistent toxic contaminants in the environment can cause a variety of developmental problems. The following are a few examples. Karmous *et al.*[693] measured dichlorodiphenyl dichloroethene (DDE) and polychlorinated biphenyls (PCB) blood concentrations in children from three regions in central Germany between 1994 and 1997. They found that DDE, a metabolite of the pesticide dichlorodiphenyl trichloroethane (DDT), was associated with a growth reduction for girls, but not boys, through age eight years. Prior studies showed that DDE was associated with higher weight and height in boys during puberty, whereas PCB levels were associated with increased weight in girls.[694] Others[695] reported that hexachlorobenzene was associated with undescended testes.

In recent years, the more subtle effects of exposures to environmental neurotoxicants have been reported. These include reduced intelligence, impairment in reasoning ability, shortening of attention span and behavior alteration.[696] The estimated annual cost for neurobehavioral disorders is US$9.2 billion,[697] an estimate that is likely to be low because it "ignores costs of pain and suffering and does not include late complications for which etiologic associations are poorly quantified." Others[698] recently suggested that exposure to selective dithiocarbamate pesticides may be a risk factor for Parkinson's disease. Unfortunately, less than 10% of the 70,000 chemicals in commercial use have been evaluated for neurotoxicity.

Recent studies have shown that many pesticides also cause impairment or suppression of the immune system.[699] In studies involving organochlorine organophosphate and carbamate compounds, Banerjee[700] reported the following: (1) the immune system is more susceptible to the toxic effect of pesticides when dietary protein intake is deficient; (2) suppression of immune responses by the immediate metabolites is an important determinant of the toxicity of the parent compound; and (3) the type and duration of physical and emotional stress and possible involvement of oxidative stress (i.e. free radical production) are important in pesticide-induced immune toxicity.

Trace elements

All biologic fluids and tissues normally contain low concentrations of various trace elements. Although the body requires daily intake of many of these elements, increased exposure interferes with biologic activity. The following 15 elements are considered essential:[701] arsenic, chromium, cobalt, copper, fluorine, iodine, iron, manganese, molybdenum, nickel, selenium, silicon, tin, vanadium and zinc. However, the concentrations required for optimal biologic function vary considerably, although a well-balanced diet usually provides an adequate supply. Unfortunately, many people become exposed to excessive levels, at which time some of these elements become poisons. In a study of 2000 people aged five to 85 years, Campbell[702] reported that the most common metals present in toxic amounts were lead, cadmium, arsenic, mercury and aluminum.

(1) Aluminum

Aluminum is among the most abundant metals on earth. Hence, the average daily intake from food and water ranges from 2 mg to 15 mg. However, only a very small amount of ingested aluminum is normally absorbed. As a result, aluminum poisoning is relatively uncommon. Nevertheless, increased exposure may occur in persons receiving some buffered medications, are on dialysis, or receiving intravenous fluids. Those at greatest risk are diabetics, dialysis patients, those who have undergone parathyroidectomy or transplant surgery, are iron deficient and children.[603] Occupational exposure to high aluminum levels may also occur. For example, numerous workers in an aluminum smelting operation developed Alzheimer-like symptoms.[604] Other common sources that may lead to increased aluminum intake include aluminum cookware, especially when used to cook acid-foods, coffee makers, beer and soft drink cans, baking powder, antacids, buffered aspirin, tea, bleached flour, pancake and cake mixes, non-dairy creamers, nasal sprays, cigarette filters, food coloring and Kaopectate.[705]

(2) Arsenic

Arsenic has been used for centuries, both as a medicine and a poison. For example, Hippocrates and Galen recommended arsenic sulfide to treat ulcers. Later, arsenic was commonly used to treat fevers, headache and syphilis. During the first 50 years of the 20th century, arsenic was still widely used in medicines, as well as for pest control, and is currently used to treat some parasitic infections and cancer. However, most recent attention has focused on its possible use as a terrorism agent (e.g. Lewisite and arsine gas), increased awareness of exposure from decks and playground equipment constructed from timber treated with chromated copper arsenate, and the publicity associated with lowering the arsenic levels in drinking water.

Persons currently at risk for arsenic poisoning are workers in industries that either produce or use arsenic-containing compounds, those whose water supply contains high levels, and those living near sources of high ambient air levels. More specifically, arsenic may be released into the environment as a by-product in the mining and smelting of lead, copper and zinc.[706] It is also released into the atmosphere when fuel oils and coal are burned. Moreover, arsenic compounds are used in pesticides, herbicides, wood preservatives, batteries, rat poisons, and as growth promoters in poultry and livestock.

Arsenic may also contaminate water due to leaching from rocks, etc. into groundwater and/or runoff from surface water, especially in Asia and South America. Significant contamination has been reported in China, Taiwan, Vietnam, Cambodia, Pakistan, Nepal, Mongolia, Chile and India.[706] Indeed, over 4000 villages in Bangladesh and India are exposed to increased arsenic levels and 20% or more of the population have symptoms of arsenic poisoning.

Arsenic may also be a risk factor for several cancers, as indicated by the following examples. Koragas *et al.*[707] recently confirmed that the measurement of arsenic in toenails is a reliable indicator of arsenic exposure. In a study of 687 basal cell and 284 squamous cell skin cancers, these workers reported odds ratios for squamous cell and basal cell carcinomas of 2.07 and 1.44 for individuals whose arsenic concentrations were above the 97th percentile compared with those with levels are at or below the median value.[708] In another study, Kurttio *et al.*[709] measured the arsenic levels in drilled wells in Finland and studied the association of arsenic exposure with the risk of kidney and bladder cancers. Although none of the exposure indicators (i.e. arsenic concentration in wells, daily and cumulative doses) were significantly associated with kidney cancer risk, bladder cancer was significantly associated with arsenic concentrations and daily dose during the third and ninth years prior to cancer diagnosis.

(3) Lead
Greek physicians recognized the association between lead exposure and disease over 2000 years ago. Although the sources of lead have

changed since then, and exposure is largely preventable, lead poisoning remains among the most studied health problems. As such, it is critical that physicians are aware of the environmental sources of lead that can cause illness in persons at high risk. Although lead exposure has decreased over the past several decades, it remains the most common environmental illness among children in the US. Indeed, chronic lead exposure continues to be a problem even though the accepted blood levels have decreased from 60 ug/dL in 1950 to 10 ug/dL in 2000.[710] Lead poisoning also remains extremely expensive, the recently estimated total annual cost being US$43.4 billion.[697]

In 1990, three to four million American children (about 17%) were considered at risk of lead poisoning.[711] Campbell reported that 3% of 2000 persons aged five to 85 years had increased blood levels.[702] A child is generally considered to have lead poisoning when the lead blood level is 10 ug/dL or greater. Based on previous US Centers for Disease Control (CDC) studies that examined lead levels during 1991–1994, 4.4% of children aged one to five years had blood levels greater than 10 ug/dL. A more recent report, however, showed that this had decreased to 2.2%.[712] Nevertheless, "current evidence suggests that there is no threshold blood level at which lead has no adverse effect on health."[713] Importantly, exposure of children who live in older homes that often contain lead-based paint and lead-contaminated dust remains a serious problem. In addition, soil contamination by emissions from leaded fuel also remains an environmental lead source. Thus, as with other toxic contaminants, those living in inner cities are particularly vulnerable. Nevertheless, no economic or racial subgroup of children is free from the adverse effects of lead.

Children less than three years of age have an increased risk of lead's entry into the developing nervous system. Moreover, children absorb and retain more lead in proportion to body weight than do adults. Young children also have a greater prevalence of iron deficiency, a disorder that can increase the gastrointestinal absorption of lead. Those at risk, in addition to children, are the developing fetus (blood lead readily crosses the placenta) and industrial workers and their families, since workers may bring lead dust home on their skin and clothes.

Acute lead poisoning is characterized by abdominal pain ("lead colic"), cognitive deficits, peripheral neuropathy, arthralgias, decreased libido and anemia. Children are especially at risk for developmental and long-term cognitive deficits. Chronic lead exposure may also lead to serious medical problems. Several recent studies have shown that blood lead levels of 10 ug/dL or below in children may still lead to serious problems. Canfield and associates[714] measured blood lead levels in children at six, 12, 18, 24, 36, 48 and 60 months of age and tested their intellectual abilities at three and five years (Standford-Binet Intelligence Scale). Their results showed that blood lead levels "even those below 10 ug per deciliter, are inversely associated with children's IQ scores at three and five years of age...." Early studies also suggested that increased lead exposure is related to aggressive and violent behavior. In a recent cross-sectional ecological study from all counties in the contiguous American 48 states, the homicide incidence rate ratio was 4.12 for the highest air lead level compared with the lowest level.[715]

Exposure to various environmental contaminants, such as polybrominated biphenyl[716] and polychlorinated aromatic hydrocarbons,[717] have been reported to accelerate or delay pubertal development in girls. Moreover, Selevan *et al.*[718] found that blood lead levels of 3.0 ug/dL were associated with significant delays in breast and pubic-hair development in African-American and Mexican-American girls, but not non-Hispanic white girls. In addition, as compared with levels of 1.0 ug/dL, lead levels of 3.0 ug/dL were associated with decreased height after adjustment for age, race and other factors but not with BMI or weight.

Over the past two decades, studies have suggested that low levels of lead exposure among adults may increase the risk of increased blood pressure and hypertension.[719,720] More recently, Nash and coworkers[721] studied a cross-sectional sample of 2165 women aged 40 to 55 years from 1988 to 1994. Their results showed that a change in blood lead levels from the lowest quartile (0.5–1.6 ug/dL) to the highest quartile (4.0–31.1 ug/dL) was associated with a statistically significant increase in both systolic and diastolic blood pressures. Women in the highest quartile had increased risks of both diastolic (>90 mmHg) hypertension (odds ratio, 3.4) and systolic (>140 mmHg) hypertension (odds ratio, 1.5). However, the association between blood lead levels and hypertension was even stronger in postmenopausal women. Here, the adjusted odds ratios for diastolic hypertension increased with increasing quartile of blood lead level compared with the lowest quartile (4.6, 5.9 and 8.1, respectively). Thus, at levels below the current US occupational exposure guidelines (40 ug/L), the blood lead level was positively associated with both systolic and diastolic hypertension.

Studies have also suggested that environmental lead exposure is associated with age-related decreases in kidney function. To further evaluate this association, Lin *et al.*[722] studied a group of patients with chronic renal insufficiency (serum creatinine 1.5–3.9 mg/dL). Non-diabetic subjects with an elevated body lead burden were randomly assigned to either a chelation or control group. Patients in the chelation group received lead-chelation therapy (calcium disodium EDTA); the control group received placebo. During the following 24 months, repeated chelation therapy was administered weekly to patients with a high-normal body lead burden. The controls received weekly placebo infusions. The results showed that the glomerular filtration rate in patients receiving chelation therapy improved significantly compared with the control group (mean change 2.1 ± 5.7 ml/minute per 1.73 m^2 body-surface area compared with 6.0 ± 5.8 ml/minute per 1.73 m^2 body-surface area).

(4) Mercury
Mercury has been used for centuries for both medicinal purposes and as a poison. It is currently used in various commercial areas. In 1973, more than 500 people in Iraq died and more than 600 were hospitalized after eating bread prepared from wheat treated with a mercury-containing fungicide.[723] In the mid-1980s, mass poisoning occurred in Japan due to fish contamination where mercury compounds were dumped into the ocean. About 80% of the mercury in fish is in the form of methylmercury, which is significantly more toxic than elemental or inorganic mercury. Because of these and other

events, attention is currently focused on the poisonous effects of mercury-contaminated seafood, use in dental amalgams, vaccine administration to infants, and in some folk remedies.[724]

Overall, environmental mercury is primarily from natural sources (soil erosion and degassing of the earth's crust), fossil fuel combustion, waste incineration, mercury spills and smelting processes.[701,725] Since elemental mercury is a liquid, it readily vaporizes at room temperature and can readily enter the body through the lungs. Indeed, about 70% to 85% is absorbed through the lungs whereas less than 3% is absorbed through the skin.[725] Moreover, less than 0.1% of ingested elemental mercury is absorbed from the gastrointestinal tract. In addition, mercury is lipid soluble, a fact that facilitates its passage into the lungs, central nervous system and placenta.

Interpretation of mercury blood levels is somewhat complicated due to the wide range of values found in presumably healthy populations. However, for populations consuming moderate amounts of seafood, the blood levels are generally 5.0 ug/L or less, a value well below the US Environmental Protection Agency's recommended upper level of 5.8 ug/L in which exposures are considered benign.[726] In a recent study of 1250 children aged one to five years and 2314 women aged 16 to 49 years, blood mercury levels were about three-fold higher in women compared with children.[718] In women who ate three or more servings of fish in the previous 30 days, blood mercury levels were four-fold higher than those who ate no fish during this time period. Importantly, 8% of the women had blood concentrations greater than 5.8 ug/L.

In communities with increased exposure to contaminants, such as methylmercury in seafood, risks of decreased height and weight, as well as neurobehavioral dysfunction, must be considered in children who are breast-fed. For example, Grandjean *et al.*[727] reported a doubling of the mercury concentration in cord blood was associated with a decrease in both height and weight at 18 months of age in children who were breast-fed. This group also recently reported that maternal mercury exposure during pregnancy was associated with detectable neuropsychological deficits at age seven years,[728] a finding that supported earlier studies.[729–731]

Increased mercury levels may also be a risk factor for coronary heart disease and myocardial infarction. In a prospective cohort study of men in eastern Finland, fish consumption and mercury levels in hair were positively associated with coronary heart disease and myocardial infarction.[732] Similarly, a recent case-control study conducted in eight European countries and Israel indicated that toenail mercury levels were directly associated with the risk of myocardial infarction.[733] The authors concluded that "high mercury content may diminish the cardioprotective effect of fish intake." However, in the same journal issue, others concluded from their nested case-control study that although toenail mercury levels significantly correlated with fish consumption, their "findings do not support an association between total mercury exposure and the risk of coronary heart disease, but a weak relation cannot be ruled out."[734] Thus, further studies are needed to clarify the association between mercury levels and coronary heart disease.

(5) Cadmium

Background levels of cadmium in food, water and ambient air are not a health concern for most people in North America. Typical dietary intake is approximately 30 ug/day, a rate about ten times lower than that required to cause kidney damage.[735] However, environmental cadmium contamination from industrial processes, fossil fuel combustion and cadmium-containing wastes is of significant importance.[736] Indeed, since there are no known biologic benefits of cadmium, even very low levels might be considered toxic. In 1992, over 500,000 American adults were occupationally exposed to cadmium levels that may be harmful.[737] These include alloy makers, auto mechanics, battery makers, cable trolley wire makers, cadmium platers, dental amalgam makers and smelterers, among various others.[735] Importantly, the allowable exposure limits for workplace air decreased from 1000 ug/m^3 in 1941 to 5.0 ug/m^3 in 1992. Cadmium concentrations in air samples from various American cities currently range from 0.002 ug/m^3 to 0.05 ug/m^3. Although these levels seem very low, the biologic half-life for cadmium is ten to 30 years. Hence, the body burden increases throughout life so that the cumulative effect can be significant even in persons not occupationally exposed to cadmium. Moreover, cigarette smoking further contributes to cadmium intake since blood levels reportedly increase about 1.6% for each cigarette smoked per day.[701]

Cadmium-induced renal tubular and glomerular damage is generally irreversible and may progress to renal failure even after cadmium exposure has been eliminated. Cadmium has also been associated with renal cell carcinoma. Thus, in a case-control German study, the odds ratio for kidney cancer was 1.4 for men and 2.5 for women who were exposed to increased levels of cadmium over a long period of time.[738] Cadmium has also been implicated as a risk factor for pulmonary disease, hypertension and coronary heart disease,[739,740] although the evidence for coronary heart disease is limited and inconsistent.[741]

Asbestos

Asbestos is a generic term for a group of six naturally occurring fibrous minerals. The basic unit of asbestos minerals is the silicate combined with various amounts of iron, magnesium, calcium, aluminum and sodium.[742] Two classes of asbestos exist: serpentine, which contains a magnesium silicate (chrysotile), and amphiboles which include crocidolite, amosite, anthophyllite and tremolite. Chrysotile accounts for about 93% of the asbestos used worldwide.[742] Asbestos fibers may result from mining, milling and weathering of asbestos-bearing rock. These fibers also come from the manufacture, wear and disposal of asbestos-containing products. Thus, asbestos fibers are ubiquitous in the environment.

Although asbestos has been banned and voluntarily phased out since the 1970s, it is still used in construction materials. Moreover, building insulation materials stockpiled before the ban remain in many homes and commercial buildings. Interestingly, asbestos levels in schools are typically 1000 times below the permissible exposure level for work environments. However, overreaction by the public and politicians led to removal and abatement programs resulting in some facilities having higher levels of airborne asbestos after removal than before due to improper removal. Thus, as noted by Case,[743] "one problem which has been vastly overstated in the US concerns non-occupational exposure to asbestos." As he emphasized, this is not to suggest that asbestos exposure presents no environmental risk, but that the risk of this and other environmental contaminants must be put in proper context. For example, in 1990 the annual projected death rate of asbestos exposure in schools was no more than 0.1/million children whereas 10/million died playing school football and 60/million children aged one to 14 years died in home accidents.[743] Moreover, the cost of asbestos removal from buildings approached US$150 billion.[744]

In the early 1900s, it became evident that occupational exposure to asbestos causes asbestosis, a fibrotic lung disease.[745] Later, in the 1950s and 1960s, epidemiologic studies of workers showed that occupational asbestos exposure also caused lung cancer and mesothelioma,[746] a problem that still exists. For example, in a recent study of 924 consecutive cases of lung cancer without a history of occupational asbestos exposure in northwest Italy, histologic asbestosis was demonstrated in 56 cases ("definitely asbestos-related").[747] In five additional cases, asbestos bodies were not microscopically demonstrated although there was pulmonary fibrosis and increased concentration of asbestos fibers/gram dry weight. Extrapolation of their estimates on a national scale suggested that 2000 cases of asbestos-related lung cancer occur in Italy each year. However, only 281 cases of asbestos-related lung cancer were reported from all occupational causes in the years 1990–1995. Thus, when one considers the association between asbestos and lung cancer today, it is probably much larger, at least worldwide, than generally recognized.

Miscellaneous organic chemicals

A wide variety of toxic organic chemicals are produced and distributed worldwide for a host of industrial purposes. Others are products of incomplete combustion of fuels, components of paints, oils, solvents, etc. As such, they are prevalent in the environment where they enter the food chain. The toxic chemical compounds discussed here will include acrylamide, polycyclic aromatic hydrocarbons, polychlorinated biphenyl (PCB), 1,3 butadiene and dioxin. Although not addressed, other toxic chemicals such as trichloroethylene, vinyl chloride, methylene chloride and the nitrosamines are also potentially harmful and widely disseminated in the environment. The primary health problem associated with some of these chemicals is that they are potentially carcinogenic. However, as with many other substances, predicting the carcinogenicity of a complex chemical mixture on the basis of one or more of its components is difficult because of possible interactions among the components.

(1) Acrylamide

Acrylamide is a monomer of polyacrylamide, whose products are used in the manufacture of paper, water treatment and as a soil stabilizer. Although polyacrylamide is non-toxic, acrylamide is potentially toxic and reportedly produces cellular changes and tumors in both rats and mice, cellular transformation in the Syrian hamster embryo.[748] As a result of these and other studies, acrylamide has been classified by the International Agency for Research on Cancer (IARC) as a probable human carcinogen. Indeed, a recent Swedish study reported that acrylamide is present in high levels in starch-based foods cooked at high temperatures.[749,750] Here, potato chips, French fries, biscuits and crackers had the highest levels; breakfast cereals, breads and corn chips had lower amounts.

The association between acrylamide and human cancers has not been proven. In a follow-up report, Marsh *et al.*[751] studied a cohort of 8508 workers with acrylamide exposure in three US plants from 1984 to 1994. Their findings showed "little evidence for a causal relation between exposure to acrylamide and mortality from cancer sites ..." Similarly, Mucci and associates[752] reported that dietary exposure to acrylamide in amounts "typically ingested by Swedish adults in certain foods has no measureable impact on risk of three major types of cancer" (i.e. large bowel, kidney and bladder). Another recent study, however, concluded that acrylamide consumed from various cooked foods produce a background dose of acrylamide that "is associated with a considerable cancer risk."[753] Hence, future studies will be needed to clarify the question as to whether acrylamide from fried foods is a risk factor for cancer. However, since fried foods are widely recognized as being unhealthy, one should limit their consumption.

(2) Polycyclic aromatic hydrocarbons

Polycyclic aromatic hydrocarbons (PAHs), which are organic compounds consisting of three or more fused benzene rings containing only carbon and hydrogen, are ubiquitous in the environment. PAHs are produced when complex organic substances are exposed to high temperatures. Indeed, they are a natural component of most fossil fuels. Although PAHs are naturally produced by volcanoes and forest fires, most ambient air PAHs result from burning coal, wood, petroleum and oil, as well as coke production, refuse burning and motor vehicle exhaust. Moreover, PAH levels in foods vary. Charring meat or barbequing food over a charcoal fire greatly increases PAH production. Other foodstuffs that contain increased levels include cooked and smoked meats and fish, roasted peanuts, coffee and cigarette smoke.[754] Although hundreds of PAHs exist, benzopyrene is the most carcinogenic PAH studied.

Occupations at increased risk of PAH exposure include the following: workers with coal, coal products, aluminum and asphalt, machinists, auto and diesel mechanics, printers, roofers, and workers exposed to creosote, among others.[754] Long-term exposure to PAHs has been associated with an increased risk of cancer, which is further increased with the additive effect of cigarette smoke and other toxic agents. In a study of 11,103 men employed in six Norwegian aluminum plants for at least three years, the overall relative risk ratio for excess bladder cancer was 1.3. However, the relative risk increased with increasing PAH exposure to 2.0 for the upper exposure group compared with expected national figures.[755] There were also "indications of an elevated risk of kidney cancer" but no association was found with lung cancer.

(3) 1,3-Butadiene

1,3-butadiene, a major ingredient of synthetic rubber, has been shown to be carcinogenic in both mice and rats.[756,757] Importantly, cancer occurred in both species at levels equal to or below the federal standard of 1000 parts/million. Human epidemiologic studies have also shown a correlation between 1,3-butadiene exposure and cancer. Thus, an early retrospective study of 8017 male workers employed in two tire manufacturing plants in Ohio showed an increased risk for gastric cancer, as well as lymphatic and hematopoietic malignancies.[758,759] A later updated epidemiologic study of 2568 workers for at least six months at a 1,3-butadiene manufacturing plant in Texas found an increased death rate due to lymphosarcoma and reticulum cell sarcoma.[760] Similarly, an updated retrospective study of 12,113 workers employed in eight synthetic rubber plants in the US and Canada also found an excess mortality rate for lymphatic and hematopoietic malignancies in both black and white production workers.[761] Thus, occupational exposure to 1,3-butadiene is a probable significant cancer risk factor, especially for lymphatic and hematopoietic malignancies. The association between 1,3-butadiene exposure and carcinogenicity risk has been critically reviewed.[762]

(4) Polychlorinated biphenyls

Polychlorinated biphenyls (PCBs) are a family of 209 chemicals that vary in the number and positions of chlorine atoms attached to two connected benzene rings. Commercial PCBs are mixtures of these compounds and are usually contaminated with small amounts of furans (polychlorinated dibenzofurans) and dioxins (polychlorinated dibenzodioxins). PCBs persist in the environment, concentrating in the food chain. As such, the major non-occupational exposure to PCBs is from various foods, especially fish from contaminated water and animal fat. Although PCBs are no longer manufactured in the US, there is still a potential for workplace exposure. Workers at increased risk include those employed in electric cable repair, electroplating, fire fighting, hazardous wastes, heat exchange equipment repair, maintenance cleaning, metal finishing, roofing and pipefitting/plumbing, among others.[763]

Fetuses and neonates appear to be more sensitive to PCBs and other chemical contaminants than adults. Indeed, some environmental contaminants have been reported to alter the sex ratio of offspring at birth. Since fish from the Great Lakes of the US are contaminated with PCBs, Weisskopf *et al.*[764] examined parental serum PCB levels in relation to the sex ratio of children of mothers and fathers in the Great Lakes region between 1970 and 1995. Their findings showed that the odds ratio for having a male child among mothers in the highest quintile compared with the lowest quintile of PCB concentration was 0.18. However, there was little evidence of an association with paternal exposure.

(5) Dioxin

Dioxin (polychlorinated dibenzo-p-dioxins) and furans (dibenzofurans) produce similar health effects and coexist in various materials. There are 75 dioxin isomers, of which 2,3,7,8-tetrachlorodibenzo-p-dioxin (TCDD) is the most studied. The food chain is the major route of dioxin exposure, although other sources are diesel exhaust, chlorine-bleached paper products and incineration gases. Other potential dioxin sources include emissions from coal-burning power plants, diesel exhausts and incomplete burning of wastes containing chlorine; smaller amounts come from volcanoes and forest fires.

Several large human populations have been exposed to dioxin, resulting in extensive publicity and considerable public health concerns. One of the most publicized events involved Vietnam veterans who were potentially exposed to dioxins by military use of the defoliant Agent Orange. In addition, different areas of the US have been contaminated as a result of industrial discharges of spraying of dirt roads with dioxin-contaminated waste oils.[765] The areas that received the most attention were in Niagra Falls, New York (Love Canal), Times Beach, Missouri and Newark, New Jersey. However, the most extensive accident exposing a residential population (more than 37,000 people) was an explosion at a chemical plant in Seveso, Italy in 1976.[766,767] Importantly, no deaths from acute poisoning occurred in any of these disasters. However, in 1988 Italian and American scientists convened to further examine the Seveso dioxin incident. They measured the TCDD levels in over 30,000 serum or plasma samples collected from residents during the period 1976–1985.[766] Some TCDD levels were the highest ever reported in humans. In general, however, the serum/plasma concentrations were of the same magnitude as those found in occupational studies.

Bertazzi *et al.*[767] carried out a ten-year mortality study of the population involved in the Seveso incident and compared the findings with a referent cohort of 167,391 subjects who lived "in the immediate surroundings." They found that biliary (females only) and brain cancers, as well as lymphatic and hematopoietic neoplasms (especially leukemia in males) were significantly increased in the dioxin-exposed residents. The authors concluded that these findings "did not appear to result from chance, confounding, or information/comparison bias." The findings were also "suggestive" of an increase in soft tissue tumors and melanoma. Certainly, dioxin has been shown to be carcinogenic in numerous studies involving laboratory animals. Prior to this study, only two negative effects of dioxin industrial exposure had been confirmed: chloracne lesions (pale yellow cysts) which appear one to three weeks after exposure and transient mild hepatotoxicity.

Except for rare major industrial accidents, those most at risk for exposure to dioxin are chemical industry workers, and possibly fetuses and breast-fed infants if the mothers have been exposed.

(6) Radon
Radon is a colorless and odorless radioactive gas that forms from naturally occurring radioactive uranium. Since uranium occurs worldwide in soil and rock, radon exposure is also universal. Thus, radon exposure in humans is primarily due to radon-contaminated gas rising from the soil. The suspicion that working in underground mines is associated with cancer was suspected even before radon was identified as an element. Indeed, in 1556 Agricola, a German scholar, reportedly wrote about the high mortality of miners in Eastern Europe.[768] About 300 years later, autopsy studies demonstrated that lung cancer was common among miners in this region. In the early 1900s, these mines were shown to contain high levels of radon and in the 1950s and 1960s, epidemiologic studies confirmed the association between radon exposure and lung cancer.[769]

Radon has been extensively studied over the past four decades and shown to be an important environmental carcinogen, affecting not only miners but workers in various occupations. Radon has also been associated with lung cancer in some general populations, especially in areas where the soil concentration is high.[769] In this latter group, radon levels are usually highest in home basements due to its proximity to the ground from which the gas diffuses.[770] Hence, those who spend considerable time in basement rooms, either at work or home, are at a greater risk for exposure. Indeed, the Environmental Protection Agency estimated that as many as eight million homes in the US have elevated radon levels.[771]

With respect to the association between lung cancer and radon exposure, it has been estimated that between 3000 and 33,000 radon-associated deaths occur in the US each year, with central estimates of 15,400 or 21,800 depending on the model used.[769] Thus, after smoking, radon is the second leading cause of lung cancer in the US. Moreover, an estimated one-third of lung cancer cases could be avoided if homes with radon levels of 4.0 pC/L or greater were reduced.

Seasonal temperature changes

Extreme environmental temperatures have been arbitrarily defined as hot ($>30°C$; $86°F$) or cold ($<0°C$; $<32°F$).[772] Prolonged periods of work, recreation, or being confined at home can lead to negative energy and nitrogen balances and dehydration. These, in turn, can lead to impaired thermoregulation, ketosis, altered acid-base and electrolyte balance, depleted glycogen stores, impaired motor coordination and diminished work capacity.[772] Thus, mortality rates are affected by both elevated and low temperatures.

Hypothermia is defined as the unintentional lowering of the core body temperatures below $35.0°C$ ($95.0°F$). Hypothermia may be mild ($90.0°F–<95.0°F$; $32.2°C–<35.0°C$), moderate ($82.5°F–<90.0°F$; $28.0°C–<32.2°C$), or severe ($<82.5°F$; $<28°C$). Common risk factors for hypothermia include exposure to cold temperatures while under the influence of alcohol, drugs, altered mental status, and immersion in cold water. Between 1979 and 1998, there were an estimated 700 annual deaths in the US attributed to cold weather.[773]

There is a substantial annual temperature change in most areas of the US, as well as in various other countries. Seasonal variations in mortality have been associated with age, outdoor temperature and influenza. The increased winter death rate has also been associated with socioeconomic status and increasing age. Essentially all cities with daily temperatures in July exceeding 30°C have January temperatures near the freezing point. Conversely, even where the January temperatures are colder than $-10°C$, the maximum afternoon temperatures in July usually exceed 30°C. Interestingly, death during the winter is reportedly more common in the UK than in most other countries in Western Europe.[774] This excess mortality rate has been attributed primarily to coronary heart disease, stroke and respiratory diseases. Laake *et al.*[774] compared winter mortality between Norway and England/Wales. They found that winter mortality in England and Wales was nearly two-fold greater in old and middle-aged people and also "markedly higher than in Norway…" However, deaths related to influenza were similar. In Britain and Wales, there were about 3500 annual deaths in persons aged 45 years and older for each 1°C reduction in winter temperature, after adjustment for age and influenza.

Increased mortality due to coronary heart disease is particularly well known to be significantly higher in the winter than in the summer. As noted in Chapter 1, coronary heart disease is associated with increased blood levels of fibrinogen and other coagulation factors. Importantly, fibrinogen levels are inversely associated with both environmental and body temperatures, as least in elderly subjects.[775]

Most anesthetics impair thermoregulation, which in combination with the cold operating room environment, open body cavities, and intravenous fluid and blood administration often lead to hypothermia. Frank *et al.*[776] carried out a randomized clinical trial to assess the association between body temperature and cardiac mortality during the postoperative period. Their results showed that in patients with risk factors for coronary heart disease who undergo non-cardiac surgery, "the perioperative maintenance of normothermia is associated with a reduced incidence of morbid cardiac events and ventricular tachycardia."

An increased environmental temperature is also a risk factor for mortality, especially among the elderly. In a 1993–1994 study from the Netherlands, the number of deaths among nursing-home patients during a 100-week study period was 38,861.[777] The lowest mortality rates were in weeks with average outside temperatures between 15°C and 19.9°C. In the hottest weeks (25.0°C–29.9°C), the mortality rate was 50% higher than the minimum rate (relative risk, 1.50), and the mortality risk for women was higher than for men. Since air-conditioning is apparently not commonly available in these nursing homes, the authors strongly recommended their availability during time of increased outside temperature. Indeed, the seasonal patterns of coronary mortality have changed significantly in the US over the past several decades, presumably due to the "gradual expansion of adequate heating and increased use of air-conditioning."[778] Similarly, Diaz et al.[779] studied the association between summer temperatures and mortality rates in Seville, Spain from 1986 to 1997. They found that mortality from all causes increased up to 51% above the mean in people aged 75 years and older for each degree Celsius above 41°C. This effect was primarily due to cardiovascular disease and, as noted above, was also more common in women than in men.

Chapter Summary

The major causes of human morbidity and mortality and the extensive associated financial costs are, to a highly significant degree, due to self-imposed lifestyles. Indeed, in addition to physical inactivity, overweight/obesity and poor nutrition, personal habits and addiction to tobacco, alcohol, and both illicit and prescription drugs are extremely costly to the involved individual, their family and to society. In addition, humans are commonly over-exposed to sunlight, artificial radiation and environmental temperature changes. Moreover, exposure to an extensive variety of potentially toxic chemicals which have contaminated our food supply, drinking water and the air we breathe is also very common. While most of these risk factors could be significantly decreased by more general public and school education, personal commitment, and medical consultation and professional counseling, the potential danger of environmental and occupational contaminants must be more fully addressed by local and federal governments, as well as the companies that produce them.

References

1. National Center for Health Statistics. *Advance Report of Final Mortality Statistics, 1990.* US Department of Health and Human Services, Hyattsville, MD, 1993, Monthly Vital Statistics Report, Vol. 41, No. 7.
2. McGinnis JM, Foege WH. Actual causes of death in the United States. *JAMA* 1993;270:2207–2212.
3. CDC. Annual smoking attributable mortality, year of potential life lost, and economic costs — United States, 1995–1999. *MMWR* 2002; 51:300–303.
4. CDC. Tobacco use — United States, 1900–1999. *JAMA* 1999; 282:2202–2204.
5. Mitka M. Surgeon Generals' newest report on tobacco. *JAMA* 2000; 284:1366–1369.
6. CDC. Tobacco use — United States, 1900–1999. *MMWR* 1999; 48:986–993.
7. CDC. Cigarette smoking among adults — United States, 1997. *MMWR* 1999;48:993–996.
8. Nelson DE, Kirkendall RS, Lawton RL, *et al.* Surveillance for smoking — attributable mortality and years of potential life lost, by state — United States, 1990. *MMWR* 1994;43:1–8.
9. Peto R, Chen ZM, Boreham J. Tobacco — the growing epidemic. *Nat Med* 1999;5:15–17.
10. Yu JJ, Mattson ME, Boyd GM, *et al.* A comparison of smoking patterns in the People's Republic of China with the United States. *JAMA* 1990;264:1575–1579.
11. Gong YL, Koplan JP, Feng W, *et al.* Cigarette smoking in China: prevalence, characteristics and attitudes in Minhang District. *JAMA* 1995;274:1232–1234.
12. Yang G, Fan L, Tan J, *et al.* Smoking in China: findings of the 1996 National Prevalence Survey. *JAMA* 1999;282:1247–1253.

13. Abundis J, Lynn G. World smoking-related deaths. *USA Today*, World Health Report, World Health Organization, 1999.

14. Chen ZM, Xu Z, Collins R, *et al.* Early health effects of the emerging tobacco epidemic in China. *JAMA* 1997;278:1500–1504.

15. Lam TH, He Y, Li LS, *et al.* Mortality attributable to cigarette smoking in China. *JAMA* 1997;278:1505–1508.

16. Lam TH, Ho Sy, Hedley AJ, *et al.* Mortality and smoking in Hong Kong: case-control study of all adult deaths in 1998. *BMJ* 2001;323:361–362.

17. Peto R, Lopez AD, Boreham J, *et al.* Mortality from smoking worldwide. *Br Med Bull* 1996;52:12–21.

18. Ohida T, Sakurai H, Mochizuki Y, *et al.* Smoking prevalence and attitudes toward smoking among Japanese physicians. *JAMA* 2001;285:2643–2648.

19. Doll R, Peto R, Wheatley K, *et al.* Mortality in relation to smoking: 40 years' observations on male British doctors. *BMJ* 1994;309:901–911.

20. CDC. Tobacco use preventing tobacco use among young people — United States, 1900–1999. *MMWR* 1999;48:986–993.

21. CDC. Tobacco use among high school students — United States, 1997. *MMWR* 1998;47:229–233.

22. CDC. *Preventing Tobacco Use Among Young People: Report of the Surgeon General.* US Department of Health and Human Services, Public Health Service, CDC, National Center of Chronic Disease Prevention and Health Promotion, Office on Smoking and Health, Atlanta, Georgia, 1999;48:986–993.

23. CDC. Tobacco use among middle and high school students — United States, 1999. *MMWR* 2000;49:49–53.

24. CDC. Trends in cigarette smoking among high school students — United States, 1991–2001. *MMWR* 2002;51:409–412.

25. Wechsler H, Rigotti NA, Gledhill-Hoyt J, Lee H. Increased levels of cigarette use among college students. *JAMA* 1998;280:1673–1678.

26. CDC. Prevalence of cigarette smoking among secondary school students—Budapest, Hungary, 1995 and 1999. *MMWR* 2000;49:438–441.

27. Pirkle JL, Flegal KM, Bernert JT, *et al.* Exposure of the US population to environmental tobacco smoke. *JAMA* 1996;275:1233–1240.

28. Lam TH, Ho LM, Hedley AJ, *et al.* Environmental tobacco smoke exposure among police officers in Hong Kong. *JAMA* 2000;284:256–263.

29. Department of Health and Human Services. *The Health Benefits of Smoking Cessation: A Report of the Surgeon General.* Government

Printing Office, Washington, DC, 1990 [DHHS Publication No. (CDC) 90-8416].

30. A clinical practice guideline for treating tobacco use and dependence: a US Public Health Service report. *JAMA* 2000;283:3244–3254.

31. Diagnostic and Statistical Manual of Mental Disorders, 4th Ed.: DSM-IV. American Psychiatric Association, Washington, DC,1994.

32. Rigotti NA. Treatment of tobacco use and dependence. *N Engl J Med* 2002;346:506–512.

33. O'Brien CP, McLellan AT. Myths about the treatment of addiction. *Lancet* 1996;347:237–240.

34. Council on Scientific Affairs. Smoking and health. *JAMA* 1980;243:779–781.

35. Anda RF, Remington PL, Sienko DG, Davis RM. Are physicians advising smokers to quit? The patient's perspective. *JAMA* 1987; 257:1916–1919.

36. Frank E, Winkleby MA, Altman DG, *et al.* Predictors of physicians' smoking cessation advice. *JAMA* 1991;266:3139–3144.

37. Pearson TA, McBride PE, Miller NH, Smith SC. 27th Bethesda conference: matching the intensity of risk factor management with the hazard for coronary events (task force 8) — organization of preventive cardiology service. *J Am Coll Cardiol* 1996;27:1039–1047.

38. Spangler JG, George G, Foley KL, Crandall SJ. Tobacco intervention training: current efforts and gaps in US medical schools. *JAMA* 2002;288:1102–1109.

39. Fiore MC, Bailey WC, Cohen SJ, *et al. Smoking Cessation: Clinical Practice Guideline No. 18.* US Department of Health and Human Services, Public Health Service, Agency for Health Care Policy and Research, Rockville, MD, 1996, AHCPR Publication 96-0692.

40. Fiore MC, Bailey WC, Cohen SJ, *et al. Treating Tobacco Use and Dependence.* Department of Health and Human Services, Public Health Service, Rockville MD, 2000.

41. Ossip-Klein DJ, McIntosh S, Utman C, *et al.* Smokers ages 50+:who gets physician advice to quit? *Prev Med* 2000;31:364–369.

42. Hughes JR, Goldstein MG, Hurt RD, Schiffman S. Recent advances in the pharacotherapy of smoking. *JAMA* 1999;281:72–76.

43. Pierce JP, Gilpin EA. Impact of over-the-counter sales on effectiveness of pharmaceutical aids for smoking cessation. *JAMA* 2002;288:1260–1264.

44. Ockene IS, Houston N. Cigarette smoking, cardiovascular disease and stroke: a statement for healthcare professionals from the American Heart Association. *Circulation* 1997;96:3243–3247.

45. Thorndike AN, Rigotti NA, Stafford RS, Singer DE. National patterns in the treatment of smokers by physicians. *JAMA* 1998;279:604–608.

46. Sargent JD, Dalton M. Does parental disapproval of smoking prevent adolescents from becoming established smokers? *Pediatrics* 2001; 108:1256–1262.

47. Farkas AJ, Gilpin EA, White MA, Pierce JP. Association between household and workplace smoking restrictions and adolescent smoking. *JAMA* 2000;284:717–722.

48. Pierce JP, Distefan JM, Jackson C, *et al.* Does tobacco marketing undermine the influence of recommended parenting in discouraging adolescents from smoking? *Am J Prev Med* 2002;23:73–81.

49. Sargent JD, Beach ML, Dalton MA, *et al.* Effect of seeing tobacco use in films on trying smoking among adolescents: cross sectional study. *BMJ* 2001;323:1394–1397.

50. Tickle JJ, Sargent JD, Dalton MA, *et al.* Favorite movie stars, their tobacco use in contemporary movies, and its association with adolescent smoking. *Tob Control* 2001;10:16–22.

51. Dalton MA, Tickle JJ, Sargent JD, *et al.* The incidence and context of tobacco use in popular movies from 1988 to 1997. *Prev Med* 2002;34:1516–1523.

52. Bauer UE, Johnson TM, Hopkins RS, Brooks RG. Changes in youth cigarette use and intentions following implementation of a tobacco control program. *JAMA* 2000;284:723–728.

53. Madarri DH. *The Costs and Benefits of Smoking Restrictions: An Assessment of the Smoke-Free Environment Act of 1993 (H.R. 3434).* Indoor Air Division, Office of Air and Radiation, Environmental Protection Agency, Washington, DC, 1994.

54. Longo DR, Brownson RC, Johnson JC, *et al.* Hospital smoking bans and employee smoking behavior. *JAMA* 1996;275:1252–1257.

55. Stillman FA, Becker DM, Swank RT, *et al.* Ending smoking at the Johns Hopkins Medical Institutions. *JAMA* 1990;264:1565–1569.

56. Knight JA. *Free Radicals, Antioxidants, Aging and Disease.* AACC Press, Washington, DC, 1999.

57. Church DF, Pryor WA. Free-radical chemistry of cigarette smoke and its toxicological implications. *Environ Health Perspect* 1985; 64:111–126.

58. Pryor WA, Stone K. Oxidants in cigarette smoke: radicals, hydrogen peroxide, peroxynitrate, and peroxynitrite. *Ann NY Acad Sci* 1993; 686:12–27.

59. Reddy S, Finkelstein EI, Wong PS-Y, *et al.* Identification of glutathione modifications by cigarette smoke. *Free Rad Biol Med* 2002;33: 1490–1498.

60. Reznick AZ, Klein I, Eiserich JP, *et al.* Inhibition of oral peroxidase activity by cigarette smoke: *in vivo* and *in vitro* studies. *Free Rad Biol Med* 2003;34:377–384.

61. Marangon K, Herbeth B, Lecomte E, *et al.* Diet, antioxidant status, and smoking habits in French men. *Am J Clin Nutr* 1998;67: 231–239.

62. Traber MG, Winklhofer-Roob BM, Roob JM, *et al.* Vitamin E kinetics in smokers and non-smokers. *Free Rad Biol Med* 2001; 31:1368–1374.

63. Tribble DL, Giuliano LG, Formann SP. Reduced plasma ascorbic acid concentrations in non-smokers regularly exposed to environmental tobacco and smoke. *Am J Clin Nutr* 1993;58:886–890.

64. Strauss RS. Environmental tobacco smoke and serum vitamin C levels in children. *Pediatrics* 2001;107:540–542.

65. Reilly M, Delanty N, Lawson JA, FitzGerald GA. Modulation of oxidant stress *in vivo* in chronic cigarette smokers. *Circulation* 1996;94:19–25.

66. Krupski NC. The peripheral vascular consequences of smoking. *Ann Vasc Surg* 1991;5:291–304.

67. McBride PE. The health consequences of smoking: cardiovascular diseases. *Med Clin North Am* 1992;76:333–353.

68. Shah PK, Helfant RH. Smoking and coronary artery disease. *Chest* 1988;98:449–452.

69. The health benefits of smoking cessation: a report of the Surgeon General. Department of Health and Human Services, Rockville, MD, 1990 [DHHS Publication No. (CDC) 90-8416].

70. Muscat JE, Harris RE, Haley NJ, Wynder EL. Cigarette smoking and plasma cholesterol. *Am Heart J* 1991;121:141–147.

71. Steinbrecher UP, Zhang HG, Lougheed M. Role of oxidatively modified LDL in atherosclerosis. *Free Rad Biol Med* 1990;9: 155–168.

72. Witztum JL. The oxidation hypothesis of atherosclerosis. *Lancet* 1994;344:793–795.

73. Hoyert DL, Freedman MA, Strobino DM, Guyer B, *et al.* Annual summary of vital statistics: 2000. *Pediatrics* 2001;108:1241–1255.

74. English JP, Willius FA, Berkson J. Tobacco and coronary disease. *JAMA* 1940;115:1327–1329.

75. Reducing the health consequences of smoking: 25 years of progress. A report of the Surgeon General: executive summary. Department of Health and Human Services, Rockville, MD, 1989 [DHHS publication No. (CDC) 89-8411].

76. Al-Delaimy WK, Manson JE, Solomon CG, *et al.* Smoking and risk of coronary heart disease among women with type 2 diabetes mellitus. *Arch Intern Med* 2002;162:273–279.

77. Ayanian JZ, Cleary PD. Perceived risks of heart disease and cancer among cigarette smokers. *JAMA* 1999;281:1019–1021.

78. Wenger NK, Speroff L, Packard B. Cardiovascular health and disease in women. *N Engl J Med* 1993;329:247–256.

79. Wenger NK. Coronary heart disease: an older woman's major health risk. *BMJ* 1997;315:1085–1090.

80. McGill HC, McMahan A, Malcom GT, *et al.* Effects of serum lipoproteins and smoking on atherosclerosis in young men and women. *Arterioscler Thromb Vasc Biol* 1997;17:95–106.

81. Jacobs EJ, Thun MJ, Apicella LF. Cigar smoking and death from coronary heart disease in a prospective study of US men. *Arch Intern Med* 1999;159:2413–2418.

82. Baker F, Ainsworth SR, Dye JT, *et al.* Health risks associated with cigar smoking. *JAMA* 2000;284:735–740.

83. Glantz SA, Parmley WW. Passive smoking and heart disease: epidemiology, physiology, and biochemistry. *Circulation* 1991;83:1–12.

84. Glantz SA, Parmley WW. Passive smoking and heart disease: mechanisms and risk. *JAMA* 1995;273:1047–1053.

85. Kawachi I, Colditz GA, Speizer FE, *et al.* A prospective study of passive smoking and coronary heart disease. *Circulation* 1997;95:2374–2379.

86. Howard G, Wagenknecht LE, Burke GL, *et al.* Cigarette smoking and progression of atherosclerosis. *JAMA* 1998;279:119–124.

87. Otsuka R, Watanabe H, Hirata K, *et al.* Acute effects of passive smoking on the coronary circulation in healthy young adults. *JAMA* 2001;286:436–441.

88. Pennington JC, Tecce MA, Segal BL. Heart protection: controlling risk factors for cardiovascular disease. *Geriatrics* 1997;52:40–50.

89. Critchley JA, Capewell S. Mortality risk reduction associated with smoking cessation in patients with coronary heart disease. A systematic review. *JAMA* 2003;290:86–97.

90. Wilson K, Gibson N, Willan A, Cook D. Effect of smoking cessation on mortality after myocardial infarction: meta-analysis of cohort studies. *Arch Intern Med* 2000;160:939–944.

91. Robbins AS, Manson JE, Lee I-M, *et al.* Cigarette smoking and stroke in a cohort of US male physicians. *Ann Intern Med* 1994;120:458–462.

92. Howard G, Evans GW, Toole JF. Silent cerebral infarction in transient ischemic attack populations: implications of advancing technology. *J Stroke Cerebrovasc Dis* 1994;4:547–550.

93. Howard G, Wagenknecht LE, Cai J, *et al.* Cigarette smoking and other risk factors for silent cerebral infarction in the general population. *Stroke* 1998;29:913–917.

94. Bonita R, Scragg R, Stewart A, *et al.* Cigarette smoking and risk of premature stroke in men and women. *BMJ* 1986;293:6–8.

95. Shaper AG, Phillips AN, Pocock AJ, *et al.* Risk factors for stroke in middle-aged British men. *BMJ* 1991;302:1111–1115.

96. Wannamethee SG, Shaper AG, Whincup PH, *et al.* Smoking cessation and the risk of stroke in middle-aged men. *JAMA* 1995; 274:155–160.

97. Kurth T, Kase CS, Berger K, *et al.* Smoking and the risk of hemorrhagic stroke in men. *Stroke* 2003;34:1151–1155.

98. Parkin DM, Pisani P, Ferlay J. Estimates of the worldwide incidence of 25 major cancers in 1990. *Int J Cancer* 1999;80:827–841.

99. Pisani P, Parkin DM, Bray F, Ferlay J. Estimates of the worldwide mortality from 25 cancers in 1990. *Int J Cancer* 1999;83:18–19.

100. The health consequences of smoking: cancer: a report of the Surgeon General. Department of Health and Human Services, Rockville, MD, 1982 [DHHS Publication No. (PHS) 82-50179].

101. Rosenow EC III. Symposium on intrathoracic neoplasms: introduction. *Mayo Clin Proc* 1993;68:168–169.

102. Kuper H, Ho A, Boffetta P. Tobacco use, cancer causation and public health impact. *J Intern Med* 2002;251:455–466.

103. Jemal A, Thomas A, Murray T, Thun M. Cancer statistics, 2002. *CA Cancer J Clin* 2002;52:23–47.

104. Bartecchi CE, MacKenzie TD, Schrier RW. The human costs of tobacco use. *N Engl J Med* 1994;330:907–912.

105. Janerich DT, Thompson WD, Varela LR, *et al.* Lung cancer and exposure to tobacco smoke in the household. *N Engl J Med* 1990;323:632–636.

106. Environmental Protection Agency. *Respiratory Health Effects of Passive Smoking: Lung Cancer and Other Disorders.* Office of Health and Environmental Assessment, Washington, DC, 1992.

107. Ghafoor A, Jemal A, Cokkinides V, *et al.* Cancer statistics for African Americans. *CA Cancer J Clin* 2002;52:326–341.

108. Blot WJ, McLaughlin JK, Winn DM, *et al.* Smoking and drinking in relation to oral and pharyngeal cancer. *Cancer Res* 1988;48:3282–3287.

109. Smokeless tobacco or health: and international perspective. Department of Health and Human Services, Rockville, MD, 1992 [NIH Publication No. 92-3461].

110. Newcomb PA, Carbone PP. The health consequences of smoking: cancer. *Med Clin North Am* 1992;76:305–331.

111. Giovannucci E, Martinez ME. Tobacco, colorectal cancer, and adenomas: a review of the evidence. *J Natl Cancer Inst* 1996;88: 1717–1730.

112. Heineman EF, Zahm SH, McLaughlin JK, Vaught JB. Increased risk of colorectal cancer among smokers: results of a 26-year follow-up of US veterans and a review. *Int J Cancer* 1994;59:728–738.

113. Chao A, Thun MJ, Jacobs EJ, *et al.* Cigarette smoking and colorectal cancer mortality in the Cancer Prevention Study II. *J Natl Cancer Inst* 2000;92:1888–1896.

114. Slattery ML, Potter JD, Friedman GD, *et al.* Tobacco use and colon cancer. *Int J Cancer* 1997;70:259–264.

115. Giovannucci E, Rimm EB, Stampfer MJ, *et al.* A prospective study of cigarette smoking and risk of colorectal adenoma and colorectal cancer in US men. *J Natl Cancer Inst* 1994;86:183–191.

116. Terry PD, Miller AB, Rohan TE. Prospective cohort study of cigarette smoking and colorectal cancer risk in women. *Int J Cancer* 2002;99:480–483.

117. Holmes E, Borek D, Owen-Kummer M, *et al.* Anal cancer in women. *Gastroenterology* 1988;95:107–111.

118. Daling JR, Sherman KJ, Hislop TG, *et al.* Cigarette smoking and the risk of anogenital cancer. *Am J Epidemiol* 1992;135:180–189.

119. Silverman DT, Dunn JA, Hoover RN, *et al.* Cigarette smoking and pancreas cancer: a case-control study based on direct interviews. *J Natl Cancer Inst* 1994;86:1510–1516.

120. Stolzenberg-Solomon RZ, Albanes D, Nieto FJ, *et al.* Pancreatic cancer risk and nutrition-related methyl group availability indicators in male smokers. *J Natl Cancer Inst* 1999;91:535–541.

121. Stolzenberg-Solomon RZ, Pietinen P, Barrett MJ, *et al.* Dietary and other methyl group availability factors and pancreatic cancer risk in a cohort of male smokers. *Am J Epidemiol* 2001;153:680–687.

122. Lin Y, Tamakoshi A, Kawamura T, *et al.* A prospective cohort study of cigarette smoking and pancreatic cancer in Japan. *Cancer Causes Control* 2002;13:249–254.

123. Yu MC, Ross RK. Epidemiology of bladder cancer. In: *Carcinoma of the Bladder: Innovations in Management*. Z Petrovich, L Baert, IW Brady (eds.). Springer-Verlag, Berlin, 1998, pp. 1–13.

124. US Department of Health and Human Services. *The Health Consequences of Smoking: 25 Years of Progress. A Report of the Surgeon General*. US Department of Health and Human Services, Public Health Service, Centers for Disease Control, Center for Chronic Disease Prevention and Health Promotion, Office of Smoking and Health [DHHS Publication No. (CDC) 89-8411, 1989].

125. Chiu BC, Lynch CF, Cerehan JR, Cantor KP. Cigarette smoking and risk of bladder, pancreas, kidney and colorectal cancers in Iowa. *Ann Epidemiol* 2001;11:28–37.

126. Castelao JE, Yuan J-M, Skipper PL, *et al.* Gender- and smoking-related bladder cancer risk. *J Natl Cancer Inst* 2001;93:538–544.

127. Tripathi A, Folsom AR, Anderson KE. Risk factors for urinary bladder carcinoma: postmenopausal women. The Iowa Women's Health Study. *Cancer* 2002;95:2316–2323.

128. McLaughlin JK, Lipworth L. Epidemiologic aspects of renal cell cancer. *Semin Oncol* 2000;27:115–123.

129. Moyad MA. Review of potential risk factors for kidney (renal cell) cancer. *Semin Urol Oncol* 2001;19:280–293.

130. Newcomb PA, Carbone PP. The health consequences of smoking. *Med Clin North Amer* 1992;76:305–331.

131. Oh WK, Manola J, Renshaw AA, *et al.* Smoking and alcohol use may be risk factors for poorer outcome in patients with clear cell renal carcinoma. *Urology* 2000;55:31–35.

132. Winkelstein W. Smoking and cancer of the uterine cervix: hypothesis. *Am J Epidemiol* 1977;106:257–259.

133. Slattery ML, Robison LM, Schuman KL, *et al.* Cigarette smoking and exposure to passive smoke are risk factors for cervical cancer. *JAMA* 1989;261:1593–1598.

134. Cancer Facts and Figures — 1993. American Cancer Society, New York, 1993.

135. Brinton L, Barrett R, Berman M, *et al.* Cigarette smoking and the risk of endometrial cancer. *Am J Epidemiol* 1993;137:281–291.

136. London S, Colditz G, Stampfer M, *et al.* Prospective study of smoking and the risk of breast cancer. *J Natl Cancer Inst* 1989;81:1625–1631.

137. Egan KM, Stampfer MJ, Hunter D, *et al.* Active and passive smoking in breast cancer: prospective results from the Nurses' Health Study. *Epidemiology* 2002;13:138–145.

138. Brownson RC, Novotny TE, Perry MC. Cigarette smoking and adult leukemia: a meta-analysis. *Arch Intern Med* 1993;153:469–475.
139. Mills PK, Newell CR, Beeson WL, *et al.* History of cigarette smoking and risk of leukemia and myeloma: results from the Adventists Health Study. *J Natl Cancer Inst* 1990;82:1832–1836.
140. Severson RK. Cigarette smoking and leukemia. *Cancer* 1987;60:141–144.
141. Speer SA, Semenza JC, Kurosaki T, Anton-Culver H. Risk factors for acute myeloid leukemia and multiple myeloma: a combination of GIS and case-control studies. *J Environ Health* 2002;64:9–16.
142. Pogoda JM, Preston-Martin S, Nichols PW, Ross RK. Smoking and risk of acute myeloid leukemia: results from a Los Angeles County case-control study. *Am J Epidemiol* 2002;155:546–553.
143. Bjork J, Albin M, Mauritzson N, *et al.* Smoking and acute myeloid leukemia: associations with morphology and karyotypic patterns and evaluation of dose-response relations. *Leuk Res* 2001;25:865–872.
144. Moorman AV, Roman E, Cartwright RA, Morgan GJ. Smoking and the risk of myeloid leukemia in cytogenetic subgroups. *Br J Cancer* 2002;86:60–62.
145. Wallace L, Pellizzari E, Hartwell TD, *et al.* Exposure to benzene and other volatile compounds from active and passive smoking. *Arch Environ Health* 1987;42:272–279.
146. Korte JE, Hertz-Picciotto I, Schulz MR, *et al.* The contribution of benzene to smoking-induced leukemia. *Environ Health Perspect* 2000;108:333–339.
147. Bjork J, Albin M, Mauritzson N, *et al.* Smoking and myelodysplastic syndromes. *Epidemiology* 2000;11:285–291.
148. Stagnaro E, Ramazzotti V, Crosignani P, *et al.* Smoking and hematolymphopoietic malignancies. *Cancer Causes Control* 2001;12:325–334.
149. Taylor DH Jr, Hasselblad V, Henley SJ, *et al.* Benefits of smoking cessation for longevity. *Am J Pub Health* 2002;92:990–996.
150. Doll R, Peto R, Wheatley K, *et al.* Mortality in relation to smoking: 40 years' observation on male British doctors. *Br Med J* 1994;309:901–910.
151. Ferrucci L, Izmirlian G, Leveille S, *et al.* Smoking, physical activity, and active life expectancy. *Am J Epidemiol* 1999;149:645–653.
152. Model D. Smokers face: an underated clinical sign? *BMJ* 1985;291:1760–1762.
153. Daniell H. Smoker's wrinkles. A study of the epidemiology of "crow's feet." *Ann Intern Med* 1971;75:873–880.

154. Kadunce DP, Burr R, Gress R, *et al.* Cigarette smoking: risk factors for premature facial wrinkling. *Ann Intern Med* 1991; 114:840–844.

155. Grady D, Ernster V. Does cigarette smoking make you ugly and old? *Am J Epidemiol* 1992;135:839–842.

156. Demierre MF, Brooks D, Koh HK, Geller AC. Public knowledge, awareness, and perceptions of the association between skin aging and smoking. *J Am Acad Dermatol* 1999;41:27–30.

157. Koh JS, Kang H, Choi SW, Kim HO. Cigarette smoking associated with premature facial wrinkling: image analysis of facial skin replicas. *Int J Dermatol* 2002;41:21–27.

158. Mosely JG, Gibbs ACC. Premature grey hair and hair loss among smokers: a new opportunity for health education? *BMJ* 1996; 313:1616.

159. Niessen LC, Jones JA. Oral health changes in the elderly: their relationship to nutrition. *Postgrad Med* 1984;75:231–237.

160. Massler M. Geriatric nutrition: the role of taste and smell in appetite. *J Prosthet Dent* 1980;43:247–250.

161. Winkler S, Garg AK, Mekayarajjananonth T, *et al.* Depressed taste and smell in geriatric patients. *JADA* 1999;130:1759–1765.

162. Faulkner MA, Hilleman DE. The economic impact of chronic obstructive pulmonary disease. *Expert Opin Pharmacother* 2002;3:219–228.

163. Mannino DM, Homa DM, Akinbami LJ, *et al.* Chronic obstructive pulmonary disease surveillance — United States, 1971–2000. *MMWR* 2002;51:1–10.

164. Sullivan SD, Ramsey SD, Lee TA. Economic burden of COPD. *Chest* 2000;117(Suppl 2):5S–9S.

165. Rennard SI. Overview of causes of COPD: new understanding of pathogenesis and mechanisms can guide future therapy. *Postgrad Med* 2002;111:28–30,33–34,37–38.

166. Sashidhar K, Gulati M, Gupta D, *et al.* Emphysema in heavy smokers with normal chest radiography: detection and quantitation by HCRT. *Acta Radiol* 2002;43:60–65.

167. Plouffe JE, Breiman RF, Facklam RR. Bacteremia with *Streptococcus pneumoniae*: implications for therapy and prevention. *JAMA* 1996;275:194–198.

168. Pastor P, Medley F, Murphy TV. Invasive pneumococcal disease in Dallas County, Texas: results from population-based surveillance in 1995. *Clin Inf Dis* 1998;26:590–595.

169. Breiman RF, Spika JS, Navarro VJ, *et al.* Pneumococcal bacteremia in Charleston County, South Carolina: a decade later. *Arch Intern Med* 1990;150:1401–1405.

170. Nuorti JP, Butler JC, Farley MM, *et al.* Cigarette smoking and invasive pneumococcal disease. *N Engl J Med* 2000;342:681–689.

171. West SK, Munoz BE, Emmet EA, Taylor HR. Cigarette smoking and risk of nuclear cataracts. *Arch Ophthalmol* 1989;107:1166–1169.

172. Leske MC, Chylack LT, Wu, SY. The Lens Opacity Case-Control Study: risk factors for cataract. *Arch Ophthalmol* 1991;109:244–251.

173. Klein BEK, Klein R, Linton KLP, Franke T. Cigarette smoking and lens opacities: the Beaver Dam Eye Study. *Am J Prev Med* 1993; 9:27–30.

174. Christen WG, Manson JE, Seddon JM, *et al.* A prospective study of cigarette smoking and risk of cataract in men. *JAMA* 1992;268: 989–993.

175. Hankinson SE, Willett WC, Colditz GA, *et al.* A prospective study of cigarette smoking and risk of cataract surgery in women. *JAMA* 1992;268:994–998.

176. Hiller R, Sperduto RD, Podgor MJ, *et al.* Cigarette smoking and risk of development of lens opacities. *Arch Ophthalmol* 1997;115:1113–1118.

177. Christen WG, Glynn RJ, Ajani UA, *et al.* Smoking cessation and risk of age-related cataract in men. *JAMA* 2000;284:713–716.

178. National Advisory Eye Council. *Vision Research, A National Plan, 1994–1998.* National Institutes of Health, Bethesda, MD, 1993. National Institutes of Health Publication 93-3186.

179. Christen WG, Glynn RJ, Manson JE, *et al.* A prospective study of cigarette smoking and age-related macular degeneration in men. *JAMA* 1996;276:1147–1151.

180. Seddon JM, Willett WC, Speizer FE, Hankinson SE. A prospective study of cigarette smoking and age-related macular degeneration in women. *JAMA* 1996;276:1141–1146.

181. Mitchell P, Wang JJ, Smith W, Leeder SR. Smoking and the five-year incidence of age-related maculopathy: the Blue Mountains Eye Study. *Arch Ophthal* 2002;120:1357–1363.

182. Goldhaber SZ, Grodstein F, Stampfer MJ, *et al.* A prospective study of risk factors for pulmonary embolism in women. *JAMA* 1997;277:642–645.

183. Cummings SR, Black DM, Rubin SM. Lifetime risk of hip, Colles', or vertebral fracture and coronary heart disease among white postmenopausal women. *Am J Pub Health* 1988;78:1554–1558.

184. Kato I, Toniolo P, Zeleniuch-Jacquotte A, *et al.* Diet, smoking and anthropometric indices and postmenopausal bone factures: a prospective study. *Int J Epidemiol* 2000;29:85–92.
185. Law MR, Hackshaw AK. A meta-analysis of cigarette smoking, bone mineral density and risk of hip fracture: recognition of a major effect. *BMJ* 1997;315:841–846.
186. Baron JA, Farahmand BY, Weiderpass E, *et al.* Cigarette smoking, alcohol consumption, and risk of hip fracture in women. *Arch Intern Med* 2001;161:983–988.
187. Hopper JL, Seeman E. The bone density of female twins discordant for tobacco use. *N Engl J Med* 1994;330:387–392.
188. Krall EA, Dawson HB. Smoking increases bone loss and decreases intestinal calcium absorption. *J Bone Mineral Res* 1999;14:215–220.
189. McKinlay SM, Bifano NL, McKinlay JB. Smoking and age at menopause in women. *Ann Intern Med* 1985;103:350–356.
190. Weisberg E. Smoking and reproductive health. *Clin Reprod Fertil* 1985;3:175–186.
191. Mocarelli P, Gerthoux PM, Ferrari E, *et al.* Paternal concentrations of dioxin and sex ratio of offspring. *Lancet* 2000;355:1858–1863.
192. Sakamoto M, Nakano PM, Akagi H. Declining Minamata male birth ratio associated with increased male fetal death due to heavy methylmercury pollution. *Environ Res* 2001;87:92–97.
193. Fukuda M, Fukuda K. Shimizu T, *et al.* Parental periconceptional smoking and male:female ratio of newborn infants. *Lancet* 2002;359:1407–1408.
194. Kramer MS. Socioeconomic determinants of intrauterine growth retardation. *Eur J Clin Nutr* 1998;52(suppl 1):529–533.
195. Wang X, Zukerman B, Pearson C, *et al.* Maternal cigarette smoking, metabolic gene polymorphism, and infant birth weight. *JAMA* 2002;289:195–202.
196. Hernan MA, Olek MJ, Asherio A. Cigarette smoking and incidence of multiple sclerosis. *Am J Epidemiol* 2001;154:69–74.
197. Villard-Mackintosh L, Vessey MP. Oral contraceptives and reproductive factors in multiple sclerosis incidence. *Contraception* 1993;47:167–168.
198. Thorogood M, Hannaford PC. The influence of oral contraceptives as the risk of multiple sclerosis. *Br J Obstet Gynecol* 1998;105:1296–1299.
199. Muller B, Zulewski H, Huber P, *et al.* Impaired action of thyroid hormone associated with smoking in women and hypothyroidism. *N Engl J Med* 1995;333:964–969.

200. Nakanishi N, Nakamura K, Matsuo Y, *et al.* Cigarette smoking and risk for impaired fasting glucose and type 2 diabetes in middle-aged Japanese men. *Ann Intern Med* 2000;133:183–191.

201. Smith JR, Landaw SA. Smoker's polycythemia. *N Engl J Med* 1978;314:6–10.

202. Nordenberg D, Yip R, Binkin NJ. The effect of cigarette smoking on hemoglobin levels and anemia screening. *JAMA* 1990;264:1556–1559.

203. LaCroix AZ, Guralnik JM, Berkman LF, *et al.* Maintaining mobility in late life, II: smoking, alcohol consumption, physical activity, and body mass index. *Am J Epidemiol* 1993;137:858–869.

204. Nelson HD, Nevitt MC, Scott JC, *et al.* Smoking, alcohol, and neuromuscular and physical function in older women. *JAMA* 1994;272:1825–1831.

205. Waal-Manning HJ, de Hamel FA. Smoking habit and psychometric scores: a community study. *N Z Med J* 1978;88:188–191.

206. Kandel DB, Davies M. Adult sequelae of adolescent depressive symptoms. *Arch Gen Psychiatry* 1986;43:255–262.

207. Hughes RJ, Hatsukami DK, Mitchell JE, Dahlgren LA. Prevalence of smoking among psychiatric outpatients. *Am J Psychiatry* 1986;143:993–997.

208. Glassman AH, Helzer JE, Covey LS, *et al.* Smoking, smoking cessation, and major depression. *JAMA* 1990;264:1546–1549.

209. Anda RF, Williamson DF, Escobedo LG, *et al.* Depression and the dynamics of smoking: a national perspective. *JAMA* 1990; 264:1541–1545. SM, *et al.* Interrelationship of smoking and alcohol dependence: use and urges to use. *J Stud Alcohol* 1995;56;202–206.

210. Petry NM, Oncken C. Cigarette smoking is associated with increased severity of gambling problems in treatment-seeking gamblers. *Addiction* 2002;97:745–753.

211. Angell M, Kassirer JP. Alcohol and other drugs — toward a more rational and consistent policy. *N Engl J Med* 1994;331:537–539.

212. Kalmijn S, van Boxtel MPJ, Verschuren MWM, *et al.* Cigarette smoking and alcohol consumption in relation to cognitive performance in middle age. *Am J Epidemiol* 2002;156:936–944.

213. Richards M, Jarvis MJ, Thompson N, Wadsworth MEJ. Cigarette smoking and cognitive decline in midlife: evidence from a perspective birth cohort study. *Am J Pub Health* 2003;93:994–998.

214. Harwood H. *Updating Estimates of the Economic Costs of Alcohol Abuse in the United States: Estimates, Update Methods and Data.* The Lewin Group for the National Institute on Alcohol Abuse and Alcoholism, Fall Church, VA, 2000.

215. Gulliver SB, Rohsenow DJ, Colby SM, *et al*. Interrelationship of smoking and alcohol dependence: use and urges to use. *J Stud Alcohol* 1995;56:202–206.

216. Foster SE, Vaughan RD, Foster WH, Califano JA. Alcohol consumption and expenditures for underage drinking and adult excessive drinking. *JAMA* 2003;289:989–995.

217. Adams WL, Yuan Z, Barboriak JJ, Rimm AA. Alcohol-related hospitalizations of elderly people. *JAMA* 1993;270:1222–1225.

218. Cryer CP, Jenkins LM, Cook AC, *et al*. The use of acute and preventive medical services by a general population: relationship to alcohol consumption. *Addiction* 1999;94:1523–1532.

219. American Medical Association. *Alcoholism in the Elderly: Diagnosis, Treatment and Prevention: Guidelines for Primary Care Physicians*. AMA, Chicago, 1995.

220. AMA Report. Alcoholism is a "hidden" epidemic of older Americans. *Geriatrics* 1995;50:12.

221. Caetano R, Clark CL. Trends in alcohol consumption patterns among whites, blacks, and Hispanics: 1984 and 1995. *J Studies Alcohol* 1998;59:656–668.

222. Naimi TS, Brewer RD, Mokdad A, *et al*. Binge drinking among US adults. *JAMA* 2003; 289:70–75.

223. Clark WD. Alcoholism: blocks to diagnosis and treatment. *Am J Med* 1981;71:271–286.

224. Moore RD, Bone LR, Geller G, *et al*. Prevalence, detection, and treatment of alcoholism in hospitalized patients. *JAMA* 1989;261:403–407.

225. Wallace P, Cutler S, Haines A. Randomized controlled trial of general practitioners interventions in patient with excessive alcohol consumption. *BMJ* 1988;297:663–668.

226. World Health Organization Brief Intervention Study Group. Across national trial of brief intervention with heavy drinkers. *Am J Pub Health* 1996;86:948–955.

227. Fleming MF, Barry KL, Manwell LB, *et al*. Brief physician advice for problem alcohol drinkers: a randomized controlled trial in community-based primary care practices. *JAMA* 1997;277:1039–1045.

228. Ewing JA. Detecting alcoholism: the CAGE questionnaire. *JAMA* 1984;252:1905.

229. Naik PC, Jones RG. Alcohol histories taken from elderly people on admission. *BMJ* 1994;309:248.

230. Gambert SR. Alcohol abuse: medical effects of heavy drinking in late life. *Geriatrics* 1997;52:30–37.

231. Adams WL, Barry KL, Fleming MF. Screening for problem drinking in older primary care patients. *JAMA* 1996;276:1964–1967.

232. Schneekloth TD, Morse RM, Herrick LM, *et al.* Point prevalence of alcoholism in hospitalized patients: continuing challenges of detection, assessment, and diagnosis. *Mayo Clin Proc* 2001;76:460–466.

233. Salaspuro M. Characteristics of laboratory markers in alcohol-related organ damage. *Scand J Gastroenterol* 1989;24:769–780.

234. Bell H, Tallaksen CME, Try K, Haug E. Carbohydrate deficient transferrin (CDT) and other markers of high alcohol consumption: a study of 502 patients admitted consecutively to a medical department. *Alcohol Clin Exp Res* 1994;18:1103–1108.

235. Gronbaek M, Deis A, Sorensen TJA, *et al.* Influence of sex, age, body mass index, and smoking on alcohol intake and mortality. *BMJ* 1994;308:302–306.

236. Doll R, Peto R, Hall E, *et al.* Mortality in relation to consumption of alcohol: 13 years' observations on male British doctors. *BMJ* 1994;309:911–918.

237. Thun MJ, Peto R, Lopez AD, *et al.* Alcohol consumption and mortality among middle-aged and elderly US adults. *N Engl J Med* 1997;337:1705–1714.

238. Gronbaek M, Becker U, Johansen D, *et al.* Type of alcohol consumed and mortality from all causes, coronary heart disease, and cancer. *Ann Intern Med* 2000;133:411–419.

239. Boffetta P, Farfinkel L. Alcohol drinking and mortality among men enrolled in an American Cancer Society prospective study. *Epidemiology* 1990;1:342–348.

240. Klatsky AL, Armstrong MA, Friedman GD. Alcohol and mortality. *Ann Intern Med* 1992;117:546–654.

241. Fuchs CS, Stampfer MJ, Colditz GA, *et al.* Alcohol consumption and mortality among women. *N Engl J Med* 1995;332:1245–1250.

242. Andreasson S, Allebeck P, Romelsjo A. Alcohol and mortality among young men: longitudinal study of Swedish conscripts. *BMJ* 1988;296:1021–1025.

243. Hingson RW, Heeren T, Zakocs RC, *et al.* Magnitude of alcohol-related mortality and morbidity among US college students ages 18–24. *J Stud Alcohol* 2002;63:136–144.

244. Fleming KC, Evans JM, Weber DC, Chutka DS. Practical functional assessment of elderly persons: a primary-care approach. *Mayo Clin Proc* 1995;70:890–910.

245. Lieber CS. Perspectives: do alcohol calories count? *Am J Clin Nutr* 1991;54:976–982.

246. Saul SH. Liver. In: *Pathology*, 3rd Ed. VA LiVoisi, MJ Merino, JS Brooks, SH Saul, JE Tomaszewski (eds.) Harwal Publishing, Philadelphia, 1994.
247. Lieber CS (ed.) *Medical and Nutritional Complications of Alcoholism: Mechanisms and Management*. Plenum Press, New York, 1992.
248. DiLuzio NR. A mechanism of the acute ethanol-induced fatty liver and the modification of liver injury by antioxidants. *Lab Invest* 1966;15:50–63.
249. Nordmann R, Ribiere C, Rouach H. Implications of free radical mechanisms in ethanol-induced cellular injury. *Free Rad Biol Med* 1992;12:219–240.
250. Hennekins CH, Willett W. Rosher B, *et al.* Effects of beer, wine, and liquor in coronary deaths. *JAMA* 1979;242:1973–1974.
251. Mukamal KJ, Maclure M, Muller JE, *et al.* Prior alcohol consumption and mortality following acute myocardial infarction. *JAMA* 2001;285:1965–1970.
252. Camargo CA, Stampfer MJ, Glynn RJ, *et al.* Prospective study of moderate alcohol consumption and risk of peripheral arterial disease in US male physicians. *Circulation* 1997;95:577–580.
253. Parks DA, Booyse FM. Cardiovascular protection by alcohol and polyphenols: role of nitric oxide. *Ann NY Acad Sci* 2002;957:115–121.
254. Mukamal KJ, Conigrave KM, Mittleman MA, *et al.* Roles of drinking pattern and type of alcohol consumed in coronary heart disease in men. *N Engl J Med* 2003;2003;348:109–118.
255. de Gaetano G, Cerletti C. European project FAIR CT 973261 Project participants. Wine and cardiovascular disease. *Nutr Metab Cardiovasc Dis* 2001;11(Suppl 4):47–50.
256. Ruidavets JB, Ducimetiere P, Arveiler D, *et al.* Types of alcoholic beverages and blood lipids in a French population. *J Epidemiol Commun Health* 2002;56:24–28.
257. Valmadrid CT, Klein R, Moss SE, *et al.* Alcohol intake and the risk of coronary heart disease mortality in persons with older-onset diabetes mellitus. *JAMA* 1999;282:239–246.
258. Criqui MH, Golomb BA. Should patients with diabetes drink to their health? *JAMA* 1999;282:279–280.
259. Klatsky AL. Cardiovascular effects of alcohol. *Sci Am Sci Med* 1995;March/April:28–37.
260. Bollinger O. Ueber die Haufigkeit und Ursachen der idiopathischen Herzhypertrophie in Munchen. *Dtsch Med Wochenschr* 1884;10:180–181.

261. Piano MR. Alcoholic cardiomyopathy: incidence, clinical characteristics, and pathophysiology. *Chest* 2002;121:1638–1650.

262. Urbano-Marquez A, Estruch R, Navarro-Lopez F, *et al.* The effects of alcoholism on skeletal and cardiac muscle. *N Engl J Med* 1989;320:409–415.

263. Urbano-Marquez A, Estruch R, Fernandez-Sola J, *et al.* The greater risk of alcoholic cardiomyopathy and myopathy in women compared with men. *JAMA* 1995;274:149–154.

264. Fernandez-Sola J, Nicolas-Arfelis JM. Gender differences in alcoholic cardiomyopathy. *J Gend Specif Med* 2002;5:41–47.

265. Fauchier L, Babuty D, Poret P, *et al.* Comparison of long-term outcome of alcoholic and idiopathic dilated cardiomyopathy. *Eur Heart J* 2000;21:306–314.

266. Lian C. L'alcoholisme, cause d'hypertension arterielle. *Bull Acad Natl Med (Paris)* 1915;74:525–528.

267. Jenei Z, Pall D, Katona E, *et al.* The epidemiology of hypertension and its associated risk factors in the city of Debrecen, Hungary. *Public Health* 2002;116:138–144.

268. Thadhani R, Camargo CA, Stampfer MJ, *et al.* Prospective study of moderate alcohol consumption and risk of hypertension in young women. *Arch Intern Med* 2002;162:569–574.

269. Klatsky AL. Alcohol and hypertension. *Clin Chim Acta* 1996;246: 91–105.

270. American Heart Association. *2002 Heart and Stroke Statistical Update.* American Heart Association, Dallas, TX, 2001.

271. Gorelick PB, Sacco RL, Smith DB, *et al.* Prevention of a first stroke: a review of guidelines and a multidisciplinary consensus statement from the National Stroke Association. *JAMA* 1999;281:1112–1120.

272. Sacco RL, Elkind M, Boden-Albala B, *et al.* The protective effect of moderate alcohol consumption on ischemic stroke. *JAMA* 1999; 281:53–60.

273. Berger K, Ajani UA, Kase CS, *et al.* Light-to-moderate alcohol consumption and the risk of stroke among US male physicians. *N Engl J Med* 1999;341:1557–1564.

274. Calandre L, Arnal C, Ortega F, *et al.* Risk factors for spontaneous cerebral hematomas: case-control study. *Stroke* 1988;17:1126–1128.

275. Niizuma H, Suzuki J, Yonemitsu T, Otsuki T. Spontaneous intracerebral hemorrhage and liver dysfunction. *Stroke* 1988;19:852–856.

276. Camargo CA Jr. Moderate alcohol consumption and stroke: the epidemiologic evidence. *Stroke* 1989;20:1611–1626.

277. Reynolds K, Lewis LB, Nolen JDL, *et al.* Alcohol consumption and risk of stroke: a meta-analysis. *JAMA* 2003;289:579–588.

278. Sun AY, Simonyi A, Sun GY. The "French Paradox" and beyond: neuroprotective effects of polyphenols. *Free Rad Biol Med* 2002; 32:314–318.

279. Longnecker MP. Alcoholic beverage consumption in relation to risk of breast cancer: meta-analysis and review. *Cancer Causes Control* 1994;5:73–82.

280. Smith-Warner SA, Spiegelman D, Shaw-Shyuan Y, *et al.* Alcohol and breast cancer in women: a pooled analysis of cohort studies. *JAMA* 1998;279:535–540.

281. Smith-Warner SA, Spiegelman D, Willett WC, *et al.* Alcohol consumption and breast cancer risk. *JAMA* 1998;280:1138–1139.

282. Sellers TA, Kushi LH, Cerhan JR, *et al.* Dietary folate intake, alcohol, and risk of breast cancer in a prospective study of postmenopausal women. *Epidemiology* 2001;12:420–428.

283. Yu H. Alcohol consumption and breast cancer risk. *JAMA* 1998; 280:1138.

284. Wright RM, McManaman JL, Repine JE. Alcohol-induced breast cancer: a proposed mechanism. *Free Rad Biol Med* 1999;26:348–354.

285. Singletary KW, Gapstur SM. Alcohol and breast cancer: review of epidemiologic and experimental evidence and potential mechanisms. *JAMA* 2001;286:2143–2151.

286. Gavaler JS, Deal SR, van Thiel DN, *et al.* Alcohol and estrogen levels in postmenopausal women: the spectrum of effect. *Alcohol Clin Exp Res* 1993;17:786–790.

287. Ginsburg ES, Mello NK, Mendelson JH, *et al.* Effects of alcohol ingestion on estrogens in postmenopausal women. *JAMA* 1996;276:1747–1751.

288. Chen WY, Colditz GA, Rosner B, *et al.* Use of postmenopausal hormones, alcohol, and risk of invasive breast cancer. *Ann Intern Med* 2002;137:798–804.

289. Hellerbrand C, Hartmann A, Richter G, *et al.* Hepatocellular carcinoma in southern Germany: epidemiological and clinicopathological characteristics and risk factors. *Dig Dis* 2001;19:345–351.

290. Meyer F, White E. Alcohol and nutrients in relation to colon cancer in middle-aged adults. *Am J Epidemiol* 1993;138:225–236.

291. Jacobs EJ, Connell CJ, Patel AV, *et al.* Multivitamin use and colon cancer mortality in the Cancer Prevention Study II cohort (United States). *Cancer Causes Control* 2001;12:927–934.

292. Jedrychowski W, Steindorf K, Popiela T, *et al.* Alcohol consumption and the risk of colorectal cancer at low levels of micronutrient intake. *Med Sci Monit* 2002;8:CR357–CR363.

293. Wolk A, Gridley G, Niwa S, *et al.* International renal cell cancer study. VII. Role of diet. *Int J Cancer* 1996;65:67–73.

294. Parker AS, Cerhan JR, Lynch CF, *et al.* Gender, alcohol consumption, and renal cell carcinoma. *Am J Epidemiol* 2002;155:455–462.

295. Kato I, Nomura AMY, Stemmermann GN, Chyou PH. Prospective study of the association of alcohol with cancer of the upper aerodigestive tract and other sites. *Cancer Causes Control* 1992;3:145–151.

296. Gao Y-T, McLaughlin JK, Blot WJ, *et al.* Risk factors for esophageal cancer in Shanghai, China. I. Role of cigarette smoking and alcohol drinking. *Int J Cancer* 1994;58:192–196.

297. Gronbaek M, Becker U, Johansen D, *et al.* Population based cohort study of the association between alcohol intake and cancer of the upper digestive tract. *BMJ* 1998;317:844–848.

298. Launoy G, Milan C, Day NE, *et al.* Oesophageal cancer in France: potential importance of hot alcoholic drinks. *Int J Cancer* 1997;71:917–923.

299. Ye W, Lagergren J, Weiderpass E, *et al.* Alcohol abuse and the risk of pancreatic cancer. *Gut* 2002;51:236–239.

300. Lin Y, Tamakoshi A, Kawamura T, *et al.* Risk of pancreatic cancer in relation to alcohol drinking, coffee consumption and medical history: findings from the Japan collaborative cohort study for evaluation of cancer risk. *Int J Cancer* 2002;99:742–746.

301. Stampfer MJ, Colditz GA, Willett WC, *et al.* A prospective study of moderate alcohol drinking and risk of diabetes in women. *Am J Epidemiol* 1988;128:549–558.

302. Lazarus R, Sparrow D, Weiss ST. Alcohol intake and insulin levels. *Am J Epidemiol* 1997;145:909–916.

303. Kiechl S, Willett J, Poewe W, *et al.* Insulin sensitivity and regular alcohol consumption. *BMJ* 1996;313:1040–1044.

304. de Vegt F, Dekker JM, Groeneveld WJ, *et al.* Moderate alcohol consumption is associated with lower risk for incident diabetes and mortality: the Hoorn Study. *Diabetes Res Clin Pract* 2002;57: 53–60.

305. Davies MJ, Baer DJ, Judd JT, *et al.* Effects of moderate alcohol intake on fasting insulin and glucose concentrations and insulin sensitivity in postmenopausal women: a randomized controlled trial. *JAMA* 2002;287:2559–2562.

306. Uppal R, Lateef SK, Korsten MA, *et al.* Chronic alcoholic gastritis: roles of alcohol and *Helicobacter pylori*. *Arch Intern Med* 1991; 151:760–764.

307. Gambert SR. Alcohol abuse: medical effects of heavy drinking in late life. *Geriatrics* 1997;52:30–37.

308. Perlow W, Baraona E, Lieber CS. Symptomatic intestinal disacchari-dase deficiency in alcoholics. *Gastroenterology* 1977;72:680–684.

309. Jacobs EA, Copperman SM, Jeffe A, Kulig J. Fetal alcohol syndrome and alcohol related neurodevelopmental disorders. *Pediatrics* 2000;106:358–361.

310. CDC. Alcohol consumption among pregnant and childbearing-aged women — United States, 1991 and 1995. *MMWR* 1997;46:346–350.

311. CDC. Alcohol use among women of childbearing age — United States, 1991–1999. *MMWR* 2002;51:273–276.

312. Jones KL, Smith DW. Recognition of the fetal alcohol syndrome in early infancy. *Lancet* 1973;2:999–1001.

313. Institute of Medicine. *Fetal Alcohol Syndrome: Diagnosis, Epidemi-ology, Prevention and Treatment*. National Academy Press, Wash-ington, DC, 1996.

314. CDC. Fetal alcohol syndrome — Alaska, Arizona, Colorado, and New York, 1995–1997. *MMWR* 2002;51:433–435.

315. Weber MK, Floyd RL, Riley EP, Snider DE Jr. National Task Force on fetal alcohol syndrome and fetal alcohol effect: defining the national agenda for fetal alcohol syndrome and other prenatal alcohol-related effects. *MMWR* 2002;51:9–12.

316. Jagust W. Untangling vascular dementia. *Lancet* 2001;358:2097–2098.

317. Ruitenberg A, van Swieten JC, Witteman JC, *et al.* Alcohol consumption and risk of dementia: the Rotterdam Study. *Lancet* 2002;359:281–286.

318. Mukamal KJ, Kuller LH, Fitzpatrick AL, *et al.* Prospective study of alcohol consumption and risk of dementia in older adults. *JAMA* 2003;289:1405–1413.

319. Zuccala G, Onder G, Pedone C, *et al.* Dose-related impact of alcohol consumption on cognitive function in advanced age: results of a multicenter survey. *Alcohol Clin Exp Res* 2001;25:1743–1748.

320. Thomas VS, Rockwood KJ. Alcohol abuse, cognitive impairment, and mortality among older persons. *J Am Geriatr Soc* 2001;49:415–420.

321. Wuethrich B. Does alcohol damage female brains more? *Science* 2001;2077–2079.

322. Hommer DW, Momenan R, Kaiser E, Rawlings RR. Evidence for a gender-related effect of alcoholism on brain volumes. *Am J Psychia-try* 2001;158:198–204.

323. Pfefferbaum A, Rosenbloom M, Deshmukh A, Sullivan EV. Sex differences in the effect of alcohol on brain structure. *Am J Psychiatry* 2001;158:188–197.

324. CDC. Involvement by young drivers in fatal alcohol-related motor-vehicle crashes — United States, 1982–2001. *MMWR* 2002;51:1089–1091.

325. Rossow I, Amundsen A. Alcohol abuse and mortality: a 40-year prospective study of Norwegian conscripts. *Soc Sci Med* 1997; 44:261–267.

326. Zador PL. Alcohol-related relative risk of fatal driver injuries in relation to driver age and sex. *J Stud Alcohol* 1991;52:302–310.

327. CDC. Behavioral Risk Factor Surrveillance System survey data. US Department of Health and Human Services, CDC, Atlanta, Georgia, 1999.

328. National Highway Traffic Safety Administration. *Traffic Safety Facts 2000: Alcohol.* US Department of Transportation, National Highway Traffic Safety Administration, National Center for Statistics and Analysis, Washington, DC, 2001.

329. Zador PL. Alcohol-related relative risk of fatal driver injuries in relation to driver age and sex. *J Stud Alcohol* 1991;52:302–310.

330. Zador PL, Krawchuck SA, Voas RB. Alcohol-related relative risk of driver fatalities and driver involvement in fatal crashes in relation to driver age and gender: an update using 1996 data. *J Stud Alcohol* 2000;61:387–395.

331. Andersson AL, Bunketorp O. Cycling and alcohol. *Injury* 2002; 33:467–471.

332. Smith GS, Keyl PM, Hadley JA, *et al.* Drinking and recreational boating fatalities: a population-based case-control study. *JAMA* 2001;286:2974–2980.

333. Bell NS, Amoroso PJ, Yore MM, *et al.* Alcohol and other risk factors for drowning among male active duty US army soldiers. *Aviat Space Environ Med* 2001;72:1086–1095.

334. Schuckit MA. New findings in the genetics of alcoholism. *JAMA* 1999;281:1875–1876.

335. Murayama M, Matsushita S, Muramatsu T, Higuchi S. Clinical characteristics and disease course of alcoholics with inactive aldehyde dehydrogenase-2. *Alcohol Clin Exp Res* 1998;22:524–527.

336. Neumark YD, Friedlander Y, Thomasson HR, Li TK. Association of the ADH2*2 allele with reduced ethanol consumption in Jewish men in Israel: a pilot study. *J Stud Alcohol* 1998;59:133–139.

337. Lieber CS, DeCarli LM. Hepatic microsomal ethanol-oxidizing system: *in vitro* characteristics and adaptive properties *in vivo. J Biol Chem* 1970;245:2505–2512.

338. Lieber CS (ed.) *Medical and Nutritional Complications of Alcoholism: Mechanisms and Management.* Plenum Press, New York, 1992.

339. Lieber CS. Medical disorders of alcoholism. *N Engl J Med* 1995; 333:1058–1065.

340. Whitcomb DC, Block GD. Association of acetaminophen hepatotoxicity with fasting and ethanol use. *JAMA* 1994;272:1845–1850.

341. Leo MA, Rosman A, Lieber CS. Differential depletion of carotenoids and tocopherol in liver disease. *Hepatology* 1993;17:977–986.

342. Kumar S, Rex DK. Failure of physicians to recognize acetaminophen hepatotoxicity in chronic alcoholics. *Arch Intern Med* 1991;151:1189–1191.

343. Schiodt FV, Lee WM, Bondesen S, *et al.* Influence of acute and chronic alcoholic intake on the clinical course and outcome in acetaminophen overdose. *Aliment Pharacol Ther* 2002;16:707–715.

344. Schmidt LE, Dalhoff K, Poulsen HE. Acute versus chronic alcohol consumption in acetaminophen-induced hepatotoxicity. *Hepatology* 2002;35:876–882.

345. Kuffner EK, Dart RC, Bogdan GM, *et al.* Effect of maximal daily doses of acteminophen on the liver of alcoholic patients: a randomized, double-blind, placebo-controlled trial. *Arch Intern Med* 2001;161:2247–2252.

346. Eisenberg DM, Davis RB, Ettner SL, *et al.* Trends in alternative medicine use in the United States, 1990–1997. *JAMA* 1998;280:1569–1575.

347. Health Agencies Update. Dietary supplement framework. *JAMA* 2002;288:823.

348. Gulla J, Singer AJ. Use of alternative therapies among emergency department patients. *Ann Emerg Med* 2000;35:226–228.

349. Lanski SL, Greenwald M, Perkins A, Simon HK. Herbal use in a pediatric emergency department population: expect the unexpected. *Pediatrics* 2003;111:981–985.

350. Dasgupta A. Review of abnormal laboratory test results and toxic effects due to use of herbal medicines. *Am J Clin Pathol* 2003;120:127–137.

351. Raffa R. Screen of receptor and uptake site activity of hypericin components of St. John's wort reveal sigma receptor binding. *Life Sci* 1998;62:PL265–PL270.

352. Wagner PJ, Jester D, LeClair B, *et al.* Taking the edge off: why patients choose St. John's wort. *J Fam Pract* 1999;48:615–619.

353. Bowman M, Nicklin DE. St. John's wort as an antidepressant. *JAMA* 1998;279:1438.

354. Kessler RC, McGonagle KA, Zhao S, *et al.* Lifetime and 12-month prevalence of DSM-III-R psychiatric disorders in the United States results from the national comorbidity study. *Arch Gen Psychiatry* 1994;51:8–19.

355. Linde K, Ramirez G, Mulrow CD, *et al.* St. John's wort for depression — an overview and meta-analysis of randomised clinical trials. *BMJ* 1996;313:253–257.

356. Woelk H. Comparison of St. John's wort and imipramine for treating depression: randomised controlled trial. *BMJ* 2000;321:536–539.

357. Shelton RC, Keller MB, Gelenberg A, *et al.* Effectiveness of St. John's wort in major depression: a randomized controlled trial. *JAMA* 2001;285:1978–1986.

358. Hypericum Depression Trial Study Group. Effect of *Hypericum perforatum* (St. John's wort) in major depressive disorder: a randomized controlled trial. *JAMA* 2002;287:1807–1814.

359. Stevinson C, Ernst E. Safety of *Hypericum* in patients with depression. *CNS Drugs* 1999;11:125–132.

360. Ernst E. Second thoughts about safety of St. John's wort. *Lancet* 1999;354:2014–2016.

361. Piscitelli SC, Burstein AH, Chaitt D, *et al.* Indinavir concentrations and St. John's wort. *Lancet* 2000;355:547–548.

362. Henney JE. Risk of drug interactions with St. John's wort. *JAMA* 2000;283:1679.

363. Ruschitzka F, Meier PJ, Turina M, *et al.* Acute heart transplant rejection due to Saint John's wort. *Lancet* 2000;355:548–549.

364. Barone GW, Gurley BJ, Ketel BL, *et al.* Drug interaction between St. John's wort and cyclosporine. *Ann Pharmacother* 2000;34:1013–1016.

365. Lal S, Iskandar H. St. John's wort and schizophrenia. *CMAJ* 2000;163:262–263.

366. Patel S, Robinson R, Burk M. Hypertensive crisis associated with St. John's wort. *Am J Med* 2002;112:507–508.

367. Brown TM. Acute St. John's wort toxicity. *Am J Emerg Med* 2000;18:531–532.

368. Bove GM. Acute neuropathy after exposure to sun in a patient treated with St. John's wort. *Lancet* 1998;352:1121–1122.

369. Nierenberg AA, Burt T, Matthews J, Weiss AP. Mania associated with St. John's wort. *Biol Psych* 1999;46:1707–1708.

370. Gordon JB. SSRIs and St. John's wort: possible toxicity. *Am Fam Physician* 1998;57:950–953.
371. Yoshikawa T, Naito Y, Kondo M. *Ginkgo biloba* leaf extract: review of biological actions and clinical applications. *Antiox Redox Signal* 1999;1:469–480.
372. Bastianetto S, Quirion R. Natural extracts as possible protective agents of brain aging. *Neurobiol Aging* 2002;23:891–897.
373. Tang F, Nag S, Shiu SY, Pang SF. The effects of melatonin and *Ginkgo biloba* extract on memory loss and choline acetytransferase activities in the brain of rats infused intracerebroventricularly with beta-amyloid 1-40. *Life Sci* 2002;71:2625–2631.
374. Luo Y, Smith JV, Paramasivam V, *et al*. Inhibition of amyloid-beta aggregation and caspase-3 activation by the *Ginkgo biloba* extract EGb761. *Proc Natl Acad Sci USA* 2002;99:12197–12202.
375. Kleijnen J, Knipschild P. *Ginkgo biloba* for cerebral insufficiency. *Br J Clin Pharmacol* 1992;34:352–358.
376. Solomon PR, Adams F, Silver A, *et al*. Ginkgo for memory enhancement: a randomized controlled trial. *JAMA* 2002;288:835–840.
377. Wettstein A. Cholinesterase inhibitors and ginkgo extracts — are they comparable in treatment of dementia? Comparison of published placebo efficacy of at least six months duration. *Phytomedicine* 2000;6:693–401.
378. Allain H, Raoul P, Lieury A, *et al*. Effect of two doses of *Ginkgo biloba* extract (EGb761) on dual-coding test in elderly subjects. *Clin Ther* 1993;15:549–557.
379. LeBars PL, Katz MM, Berman N, *et al*. A placebo-controlled, double-blind, randomized trial of an extract of *Ginkgo biloba* for dementia. *JAMA* 1997;278:1327–1332.
380. Oken BS, Storzbach DM, Kaye JA. The efficacy of *Ginkgo biloba* on cognitive function in Alzheimer disease. *Arch Neurol* 1998;55:1409–1415.
381. van Dongen M, van Rossum E, Kessels A, *et al*. The efficacy of *Ginkgo biloba* for elderly people with dementia and age-associated memory impairment: new results of a randomized clinical trial. *J Am Geriatr Soc* 2000;48:1183–1194.
382. Grundman M, Grundman M, Delaney P. Antioxidant strategies for Alzheimer's disease. *Proc Nutr Soc* 2002;61:191–202.
383. Pittler MH, Ernst E. *Ginkgo biloba* extract for the treatment of intermittent claudication: a meta-analysis of randomized trials. *Am J Med* 2000;108:276–281.

384. Ernst E, Stevinson C. *Ginkgo biloba* for tinnitus: a review. *Clin Otolaryngol* 1999;24:164–167.
385. Morgenstern C, Biermann E. The efficacy of *Ginkgo* special extract EGb761 in patients in tinnitus. *Int J Pharmacol Ther* 2002;40:188–197.
386. Rowin J, Lewis SL. Spontaneous bilateral subdural hematomas associated with chronic *Ginkgo biloba* ingestion. *Neurology* 1996; 46:1775–1776.
387. Gilbert GJ. *Gingko biloba. Neurology* 1997;48:1137 (Letter).
388. Fessenden JM, Wittenborn W, Clarke L. *Gingko biloba*: a case report of herbal medicine and bleeding postoperatively from a laparoscopic cholecystectomy. *Am Surg* 2001;67:33–35.
389. Miwa H, Iijima M, Tanaka S, Mizuno Y. Generalized convulsion after consuming a large amount of ginkgo nuts. *Epilepsia* 2001;42:280–281.
390. Rosenblatt M, Mindel J. Spontaneous hyphema associated with ingestion of *Ginkgo biloba* extract. *N Engl J Med* 1997;336:1108 (Letter).
391. Hauser D, Gayowski T, Singh N. Bleeding complications precipitated by unrecognized *Gingko biloba* use after liver transplantation. *Transpl Int* 2002;15:377–379.
392. Miman MC, Ozturan O, Iraz M, *et al.* Amikacin ototoxicity enhanced by *Ginkgo biloba* extract (EGb761). *Hear Res* 2002;169:121–129.
393. Chong SK, Oberholzer VG. Ginseng — is there a use in clinical medicine? *Postgrad Med J* 1988;64:841–846.
394. Ernst E. The risk-benefit profile of commonly used herbal therapies: *Ginkgo biloba*, St. John's wort, ginseng, echinacea, saw palmetto and kava. *Ann Intern Med* 2002;136:42–53.
395. Cupp MJ. Herbal remedies: adverse effects and drug interactions. *Am Fam Phys* 1999;59:1239–1244.
396. Lewis W. In: *Plants in Indigenous Medicine and Diet: Behavioral Approaches.* NL Etkin (ed.) Redgrove Publishing Co., Bedford Hills, NY, 1986, pp. 290–305.
397. Vasquez I, Aguera-Ortiz LF. Herbal products and serious side effects: a case of ginseng-induced manic episode. *Acta Psychiatr Scand* 2002;105:76–77.
398. Vuksan V, Sievenpiper JL, Koo VY, *et al.* American ginseng (*Panox quinquefolius*) reduces postprandial hypoglycemia in non-diabetic subjects and subjects with type 2 diabetes mellitus. *Arch Intern Med* 2000;160:1009–1013.
399. Janetzky K, Morreale AP. Probable interaction between ginseng and warfarin. *Am J Health Syst Pharm* 1997;54:692–693.

400. van Berkel GJ, Quirke JM, Tigani RA, *et al.* Derivatization for electrospray ionization mass spectrometry: three electrochemically ionizable derivatives. *Anal Chem* 1998;70:1544–1554.

401. Shimada H, Tyler VE, McLaughlin JL. Biologically active acylglycerides from the berries of saw palmetto. *J Nat Prod* 1997; 60:417–418.

402. Feifer AH, Fleshner NE, Klotz L. Analytical accuracy and reliability of commonly used nutritional supplements in prostate disease. *J Urol* 2002;168:150–154.

403. Carraro JC, Rayaud JP, Koch G. Comparison of phytotherapy (Permixon) with finasteride in the treatment of benign prostate hyperplasia: a randomized international study of 1098 patients. *Prostate* 1996;29:231–240.

404. Wilt TJ, Ishani A, Stark G, *et al.* Saw palmetto extracts for treatment of benign prostatic hyperplasia; a systematic review. *JAMA* 1998;280:1604–1609.

405. Melchart WE, Linde K, Brandmeier R, Lersch C. Echinacea root extracts for the prevention of upper respiratory tract infections — a double-blind, placebo-controlled randomized trial. *Arch Fam Med* 1998;7:541–545.

406. Grimm W, Muller H-H. A randomized controlled trial of the effect of fluid extract of *Echinacea purpurea* on the incidence and severity of colds and respiratory infections. *Am J Med* 1999; 106:138–143.

407. Barrett B, Vohmann M, Calabrese C. Echinacea for upper respiratory infection. *J Fam Pract* 1999;48:628–635.

408. Mullins RJ. Echinacea-associated anaphylaxis. *Med J Aust* 1998;168:170–171.

409. Jamieson DD, Duffield PH, Cheng D, Duffield AM. Composition of central nervous system activity of the aqueous and lipid extracts of kava (*Piper mesthysticum*). *Arch Int Pharmacodyn* 1989;301:66–80.

410. Lindenberg D, Pitule-Schodel H. D, L-kavain in comparison with oxazepam in anxiety disorders: a double-blind study of clinical effectiveness. *Fortschr Med* 1990;108:49–50.

411. Scherer J. Kava-kava extract in anxiety disorders: an outpatient observational study. *Adv Ther* 1998;15:261–269.

412. Pittler MH, Ernst E. Efficacy of kava extract for treating anxiety: systematic review and meta-analysis. *J Clin Psychopharmacol* 2000;20:84–89.

413. De Leo V, Ia Marca A, Morgante G, *et al.* Evaluation of combining kava extract with hormone replacement therapy in the treatment of postmenopausal anxiety. *Maturitas* 2001;39:185–188.

414. Jappe U, Frankle I, Reinhold D, Gollnick HP. Sebotropic drug reaction resulting from kava-kava extract therapy: a new entity? *J Am Acad Dermatol* 1998;38:104–106.

415. Norton SA, Ruze P. Kava dermopathy. *J Am Acad Dermatol* 1994;31:89–97.

416. Escher M, Desmeules J. Hepatitis associated with kava, and herbal remedy. *BMJ* 2001;322:139.

417. CDC. Hepatic toxicity possibly associated with kava-containing products — United States, Germany and Switzerland, 1999–2002. *MMWR* 2002;51:1065–1067.

418. Mar C, Bent S. An evidence-based review of the 10 most commonly used herbs. *West J Med* 1999;171:168–171.

419. Chan TY, Tang CH, Critchley JA. Poisoning due to an over-the-counter hypnotic, Sleep-Qik (hyoscine, cyproheptadine, valerian). *Postgrad Med J* 1995;71:227–228.

420. Borek C. Antioxidant health effects of aged garlic extract. *J Nutr* 2001;131:1010S–1015S.

421. Lau BHS. Suppression of LDL oxidation by garlic. *J Nutr* 2001;131:985S–988S.

422. Fleischauer AT, Arab L. Garlic and cancer: a critical review of the epidemiologic literature. *J Nutr* 2001;131:1032S–1040S.

423. Jonkers D, van den Broek E, van Dooren I, *et al.* Antibacterial effect of garlic and omeprazole on *Helicobacter pylori*. *J Antimicrob Chemother* 1999;43:837–839.

424. Lau BHS, Lam F, Wang-Cheng R. Effect of odor modified garlic preparation on blood lipids. *Nutr Res* 1987;7:139–149.

425. Warshafsky S, Kamer RS, Sivak SL. Effect of garlic on total serum cholesterol: a meta-analysis. *Ann Intern Med* 1993;119:599–605.

426. Stevinson C, Pittler MH, Ernst E. Garlic for treating hypercholesterolemia: a meta-analysis of randomized clinical trials. *Ann Intern Med* 2000;133:420–429.

427. Berthold HK, Sudhop T, von Bergmann K. Effect of garlic oil preparation on serum lipoproteins and cholesterol metabolism: a randomized controlled trial. *JAMA* 1998;279:1900–1902.

428. Isaacsohn JL, Moser M, Stein EA, *et al.* Garlic powder and plasma lipids and lipoproteins: a multicenter, randomized, placebo-controlled trial. *Arch Intern Med* 1998;158:1189–1194.

429. Banerjee S, Maulik S. Effect of garlic on cardiovascular disorders: a review. *Nutr J* 2002;1:4 (http//www.nutritionj.com/content/1/1/4).

430. Silagy CA, Neil HAW. A meta-analysis of effect of garlic on blood pressure. *J Hypertension* 1994;12:463–468.

431. Hsing AW, Chokkalingam AP, Gao YT, *et al.* Allium vegetables and risk of prostate cancer: a population-based study. *J Natl Cancer Inst* 2002;94:1648–1651.

432. Fleischauer AT, Poole C, Arab L. Garlic consumption and cancer prevention: meta-analysis of colorectal and stomach cancers. *Am J Clin Nutr* 2000;72:1047–1052.

433. Lamm DL, Riggs DR. Enhanced immunocompetence by garlic: role in bladder cancer and other malignancies. *J Nutr* 2001;131:1067S–1070S.

434. Fleischauer AT, Arab L. Garlic and cancer: a critical review of the epidemiologic literature. *J Nutr* 2001;131:1032S–1040S.

435. Clark F. Chaparral-induced toxic hepatitis: California and Texas, 1992. *MMWR* 1992;41:812–814.

436. Gordon DW, Rosenthal G, Hart J, *et al.* Chaparral ingestion: the broadening spectrum of liver injury caused by herbal medications. *JAMA* 1995;273:489–490.

437. Alderman S, Kailas S, Goldfarb S, *et al.* Cholestatic hepatitis after ingestion of chaparral leaves: confirmation by endoscopic retrograde cholangiopancreatography and liver biopsy. *J Clin Gastroenterol* 1994;19:242–247.

438. Sheikh NM, Philen RM, Love LA. Chaparral-associated hepatotoxicity. *Arch Intern Med* 1997;157:913–919.

439. Koff RS. Herbal hepatotoxicity: revisiting a dangerous alternative. *JAMA* 1995;273:502 (Editorial).

440. Street drug alternative with ephedra. *FDA Consumer* 1996;30:4.

441. Shekelle PG, Hardy ML, Morton SC, *et al.* Efficacy and safety of ephedra and ephedrine for weight loss and athletic performance: a meta-analysis. *JAMA* 2003;289:1537–1545.

442. Holler Ca, Benowitz ML. Adverse and central nervous system events associated with dietary supplements containing ephedra alkaloids. *N Engl J Med* 2000;343:1833–1838.

443. Samenuk D, Link MS, Homoud MK, *et al.* Adverse cardiovascular events temporally associated with ma huang, an herbal source of ephedrine. *Mayo Clin Proc* 2002;77:12–16.

444. Bent S, Tiedt TN, Odden MC, Shlipak MG. The relative safety of ephedra compared with other herbal products. *Ann Intern Med* 2003;138:468–471.

445. Verduin ML, Labbate LA. Psychosis and delirium following Metabolife use. *Psychopharmacol Bull* 2002;36:42–45.

446. Zaacks SM, Klein L, Tan CD, *et al.* Hypersensitivity myocarditis associated with ephedra use. *J Toxicol Clin Toxicol* 1999;37: 485–489.

447. Nadir A, Agrawal S, King PD, Marshall JB. Acute hepatitis associated with the use of a Chinese herbal product, ma-huang. *Am J Gastroenterol* 1996;91:2647–2648.

448. Wolfe SM, Ephedra — scientific evidence versus money/politics. *Science* 2003;300:437.

449. Neergaard L. *Criminal Probe Targets Metabolife, Ephedra.* Desert News, Salt Lake City, 16 August 2002.

450. Phillips S, Ruggier R, Hutchinson SE. *Zingiber officinale* (ginger) — an antiemetic for day care surgery. *Anesthesia* 1993;48: 715–717.

451. Arfeen Z, Owen R, Plummer J, *et al.* A double-blind random controlled tiral of ginger for the prevention of postoperative nausea and vomiting. *Anesth Intensive Care* 1995;23:449–452.

452. Visalyaputra S, Petchpaisit N, Somcharoen K, Choavaratana R. The efficacy of ginger root in the prevention of postoperative nausea and vomiting after outpatient gynaecological laparoscopy. *Anaesthesia* 1998;53:506–510.

453. Grontved A, Brask T, Kambskard J, Hentzer E. Ginger root against seasickness. A controlled trial on the open sea. *Acta Otolaryngol* 1988;105:45–49.

454. Grontved A, Hentzer E, Vertigo-reducing effect of ginger root. A controlled clinical study. *ORL J Otorhinolaryngol Relat Spec* 1986;48:282–286.

455. Mowbrey D, Clayson D. Motion sickness, ginger, and psycophysics. *Lancet* 1982;1:656–657.

456. Stewart J, Wood M, Wood C, Mims M. Effects of ginger on motion sickness susceptibility and gastric function. *Pharmacology* 1991;42:111–120.

457. Syed Ta, Afzal M, Ashfaq AS, *et al.* Management of genital herpes with 0.5% Aloe vera extract in a hydrophilic cream: a placebo-controlled, double-blind study. *J Dermatol Treatment* 1997;8:99–102.

458. Syed TA, Ahmud SA, Holt AH, *et al.* Management of psoriasis with aloe vera extract in hydrophilic cream: a placebo-controlled, drouble-blind study. *Trop Med Int Health* 1996;1:505–509.

459. Hayes SM. Lichen planus — report of successful treatment with aloe vera. *Gen Dent* 1999;47:268–272.

460. Williams MS, Burk M, Loprinzi CI, *et al.* Phase III double-blind evaluation of an Aloe vera gel as a prophylactic agent for radiation-induced skin toxicity. *Int J Radiat Oncol Biol Phys* 1996;36:345–349.

461. Schmidt JM, Greenspoon JS. Aloe vera dermal wound gel is associated with delay in wound healing. *Obstet Gynecol* 1991;78:115–117.

462. Agarwal OP. Prevention of atheromatous heart disease. *Angiology* 1985;36:485–492.

463. Davila J, Lenher A, Acosta D. Protective effect of flavonoids on drug-induced hepatotoxicity *in vitro. Toxicology* 1989;57:257–286.

464. Muriel P, Garciapina T, Perez-Alvarez V, Mourelle M. Silymarin protects against paracetamol-induced lipid peroxidation and liver damage. *J Appl Toxicol* 1992;12:439–442.

465. Letteron P, Labbe G, Cegott C, *et al.* Mechanisms for the protective effects of silymarin against carbon tetracholoride-induced lipid peroxidation and hepatotoxicity in mice. *Biochem Pharmacol* 1990;39:2027–2034.

466. Lawrence Review of Natural Products. *Milk Thistle.* Facts and Comparisons, St. Louis, MO, 1994.

467. Wang MJ, Lin WW, Chen HL, *et al.* Silymarin protects dopaminergic neurons against lipopolysaccharide-induced neurotoxicity by inhibiting microglia activation. *Eur J Neurosci* 2002;16:2103–2112.

468. Katiyar SK. Treatment of silymarin, a plant flavonoid, prevents ultraviolet light-induced immune suppression and oxidative stress in mouse skin. *Int J Oncol* 2002;21:1213–1222.

469. Tyagi A, Bhatia N, Condon MS, *et al.* Antiproliferative and apoptotic effects of silibinin in rat prostrate cancer cells. *Prostrate* 2002;53: 211–217.

470. Ferenci P, Dragosics B, Dittrich H, *et al.* Randomized controlled trial of silymarin treatment in patients with cirrhosis of the liver. *J Hepatol* 1989;9:105–113.

471. Pares A, Planas R, Torres M, *et al.* Effects of silymarin in alcoholic cirrhosis of the liver: results of a controlled, double-blind, randomized and multicenter trial. *J Hepatol* 1998;28:615–621.

472. Velussi M, Cernigoi A, Viezzoli L, *et al.* Silymarin reduced hyperinsulinemia, malondialdehyde levels and daily insulin need in cirrhotic diabetic patients. *Curr Ther Res* 1993;53:533–545.

473. De Smet PAGM. Health risks of herbal remedies. *Drug Saf* 1995; 13:81–93.

474. Adverse Event Reporting for Dietary Supplements: An Inadequate Safety Valve. Office of Inspector General, Washington, DC, April 2001 (Report No. OEI-01-00-00180).

475. Palmer ME, Haller C, McKinney PE, *et al.* Adverse events associated with dietary supplements: an observational study. *Lancet* 2003;361:101–106.
476. Marcus DM, Grollman AP. Botanical medicines — the need for new regulations. *N Engl J Med* 2002;347:2073–2076.
477. Rice DP, Kelman S, Miller LS. Estimates of economic costs of alcohol and drug abuse and metnal illness, 1985 and 1988. *Public Health Rep* 1991;106:280–292.
478. Rice DP. Economic costs of substance abuse, 1995. *Proc Assoc Am Physicians* 1999;111:119–125.
479. Hurwitz N, Wade OL. Intensive hospital monitoring of adverse reactions to drugs. *BMJ* 1969;531–535.
480. Hurwitz N. Predisposing factors in adverse reactions to drugs. *BMJ* 1969;1:536–539.
481. Williamson J, Chopin JM. Adverse reactions to prescribed drugs in the elderly: a multicentre investigation. *Age Ageing* 1980;9:73–80.
482. Nolan L, O'Malley K. Prescribing for the elderly: Part 1: Sensitivity of the elderly to adverse drug reactions. *J Am Geriatr Soc* 1988;36:142–149.
483. Willcox SM, Himmelstein DU, Woodhandler S. Inappropriate drug prescribing for the community-dwelling elderly. *JAMA* 1994;272:292–296.
484. Zhan C, Sangl J, Bierman AS, *et al.* Potentially inappropriate medication use in the community-dwelling elderly: findings from the 1996 Medical Expenditure Panel Survey. *JAMA* 2001;286:2823–2829.
485. Gandhi TK, Weingart SN, Borus J, *et al.* Adverse drug events in ambulatory care. *N Engl J Med* 2003;348:1556–1564.
486. Phillips DP, Bredder CC. Morbidity and mortality from medical errors: an increasingly serious public health problem. *Annu Rev Pub Health* 2002;23:135–150.
487. Lazarou J, Pomeranz BH, Corey PN. Incidence of adverse drug reactions in hospitalized patients: a meta-analysis of prospective studies. *JAMA* 1998;279:1200–1205.
488. Hoyert DL, Freedman MA, Strobino DM, Guyer B. Annual summary of vital statistics: 2000. *Pediatrics* 2001;108:1241–1255.
489. Vargas E, Terleira A, Hernando F, *et al.* Effect of adverse drug reactions on length of stay in surgical intensive care units. *Crit Care Med* 2003;31:694–698.
490. Hohl CM, Dankoff J, Colacone A, Afilalo M. Polypharmacy, adverse drug-related events and potential adverse drug interactions in elderly

patients presenting to an emergency department. *Ann Emerg Med* 2001;38:666–671.

491. Gurwitz JH, Field TS, Harrold LR, *et al.* Incidence and preventability of adverse drug events among older persons in the ambulatory setting. *JAMA* 2003;289:1107–1116.

492. Phillips KA, Veenstra DL, Oren E, *et al.* Potential role of pharmacogenomics in reducing adverse drugs reactions: a systematic review. *JAMA* 2001;286:2270–2279.

493. Weinshilboum R. Inheritance and drug responses. *N Engl J Med* 2003;346:529–537.

494. Block RI, Erwin WJ, Ghoneim MM. Chronic drug use and cognitive impairments. *Pharmacol Biochem Behav* 2002;73:491–504.

495. Brook DW, Brook JS, Zhang C, *et al.* Drug use and risk of major depressive disorder, alcohol dependence, and substance use disorders. *Arch Gen Psychiatry* 2002;59:1039–1044.

496. Meyer RE. The disease called addiction: emerging evidence in a 200-year debate. *Lancet* 1996;347:162–165.

497. Robeznieks A. Prescription drug abuse deadlier than the use of illegal drugs. *Am Med News* 2002;December 16:17.

498. Landers SJ. Prescriptions drug abuse by teens increasing. *Am Med News* 2003;February 10:26.

499. Hemmelgarn B, Suissa S, Huang A, *et al.* Benzodiazepine use and the risk of motor vehicle crash in the elderly. *JAMA* 1997;278:27–31.

500. Rao R, Desai NS. OxyContin and neonatal abstinence syndrome. *J Perinatol* 2002;22:324–325.

501. Rischitelli DG, Karbowicz SH. Safety and efficacy on controlled-release oxycodon: a systematic literature review. *Pharmacotherapy* 2002;22:898–904.

502. Widlitz M, Marin DB. Substance abuse in older adults: an overview. *Geriatrics* 2002;57(12):29–34.

503. Jinks MJ, Raschko RR. A profile of alcohol and prescription drug abuse in a high-risk community-based elderly population. *DICP* 1990;24:971–975.

504. Edgell RC, Kunik ME, Molinari VA, *et al.* Nonalcohol-related use disorders in geropsychiatric patients. *J Geriatr Psychiatry Neurol* 2000;13:33–37.

505. Office of Applied Studies. *Year-end 1999 Emergency Department Data from Drug Abuse Warning Network.* Substance Abuse and Mental Health Services Administration, Rockville, MD, August 2000 [DHHS Publication No. (SMA) 00-3462].

506. Lange RA, Hillis LD. Cardiovascular complications of cocaine use. *N Engl J Med* 2001;345:351–358.

507. Grunbaum J, Kann L, Kinchen SA, *et al.* Youth risk behavior surveillance — United States, 2001. *MMWR* 2002;51(SS-4):1–21.

508. Kloner RA, Rezkalla SH. Cocaine and the heart. *N Engl J Med* 2003;348:487–488.

509. Coleman DL, Ross TF, Naughton JL. Mycardial ischemia and infarction related to recreational cocaine use. *West J Med* 1982;136:444–446.

510. Hollander JE, Hoffman RS, Burstein JL, *et al.* Cocaine-associated myocardial infarction: mortality and complications. *Arch Intern Med* 1995;155:1081–1086.

511. Seigel AJ, Sholar MB, Mendelson JH, *et al.* Cocaine-induced erythrocytosis and increase in von Willebrand factor: evidence for drug-related blood doping and prothrombotic effects. *Arch Intern Med* 1999;159:1925–1930.

512. Mittleman MA, Mintzer D, Maclure M, *et al.* Triggering of myocardial infarction by cocaine. *Circulation* 1999;99:2737–2741.

513. Silva MO, Roth D, Reddy KR, *et al.* Hepatic dysfunction accompanying acute cocaine intoxication. *J Hepatol* 1991;12:312–315.

514. Gottschalk P, Kosten T. Cerebral perfusion defects in combined cocaine and alcohol dependence. *Drug Alcohol Depend* 2002;68:95.

515. Hsue PY, Salinas CL, Bolger AF, *et al.* Acute aortic dissection related to crack cocaine. *Circulation* 2002;105:1592–1595.

516. Martinez M, Davenport L. Saussy J, Martinez J. Drug-associated heat stroke. *South Med J* 2002;95:799–802.

517. Singer LT, Arendt R, Minnes S, *et al.* Cognitive and motor outcomes of cocaine-exposed infants. *JAMA* 2002;287:1952–1960.

518. Solowij N, Stephens RS, Roffman RA, *et al.* Cognitive functioning of long-term heavy cannabis users seeking treatment. *JAMA* 2002;287:1123–1131.

519. von Sydow K, Lieb R, Pfister H, *et al.* What predicts incident use of cannabis and progression to abuse and dependence? A four-year prospective examination of risk factors in a community sample of adolescents and young adults. *Drug Alcohol Depend* 2002;68:49–64.

520. Pope HG, Gruber AJ, Yurgelun-Todd D. The residual neuropsychological effects of cannabis: the current status of research. *Drug Alcohol Depend* 1995;38:25–34.

521. Roeloffs CA, Wells KB, Ziedonis D, *et al.* Problem substance use among depressed patients in managed primary care. *Psychosomatics* 2002;43:405–412.

522. Patton GC, Coffey C, Carlin JB, *et al.* Cannabis use and mental health in young people: a cohort study. *BMJ* 2002;325:1195–1198.

523. Zammit S, Allebeck P, Andreasson S, *et al.* Self-reported cannabis use as a risk factor for schizophrenia in Swedish conscripts of 1969: historical cohort study. *BMJ* 2002;325:1199–1201.

524. Arseneault L, Cannon M, Poulton R, *et al.* Cannabis use in adolescence and risk for adult psychosis: longitudinal prospective study. *BMJ* 2002;325:1212–1213.

525. Rey JM, Tennant CC. Cannabis and mental health: more evidence establishes clear link between use of cannabis and psychiatric illness. *BMJ* 2002;325:1183–1184.

526. Buhler B, Hambrecht M, Loffler W, *et al.* Precipitation and determination of the onset and course of schizophrenia by substance abuse — a retrospective and prospective study of 232 population-based first illness episodes. *Schizophr Res* 2002;54:243–251.

527. Nunez LA, Gurpegui M. Cannabis-induced psychosis: a cross-sectional comparison with acute schizophrenia. *Acta Psychiatr Scand* 2002;105:173–178.

528. Mittleman MA, Lewis RA, Maclure M, *et al.* Triggering myocardial infarction by marijuana. *Circulation* 2001;103:2805–2809.

529. Bachs L, Morland H. Acute cardiovascular fatalities following cannabis use. *Forensic Sci Int* 2001;124:200–203.

530. McLeod AL, McKenna CJ, Northridge DB. Myocardial infarction following combined recreational use of viagra and cannabis. *Clin Cardiol* 2002;25:133–134.

531. Jones RT. Cardiovascular system effects of marijuana. *J Clin Pharmacol* 2002;42:58S–63S.

532. Klein TW, Friedman H, Specter S. Marijuana, immunity and infection. *J Neuroimmunol* 1998;83:102–115.

533. Friedman H, Klein TW. Marijuana and immunity. *Sci Med* 1999;March/April:12–21.

534. Kandel DB. Does marijuana use cause the use of other drugs? *JAMA* 2003;289:482–483.

535. Kandel DB (ed.) *Stages and Pathways of Drug Involvement: Examining the Gateway Hypothesis.* Cambridge University Press, Cambridge, England, 2002.

536. Lynskey MT, Heath AC, Bucholz KK, *et al.* Escalation of drug use in early-onset cannabis users versus co-twin controls. *JAMA* 2003;289:427–433.

537. Kalant H. Medicinal use of cannabis: history and current status. *Pain Res Manag* 2001;6:80–91.

538. Grundy RI. The therapeutic potential of cannabinoids in neuroprotection. *Expert Opin Investig Drugs* 2002;11:1365–1374.

539. Croxford JL. Therapeutic potential of cannabinoids in CNS disease. *CNS Drugs* 2003;17:179–202.

540. Ware MA, Gamsa A, Persson J, Fitzcharles MA. Cannabis for chronic pain: case series and implications for clinicians. *Pain Res Manag* 2002;7:95–99.

541. Campbell FA, Tramer MR, Carroll D, *et al.* Are cannabinoids an effective safe treatment option in the management of pain? A qualitative systematic review. *BMJ* 2001;323:13–16.

542. Fliegel SE, Roth MD, Kleerup EC, *et al.* Tracheobronchial histopathology in habitual smokers of cocaine, marijuana, and/or tobacco. *Chest* 1997;112:319–326.

543. Barsky SH, Roth MD, Kleerup EC. Histopathologic and molecular alterations in bronchial epithelium in habitual smokers of marijuana, cocaine, and/or tobacco. *J Natl Cancer Inst* 1998;90:1198–1205.

544. Gibson DR, Leamon MH, Flynn N. Epidemiology and public health consequences of methamphetamine use in California's Central Valley. *J Psychoactive Drugs* 2002;34:313–319.

545. Wilkins C, Bhatta K, Casswell S. The emergence of amphetamine use in New Zealand: findings from the 1998 and 2001 Nation Drug Surveys. *N Z Med J* 2002;11:U256.

546. Topp L, Degenhardt L, Kaye S, Darke S. The emergence of potent forms of methamphetamine in Sydney, Australia: a case study of IDRS as a strategic early warning system. *Drug Alcohol Rev* 2002;21:341–348.

547. Farabee D, Prendergast M, Cartier J. Methamphetamine use and HIV risk among substance-abusing offenders in California. *J Psychoactive Drugs* 2002;34:295–300.

548. Guavirat A, Page-Shafer K, van Griensuen GJ, *et al.* Risk of prevalent HIV infection associated with incarceration among injecting drug users in Bangkok, Thailand: case-control study. *BMJ* 2003;326:308–310.

549. Wohl AR, Johnson DF, Lu S, *et al.* HIV risk behaviors among African American men in Los Angeles County who self-identify as heterosexual. *J Acquir Immune Defic Syndr* 2002;31:354–360.

550. Nemoto T, Operario D, Soma T. Risk behaviors of Filipino methamphetamine users in San Francisco: implications for prevention and

treatment of drug use and HIV. *Public Health Rep* 2002; 117(Suppl 1):S30–S38.

551. Inamasu J, Nakamura Y, Saito R, *et al.* Subcortical hemorrhage caused by methamphetamine abuse: efficacy of the triage system in the differential diagnosis — case report. *Neural Med Chir (Tokyo)* 2003; 43:82–84.

552. Smith L, Yonekura ML, Wallace T, *et al.* Effects of prenatal methamphetamine exposure on fetal growth and drug withdrawal symptoms in infants born at term. *J Dev Behav Pediatr* 2003;24:17–23.

553. Strote J, Lee JE, Wechsler H. Increasing MDMA use among college students: results of a national survey. *J Adolesc Health* 2002;30:64–72.

554. Ricaurte GA, Yuan J, Hatzidimitriou G, *et al.* Severe dopaminergic neurotoxicity in primates after a common recreational dose regimen of MDMA ("Ecstasy"). *Science* 2002;297:2260–2263.

555. Soar K, Turner JJ, Parrott AC. Psychiatric disorders in Ecstasy (MDMA) users: a literature review focusing on personal predisposition and drug history. *Hum Psychopharmacol* 2001;16:641–645.

556. Heffernan TM, Ling J, Scholey AB. Subjective ratings of prospective memory deficits in MDMA ("ecstasy") users. *Hum Psychopharmacol* 2001;16:339–344.

557. Heffernan TM, Jarvis H, Rodgers J, *et al.* Prospective memory, everyday cognitive failure and central executive function in recreational users of Ecstasy. *Hum Psychopharmacol* 2001;16:607–612.

558. Parrott AC. Human psychopharmacology of Ecstasy (MDMA): a review of 15 years of empirical research. *Hum Psychopharmacol* 2001;16:557–577.

559. Gowing LR, Henry-Edwards SM, Irvine RJ, Ali RL. The health effects of ecstasy: a literature review. *Drug Alcohol Rev* 2002;21:53–63.

560. Auer J, Berent R, Weber T, *et al.* Subarachnoid haemorrhage with "Ecstasy" abuse in a young adult. *Neurol Sci* 2002;23:199–201.

561. Lange-Brock N, Berg T, Muller AR, *et al.* Acute liver failure following the use of ecstasy (MDMA). *Z Gastroenterol* 2002;40:581–586.

562. Henry JA, Jeffreys KJ, Dawling S. Toxicity and deaths from 3,4-methylenedioxy-methamphetamine ("ecstasy"). *Lancet* 1992; 340:384–387.

563. Schifano F, Oyefeso A, Webb L, *et al.* Review of deaths related to taking ecstasy, England and Wales, 1997–2000. *BMJ* 2003;326:80–81.

564. Weinbroum AA. Importance of early identification of methylenedioxymethamphetamine ("ecstasy") ingestion in victims of motor vehicle accidents. *Eur J Emerg Med* 2003;10:19–22.

565. London LE. UK government approves heroin use on prescription. *BMJ* 2002;325:1321.

566. D'Aunno T, Pollack HA. Changes in methadone treatment practices: results from a national panel study, 1988–2000. *JAMA* 2002;288: 850–856.

567. Sporer KA. Acute heroin overdose. *Ann Intern Med* 1999;130: 584–590.

568. Sporer KA. Strategies for preventing heroin overdose. *BMJ* 2003; 326:442–444.

569. Oxman GL, Kowalski S, Drapela L, *et al.* Heroin overdose deaths — Multnomah County, Oregon, 1993–1999. *MMWR* 2000;49:633–636.

570. Hall WD, Ross JE, Lynskey MT, *et al.* How many dependent heroin users are there in Australia? *Med J Aust* 2000;173:528–531.

571. Hall WD, Degenhardt LJ, Lynskey MT. Opioid overdose mortality in Australia, 1964–1997: birth cohort trends. *Med J Aust* 1999;171: 34–37.

572. Davoli M, Perucci CA, Forastiere F, *et al.* Risk factors for overdose mortality: a case-control study within a cohort of intravenous drug users. *Int J Epidemiol* 1993;22:273–277.

573. Oliver P, Keen J. Concomitant drugs of misuse and drug using behaviors associated with fatal opiate-related poisonings in Sheffield, UK, 1997–2000. *Addiction* 2003;98:191–197.

574. Gyarmathy VA, Neaigus A, Miller M, *et al.* Risk correlates of prevalent HIV, hepatitis B virus, and hepatitis C virus infections among noninjecting heroin users. *J Acquir Immune Defic Syndr* 2002; 30:448–456.

575. Miller CL, Johnson C. Spittal PM, *et al.* Opportunities for prevention: hepatitis C prevalence and incidence in a cohort of young injection drug users. *Hepatology* 2002;36:737–742.

576. Sanchez-Carbonell X, Vilaregut A. A 10-year follow-up study on the health status of heroin addicts based on official registers. *Addiction* 2001;96:1777–1786.

577. AIDS cases rise in China. *AIDS Wkly* 2000;April 10:15.

578. Jones JA, Salmon JE, Djuretic T, *et al.* An outbreak of serious illness and death among injecting drugs users in England during 2000. *J Med Microbiol* 2002;51:978–984.

579. McGuigan CC, Penrice GM, Gruer L, *et al.* Lethal outbreak of infection with *Clostridium novyi* type A and other spore-forming organisms in Scottish injecting drug users. *J Med Microbiol* 2002;51:971–977.

580. Gacouin A, Lavoue S, Signouret T, *et al.* Reversible spongioform leucoencephalopathy after inhalation of heated heroin. *Intensive Case Med* 2003;29:1012–1015.

581. Shahidi NT. A review of the chemistry, biological action, and clinical application of anabolic-androgenic steroids. *Clin Ther* 2001;23: 1355–1390.

582. Rambaldi A, Laquinto G, Gluud C. Anabolic-androgenic steroids for alcoholic liver disease: a Cochrane review. *Am J Gastroenterol* 2002;97:1674–1681.

583. Wichstrom L, Pedersen W. Use of anabolic-androgenic steroids in adolescence: winning, looking good or being bad? *J Stud Alcohol* 2001;62:5–13.

584. Kindlundh AM, Hagekull B, Osacson DG, Nyberg F. Adolescent use of anabolic-androgenic steroids and relations to self-reports of social, personality and health aspects. *Eur J Public Health* 2001;11: 322–328.

585. Tamaki T, Uchiyama S, Uchiyama Y, *et al.* Anabolic steroids increase exercise tolerance. *Am J Physiol Endocrinol Metab* 2001;280:E973–E981.

586. Lindqvist AS, Johansson-Steensland P, Nyberg F, Fahike C. Anabolic androgenic steroids affect competitive behaviour, behavioural response to ethanol and brain serotonin levels. *Behav Brain Res* 2002;133:21–29.

587. Bahrke MS, Wright JE, Strauss RH, Catlin DH. Psychological moods and subjectively perceived behavioral and somatic changes accompanying anabolic-androgenic steroid use. *Am J Sports Med* 1992;20:717–724.

588. Yesalis CE, Wright JE, Lombardo JA. Anabolic steroids in athletes. *Wien Med Wochenschr* 1992;142:298–308.

589. Thiblin I, Parlklo T. Anabolic androgenic steroids and violence. *Acta Psychiatr Scand Suppl* 2002;412:125–128.

590. Midgley SJ, Heather N, Davies JB. Levels of aggression among a group of anabolic-androgenic steroid users. *Med Sci Law* 2001;41:309–314.

591. Brower KJ. Anabolic steroid abuse and dependence. *Curr Psychiatry Rep* 2002;4:377–387.

592. Brower KJ, Blow FC, Young JP, Hill EM. Symptoms and correlates of anabolic-androgenic steroid dependence. *Br J Addict* 1991;86: 759–768.

593. Kanayama G, Cohane GH, Weiss RD, Pope HG. Post anabolic-androgenic steroid use among men admitted for substance abuse

treatment: an underrecognized problem? *J Clin Psychiatry* 2003; 64:156–160.

594. Aitken C, Delalande C, Stanton K. Pumping iron, risking infection? Exposure to hepatitis C, hepatitis B and HIV among anabolic-androgenic steroid injectors in Victoria, Australia. *Drug Alcohol Depend* 2002;65:303–308.

595. Braseth NR, Allison EJ Jr, Gough JE. Exertional rhabdomyolysis in a body builder abusing anabolic-androgenic steroids. *Eur J Emerg Med* 2001;8:155–157.

596. Newman LS. Occupational illness. *N Engl J Med* 1995;333:1128–1134.

597. Leigh JP, Markowitz SB, Fahs M, *et al.* Occupational injury and illness in the United States. Estimates of costs, mobidity, and mortality. *Arch Intern Med* 1997;157:1557–1568.

598. Leigh JP, McCurdy SA, Schenker MB. Costs of occupational injuries in agriculture. *Public Health Rep* 2001;116:235–248.

599. Leigh JP, Cone JE, Harrison R. Costs of occupational injuries and illnesses in California. *Pre Med* 2001;32:393–406.

600. Leigh JP, Seavey W, Leistikow B. Estimating the costs of job related arthritis. *J Rheumatol* 2001;28:1647–1654.

601. Leigh JP, Miller TR. Occupational illnesses within two national data sets. *Int J Occup Environ Health* 1998;4:99–113.

602. Leigh JP, Miller TR. Ranking occupations based upon the costs of job-related injuries and diseases. *J Occup Environ Med* 1997;39: 1170–1182.

603. Beckett WS. Occupational respiratory diseases. *N Engl J Med* 2000;342:406–413.

604. Simoes E, Phillips P, Maley R, Kreiss K. Fixed obstructive lung disease in workers at a microwave popcorn factory — Missouri, 2000–2002. *MMWR* 2002;51:345–347.

605. Beckett WS, Pope CA, Xu XP, Christiani DC. Women's respiratory health in the cotton textile industry: an analysis of respiratory symptoms in 973 non-smoking female workers. *Occup Environ Med* 1994;51:14–18.

606. Cowie RL. The influence of silicosis on deteriorating lung function in gold miners. *Chest* 1998;113:340–343.

607. *Report on Carcinogens*, 8th ed. National Toxicology Program, Research Triangle Park, NC, 1998.

608. Doll R, Peto R. The causes of cancer: quantitative estimates of avoidable risks of cancer in the United States today. *J Natl Cancer Inst* 1981;66:1191–1308.

609. Steenland K, Loomis D, Shy C, Simonsen N. Review of occupational lung carcinogens. *Am J Ind Med* 1996;29:474–490.

610. Rosenstock L, Rest KM, Benson JA, *et al.* Occupational and environmental medicine: meeting the growing need for clinical services. *N Engl J Med* 1991;325:924–927.

611. Lax MB, Grant WD, Manetti FA, Klein R. Recognizing occupational disease — taking an effective occupational history. *Am Fam Phys* 1998;58:935–944.

612. Taylor CR, Stern RS, Leyden JJ, Hilchrest BA. Photoaging/photodamage and photoprotection. *J Am Acad Dermatol* 1990; 22:1–15.

613. Knight JA. *Free Radicals, Antioxidants, Aging and Disease*. AACC Press, Washington DC, 1999, p. 361.

614. Greenlee RT, Murray T, Bolden S, Wingo PA. Cancer statistics, 2000. *CA Cancer J Clin* 2000;50:7–30.

615. International Agency for Research on Cancer. Monograph on the evaluation of carcinogenic risks to humans: solar and ultraviolet radiation. *WHO* 1992;28:645–647.

616. Karagas MR, Greenberg ER, Spencer SK, *et al.* Increase in incidence rates of basal cell and squamous cell skin cancer in New Hampshire, USA. New Hampshire Skin Cancer Study Group. *Int J Cancer* 1999;81:555–559.

617. American Cancer Society. *Cancer Prevention and Early Detection — Cancer Facts and Figures 2002*. American Cancer Society, Atlanta, CA, 2002.

618. Glanz K, Saraiya M, Wechsler H. Guidelines for school programs to prevent skin cancer. *MMWR* 2002;51:1–16.

619. Karagas MR, Stannard LA, Mott LA, *et al.* Use of tanning devices and risk of basal cell and squamous cell skin cancers. *J Natl Cancer Inst* 2002;94:224–226.

620. Miller SA, Hamilton SL, Wester UG, Cyr WH. An analysis of UVA emissions from sunlamps and the potential importance for melanoma. *Photochem Photobiol* 1998;68:63–70.

621. Spencer JM, Amonette RA. Indoor tanning: risks, benefits, and future trends. *J Am Acad Dermatol* 1995;33:288–298.

622. Thylefors B, Negrel AD, Pararajasegaram R, Dadzie KY. Available data on blindness (update 1994). *Ophthalmic Epidemiol* 1994;2: 5–39.

623. Steinberg EP, Javitt JC, Sharkey PD, *et al.* The content and cost of cataract surgery. *Arch Ophthalmol* 1993;111:1041–1049.

624. Taylor HR. The environment and the lens. *Br J Ophthalmol* 1980;64:303–310.

625. Hollows F, Moran D. Cataract — the ultraviolet risk factor. *Lancet* 1981;2:1249–1250.

626. Taylor HR, West SK, Rosenthal FS, *et al.* Effect of ultraviolet radiation on cataract formation. *N Engl J Med* 1988;319:1429–1433.

627. West SK, Duncan DD, Munoz B, *et al.* Sunlight exposure and risk of lens opacities in a population-based study. The Salisbury Eye Evaluation Project. *JAMA* 1998;280:714–718.

628. West S. Ocular ultraviolet B exposure and lens opacities: a review. *J Epidemiol* 1999;9(Suppl 6):S97–S101.

629. McCarty CA, Taylor HR. A review of the epidemiologic evidence linking ultraviolet radiation and cataracts. *Dev Ophthalmol* 2002;35:21–31.

630. Giblin FJ, Leverenz VR, Padgaonkar VA, *et al.* UVA light *in vivo* reaches the nucleus of the guinea pig lens and produces deleterious oxidative effects. *Exp Eye Res* 2002;75:445–458.

631. Dillon J, Zheng L, Merriam JC, Gaillard FR. The optical properties of the anterior segment of the eye: implications for cortical cataract. *Exp Eye Res* 1999;68:785–795.

632. Knight JA. *Free Radicals, Antioxidants, Aging and Disease.* AACC Press, Washington, DC, 1999, pp. 192–197.

633. Gupta SK, Halder N, Srivastava S, *et al.* Green tea (*Camellia sinesis*) protects against selenite-induced oxidative stress in experimental cataractogenesis. *Ophthalmic Res* 2002;34:258–263.

634. Cornish KM, Williamson G, Sanderson J. Quercetin metabolism in the lens: role in inhibition of hydrogen peroxide induced cataract. *Free Radic Biol Med* 2002;33:63–70.

635. Li ZR, Reiter RJ, Fujimori O, *et al.* Cataractogenesis and lipid peroxidation in newborn rats treated with buthionine sulfoximine: preventive actions of melatonin. *J Pineal Res* 1997;22:117–123.

636. Seddon JM, Christen WG, Manson JE, *et al.* The use of vitamin supplements and risk of cataract among US male physicians. *Am J Public Health* 1994;84:788–792.

637. Jaques PF, Chylack LT Jr. Epidemiologic evidence for a role for the antioxidant vitamins and carotenoids in cataract prevention. *Am J Clin Nutr* 1991;53(Suppl):352S–355S.

638. Garland DL. Ascorbic acid and the eye. *Am J Clin Nutr* 1991; 54(Suppl):1198S–1202S.

639. Taylor A, Jacques PF, Epstein EM. Relations among aging, antioxidant status, and cataract. *Am J Clin Nutr* 1995;62(Suppl):1439S–1447S.

640. Spector A. Oxidative stress-induced cataract: mechanism of action. *FASEB J* 1995;9:1173–1182.

641. Klein R, Klein BEK, Linton KLP. Prevalence of age-related maculopathy: The Beaver Dam Eye Study. *Ophthalmology* 1992;99:933–943.

642. Gerster H. Review: antioxidant protection of the ageing macula. *Age Ageing* 1991;20:60–69.

643. Young RW. Solar radiation and age-related macular degeneration. *Surv Ophthalmol* 1988;32:252–269.

644. Goldberg J, Flowerdew G, Smith E, *et al.* Factors associated with age-related macular degeneration: an analysis of data from the first National Health and Nutrition Examination Survey. *Am J Epidemiol* 1988;128:700–710.

645. West S, Vitale S, Hallfrisch J, *et al.* Are antioxidants or supplements protective for age-related macular degeneration? *Arch Ophthalmol* 1994;112:222–227.

646. Seddon JM, Ajani UA, Sperduto RD, *et al.* Dietary carotenoids, vitamins A, C, and E, and advanced age-related macular degeneration. *JAMA* 1994;272:1413–1420.

647. Eye Disease Case-Control Study Group. Antioxidant status and neovascular age-related macular degeneration. *Arch Ophthalmol* 1993;111:104–109.

648. Ministry of Health. *Mortality and Morbidity During the London Fog of December 1952.* Reports on Public Health and Medical Subjects No. 95. HMSO, London, 1954.

649. Logan WPD. Mortality in the London fog incident, 1952. *Lancet* 1953;1:336–338.

650. Brunekreef B, Holgate ST. Air pollution and health. *Lancet* 2002;360:1233–1247.

651. Bell ML, Davis DL. Reassessment of the lethal London fog of 1952: novel indicators of acute and chronic consequences of acute exposure to air pollution. *Environ Health Perspect* 2001;109(Suppl 3):389–394.

652. Devlin RB, Raub JA, Folinsbee LJ. Health effects of ozone. *Sci Med* 1997;May/June:8–17.

653. Miller FJ, Gardner DE, Graham JA, *et al.* Size considerations for establishing a standard for inhalable particles. *J Air Poll Control Assoc* 1979;29:610–615.

654. WHO. *Health and Environment in Sustainable Development: Five Years After the Earth Summit.* World Health Organization, Geneva, 1997.

655. Working Group on Public Health and Fossil-Fuel Combustion. Short-term improvements in public health from global-climate policies on fossil-fuel combustion: an interim report. *Lancet* 1997;350: 1341–1347.

656. Dockery DW, Pope CA III. A review of the acute respiratory effects of particulate air pollution. *Annu Rev Public Health* 1994;15: 101–132.

657. Samet JM, Dominici F, Curriero FC, *et al.* Fine particulate air pollution and mortality in 20 US cities, 1987–1994. *N Engl J Med* 2000;343:1742–1749.

658. Dockery DW, Pope CA III, Xu X, *et al.* An association between air pollution and mortality in six US cities. *N Engl J Med* 1993;329:1753–1759.

659. Pope CA III, Thun MJ, Namboodiri MM, *et al.* Particulate air pollution as a predictor of mortality in a prospective study of US adults. *Am J Respir Crit Care Med* 1995;151:669–674.

660. Pope CA III, Burnett RT, Thun MJ, *et al.* Lung cancer, cardiopulmonary mortality, and long-term exposure to fine particulate air pollution. *JAMA* 2002;287:1132–1141.

661. Hoek G, Brunekreef B, Goldbohm S, *et al.* Association between mortality and indicators of traffic-related pollution in the Netherlands: a cohort study. *Lancet* 2002;360:1203–1209.

662. Kunzli N, Kaiser R, Medina S, *et al.* Public-health impact of outdoor and traffic-related air pollution: a European assessment. *Lancet* 2000;356:795–801.

663. Clancy L, Goodman P, Sinclair H, Dockery DW. Effect of air-pollution control on death rates in Dublin, Ireland: an intervention study. *Lancet* 2002;360:1210–1214.

664. Abbey DE, Lebowitz MD, Mills PK, *et al.* Long-term ambient concentrations of particulates and oxidants and development of chronic disease in a cohort of non-smoking California residents. *Inhal Toxicol* 1995;7:19–34.

665. Nyberg F, Gustavsson P, Jarup L, *et al.* Urban air pollution and lung cancer in Stockholm. *Epidemiology* 2000;11:487–495.

666. Schwartz J. Air pollution and hospital admission for heart disease in eight US counties. *Epidemiology* 1999;10:17–22.

667. Peters A, Dockery DW, Muller JE, *et al.* Increased particulate air pollution and the triggering of myocardial infarction. *Circulation* 2001;103:2810–2815.

668. Gustavsson P, Plato N, Hallqvist J, *et al.* A population-based case-referent study of myocardial infarction and occupational exposure to motor exhaust, other combustion products, organic solvents, lead and dynamite. Stockholm Heart Epidemiology Program (SHEEP) Study Group. *Epidemiology* 2001;12:222–228.
669. Zanobetti A, Schwartz J. Cardiovascular damage by airborne particles: are diabetics more susceptible? *Epidemiology* 2002;13:588–592.
670. Brook RD, Brook JR, Urch B, *et al.* Inhalation of fine particulate air pollution and ozone causes acute arterial vasoconstriction in healthy adults. *Circulation* 2002;105:1534–1536.
671. Strachan D, Sibbald B, Weiland S, *et al.* Worldwide variations in prevalence of symptoms of allergic rhinoconjunctivitis in children: the International Study of Asthma and Allergies in Childhood (ISAAC). *Pediatr Allergy Immunol* 1997;8:161–176.
672. Emanuel MB. Hay fever, a post industrial revolution epidemic: a history of its growth during the 19th century. *Clin Allergy* 1988;18: 295–304.
673. Mannino DM, Homa DM, Pertowski CA, *et al.* Surveillance for asthma — United States, 1960–1995. In: CDC Surveillance Summary, 24 April 1998. *MMWR* 1998;47(55-1):1–28.
674. Mannino DM, Homa DM, Akinbami LJ, *et al.* Surveillance for asthma — United States, 1980–1999. *MMWR* 2002;51(55-1):1–13.
675. US Department of Health and Human Services. Respiratory disease [Goal 24]. In: *Healthy People 2010* (conference ed., Vol. II). Department of Health and Human Services, Washington, DC, 2000;24:1–27.
676. Centers for Disease Control and Prevention. Measuring childhood asthma prevalence before and after the 1997 redesign of the National Health Interview Survey — United States. *MMWR* 2000; 49:908–911.
677. Murray AB, Morrison BJ. The effect of cigarette smoke from the mother on bronchial responsiveness and severity of symptoms in children with asthma. *J Allergy Clin Immunol* 1986;77:575–581.
678. Halken S, Host A, Nilsson L, Taudorf E. Passive smoking as a risk factor for development of obstructive respiratory disease and allergic sensitization. *Allergy* 1995;50:97–105.
679. Malo JL, Ghezzo H, D'Aquino C, *et al.* Natural history of occupational asthma: relevance of type of agent and other factors in the rate of development of symptoms in affected subjects. *J Allergy Clin Immunol* 1992;90:937–944.
680. Baur X. Occupational asthma due to isocyanates. *Lung* 1996;174: 23–30.

681. Pope CA 3rd. Respiratory disease associated with community air pollution and a steel mill, Utah Valley. *Am J Public Health* 1989;79:623–628.

682. Kim Y-K, Baek D, Koh Y-I, *et al.* Outdoor air pollutants derived from industrial processes may be causely related to the development of asthma in children. *Ann Allergy Asthma Immunol* 2001;86:456–460.

683. Friedman MS, Powell KE, Hutwagner L, *et al.* Impact of changes in transportation and commuting behaviors during the 1996 summer Olympic Games in Atlanta on air quality and childhood asthma. *JAMA* 2001;285:892–905.

684. Brauer M, Hoek G, van Vliet P, *et al.* Air pollution from traffic and the development of respiratory infections and asthmatic and allergic symptoms in children. *Am J Respir Crit Care Med* 2002;166:1092–1098.

685. Zemp E, Elasser S, Schindler C, *et al.* Long-term ambient air pollution and respiratory symptoms in adults (SAPALDIA study). The SAPALDIA Team. *Am J Respir Crit Care Med* 1999;159:1257–1266.

686. Wyler C, Braun-Fahrlander C, Kunzli N, *et al.* Exposure to motor vehicle traffic and allergic sensitization. The Swiss Study on air pollution and lung diseases in adults (SAPALDIA) Team. *Epidemiology* 2000;11:450–456.

687. Landrigan PJ, Goldman LR. Report of a panel on the relationship between public exposure to pesticides and cancer. *Cancer* 1998;83:1057–1058 (Letter).

688. Landrigan PJ, Claudio L, Markowitz SB, *et al.* Pesticides and inner-city children: exposures, risks, and prevention. *Environ Health Perspect* 1999:107(Suppl 3):431–437.

689. Whitemore RW, Immerman FW, Camann DE, *et al.* Non-occupational exposures to pesticides for residents in two US cities. *Arch Environ Contam Toxicol* 1994;26:47–59.

690. Lewis RG, Fortmann RC, Camann DE. Evaluation of methods for monitoring the potential exposure of small children to pesticides in the residential environment. *Arch Environ Contam Toxicol* 1994;26:37–46.

691. National Research Council. *Pesticides in the Diets of Infants and Children.* National Academy Press, Washington, DC, 1993.

692. Whyatt RM, Camann DE, Kinney PL, *et al.* Residential pesticide use during pregnancy among a cohort of urban minority women. *Environ Health Perspect* 2002;110:507–514.

693. Karmaus W, Asakevich S, Indurkhya A, *et al.* Childhood growth and exposure to dichlorodiphenyl dichloroethene and polychlorinated biphenyls. *J Pediatr* 2002;140:33–39.

694. Gladen BC, Ragan NB, Rogan WJ. Pubertal growth and development and prenatal and lactational exposure to polychlorinated biphenyls and dichlorobiphenyl dichloroethene. *J Pediatr* 2000;136:490–496.

695. Hosie S, Loff S, Witt K, *et al.* Is there a correlation between organochlorine compounds and undescended testes? *Eur J Pediatr Surg* 2000;10:304–309.

696. Landrigan PJ, Graham DG, Thomas RD. Environmental neurotoxic illness: research for prevention. *Environ Health Perspect* 1994; 102(Suppl 2):117–120.

697. Landrigan PJ, Schechter CB, Lipton JM, *et al.* Environmental pollutants and disease in American children: estimates of morbidity, mortality, and costs for lead poisoning, asthma, cancer, and developmental disabilities. *Environ Health Perspect* 2002;110:721–728.

698. Barlow BK, Thiruchelvam MJ, Bennice L, *et al.* Increased synaptosomal dopamine content and brain concentrations of paraquat produced by selective dithiocarbamates. *J Neurochem* 2003;85: 1075–1086.

699. Banerjee BD, Koner BC, Pasha ST, Ray A. Immunotoxicity of pesticides: perspective and trends. *Indian J Exp Biol* 1996;34:723–733.

700. Banerjee BD. The influence of various factors on immune toxicity assessment of pesticide chemicals. *Toxicol Lett* 1999;107:21–31.

701. Ash KO. Trace elements: when essential nutrients become poisonous. *Lab Med* 1995;26:266–271.

702. Campbell JD. Lifestyle, minerals and health. *Med Hypoth* 2001;57:521–531.

703. Abreo K, Altmann P, Boelaert JR, *et al.* Aluminum overload, consensus conference. *Nephrol Dial Transplant* 1993;1(Suppl):1–54.

704. White DM, Longstreth WT, Rosenstock L, *et al.* Neurologic syndrome in 25 workers from an aluminum smelting plant. *Arch Intern Med* 1992;152:1443–1448.

705. Perl AR, Brody RR. Alzheimer's disease. *Science* 1980;208:297–299.

706. Hammett Stabler CA, Broussard LA, Winecker RE, Ropero-Miller JD. New insights into an old poison, arsenic. *Lab Med* 2002;33: 437–447.

707. Karagas MR, Stukel TA, Tosteson TD. Assessment of cancer risk and environmental levels of arsenic in New Hampshire. *Int J Hyg Environ Health* 2002;205:85–94.

708. Kraagas MR, Stukel TA, Morris JS, *et al.* Skin cancer risk in relation to toenail arsenic concentrations in a US population-based case-control study. *Am J Epidemiol* 2001;153:559–565.

709. Kurttio P, Pukkala E, Kahelin H, *et al.* Arsenic concentrations in well water and risk of bladder and kidney cancer in Finland. *Environ Health Perspect* 1999;107:705–710.

710. Rogan WJ, Ware JH. Exposure to lead in children — how low is low enough? *N Engl J Med* 2003;348:1515–1516.

711. Royce SE. *Case Studies in Environmental Medicine. Lead Toxicity.* US Department of Health and Human Serivices, Public Health Service, Agency for Toxic Substances and Disease Registry, June 1990.

712. Stephenson J. CDC report on environmental toxins: some progress, some concern. *JAMA* 2003;289:1230–1233.

713. Marsden PA. Increased body lead burden — cause of consequence of chronic renal insufficiency? *N Engl J Med* 2003;348:345–347 (Editorial).

714. Canfield RL, Henderson CR, Cory-Slechta DHB, *et al.* Intellectual impairment in children with blood lead concentrations below 10 ug per deciliter. *N Engl J Med* 2003;348:1517–1526.

715. Stretesky PB, Lynch MJ. The relationship between lead exposure and homicide. *Arch Pediatr Adolesc Med* 2001;155:579–582.

716. Blanck HM, Marcus M, Tolbert PE, *et al.* Age at menarche and Tanner stage in girls exposed in utero and postnatally to polybrominated biphenyl. *Epidemiology* 2000;11:641–647.

717. Den Hond E, Roels HA, Hoppenbrouwers K, *et al.* Sexual maturation in relation to polychlorinated aromatic hydrocarbons: Sharpe and Skakkeback's hypothesis revisited. *Environ Health Perspect* 2002;110:771–776.

718. Seleven SG, Rice DC, Hogan KA, *et al.* Blood lead concentration and delayed puberty in girls. *N Engl J Med* 2003;348:1527–1536.

719. Pirkle JL, Schwartz J, Landis JR, Harlan, WR. The relationship between blood lead levels and blood pressure and its cardiovascular risk implications. *Am J Epidemiol* 1985;121:246–258.

720. Burt VL, Whelton P, Roccella EJ, *et al.* Prevalence of hypertension in the US adult population: results from the Third National Health Examination Survey, 1988–1991. *Hypertension* 1995;25:305–313.

721. Nash DN, Magder L, Lustberg M, *et al.* Blood lead, blood pressure and hypertension in perimenopausal and postmenopausal women. *JAMA* 2003;289:1523–1532.

722. Lin J-L, Lin-Tan D-T, Hsu K-H, Yu C-C. Environmental lead exposure and progression of chronic renal disease in patients without diabetes. *N Engl J Med* 2003;348:277–286.

723. Bakir F, Damluji SF, Amin-Zaki L, *et al.* Methylmercury poisoning in Iraq. *Science* 1973;181:230–241.

724. Broussard LA, Hammett-Stabler CA, Wirecker RE, Ropero-Miller JD. The toxicology of mercury. *Lab Med* 2002;33:614–625.
725. Hursh JB, Clarkson TW, Miles EF, *et al.* Percutaneous absorption of mercury vapor by man. *Arch Environ Health* 1989;44:120–127.
726. Schober SE, Sinks TH, Jones RL, *et al.* Blood mercury levels in US children and women of childbearing age, 1999–2000. *JAMA* 2003;289:1667–1674.
727. Grandjean P, Budtz-Jorgensen E, Steurwald U, *et al.* Attenuated growth of breast-fed children exposed to increased concentrations of methylmercury and polycholorinated biphenyls. *FASEB J* 2003; 17:699–701.
728. Grandjean P, White RF, Weihe P, Jorgensen PJ. Neurotoxic risk caused by stable and variable exposure to methylmercury from seafood. *Ambul Pediatr* 2003;3:18–23.
729. Grandjean P, Weihe P, Nielsen JB. Methylmercury: significance of intrauterine and postnatal exposures. *Clin Chem* 1994;40:1395–1400.
730. Grandjean P, Weight, White RF, *et al.* Cognitive deficit in 7-year-old children with prenatal exposure to methylmercury. *Neurotoxicol Teratol* 1997;19:417–428.
731. Steurerwald U, Weihe P, Jorgensen PJ, *et al.* Maternal seafood diet, methylmercury exposure, and neonatal neurologic function. *J Pediatr* 2000;136:599–605.
732. Salonen JT, Seppanen K, Nyyssonen K, *et al.* Intake of mercury from fish, lipid peroxidation, and the risk of myocardial infarction and coronary, cardiovascular, and any death in eastern Finnish men. *Circulation* 1995;91:645–654.
733. Guallar E, Sanz-Gallardo MI, van't Veer P, *et al.* Mercury, fish oils and the risk of myocardial infarction. *N Engl J Med* 2002;347:1747–1760.
734. Yoshikzawa K, Rimm EB, Morris JS, *et al.* Mercury and the risk of coronary heart disease in men. *N Engl J Med* 2002;347:1755–1760.
735. Grum EE, Bresnitz EA. *Case Studies in Environmental Medicine: Cadmium Toxicity.* US Department of Health and Human Services, Public Health Service, Agency for Toxic Substances and Disease Registry, June 1990.
736. OSHA. Department of Labor report on occupational exposure to cadmium. *Federal Register.* 14 September 1992;57:42102–42437.
737. Iwata K, Saito H, Moriyama M, Nakano A. Renal tubular function after reduction of environmental cadmium exposure: a ten-year follow-up. *Arch Environ Health* 1993;48:157–163.
738. Pesch B, Haerting J, Ranft U, *et al.* Occupational risk factors for renal cell carcinoma: agent-specific results from a case-control study

in Germany. MURC Study Group. Multicenter urothelial and renal cancer. *Int J Epidemiol* 2000;29:1014–1024.

739. Linder MC (ed.), *Nutritional Biochemistry and Metabolism: Clinical Applications*, 2nd Ed. Elsevier, New York, 1991, p. 268.

740. Schroeder HA. *The Trace Elements and Man: Some Positive and Negative Aspects*. Devin-Adair, Old Greenwich, Connecticut, 1973.

741. Kristensen TS. Cardiovascular disease and the work environment: a critical review of the epidemiologic literature on chemical factors. *Environ Health* 1989;15:245–264.

742. Demers R, Selikoff IJ. *Case Studies in Environmental Medicine: Asbestos Toxicity*. US Department of Health and Human Services, Public Health Service Agency for Toxic Substances and Disease Registry, June 1990.

743. Case BW. Approaching environmental medicine. *Penn Med* 1990; 93:52–55.

744. Abelson PH. The asbestos removal fiasco. *Science* 1990;247:1017 (Editorial).

745. Selikoff IJ, Greenberg M. A landmark case in asbestosis. *JAMA* 1991;265:898–901.

746. Murray R. Asbestos: a chronology of its origins and health effects. *Br J Ind Med* 1990;47:361–365.

747. Mollo F, Magnani C, Bo P, *et al.* The attribution of lung cancers to asbestos exposure: a pathologic study of 924 unselected cases. *Am J Clin Pathol* 2002;117:90–96.

748. Park J, Kamendulis LM, Friedman MA, Klaunig JE. Acrylamide-induced cellular transformation. *Toxicol Sci* 2002;65:177–183.

749. Reynolds T. Acrylamide and cancer: tunnel leak in Sweden prompted studies. *J Natl Cancer Inst* 2002;94:876–878.

750. Weiss G. Acrylamide in food: uncharted territory. *Science* 2002;297:27.

751. Marsh GM, Lucas LJ, Youk AO, Schall LC. Mortality patterns among workers exposed to acrylamide: 1994 follow-up. *Occup Environ Med* 1999;56:181–190.

752. Mucci LA, Dickman PW, Steineck G, *et al.* Dietary acrylamide and cancer of the large bowel, kidney and bladder: absence of an association in a population-based study in Sweden. *Br J Cancer* 2003;88:84–89.

753. Tareke E, Rydberg P, Karlsson P, *et al.* Acrylamide: a cooking carcinogen? *Chem Res Toxicol* 2000;13:517–522.

754. Brudzewski J. *Case Studies in Environmental Medicine: Polynuclear Aromatic Hydrocarbon (PAH) Toxicity*. US Department of Health and

Human Services, Public Health Service, Agency for Toxic Substances and Disease Registry, June 1990.

755. Romundstad P, Andersen A, Haldorsen T. Cancer incidence among workers in six Norwegian aluminum plants. *Scand J Work Environ Health* 2000;26:461–469.

756. Huff JE, Melnick RL, Solleveld HA, *et al.* Multiple organ carcinogenicity of 1,3-butadiene in B6C3F1 mice after 60 weeks of inhalation exposure. *Science* 1985;227:548–549.

757. Owen PE, Glaister JR. Inhalation toxicity and carcinogenicity of 1,3-butadiene in Sprague-Dawley rats. *Environ Health Perspect* 1990;86:19–25.

758. McMichael PJ, Spirtas R, Gamble JF, Tousey PM. Mortality among rubber workers: relationship to specific jobs. *J Occup Med* 1976; 18:178–183.

759. Meinhardt TJ, Young RJ, Hartle RW. Epidemiologic investigations of styrene-1,3-butadiene rubber production and reinforced plastics production. *Scand J Work Environ Health* 1978;4(Suppl 2):240–246.

760. Downs TD, Crane MM, Kim KW. Mortality among workers at a 1,3-butadiene facility. *Am J Ind Med* 1987;12:311–329.

761. Matanoski GM. Mortality of a cohort of workers in the styrene-1,3-butadiene polymer manufacturing industry (1948–1982). *Environ Health Perspect* 1990;86:107–117.

762. Landrigan PJ. Critical assessment of epidemiologic studies on the human carcinogenicity of 1,3-butadiene. *Environ Health Perspect* 1990;86:143–148.

763. Wabeke R, Weinstein R. *Case Studies in Environmental Medicine: Polychlorinated Biphenyl (PCB) Toxicity.* US Department of Health and Human Services, Public Health Service, Agency for Toxic Substances and Disease Registry, June 1990.

764. Weisskopf MG, Anderson HA, Hanrohan LP. Decreased sex ratio following maternal exposure to polychlorinated biphenyls from contaminated Great Lakes sport-caught fish: a retrospective study. *Environ Health* 2003;12:2–15.

765. Demers R. *Case Studies in Environmental Medicine: Dioxin Toxicity.* US Department of Health and Human Services, Public Health Service, Agency for Toxic Substances and Disease Registry, June 1990.

766. Centers for Disease Control. Preliminary Report: 2,3,7, 8-tetrachlorodibenzo-p-dioxin exposure in humans — Seveso, Italy. *JAMA* 1989;261:831–832.

767. Bertazzi PH, Zocchetti C, Pesatori AC, *et al.* Ten-year mortality study of the population involved in the Seveso incident in 1976. *Am J Epidemiol* 1989;129:1187–1200.

768. Franklin H, Samet JM. Radon. *CA, Cancer J Clin* 2001;51:337–344.

769. National Research Council, Committee on the Biological Effects of Ionizing Radiation. *Health Effects on Exposure to Low Levels of Radon (BEIR VI)*. National Academy Press, Washington, DC, 1998.

770. Marcinowshi F, Lucas RM, Yeager WM. National and regional distribution of airborne radon concentrations in US homes. *Health Phys* 1994;66:699–706.

771. Environmental Protection Agency. *Radionuclides (Uranium, Radium and Radon), 1998.* (www.epa.gov/ttuatwl/hlthef/radionucl.html).

772. Askew EW. Nutrition and performance at environmental extremes. In: *Nutrition in Exercise and Sport*, 2nd Ed. I Wolinsky, JF Hickson Jr (eds.) CRC Press, Boca Raton, FL, 1993, pp. 455–474.

773. National Center for Health Statistics. *Compressed Mortality File.* US Department of Health and Human Services, CDC, National Center for Health Statistics, Hyattsville, Maryland, 2002.

774. Laake K, Sverre JM. Winter excess mortality: a comparison between Norway and England plus Wales. *Age Ageing* 1996;25:343–348.

775. Stout RW, Crawford V. Seasonal variations in fibrinogen concentrations among elderly people. *Lancet* 1991;338:9–13.

776. Frank SM, Fleisher LA, Breslow MJ, *et al.* Perioperative maintenance of normothermia reduces the incidence of morbid cardiac events: a randomized trial *JAMA* 1997;277:1127–1134.

777. Mackenbach JP, Borst V, Schols JMGA. Heat-related mortality among nursing-home patients. *Lancet* 1997;349:1297–1298.

778. Seretakis D, Lagiou P, Lipworth L, *et al.* Changing seasonality of mortality from coronary heart disease. *JAMA* 1997;278:1012–1014.

779. Diaz J, Garcia R, Velazquez de Castro F, *et al.* Effects of extremely hot days on people older than 65 years in Seville (Spain) from 1986–1997. *Int J Biometeorol* 2002;46:145–149.

Index